VETERINARY CLINICAL PATHOLOGY SECRETS

VETERINARY CLINICAL PATHOLOGY SECRETS

Rick L. Cowell, DVM, MS, MRCVS, Dipl ACVP
Clinical Pathologist
IDEXX Laboratories, Inc.
Westbrook, Maine
Adjunct Professor
Oklahoma State University
College of Veterinary Medicine
Department of Veterinary Pathobiology
Stillwater, Oklahoma

with **178** *illustrations*

ELSEVIER
MOSBY

ELSEVIER
MOSBY

11830 Westline Industrial Drive
St. Louis, Missouri 63146

VETERINARY CLINICAL PATHOLOGY SECRETS

Library of Congress Cataloging-in-Publication Data

Cowell, Rick L.
Veterinary clinical pathology secrets / Rick L. Cowell.
p. cm. -- (The secrets series)
Includes bibliographical references (p.).
ISBN-13: 978-1-56053-633-8 ISBN-10: 1-56053-633-0
1. Veterinary clinical pathology--Examinations, questions, etc. I. Title. II. Series.

SF772.6.C68 2004
636.089'607'076--dc22 2004046548

Publishing Director: Linda L. Duncan
Managing Editor: Teri Merchant
Senior Developmental Editor: Jolynn Gower
Publishing Services Manager: Patricia Tannian
Senior Project Manager: Anne Altepeter
Book Design Manager: Gail Morey Hudson

ISBN-13: 978-1-56053-633-8
ISBN-10: 1-56053-633-0

Transferred to DIgital Printig 2011

CONTRIBUTORS

A. Rick Alleman, DVM, PhD, Dipl ACVP, ABVP
Professor, Department of Physiological Sciences, College of Veterinary Medicine, University of Florida, Gainesville, Florida

Claire B. Andreasen, DVM, PhD, Dipl ACVP
Professor, Department of Veterinary Pathology, College of Veterinary Medicine, Iowa State University, Ames, Iowa

Sylvie Beaudin, DVM
Clinical Pathologist, Antech Diagnostics, Irvine, California

Rick L. Cowell, DVM, MS, MRCVS, Dipl ACVP
Clinical Pathologist, IDEXX Laboratories, Inc., Westbrook, Maine, Adjunct Professor, Oklahoma State University, College of Veterinary Medicine, Department of Veterinary Pathobiology, Stillwater, Oklahoma

Debbie J. Cunningham
Resident, Oklahoma State University, College of Veterinary Medicine, Department of Veterinary Pathobiology, Stillwater, Oklahoma

Heather Leigh DeHeer, DVM, Dipl ACVP
Clinical Pathologist, University of Pennsylvania, School of Veterinary Medicine Philadelphia, Pennsylvania

Michel Desnoyers, DVM, PhD, Dipl ACVP
Université de Montreal, College of Veterinary Medicine, St-Hyacinthe, Québec

Karen S. Dolce, DVM
Clinical Pathology Resident, Kansas State University, Manhattan, Kansas

Karen Dorsey, DVM
Clinical Pathology Consultant, McLoud, Oklahoma

†Bernard F. Feldman, DVM, PhD
Professor, Biomedical Sciences and Pathobiology, Virginia-Maryland Regional College of Veterinary Medicine, Virginia Polytechnic Institute and State University, Blacksburg, Virginia

Stephen D. Gaunt, DVM, PhD, Dipl ACVP
Professor, Department of Pathobiologic Sciences, School of Veterinary Medicine, Louisiana State University, Baton Rouge, Louisiana

---

†Deceased.

Shannon Jones Hostetter, DVM
Adjunct Professor, Veterinary Pathology, College of Veterinary Medicine, Iowa State University, Ames, Iowa

Armando R. Irizarry-Rovira, DVM, PhD, Dipl ACVP
Senior Pathologist, Eli Lilly and Company, Greenfield Research Laboratories, Greenfield, Indiana

Tarja Juopperi, DVM, MS
Department of Pathology, Johns Hopkins Medical Institutions
Baltimore, Maryland

James H. Meinkoth, DVM, PhD, Dipl ACVP
Professor, College of Veterinary Medicine, Department of Veterinary Pathobiology, Oklahoma State University, Stillwater, Oklahoma

Theresa E. Rizzi
Resident, Oklahoma State University, College of Veterinary Medicine, Department of Veterinary Pathobiology, Stillwater, Oklahoma

Steven L. Stockham, DVM, MS, Dipl ACVP
Professor of Veterinary Clinical Pathology, Department of Diagnostic Medicine and Pathology, College of Veterinary Medicine, Kansas State University, Manhattan, Kansas

Susan J. Tornquist, DVM, PhD, Dipl ACVP
Associate Professor, Department of Biomedical Sciences, College of Veterinary Medicine, Oregon State University, Corvallis, Oregon

Ronald D. Tyler, DVM, PhD, Dipl ACVP
Adjunct Professor, Department of Veterinary Pathobiology, College of Veterinary Medicine, Oklahoma State University, Stillwater, Oklahoma

Heather L. Wamsley, DVM
Resident Clinical Pathology, Department of Physiological Sciences, College of Veterinary Medicine, University of Florida, Gainesville, Florida

Douglas J. Weiss, DVM, PhD, Dipl ACVP
Professor, Department of Veterinary Pathobiology, College of Veterinary Medicine, University of Minnesota, St. Paul, Minnesota

PREFACE

Veterinary Clinical Pathology Secrets was written for veterinary students, practitioners, and residents in the hope that it will serve as a study guide and source of relevant, useful information. As with other texts in the Secrets Series, the format of this text consists of a series of questions, with each question followed by an answer.

The authorship comprises a broad group of contributors from around the country and encompasses professionals from both academic and reference laboratory settings. Each contributing author was chosen based on his or her in-depth practical knowledge of a particular subject. All authors were limited in the number of questions they could write. Because veterinary clinical pathology has broad practical application and therefore a vast potential number of questions, this book was not intended to be all inclusive. Rather, the goal was for each author to focus on practical, current application of the subject matter so as to cover his or her topic in the allotted number of questions.

I am pleased with the outstanding job the authors did in preparing their chapters, and I thank them for sharing their time, talent, and expertise. I extend a special thanks to the staff at Elsevier for all their hard work, patience, and excellent guidance in bringing this book to fruition.

Rick L. Cowell, DVM, MS, Dipl ACVP

CONTENTS

Section I
Hematology
Erythrocytes

1. GENERAL PRINCIPLES

Shannon Jones Hostetter and Claire B. Andreasen

1. What is erythropoietin, where is it produced, and what are its principal effects?

Erythropoietin is a glycoprotein hormone produced by the peritubular capillary endothelium of the kidney in response to reduced oxygen tension (hypoxia). Erythropoietin's principal site of action is the bone marrow.

The effects of erythropoietin include stimulation of growth and differentiation of both erythroid and platelet progenitors and the induction of hemoglobin synthesis in dividing erythrocyte precursors. Increased erythropoietin release can ultimately lead to increased hematocrit, total red blood cell (RBC) numbers, and platelet count.

2. How is iron, either dietary or recycled, transported through the body?

Iron is transported in the blood by *transferrin,* a β-globulin (serum protein), from the site of absorption in the intestine or from macrophage stores to the marrow and tissues. Iron can then be incorporated into hemoglobin during heme synthesis.

3. How are aged or damaged erythrocytes normally removed from circulation?

Aged or damaged erythrocytes have changes in either their cell membranes or cytosolic enzymes that allow them to be recognized by macrophages within the spleen and liver. These erythrocytes are subsequently phagocytosed by the macrophages and removed from circulation. Additionally, a small percentage of "old" or abnormal erythrocytes are removed from circulation through intravascular hemolysis.

4. What is the average erythrocyte life span in the dog and cat?

The average RBC life span in the dog is approximately 110 days. It is significantly shorter in the cat, approximately 70 days.

5. What is methemoglobin, and how is it normally metabolized to hemoglobin?

Methemoglobin is structurally identical to hemoglobin except that the iron moiety of the heme group is in the ferric (3+) state instead of the ferrous (2+) state. Therefore, methemoglobin is oxidized hemoglobin that is no longer capable of binding oxygen. A small percentage of hemoglobin is oxidized to methemoglobin in healthy animals. Methemoglobin is continuously changed back to hemoglobin by an enzyme found within erythrocytes known as *methemoglobin reductase*. Methemoglobinemia (increased concentration of methemoglobin within the blood) can result from either excess formation of methemoglobin secondary to an oxidizing agent (e.g., nitrite) or reduced activity of methemoglobin reductase.

6. What are reticulocytes, and how do you identify them?

Reticulocytes are immature, anucleate, circulating erythrocytes that contain residual cytoplasmic ribonucleic acid (RNA), mitochondria, and organelles (also known as *reticulum*) that are visible when stained with new methylene blue. Reticulocytes appear bluish on a Romanowsky stain (Wright's, Diff-Quik) and are referred to as *polychromatophilic cells* (Figure 1-1).

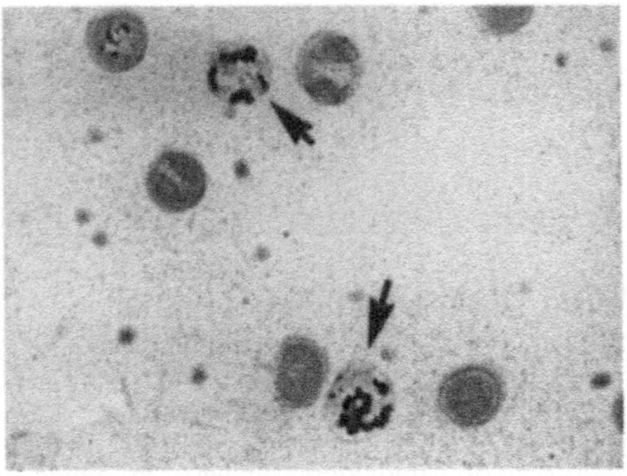

Figure 1-1 Canine peripheral blood smear stained with new methylene blue. Arrows indicate aggregate reticulocytes.

7. Approximately how long does it take for reticulocytes to be produced and released from the bone marrow?

It takes approximately 2 to 3 days for reticulocytes to be produced and released from the bone marrow in response to anemia. It takes 5 to 7 days for reticulocytes to reach a maximum response.

8. What are nucleated erythrocytes (nRBCs)?

Nucleated erythrocytes are RBC precursors that have not yet expelled their nuclei. Nucleated RBCs include metarubricytes, rubricytes, prorubricytes, and rubriblasts. Usually, nRBCs refer to metarubricytes (Figure 1-2).

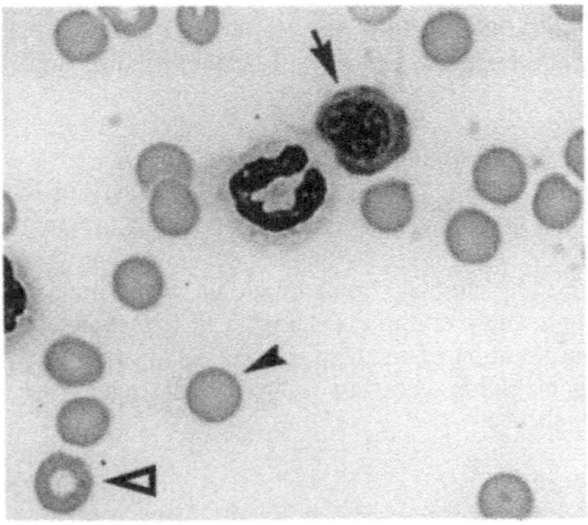

Figure 1-2 Peripheral blood smear stained with Wright's from a dog diagnosed with autoimmune hemolytic anemia. The arrow indicates a metarubricyte. The solid arrowhead identifies a spherocyte, and the open arrowhead points to an erythrocyte with normal morphology.

9. When are increased numbers of nRBCs expected in peripheral blood?

Nucleated erythrocytes are normally present in the bone marrow. Increased numbers of nRBCs can be released from the bone marrow with both strongly regenerative anemias and increased erythropoietin secretion. This condition is known as *appropriate metarubricytosis.* Appropriate metarubricytosis is accompanied by reticulocytosis.

10. Define inappropriate metarubricytosis and identify associated conditions.

Inappropriate metarubricytosis occurs when metarubricytes are released from the bone marrow, often when there is an alteration of the blood–bone marrow barrier. Reticulocytosis is not associated with inappropriate metarubricytosis.

Inappropriate metarubricytosis has been associated with several conditions, including lead toxicosis, myelodysplasia, erythroid leukemia, splenic disease/neoplasia, and endotoxemia.

2. ERYTHROCYTE MORPHOLOGY

Shannon Jones Hostetter and Claire B. Andreasen

1. What are Howell-Jolly bodies, and when do they usually occur?

Howell-Jolly bodies are remnant portions of nuclear material that are found within the cytoplasm of erythrocytes. These bodies are basophilic and spherical. Howell-Jolly bodies are usually observed with accelerated erythrocyte production or after splenectomy.

2. What are Heinz bodies, and what causes them?

Heinz bodies are precipitates of denatured hemoglobin attached to the erythrocyte membrane. These bodies occur following oxidation of hemoglobin. Heinz bodies are found in low numbers in health in certain species (e.g., cat) or may be associated with hemolytic anemias (Figure 2-1).

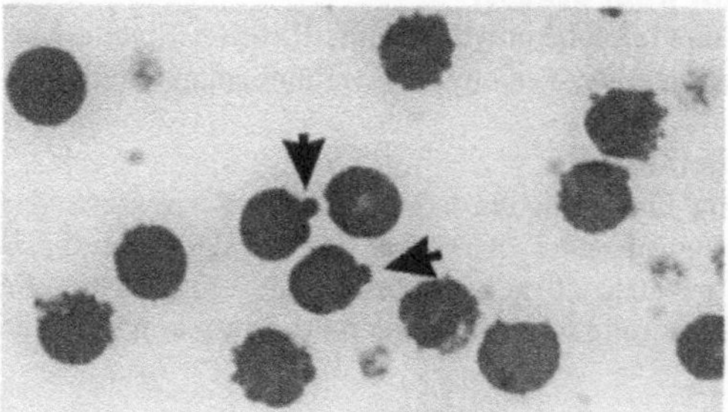

Figure 2-1 Peripheral blood smear stained with Wright's from a cat with Heinz body anemia. The arrows indicate Heinz bodies on the erythrocyte surface.

3. How are Howell-Jolly and Heinz bodies distinguished morphologically?

Although both structures are round, Howell-Jolly bodies are basophilic and located deeper within the cytoplasm than Heinz bodies, which protrude from the red blood cell (RBC) surface. Also, Heinz bodies on Wright's stain are the same color as the erythrocyte's cytoplasm because they are derived from hemoglobin.

4. What is the cause of basophilic stippling in erythrocytes, and when does it occur?

Basophilic stippling results from minute aggregations of residual ribonucleic acid (RNA) that collect within the cytoplasm of the erythrocyte and is an indicator of RBC immaturity. Stippling is readily observed with either Wright's or Diff-Quik staining. Basophilic stippling is occasionally observed in anemic cats and indicates a regenerative response. Basophilic stippling with polychromasia and anemia may be an appropriate response to the anemia. An inappropriate basophilic stippling response occurs in lead toxicosis, in which there is increased basophilic stippling, as well as metarubricytosis, with variable polychromasia.

5. Define anisocytosis and identify associated conditions.

Anisocytosis is variation in cell size. Although mild anisocytosis can be observed in erythrocytes from healthy dogs and cats, more pronounced anisocytosis is associated with a variety of conditions. These include regenerative anemias, some hemolytic anemias, Heinz-body anemia, and breed-associated variations in RBC size (see Question 29).

6. What are macrocytes and microcytes?

Macrocytes are larger erythrocytes of normal shape.

Microcytes are abnormally small erythrocytes.

7. What are spherocytes?

Spherocytes are small, spherical erythrocytes that lack central pallor. Spherocytes are more easily observed in the dog; dogs normally have erythrocytes that are slightly larger than other domestic animals, and dog erythrocytes have well-defined central pallor. Rare spherocytes may be seen in circulation before being removed by the liver or spleen, since immunoglobulin G (IgG) increases on the surface of "old" erythrocytes. This is the process by which old erythrocytes are removed from circulation (see Figure 1-2).

8. How are spherocytes formed?

Spherocytes are formed when macrophages within the liver and spleen remove a portion of a damaged erythrocyte's cell membrane. This generally occurs after the erythrocyte's surface has been coated with either antibody or complement. Because a portion of the membrane is removed, the resulting RBC has reduced cell membrane surface area relative to cytoplasmic volume. Therefore, spherocytes appear as smaller, dense cells that lack central pallor.

9. Spherocytes are typically associated with what disease?

Spherocytes are associated with immune-mediated hemolytic anemia (IMHA). Spherocytes also occur as part of a natural aging process, but then are seen only in low numbers in circulation.

10. Define polychromasia and explain its significance.

Polychromasia is the variation in cell staining (change to bluish gray) observed in erythrocytes stained with Romanowsky-type stains due to the presence of residual RNA. Polychromasia is used as an index of regeneration in anemia because all polychromatophilic erythrocytes are reticulocytes; however, not all reticulocytes have enough reticulin to be polychromatophilic.

11. What is a poikilocyte?

Poikilocytes are abnormally shaped erythrocytes. *Poikilocyte* is a general term used to describe any specific change in shape in an erythrocyte.

12. What are leptocytes, and with what conditions are they associated?

Leptocytes are thin erythrocytes with an increased amount of cell membrane relative to the total cell volume; thus they are folded over. Because polychromatophilic erythrocytes are often larger with more membrane, many leptocytes may be observed during increased erythrocyte turnover. Leptocytes also may be present with liver diseases such as portosystemic shunts in the dog. Target cells are a type of leptocyte (see Question 13).

13. What are target cells (codocytes), and what is their significance?

A *target cell* is a subclass of leptocyte with a distribution of hemoglobin to the center and periphery of the erythrocyte, forming a target-like structure. Codocytes are formed because of either increased membrane surface area or decreased cytoplasmic volume, such as occurs with hypochromia. Animals with liver disease, iron-lacking anemia, or immune-mediated hemolytic anemia may have increased numbers of circulating target cells (Figure 2-2).

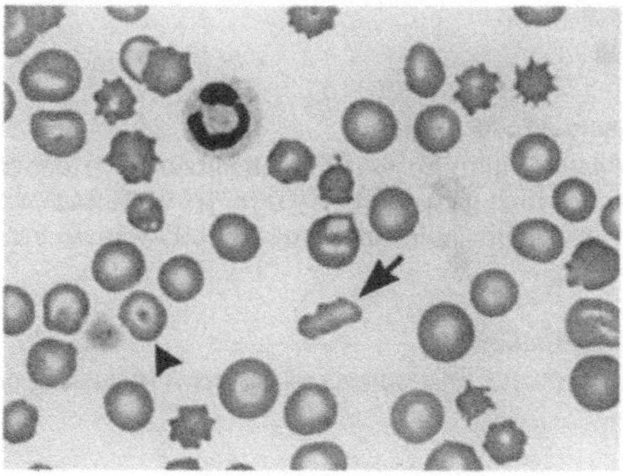

Figure 2-2 Peripheral blood smear from a dog diagnosed with splenic hemangiosarcoma. A schistocyte is identified by the arrow. The arrowhead points to a target cell.

14. What are stomatocytes, and what is their significance?

Stomatocytes are a type of leptocyte that is bowl shaped when three dimensional. When folded, however, stomatocytes appear to have a central crescentic clearing that is a slit or is mouth shaped (Figure 2-3). The inner leaf of the cell membrane is expanded. Stomatocytes may be seen in liver disease, chronic anemias, and hereditary stomatocytosis of malamutes.

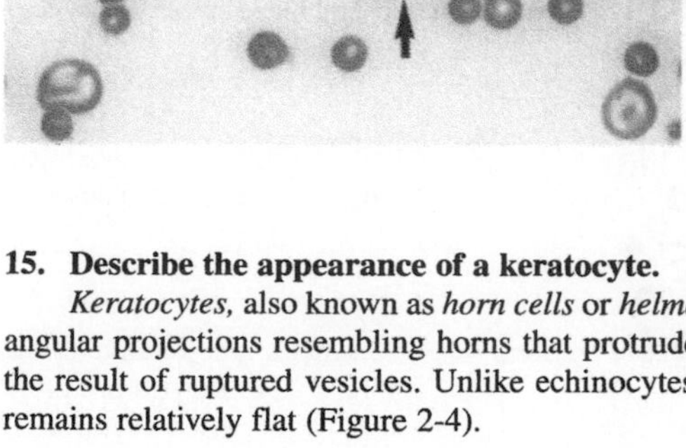

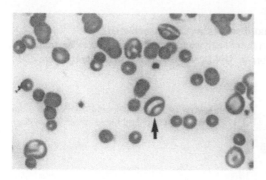

Figure 2-3 Peripheral blood smear from a dog. The arrow indicates a stomatocyte.

15. Describe the appearance of a keratocyte.

Keratocytes, also known as *horn cells* or *helmet cells,* are erythrocytes that have one or more angular projections resembling horns that protrude from the cell surface. These projections are the result of ruptured vesicles. Unlike echinocytes, the cell membrane between the projections remains relatively flat (Figure 2-4).

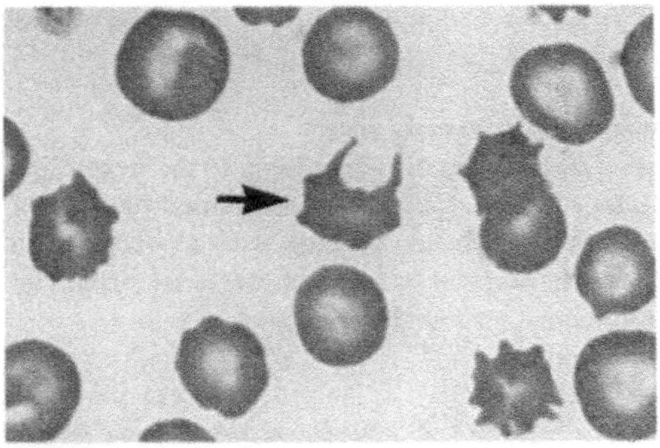

Figure 2-4 Canine peripheral blood smear stained with Wright's. The arrow indicates a keratocyte.

16. Identify conditions that can result in keratocyte formation.

Keratocytes are formed secondary to oxidative injury to the RBC membrane. Oxidative injury also may result in Heinz body formation, in which parts of the erythrocyte membrane are removed by macrophages, resulting in a keratocyte. Microangiopathy also can lead to keratocyte formation.

17. Describe the morphologic appearance of schistocytes.

Schistocytes are fragments of damaged erythrocytes that appear as crescents, triangles, or other irregular shapes (see Figure 2-2).

18. How are schistocytes formed?

Schistocytes are formed secondary to mechanical trauma in the vasculature. Physical trauma to the erythrocyte membrane as it passes through fibrin deposits within vessel walls, as seen with disseminated intravascular coagulation (DIC), can result in schistocyte formation.

19. What diseases have schistocytes been associated with in small animals?

Schistocytes have been associated with a number of fibrin-forming conditions, including hemangiosarcoma, vasculitis, congestive heart failure, DIC, myelofibrosis, microangiopathic anemia, and glomerulonephritis.

20. What are acanthocytes, and with what diseases are they associated?

Acanthocytes are erythrocytes with several unevenly spaced, irregular projections or spicules that form secondary to an altered membrane lipid and cholesterol content (Figure 2-5).

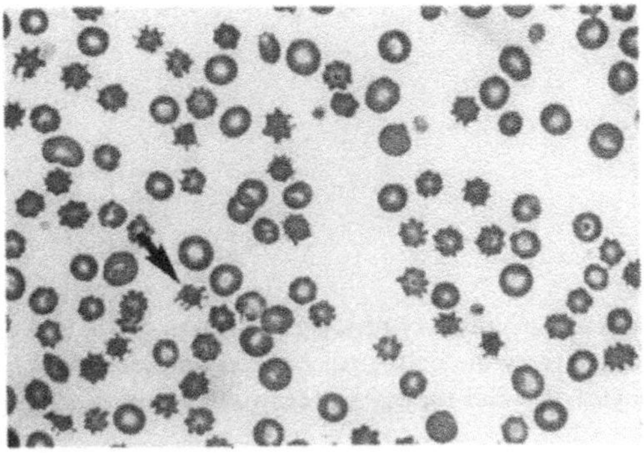

Figure 2-5 The arrow indicates an acanthocyte in this peripheral blood smear from a dog.

Acanthocytes are associated with diseases that alter lipid and cholesterol, such as liver disease, endocrine disease, malabsorptive diseases, and hemangiosarcoma, especially involving the liver.

21. What are the two major forms of echinocytes, and how are they formed?

The two major forms of echinocytes are crenated erythrocytes (*type I* echinocytes) and Burr cells (*type III* echinocytes) (Figure 2-6). *Crenated erythrocytes* have projections only along the outer perimeter of the erythrocyte that is in contact with the glass slide. Crenation is an artifact associated with blood smear preparation and caused by temperature, pH, and drying time. In contrast, *Burr cells* are formed in vivo, often as a result of changes in electrolyte concentration. Burr cells have projections over their entire surface.

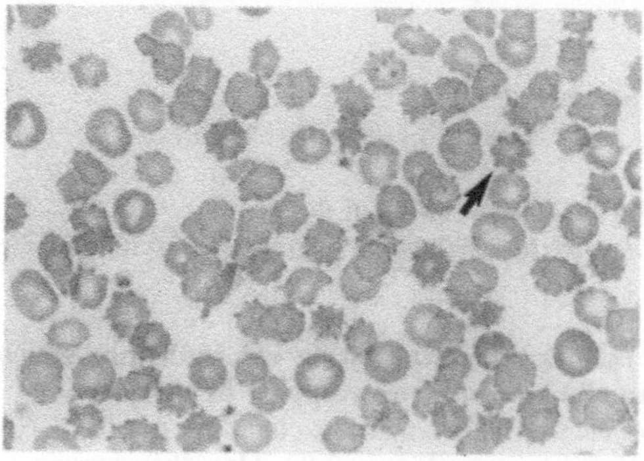

Figure 2-6 Peripheral blood smear from a dog. The arrow identifies an echinocyte.

22. Describe the morphologic features that distinguish an echinocyte from an acanthocyte.

As with acanthocytes, echinocytes are characterized by the presence of multiple projections along the erythrocyte surface. However, echinocyte spicules are uniform and evenly spaced along the cell surface (see Figure 2-6), whereas acanthocyte spicules are unevenly spaced and irregular (see Figure 2-5).

23. What are eccentrocytes, and how are they formed?

Eccentrocytes, also known as *hemighost erythrocytes,* contain a clear-staining area (blister) in their cytoplasm that results from redistribution of hemoglobin concentration. Eccentrocytes are formed secondary to oxidative injury to the erythrocyte.

24. Define hypochromia and explain its significance.

Hypochromia is reduced cytoplasmic staining with increased central pallor in the erythrocyte (Figure 2-7). This is a result of decreased amounts of hemoglobin within the RBC. Normally in the dog, central pallor is a light-pale area in the central one third to one half of the erythrocyte. Extension beyond this area can subjectively indicate hypochromasia. Any factor that interferes with the production of hemoglobin can result in hypochromia, including iron deficiency and lead toxicosis. However, iron deficiency is the most common cause of hypochromia in the dog and cat.

25. What is the difference between a reticulocyte and a polychromatophilic erythrocyte?

There is no true difference between a reticulocyte and a polychromatophilic erythrocyte. Immature erythrocytes are termed *reticulocytes* when stained with new methylene blue and are termed *polychromatophilic erythrocytes* when stained with a Romanowsky stain (Wright's, Diff-Quik) because they appear as larger, bluish pink erythrocytes. Although all polychromatophilic erythrocytes are reticulocytes when stained with new methylene blue, not all reticulocytes are polychromatophilic on Wright's stain.

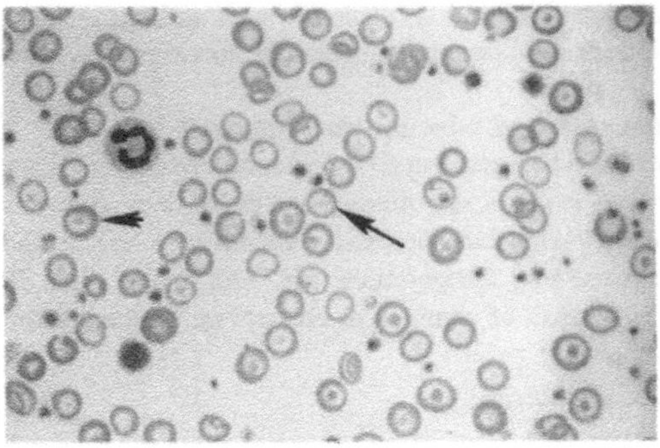

Figure 2-7 Erythrocyte hypochromasia is observed in this peripheral blood smear from a dog. The arrow indicates a hypochromic red blood cell (RBC); the arrowhead points to a normochromic RBC.

26. Do dogs have circulating reticulocytes in health?

Low numbers of reticulocytes are present in the blood of healthy dogs (<1%).

27. What type of reticulocyte is found in the peripheral blood of dogs?

Canine reticulocytes are *aggregate* reticulocytes, in which larger aggregates of reticulum are found within the cytoplasm (see Figure 1-1).

28. Identify and describe the two types of reticulocytes found in the cat, indicating which type is most useful in the determination of a bone marrow response to anemia.

a. *Punctate reticulocytes*. These reticulocytes have small, punctate clumps of residual RNA and are more mature than aggregate reticulocytes (Figure 2-8). Also, they remain in circulation for several weeks. Punctate reticulocytes are not evaluated as often in reticulocyte counts because they persist so long in circulation, and they are not considered a good index of the current bone marrow response.

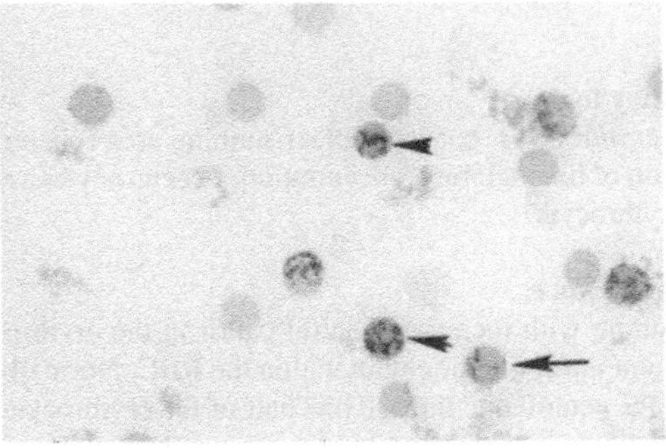

Figure 2-8 Punctate and aggregate reticulocytes stained with new methylene blue can be seen in this peripheral blood smear from a cat. The arrowheads indicate aggregate reticulocytes, and the arrow points to a punctate reticulocyte.

b. *Aggregate reticulocytes*. These reticulocytes are similar in appearance to those in the dog (see Question 27). Aggregate reticulocytes may exist in low numbers in the circulation of healthy cats (<0.4%) and are the type of reticulocyte evaluated in the determination of a bone marrow response. All polychromatophilic erythrocytes in cats are aggregate reticulocytes when stained with new methylene blue.

29. What are some normal breed variations in red cell morphology?

a. Asian dog breeds, including Akitas and Chow Chows, normally may have microcytic, normochromic erythrocytes.

b. Some miniature and toy poodles can have macrocytic, normochromic erythrocytes in health.
c. Hereditary stomatocytosis, or increased numbers of circulating stomatocytes, has been reported in the miniature schnauzer, malamute, and Drentse partrijshond.

3. EVALUATION OF ERYTHROCYTES

Shannon Jones Hostetter and Claire B. Andreasen

1. What are the major red blood cell indices used to characterize anemia in dogs and cats?

a. *Mean corpuscular volume* (MCV) is a measure of the size of the average erythrocyte and is measured in femtoliters (fl).
b. *Mean corpuscular hemoglobin concentration* (MCHC) is a measure of the concentration of hemoglobin in the average packed cell volume (PCV) unit and is expressed as grams per deciliter (g/dl).
c. *Red cell distribution width* (RDW) is a measure of the degree of size variation in erythrocytes (anisocytosis) and is expressed as a percentage.

2. List some factors that influence the mean corpuscular volume.

a. Young animals tend to have smaller erythrocytes and a corresponding low MCV.
b. MCV is most often increased as a result of reticulocytosis.
c. *Microcytosis,* or decreased MCV, can be seen in animals with portosystemic shunts.
d. Iron deficiency causes decreased MCV.
e. *Macrocytosis,* or increased MCV, has been described in cats infected with feline leukemia virus (FeLV).

3. What are some causes of hyperchromasia (increased MCHC)?

a. Absolute increases in MCHC, or actual increased hemoglobin within erythrocytes, are not usually observed and often are artifactual.
b. Intravascular or in vitro hemolysis is the most common artifact that causes increased MCHC.
c. Hyperlipidemia or Heinz bodies may cause falsely increased hemoglobin concentration due to interference.
d. Spherocytosis

4. What are some causes of hypochromia (decreased MCHC)?

a. Reticulocytosis leads to hypochromia (decreased MCHC.)
b. Iron deficiency can cause hypochromia.

5. How is new methylene blue used in erythrocyte evaluation?

New methylene blue is a stain used to identify the residual ribonucleic acid (RNA) in the cytoplasm of reticulocytes. Reticulocytes and Heinz bodies are accurately identified with this stain (see Figure 1-1).

6. What is rouleaux formation, and what is its significance in the dog and cat?

Rouleaux formations are clusters of erythrocytes that line up to resemble a stack of coins. These clusters are presumed to result from altered charge on the erythrocyte surface (Figure 3-1).

A mild degree of rouleaux formation can be observed in healthy dogs and cats. More pronounced rouleaux formation, however, has been associated with neoplastic and inflammatory disease, usually caused by increased plasma protein that alters the erythrocyte surface charge.

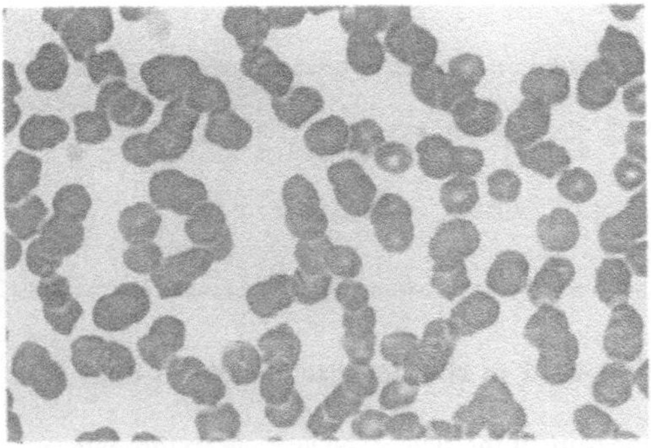

Figure 3-1 Prominent rouleaux formation is present in this peripheral blood smear from a horse.

7. Define erythrocyte autoagglutination, how it occurs, and how it is used as a diagnostic screening test.

Autoagglutination is the process by which erythrocytes adhere to each other and form cohesive aggregates that do not dissipate when mixed with equal parts of saline (Figure 3-2). Autoagglutination occurs when erythrocytes are coated with surface antibody that interacts with adjacent erythrocytes; therefore, autoagglutination indicates immune-mediated hemolytic anemia. Autoagglutination is usually associated with immunoglobulin M (IgM) antibody deposition on the erythrocyte surface because IgM is more efficient at cross-linking than any other class of antibody. High concentrations of IgG complex deposition on the erythrocyte surface also can result in autoagglutination.

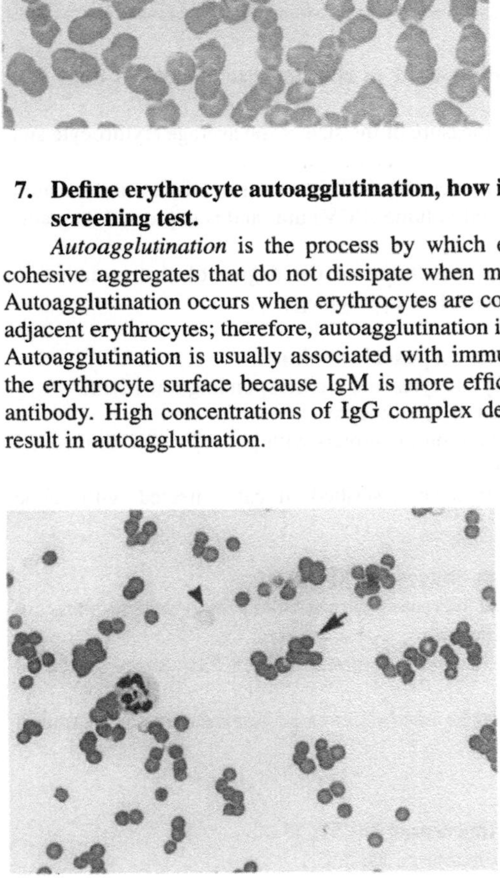

Figure 3-2 Peripheral blood smear from a dog. The arrow indicates autoagglutination. A ghost erythrocyte also is present *(arrowhead).*

8. What does the red cell distribution width measure?

The RDW is an erythrocyte index used to determine the degree of variation in red cell volume. The higher the value above the reference interval, the greater is the erythrocyte size variation. Therefore, RDW correlates to the degree of anisocytosis in the erythrocyte population.

9. What is a direct Coombs' test, and under what circumstances is it useful as a diagnostic tool?

The direct Coombs' test identifies either surface antibody or complement on erythrocytes.

The direct Coombs' test is used when immune-mediated hemolytic anemia is suspected (e.g., cases of regenerative anemia), but autoagglutination and significant spherocytosis are not observed. The Coombs' test is more sensitive and is capable of detecting lower concentrations of surface antibody and complement than autoagglutination.

10. By what methods are reticulocytes typically evaluated?

Peripheral blood smears are stained with new methylene blue, and reticulocytes are enumerated in the following ways:

a. Reticulocyte percentage
b. Corrected reticulocyte percentage
c. Absolute reticulocyte count

11. What accuracy problems exist for methods of reticulocyte evaluation?

a. The reticulocyte percentage tends to overestimate the bone marrow response for two reasons. First, less mature reticulocytes remain longer in peripheral blood than mature reticulocytes, thus falsely overestimating the current bone marrow response. Second, because anemic animals have lower numbers of mature erythrocytes in circulation, the number of reticulocytes is increased relative to mature erythrocytes.
b. Corrected reticulocyte percentage and absolute reticulocyte counts correct for the reduced red cell mass in anemia, but do not account for less mature erythrocytes.

12. How is an absolute reticulocyte count calculated, and at what value is a response considered regenerative?

Absolute reticulocyte count = Reticulocyte percentage (converted to a decimal) × Total erythrocyte count per microliter (μl)

Example: 10% reticulocytes with 1 million RBCs/μl:

$$0.1 \times 1{,}000{,}000 = 100{,}000 \text{ reticulocytes/}\mu\text{l}$$

A regenerative response is indicated by a reticulocyte count greater than 80,000/μl in the dog and greater than 60,000/μl in the cat.

13. How is the corrected reticulocyte percentage determined, and at what value is a response considered regenerative?

The corrected reticulocyte percentage is determined using the following formula:

Reticulocyte percentage × (Patient's hematocrit/Average normal hematocrit*)

*For the species: 45% in dogs, 37% in cats.

A corrected reticulocyte percentage of greater than 1% in the dog and greater than 0.4% in the cat is considered an indication of a regenerative response.

4. ANEMIA

Shannon Jones Hostetter and Claire B. Andreasen

1. Define anemia and explain the difference between relative anemia and absolute anemia.

Anemia is defined as a decrease in the hematocrit, erythrocyte count, and hemoglobin concentration. *Relative anemia* is not associated with a true reduction in the total red blood cell (RBC) mass, but rather is caused by a dilutional effect that can be observed after aggressive fluid therapy or other cause of increased plasma volume. *Absolute anemia* is considered an actual reduction in the total RBC mass.

2. What parameters are used to classify anemias in dogs and cats?

The various RBC indices, including mean corpuscular volume (MCV), mean corpuscular hemoglobin (MCH), mean corpuscular hemoglobin concentration (MCHC), and red cell distribution width (RDW) (see Chapter 3), are useful in classifying anemias as either regenerative or nonregenerative. Also, both reticulocyte count and RBC morphology are extremely important in determining if an anemia is regenerative or nonregenerative.

3. Identify some common causes of nonregenerative anemia.

a. Blood loss of less than 3 days (a regenerative anemia that has not yet had time to show a regenerative response)
b. Erythropoietic suppression
   (1) Anemia of chronic disease (anemia of inflammatory disease)
   (2) Renal failure
   (3) Metabolic disease
   (4) Drugs and toxins
c. Infections (e.g., parvoviruses)
d. Bone marrow disease:
   (1) Myelofibrosis
   (2) Pure red cell aplasia
   (3) Marrow necrosis
   (4) Neoplasia
e. Radiation

4. List the two major categories of regenerative anemia and give examples of each.

Hemorrhage

a. Acute blood loss of greater than 3 days' duration
b. Some cases of shorter term chronic blood loss anemia (but if iron deficiency develops or if a concurrent disease blunts the regenerative response, then there can be a nonregenerative anemia)

Hemolysis

a. Pyruvate kinase (PK) deficiency
b. Phosphofructokinase (PFK) deficiency
c. Immune-mediated hemolytic anemia
d. Infection-associated hemolysis (e.g., erythrocyte parasites, some bacteria)
e. Chemical/toxin-induced hemolytic anemia
f. Microangiopathic hemolytic anemia

5. Describe the characteristics of anemia from acute blood loss.

a. After acute hemorrhage, hematocrit initially is within the normal reference interval because both cellular components and plasma are lost in equal amounts. The body begins to replace plasma volume a few hours after blood loss, with total replacement of plasma volume in 2 to 3 days. Hematocrit begins to drop as plasma volume is restored as a result of hemodilution.

b. Polychromasia is an indicator of increased bone marrow production of erythrocytes and is observed within 2 to 3 days after acute blood loss.

c. Reticulocytosis is observed within 2 to 3 days of acute blood loss unless suppressed by another concurrent disease.

6. Approximately how long does it take for the hemogram to return to normal after an acute, finite period of blood loss in the dog?

It takes approximately 1 to 2 weeks for the hemogram to return to reference intervals in the dog.

7. What are the characteristics of anemia secondary to chronic blood loss?

a. Regenerative progressing to nonregenerative anemia: the anemia becomes nonregenerative as iron stores are used up leading to an iron deficiency anemia with time. This anemia is generally not as pronounced as that seen with acute blood loss.

b. Iron deficiency anemia: can develop secondary to prolonged hemorrhage.

8. What is the most reliable laboratory indicator of regenerative anemia in dogs and cats?

An absolute increase in reticulocyte numbers is the best indicator of a regenerative bone marrow response to anemia.

9. List the common erythrocyte changes that indicate a regenerative anemia.

a. Reticulocytosis

b. Polychromasia

c. Anisocytosis/increased RDW

d. Macrocytosis/hypochromasia due to reticulocytosis

10. Define extravascular hemolysis, and list common causes of extravascular hemolysis in the dog and cat.

Extravascular hemolysis is the removal and subsequent breakdown of erythrocytes by macrophages within the spleen and liver.

Causes of extravascular hemolysis include reduced RBC deformability, antibody or complement-mediated phagocytosis, hypersplenism, and altered cytoplasmic adenosine triphosphate (ATP) content.

11. What is intravascular hemolysis, and what are at least four mechanisms of this disorder in the dog and cat?

Intravascular hemolysis is the rupture of erythrocytes within the vascular system.

Mechanisms for intravascular hemolysis include the following:

a. Oxidative injury

b. Membrane alteration

c. Physical damage

d. Immune-mediated lysis

e. Parasitism (e.g., babesiosis) (Figure 4-1)

f. Traumatic rupture

g. Enzyme deficiency

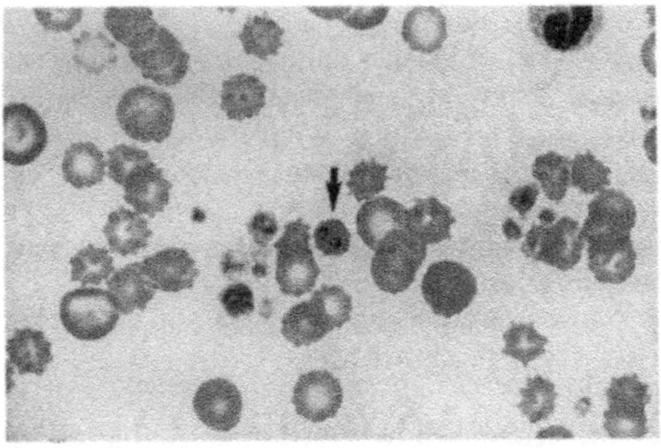

Figure 4-1 Peripheral blood smear from a dog infected with *Babesia canis*. The arrow identifies an erythrocyte containing the parasite.

12. Identify causes of Heinz body anemia in the cat and dog.

Cats are more susceptible to Heinz body formation than other species because their hemoglobin is more easily oxidized. Heinz body anemia in the cat may be associated with certain endocrine disorders (e.g., diabetes mellitus, hyperthyroidism) and certain oxidative agents (e.g., onions, acetaminophen). Heinz body anemia in the canine may result from ingestion of onions, acetaminophen, or zinc-containing foreign objects, such as pennies (see Figure 2-1).

13. What is the most common cause of iron deficiency anemia in the dog and cat?

The most common cause of iron deficiency anemia in small animals is external blood loss. Although dietary deficiency is a major cause of iron deficiency anemia in humans, this is rarely a factor in small animals except in extreme cases of inadequate nutrition. The period of blood loss is often prolonged (chronic hemorrhage) before iron deficiency anemia develops in adult animals. Although there are many potential causes of chronic blood loss, gastrointestinal (GI) hemorrhage is the most common. Internal blood loss typically does not result in iron-lacking anemia because the iron can be reabsorbed from the site of hemorrhage.

14. Define immune-mediated hemolytic anemia.

Immune-mediated hemolytic anemia (IMHA) is typically a regenerative anemia that develops when the animal produces antibody against proteins on the surface of its own erythrocytes or erythrocyte precursors (antibodies against erythrocyte precursors can result in a nonregenerative anemia). This antibody bound to the surface of the erythrocyte leads to destruction of the red cell through complement-mediated lysis and phagocytosis by splenic or hepatic macrophages. IMHAs are a form of type II hypersensitivity.

15. List potential causes of immune-mediated hemolytic anemia.

a. Idiopathic: autoimmune hemolytic anemia (AIHA)
b. Drugs (e.g., penicillin) can adhere to the erythrocyte membrane. If antibodies are produced against the drug, the erythrocyte is destroyed.
c. Paraneoplastic syndrome (multiple myeloma, lymphoma)
d. Infectious agents, such as feline leukemia virus (FeLV), *Ehrlichia* species, and *Mycoplasma haemofelis* (formerly *Haemobartonella felis*) or *Mycoplasma haemocanis* (formerly *Haemobartonella canis*) (Figure 4-2)

16. Describe the signalment and typical clinical signs associated with autoimmune hemolytic anemia.

AIHA is considered the most common cause of hemolytic anemia in the dog and most often affects young adult to middle-aged dogs.

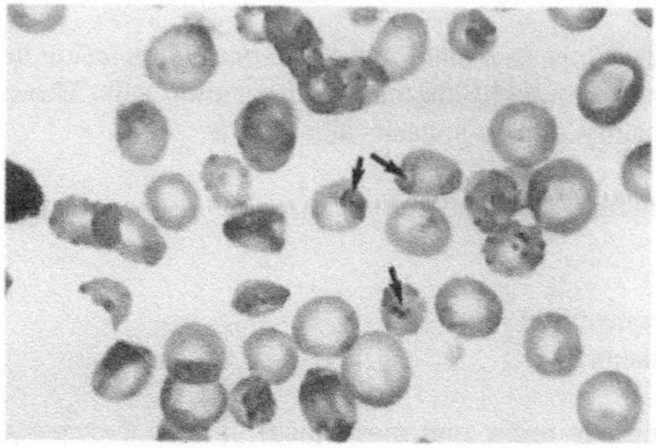

Figure 4-2 Peripheral blood smear from a dog infected with *Mycoplasma haemocanis*. The arrows identify organisms.

Clinical signs of AIHA are often associated with an acute hemolytic crisis and include the following:

a. Acute lethargy, weakness, and anorexia
b. Pallor with or without icterus
c. Fever in some dogs

In other dogs the clinical signs can be more vague and may include GI signs (vomiting, diarrhea) or owner complaints that the dog "isn't doing right."

17. What are the typical hematologic findings in a dog with autoimmune hemolytic anemia?

a. Decreased hematocrit: in dogs in an acute hemolytic crisis, hematocrit can be quite low (7%-15%). In compensated dogs not in an acute crisis, hematocrit may be only moderately decreased (20%-25%).
b. Reticulocytosis: most affected dogs have a strong regenerative response with substantially increased numbers of circulating reticulocytes (see Figure 1-1).
c. Spherocytosis: dogs may have numerous spherocytes circulating in their blood, since antibody-coated erythrocytes are partially phagocytosed by splenic and hepatic macrophages, resulting in spherocyte formation (see Figure 1-2).
d. Macrocytic, hypochromic anemia: this is a common finding caused by increased reticulocytes and indicating a regenerative response.
e. Positive Coombs' test: this can strongly support the diagnosis of AIHA. Use caution if the test is negative, however, because a percentage of AIHA patients will have a negative Coombs' test.

18. Describe the typical findings in an animal with aplastic anemia (pancytopenia), including clinical signs and laboratory findings.

Aplastic anemia is caused by decreased to absent erythropoiesis, granulopoiesis, and thrombopoiesis due to bone marrow suppression. As a result, affected animals have a nonregenerative, normocytic, normochromic anemia accompanied by leukopenia and thrombocytopenia. In cats with FeLV-induced pancytopenia, the anemia can be macrocytic, normochromic.

Affected dogs and cats often exhibit the typical clinical signs of anemia (lethargy, pallor, exercise intolerance). Additionally, these animals also may present with a bleeding disorder (secondary to the thrombocytopenia) or acute infection (secondary to the leukopenia).

19. Identify potential causes of aplastic anemia in the dog and cat.

a. Infectious agents (FeLV in cats, ehrlichiosis in dogs)
b. Irradiation
c. Certain toxicoses
d. Drugs (e.g., estrogen, phenylbutazone, chloramphenicol)

20. Define myelophthisic anemia.

Myelophthisic anemia is an anemia that develops secondary to a space-occupying lesion in the bone marrow, in which nonmarrow elements crowd out the marrow progenitor cells. These nonmarrow elements include stromal, inflammatory, and neoplastic cells.

21. List specific causes of myelophthisic anemia.

a. Myelofibrosis
b. Metastatic neoplasia
c. Severe osteomyelitis (e.g., fungal osteomyelitis)
d. Myeloproliferative disorders (e.g., leukemia)

22. Describe the disease characteristics and the most common causes of iron deficiency anemia in the dog and cat.

Chronic iron deficiency leads to ineffective erythropoiesis and subsequent anemia. Affected dogs and cats may show different clinical signs, depending on the underlying cause of the iron deficiency. Many animals with iron deficiency anemia are diagnosed by chance when a complete blood count (CBC) is performed for some other purpose.

The most common cause of iron deficiency anemia in the dog and cat is chronic blood loss. Puppies and kittens on an all-milk diet may develop transient iron deficiency and a subsequent mild anemia.

23. List the key laboratory findings in iron deficiency anemia.

a. Microcytic, hypochromic anemia. The microcytosis occurs because the erythrocytes undergo an extra division during maturation, since a sufficient concentration of hemoglobin is needed to stop cell division.
b. Decreased serum iron and decreased serum ferritin
c. Decreased iron stores noted upon bone marrow examination
d. Decreased total saturation of transferrin, the iron transport protein

24. What is anemia of chronic disease, and what are general causes of the disorder?

Anemia of chronic disease, also known as *anemia of inflammatory disease,* is a common anemia that develops secondary to a variety of chronic diseases in both dogs and cats. Excess cytokines released in inflammation, decreased erythropoietin production and efficacy, and decreased utilization of iron stores are all presumed to be involved in the development of the disorder.

A variety of infectious, inflammatory, and neoplastic diseases can result in anemia of chronic disease.

25. List the typical laboratory findings in anemia of chronic disease.

a. Mild to moderate anemia, with hematocrit usually 20% to 30%
b. Normocytic, normochromic, nonregenerative anemia
c. Normal to decreased serum iron concentration
d. Normal to increased serum ferritin

26. Which endocrine disorders in the dog can affect red cell production?

Hypothyroidism can result in a mild, nonregenerative anemia secondary to decreased demand for oxygen because of reduced metabolism.

Hypoadrenocorticism can cause a mild nonregenerative anemia because of decreased action of erythropoietin (adrenocortical hormones enhance the action of erythropoietin). Also, some dogs with hypoadrenocorticism develop a more severe anemia secondary to both GI hemorrhage and chronic disease.

Hyperestrogenism, either iatrogenic or primary, can cause bone marrow suppression and lead to nonregenerative anemia.

27. Enumerate the mechanisms by which chronic renal failure leads to anemia.

a. Loss of functional peritubular cells in the kidney leads to decreased production of erythropoietin.
b. Uremia can inhibit erythropoiesis and cause intravascular hemolysis.
c. Ulcers that develop within the GI tract secondary to uremia can bleed and further exacerbate the anemia.
d. Uremia can decrease platelet function and contribute to hemorrhage, especially in the ulcerated GI tract.

28. How does feline leukemia virus infection cause anemia in the cat?

FeLV directly infects erythroid progenitors and inhibits their differentiation, subsequently leading to decreased production of mature erythrocytes and resulting in a mild, moderate, or severe anemia. Additionally, anemia of chronic disease can further exacerbate the anemia. Infected cats that develop lymphoma involving the bone marrow also may develop anemia secondary to a myelophthistic process.

29. Which common veterinary drugs can lead to aplastic anemia in dogs and cats?

a. Estrogen (diethylstilbestrol, estradiol)
b. Phenylbutazone
c. Chloramphenicol
d. Trimethoprim-sulfadiazine
e. Albendazole
f. Many chemotherapeutic drugs

30. Define pure red cell aplasia, and identify a cause of the disorder in the dog and cat.

Pure red cell aplasia is a marked normocytic, normochromic, nonregenerative anemia caused by the selective loss of RBC precursors in the bone marrow. In the dog and cat, both primary and secondary forms of the disorder have been described. *Primary* pure red cell aplasia is presumed to result from immune-mediated destruction of erythroid precursors. *Secondary* pure red cell aplasia in the cat has been associated with FeLV infection. Parvovirus infection has been implicated as a cause of secondary pure red cell aplasia in the dog.

31. Define microangiopathic hemolytic anemia.

Microangiopathic hemolytic anemia is the destruction of erythrocytes resulting from the narrowing or obstruction of small blood vessels. This small vessel pathology causes lysis of RBCs as they pass through the affected vessel and can lead to anemia.

32. List the laboratory characteristics of microangiopathic anemia.

a. Schistocytes
b. Thrombocytopenia
c. Regenerative or nonregenerative anemia

33. Identify conditions that can lead to microangiopathic anemia.

Any process that results in deposition of fibrin in vessel lumens or vascular damage can lead to microangiopathic anemia. Specific examples include disseminated intravascular coagulation (DIC), hemangiosarcoma, vasculitis, and inflammation.

5. POLYCYTHEMIA

Shannon Jones Hostetter and Claire B. Andreasen

1. Define polycythemia, and explain the difference between relative and absolute polycythemia.

Polycythemia is defined as an increase in the hematocrit, erythrocyte count, and hemoglobin concentration.

In *relative* polycythemia, total erythrocyte mass is normal but appears to increase.

In *absolute* polycythemia, increased erythrocyte production results in a true expansion of the total erythrocyte mass.

2. What are the two types of absolute polycythemia?

Absolute polycythemia can be further divided into *primary* absolute polycythemia (normal to decreased erythropoietin levels) and *secondary* absolute polycythemia (increased erythropoietin levels).

3. What are the common causes of relative polycythemia in the dog and cat?

a. *Dehydration.* Hematocrit, erythrocyte count, and hemoglobin concentration are all relatively increased because of reduced plasma volume. The most common mechanisms of dehydration in the dog and cat include vomiting, diarrhea, diuresis, and water deprivation.
b. *Splenic contraction.* Cats in particular can have a relative polycythemia caused by release of erythrocytes from the spleen after splenic contraction. In cats, excitement causes release of epinephrine that mediates contraction of the spleen.

4. Discuss the major mechanism of primary absolute polycythemia.

Also known as *polycythemia vera* and *primary erythrocytosis,* primary absolute polycythemia is an erythrocytosis that results from a myeloproliferative disorder. Erythropoietin levels are typically normal to decreased in affected animals.

5. Identify two causes of secondary absolute polycythemia.

a. Chronic hypoxia, as seen with chronic lung disease or at high altitudes, can lead to increased production of erythropoietin, resulting in increased erythrocyte production.
b. Several diseases can lead to increased erythropoietin secretion without hypoxia, also known as *inappropriate erythropoietin secretion,* including erythropoietin-secreting neoplasms (e.g., nephroma, hepatoma), some endocrinopathies, and renal cysts.

6. ERYTHROCYTE DISORDERS

Shannon Jones Hostetter and Claire B. Andreasen

1. Identify the characteristic hematologic changes secondary to lead toxicity in small animals.

a. Normal to mildly decreased hematocrit, but usually not less than 30%
b. Basophilic stippling of erythrocytes
c. Increased nucleated red blood cells (nRBCs)
d. Poikilocytosis

2. Explain the pathogenesis of lead toxicity in dogs and cats.

Lead toxicosis in small animals usually results from ingestion of lead-containing objects, such as lead-based paint chips, batteries, and lead fishing weights. Puppies under 6 months of age are at a greater risk of toxicosis than older dogs or cats, both because they are more likely to ingest foreign objects and because they absorb more lead from the gastrointestinal (GI) tract than their adult counterparts. Dogs and cats with lead toxicity develop GI and neurologic signs as well as the hematologic changes listed above. Lead inhibits several enzymes that incorporate iron into hemoglobin, causing oxidative damage to the bone marrow, which results in increased release of nRBCs from the marrow. Lead also inhibits ribosomal breakdown in erythrocytes, leading to basophilic stippling.

3. What is methemoglobin reductase deficiency in the dog?

Methemoglobin reductase deficiency is presumed to be an inherited disorder that results in persistent methemoglobinemia. Although considered a rare disorder, it has been identified in several breeds, including poodles, Chihuahuas, Eskimo dogs, Borzoi, and English setters. Affected animals typically have a normal life expectancy and exhibit minimal clinical signs.

4. List the clinical signs and laboratory findings associated with methemoglobin reductase deficiency in the dog.

Clinical Signs

a. Persistently cyanotic mucous membranes
b. Exercise intolerance
c. No clinical signs exhibited in many animals

Laboratory Findings

a. Persistently dark-brown/red venous blood samples
b. Increased methemoglobin content in the blood (greater than 12% methemoglobin)
c. Normal oxygen tension (Po_2)
d. Normal to mildly increased hematocrit

5. What is phosphofructokinase deficiency, and what breeds are predisposed?

Phosphofructokinase (PFK) *deficiency* is a relatively uncommon disease of dogs that results from an enzyme defect. Decreased activity of PFK in affected dogs leads to decreased adenosine triphosphate (ATP) and 2,3-diphosphoglycerate (2,3-DPG) in erythrocytes.

PFK deficiency is an inherited disorder that affects different breeds, including English springer spaniels and cocker spaniels.

6. Describe the clinical signs associated with PFK deficiency.

Clinical signs associated with PFK deficiency include intermittent episodes of extreme lethargy, anorexia, pallor or icterus, and pigmentation of urine (corresponding to hemolytic episodes). These events are often initiated by periods of stress (e.g., heavy exercise, hyperthermia). Some affected dogs also exhibit an exertional myopathy.

7. List the typical laboratory findings in animals with PFK deficiency.

a. Intermittent intravascular hemolysis
b. Macrocytic, hypochromic anemia
c. Persistent reticulocytosis
d. Intermittent pigmenturia

8. What is pyruvate kinase deficiency?

Pyruvate kinase (PK) *deficiency* is an inherited disorder that has been described in humans, dogs, and cats. PK is an important enzyme in the production of ATP through the glycolytic pathway. Because erythrocytes lack mitochondria and generate all their ATP through anaerobic glycolysis, PK deficiency results in decreased production of ATP. This altered ATP production leads to erythrocyte dysfunction and premature lysis.

9. Identify the clinical signs and laboratory findings associated with PK deficiency in the dog.

Dogs with PK deficiency develop a highly regenerative anemia combined with osteosclerosis and myelofibrosis. Affected dogs seem to adapt well to the anemia and may not show the clinical signs of lethargy and inappetence associated with severe anemia.

Laboratory findings include (a) severe macrocytic, hypochromic anemia (hematocrit range typically 12% to 26%) that is strongly regenerative and (b) shortened RBC life span.

Radiographs of long bones often reveal concurrent osteosclerosis by 1 year of age.

10. Which breeds have been identified with PK deficiency?

PK deficiency has been identified in Basenjis, Chihuahuas, West Highland White terriers, Cairn terriers, Beagles, Eskimo dogs, miniature poodles, and Abyssinian and domestic shorthaired cats.

11. In which cellular locations do erythrocyte parasites reside?

a. Intracellular: within the erythrocyte
b. Epicellular: immediately beneath the cell membrane

12. Identify the various erythrocyte parasites that occur in the dog and the cat.

Dog

a. Intracellular
   (1) *Babesia canis*
   (2) *Babesia gibsoni*
b. Epicellular: *Mycoplasma haemocanis* (formerly *Haemobartonella canis*)

Cat

a. Intracellular
   (1) *Babesia felis* (not present in North America)
   (2) *Babesia cati* (not present in North America)
   (3) *Cytauxzoon felis*
b. Epicellular: *Mycoplasma haemofelis* (formerly *Haemobartonella felis*)

13. Describe the clinical and laboratory findings associated with *Mycoplasma haemofelis* infection.

Although subclinical infections are common, acutely ill cats often have anemia, lethargy, inappetence, weight loss, pallor, and splenomegaly.

Peripheral blood smears from acutely ill cats reveal parasitemia in approximately half the cases. Other laboratory findings include mild to severe anemia that is usually regenerative, except in acute cases or immunocompromised cats.

14. List the risk factors for acquiring *Mycoplasma haemofelis.*

a. Exposure to blood-sucking arthropods
b. Feline leukemia virus (FeLV) infection
c. Outdoor roaming behavior
d. Age less than 3 years
e. Anemia

15. What classification of organism causes canine babesiosis, how is the disease transmitted, and which species are found in the United States?

Canine babesiosis is caused by intraerythrocytic protozoal parasites in the genus *Babesia.* Babesiosis is transmitted by ticks and blood transfusions. Two distinct *Babesia* isolates have been identified in the United States: *Babesia gibsoni* and a small piroplasm isolate related to *B. gibsoni* that has been reported in California. In the United States there is an increased incidence of *B. gibsoni* infection in pit bull terriers.

7. LARGE ANIMAL HEMATOLOGY

Shannon Jones Hostetter and Claire B. Andreasen

1. Can reticulocyte counts be used as a measure of a regenerative response in anemia in the horse? Why or why not?

Reticulocyte counts are not used to evaluate the bone marrow response in equine anemia. Reticulocytes are not found in significant numbers in the peripheral blood of the horse in health or disease because they mature within the bone marrow.

2. How do you determine a regenerative response in equine anemias?

Because horses do not release reticulocytes from the bone marrow into circulation in significant numbers, reticulocyte counts cannot be used as an index of regeneration in this species.

Methods to evaluate bone marrow responses in horses include repeated hematocrits, bone marrow evaluation, and red cell distribution width (RDW).

3. Ingestion of bracken fern by ruminants has been associated with what hematologic abnormality?

Bracken fern toxicosis in ruminants can result in aplastic anemia.

4. **What is the average erythrocyte life span in the horse, cow, sheep, and pig?**
The average erythrocyte life span in the horse is 145 days versus 160 days in the cow and 150 days in sheep. Pig erythrocytes have a substantially shorter life span that averages approximately 86 days.

5. **Which vitamin deficiency can cause a nonregenerative anemia in swine?**
Vitamin E deficiency in swine can produce a nonregenerative anemia characterized by erythroid hyperplasia and dyserythropoiesis in the bone marrow.

6. **Erythrocytes from healthy Angora goats have what characteristic shape?**
Angora goats normally have elongate erythrocytes known as *fusocytes.*

7. **What group of domestic mammals normally has oval erythrocytes?**
Camelids, including llamas and alpacas, have oval erythrocytes often referred to as *elliptocytes.*

8. **Identify several morphologic features of normal bovine erythrocytes.**
Bovine erythrocytes average approximately 5.5 microns (μ) in diameter and have slight central pallor. Anisocytosis and crenation are common morphologic variations in erythrocytes of healthy bovines.

9. **What are the differences in erythrocyte size in ruminants?**
Sheep erythrocytes (3.2-6.0 μ) and goat erythrocytes (2.5-3.9 μ) are smaller than cattle erythrocytes (4-8 μ). This can cause difficulties in obtaining accurate erythrocyte counts with cell counters. The thresholds must be adjusted for the smaller erythrocyte size.

10. **What are the characteristic hematologic changes resulting from ingestion of red maple *(Acer rubrum)* leaves in the horse, and what is the pathogenesis of these changes?**
Red maple toxicity in the horse causes oxidative injury to erythrocytes, leading to intravascular hemolysis. The characteristic hematologic changes include anemia, Heinz body and eccentrocyte formation, methemoglobinemia, and hemoglobinemia.

11. **When do cattle have circulating reticulocytes?**
In health, cattle do not release reticulocytes from the bone marrow in significant numbers; normal erythrocyte maturation occurs in the bone marrow. Low numbers of circulating reticulocytes (approximately 1% or greater) are associated with a regenerative response to anemia.

12. **When do cattle have basophilic stippling in erythrocytes?**
During strongly regenerative anemias, cattle can have basophilic stippling in erythrocytes. These cases usually have associated reticulocytosis. Basophilic stippling in erythrocytes is not seen as often in cattle during lead poisoning, as seen in dogs.

13. **Identify several features of normal equine erythrocytes.**
Equine erythocytes are approximately 5.7 μ in diameter and lack significant central pallor. Equine erythrocytes often have rouleaux formation.

14. **How do you differentiate between regenerative and nonregenerative anemia in swine?**
Regenerative anemia in swine is characterized by reticulocytosis, significant polychromasia, and increased numbers of circulating nucleated red blood cells (nRBCs). Nonregenerative anemias do not have these characteristics of regeneration.

15. **Circulating nRBCs are common in newborns of which domestic species?**
It is common to find circulating nRBCs in young pigs.

16. Is rouleaux formation typically observed in the horse? In ruminants?

Rouleaux formation is often observed in healthy horses. Rouleaux formation is often absent in anemic and cachexic horses.

Rouleaux formation is rare in ruminants in both health and disease.

17. Identify the two species of the erythrocyte parasite *Anaplasma* that cause hemolytic anemia in cattle.

a. *Anaplasma marginale* affects cattle in tropical and subtropical climates worldwide and is capable of producing severe infection in naive cattle. This species is now considered endemic in the U.S. Southwest and West Coast.

b. *Anaplasma centrale* can cause mild disease in cattle and is endemic in the Middle East, South America, and southern Africa.

18. What are the two clinical syndromes associated with *Anaplasma marginale* infection in cattle, and what are the clinical signs associated with each?

a. *Acute anaplasmosis* is characterized by fever, hemolytic anemia, lethargy, anorexia, decrease in milk production, constipation, pallor, and icterus. Sudden death may occur, especially in cattle acquiring the infection after 2 years of age.

b. *Subclinical anaplasmosis* usually occurs if cattle are exposed to the organism as calves less than 1 year of age. Although these animals are typically asymptomatic, they can serve as a reservoir of infection for other cattle.

19. How do *Anaplasma marginale* organisms appear on Romanowsky-stained smears?

A. marginale organisms appear as basophilic bodies approximately 1 μ in diameter that are located within the erythrocyte. *A. marginale* infection is typically found along the erythrocyte margin.

20. When does poikilocytosis (variable shape) of erythrocytes occur in the peripheral blood of swine, ruminants, and horses?

Poikilocytes are typically found in healthy swine of all ages and are considered a normal finding in peripheral blood of pigs.

In cattle and goats, poikilocytes can normally be found in young animals during the switch from fetal to adult hemoglobin.

Poikilocytes are considered an abnormal hematologic finding in horses of all ages.

21. *Trichostrongylus* infection has been associated with what hematologic abnormality in ruminants?

Trichostrongylus infection can produce a nonregenerative anemia in cattle and sheep by an unknown mechanism.

22. What is the cause of bacillary hemoglobinuria in cattle?

A β toxin produced by *Clostridium haemolyticum* and *Clostridium novyi* type D produces bacillary hemoglobinuria in cattle. The β toxin is a hemolytic toxin that can rapidly lead to massive intravascular hemolysis in affected animals.

23. Describe the pertinent clinical findings in bacillary hemoglobinuria.

Bacillary hemoglobinuria causes an acute, marked hemolytic anemia that frequently results in sudden death. Clinical signs observed antemortem consist of fever, tachypnea, lethargy, and anorexia. Despite the implication in the disease's name, hemoglobinuria is an uncommon clinical finding in affected animals.

24. An abnormality of iron metabolism has been reported in what large animal species?

A hereditary condition in Salers cattle leads to iron accumulation and overload (hemochromatosis).

Erythrocytes

BIBLIOGRAPHY

1. Abkowitz JL: Retrovirus-induced feline pure red cell aplasia: pathogenesis and response to suramin, *Blood* 77(7):1442-1451, 1991.
2. Beutler E, Lichtman MA, Coller BS, et al, editors: *Williams hematology,* ed 6, New York, 2001, McGraw-Hill.
3. Brockus CW, Andreasen CB: Erythrocytes. In Duncan JR, Prasse KW, Mahaffey EA, editors: *Duncan and Prasse's veterinary laboratory medicine: clinical pathology,* ed 4, Ames, 2003, Iowa State University Press, pp 3-45.
4. Ettinger SJ, Feldman EC, editors: *Textbook of veterinary internal medicine: diseases of the dog and cat,* ed 5, 2000, Philadelphia, Saunders, pp 406-407, 1784-1816.
5. Feldman BF, Zinkl JG, Jain NC, editors: *Schalm's veterinary hematology,* ed 5, Philadelphia, 2000, Lippincott, Williams & Wilkins, pp 169-175, 197-198, 200-204, 1020-1025.
6. George LW, Divers TJ, Mahaffey EA, et al: Heinz body anemia and methemoglobinemia in ponies given red maple *(Acer rubrum L.)* leaves, *Vet Pathol* 19(5):521-533, 1982.
7. Greene CE, editor: *Infectious diseases of the dog and cat,* ed 2, Philadelphia, 1998, Saunders, pp 71-84, 166-172.
8. Grindem CB, Corbett WT, Tomkins MT: Risk factors for *Haemobartonella felis* infection in cats, *J Am Vet Med Assoc* 196(1):96-99, 1990.
9. Irizarry-Rovira AR, Stephens J, Christian J, et al: *Babesia gibsoni* infection in a dog from Indiana, *Vet Clin Pathol* 30(4):180-188, 2001.
10. McGavin MD, Carlton WW, Zachary JF, editors: Thomson's special veterinary pathology, ed 3, St Louis, 2001, Mosby, pp 325-245.
11. Means RT: Pathogenesis of the anemia of chronic disease: a cytokine-mediated anemia, *Stem Cells* 13(1):32-37, 1995.
12. Means RT, Krantz SB: Progress in understanding the pathogenesis of anemia of chronic disease, *Blood* 80(7):1639-1647, 1992.
13. Smith BP, editor: *Large animal internal medicine,* ed 2, St Louis, 1996, Mosby.

Leukocytes

8. MORPHOLOGY, FUNCTION, AND KINETICS

Stephen D. Gaunt

1. Describe the morphology of neutrophils from animals.

Neutrophils are the granulocytic leukocytes with specific granules that are usually inconspicuous or "neutral" in color. The specific granules of neutrophils from primates (including humans) stain more prominently, whereas in bovine neutrophils the cytoplasmic color is pink because of large tertiary granules. The neutrophil nucleus has darkly condensed chromatin and is segmented into three to five lobes interspersed by nuclear constrictions. In horses the individual lobes are further lobulated, producing a jagged or more segmented nuclear profile. On blood smears, neutrophils appear slightly smaller than the other granulocytic leukocytes, eosinophils and basophils (Figure 8-1).

2. What are heterophils?

In some small mammals the specific granules in neutrophils stain eosinophilic, so their neutrophils are termed *heterophils*. In rabbits the granules in heterophils are very prominent and, at first glance of a blood smear, more closely resemble eosinophils (Figure 8-2). The eosinophils

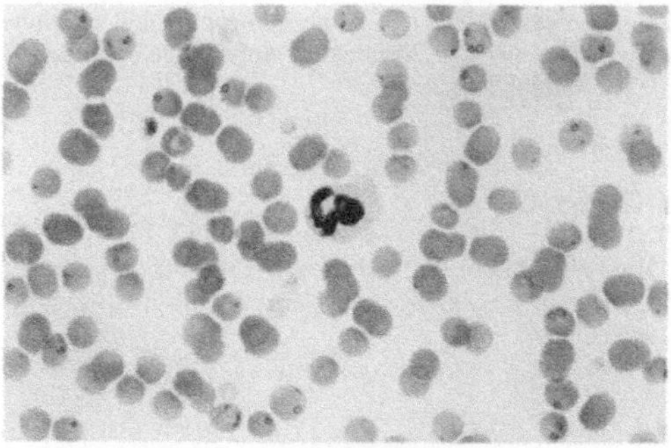

Figure 8-1 Canine neutrophil. (Wright's stain; 330×.)

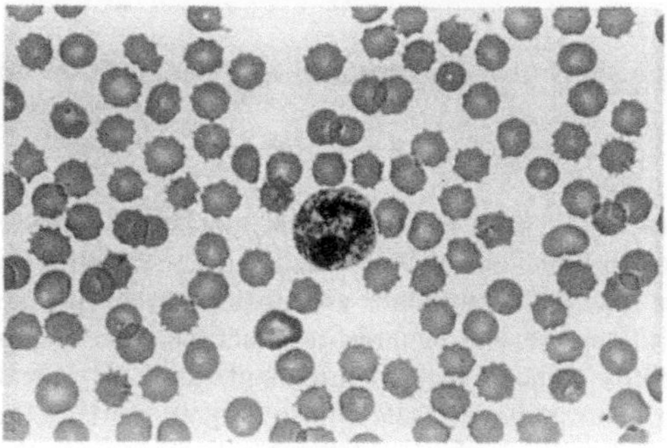

Figure 8-2 Rabbit heterophil. (Wright's stain; 330×.)

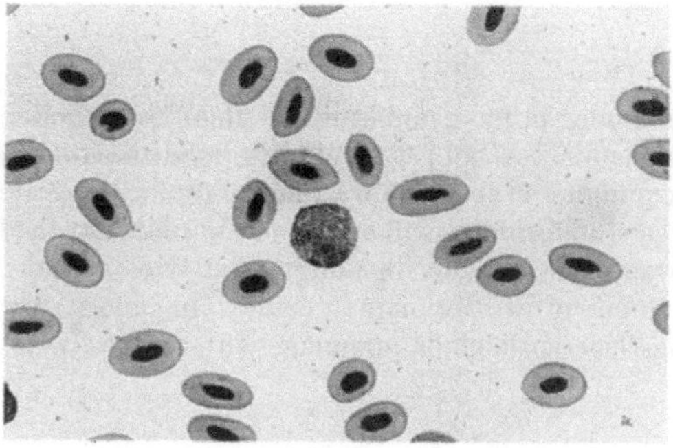

Figure 8-3 Avian heterophil. (Wright's stain; 330×.)

in rabbits are distinguished by their more intensely eosinophilic granules. In guinea pigs and hamsters the granules in heterophils are less prominent. In birds and reptiles the leukocytes considered the counterpart of neutrophils are also called heterophils. The heterophils of birds and reptiles contain large, prominent eosinophilic granules that are fusiform or round (Figure 8-3).

3. What is the "drumstick appendage"?

The drumstick appendage is a small, round nuclear lobe connected to the neutrophil nucleus by a thin filament (Figure 8-4). It is observed normally in a low percentage of the neutrophils in females and represents the inactivated second X chromosome. This structure corresponds to the Barr body found in epithelial cells of females. If observed in a significant number of the

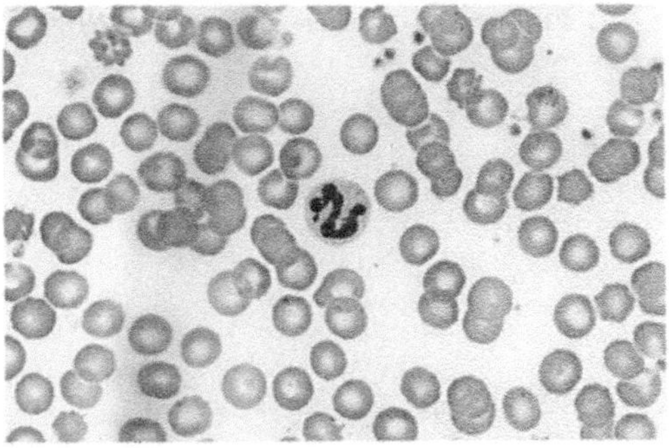

Figure 8-4 Canine neutrophil that contains the nuclear "drumstick appendage." (Wright's stain; 330×.)

neutrophils in a male, the drumstick appendage suggests a chromosomal disorder, such as the XXY syndrome in male calico cats.

4. What is the primary function of neutrophils?

Blood neutrophils are destined to enter tissues and serve as the frontline attack cell in acute inflammation. Neutrophils emigrate to sites of inflammation, where chemoattractants such as interleukin-8 (IL-8) and complement (C5a) are released. Neutrophils are most important for the phagocytosis and killing of bacteria. Neutrophils use several methods to attack bacteria within phagosomes, including the generation of oxidative radicals such as superoxide anion (O_2^-) and hydrogen peroxide (H_2O_2). The peroxidase in neutrophils interacts with hydrogen peroxide to generate hypochlorous acid ($HOCl^-$). Together, these and other oxidative products damage the lipid membranes of target cells. Neutrophils also release proteins such as defensin and lysozyme that have antibacterial activity.

5. Describe the morphology of eosinophils.

Eosinophils contain prominent specific granules in the cytoplasm that stain eosinophilic. The nucleus is lobulated as in other granulocytic leukocytes but is typically less lobulated than in neutrophils. The appearance of the cytoplasmic granules in eosinophils is unique for the domestic animals (Figures 8-5 and 8-6): rod shaped in cats, uniformly small and round in ruminants and pigs, very large and round in horses, and round but variable in number and size in dogs. Some canine eosinophils may contain as few as one or two very large granules. In contrast, the eosinophils of greyhounds and some other dogs lack eosinophilic granules, with clear vacuoles in the lightly basophilic cytoplasm.

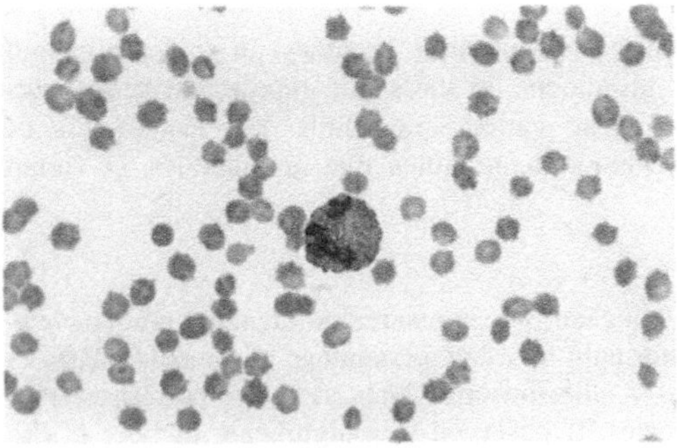

Figure 8-5 Equine eosinophil with large, round granules. (Wright's stain; 330×.)

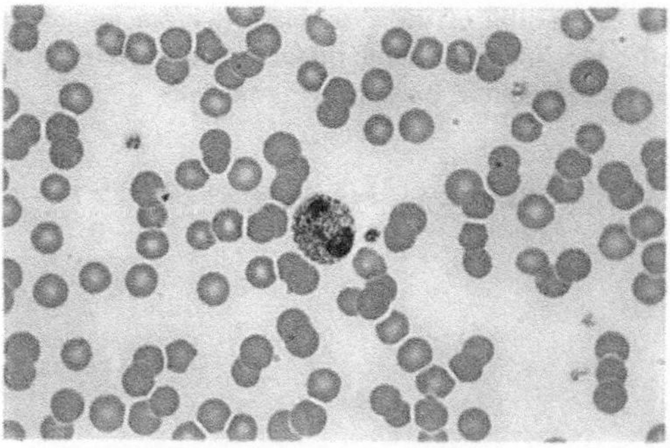

Figure 8-6 Feline eosinophil with rod-shaped granules. (Wright's stain; 330×.)

6. What are the functions of eosinophils?

Eosinophils have several functions, including the initiation of certain inflammatory responses and the suppression of immediate-type hypersensitivity responses. Eosinophils are particularly important in responding to helminthic parasites and are found in tissues (e.g., skin, respiratory, intestinal) where encounters with parasites are likely. Rather than phagocytize these large parasites, eosinophils release several cytotoxic mediators, in particular major basic protein, to the extracellular area surrounding the parasite. The myeloperoxidase in eosinophils can also generate oxidative radicals, but less effectively than neutrophils. The downside of this strategy is that during exuberant eosinophilic inflammation, the cytotoxic mediators released by eosinophils also injure host tissues.

7. Why is interleukin-5 important?

Interleukin-5 (IL-5) is a relatively specific mediator of eosinophil responses. This cytokine increases marrow eosinophilopoiesis, causes eosinophilia, and enhances the functions of mature eosinophils. IL-5 prolongs the survival of eosinophils by preventing their early demise from apoptosis. IL-5 is released by helper T lymphocytes in response to specific inflammatory or immunologic stimuli.

8. Describe the morphology of basophils.

The specific granules in basophils typically stain metachromatic (meaning "other color"), the unique color produced by hematologic stains that is purple rather than basophilic. The metachromatic staining characteristic of basophils is attributed to the proteoglycan content of their granules. The metachromatic granules in bovine, equine, and porcine basophils are numerous and can obscure the segmented nucleus (Figure 8-7). There are relatively low numbers

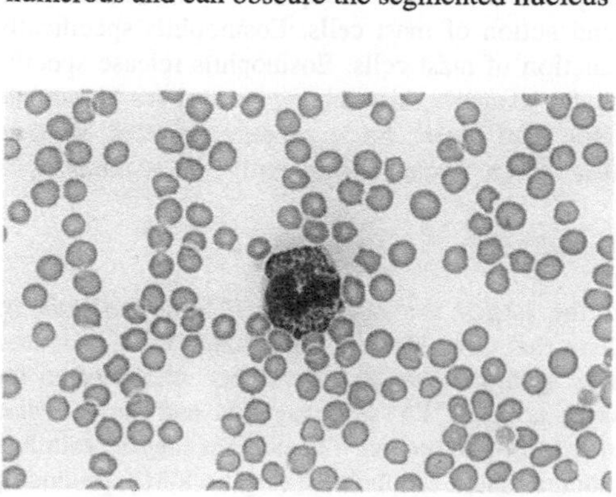

Figure 8-7 Equine basophil. (Wright's stain; 330×.)

of cytoplasmic granules in dogs, so the diffuse basophilia of the cytoplasm is more apparent. Feline basophils are unusual because the specific granules lose their metachromatic staining in basophil precursors and appear lavender or gray in the mature basophil (Figure 8-8).

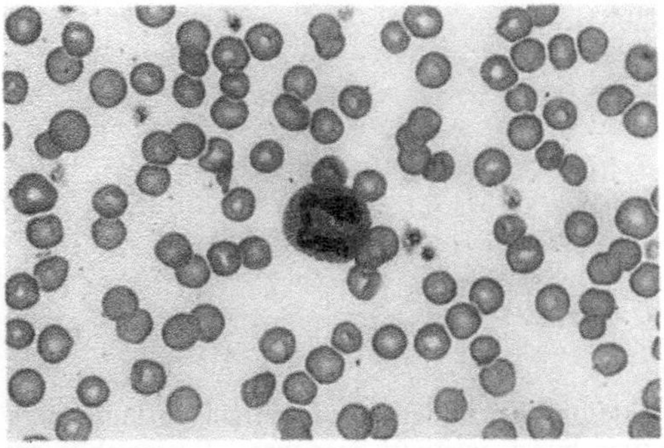

Figure 8-8 Feline basophil. (Wright's stain; 330×.)

9. What is the association between basophils and mast cells?

The basophil and mast cell share many features. Both originate from the hematopoietic stem cell in bone marrow, bear surface receptors for immunoglobulin E (IgE), participate in hypersensitivity reactions, and have metachromatic granules that contain similar mediators (e.g., histamine, heparin). However, basophils have a segmented nucleus and occur in blood, whereas mast cells are mononuclear cells that reside in tissues. Mast cells can be further categorized by biochemical features (e.g., chymase and tryptase content).

10. What are the functions of basophils?

Basophils are involved in hypersensitivity reactions to allergens that are mediated by IgE antibodies. While mast cells in tissues provide the initial response, basophils are recruited from blood to augment the allergic reaction. Basophils (and mast cells) release vasoactive mediators (e.g., histamine, leukotrienes) that increase vascular permeability and induce bronchoconstriction. These cells also release heparin, which interacts with antithrombin to inhibit coagulation locally. The hypersensitivity reactions involving basophils and mast cells are typically localized to the skin, intestines, and respiratory tract.

11. How do eosinophils counteract mast cells and basophils?

Eosinophils are important for neutralizing the immediate-type hypersensitivity mediated by mast cells and basophils. Eosinophils can phagocytose immune complexes and free mast cell granules, which diminishes the recruitment and action of mast cells. Eosinophils specifically inhibit the degranulation and leukotriene production of mast cells. Eosinophils release specific inhibitors of basophil and mast cell mediators; for example, histaminase neutralizes histamine, phospholipase inhibits platelet-activating factor, and major basic protein counters heparin. Not surprisingly, eosinophilia and basophilia often occur concurrently in animals with hypersensitivity reactions.

12. Describe the morphology of monocytes.

On blood smears, monocytes appear as the largest leukocytes. They have moderate to abundant amounts of more basophilic cytoplasm that often contains fine, azurophilic granules. Clear cytoplasmic vacuoles occur inconsistently in monocytes and have been attributed to the collection of blood in ethylenediaminetetraacetic acid (EDTA) anticoagulant and the activated status of the monocyte. The nuclear chromatin is loosely clumped. The nucleus may be round or band shaped (Figure 8-9), but more often the nuclear shape is lobulated (Figure 8-10), producing

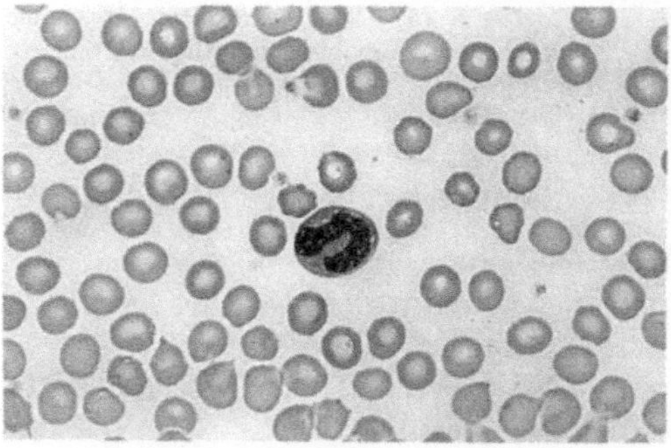

Figure 8-9 Canine monocyte with band-shaped nucleus. (Wright's stain; 330×.)

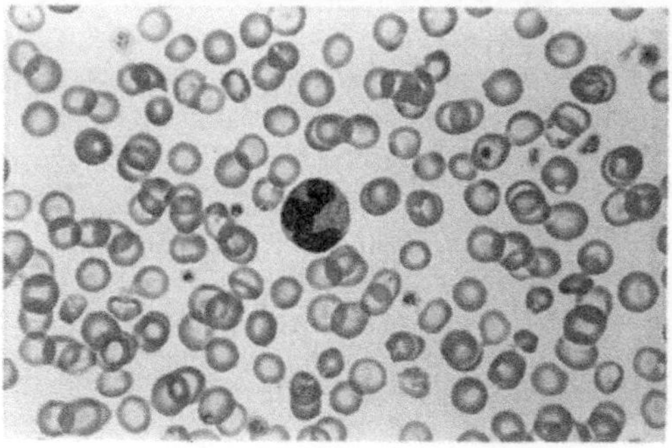

Figure 8-10 Canine monocyte with lobulated nucleus. (Wright's stain; 330×.)

many variable shapes. Monocytes in elephants are unique because the nucleus is often bilobed, and they can be mistaken as neutrophils or lymphocytes. Because the nuclear shape of monocytes is not consistent, their cytoplasmic features and cell size are more important features in differentiating them from other leukocytes. In snakes the azurophilic granules of monocytes are very prominent, and these monocytes are identified as "azurophils" by some laboratories.

13. What are the functions of monocytes?

Blood monocytes develop into macrophages at sites of inflammation or in specific tissues. Resident macrophage populations include serosal cavity macrophages, Kupffer's cells in liver, pulmonary alveolar macrophages, and macrophages in spleen and lymph nodes. Macrophages have surface receptors for immunoglobulin and complement, which enhance the phagocytosis of antibody-coated cells or organisms (especially protozoa and fungi). Macrophages also phagocytose apoptotic cells and cell debris at sites of inflammation. Macrophages function as antigen-presenting cells for humoral and cell-mediated immune responses and participate in antibody-mediated cytotoxicity against neoplastic cells by releasing tumor necrosis factor.

14. Describe the morphology of lymphocytes.

The nuclear shape of lymphocytes is characteristically round, oval, or slightly indented. The nucleus has a dense chromatin pattern and lacks a nucleolus. In most animals the blood lymphocytes are predominantly small in size, appearing smaller than neutrophils (Figure 8-11). The exception is cattle, whose lymphocytes normally include many medium-sized and large cells, often with an indented nucleus that may resemble monocytes. The nuclear/cytoplasmic (N/C) ratio of lymphocytes is usually high because the amount of cytoplasm is scant or moderate. The cytoplasm stains lightly basophilic and typically lacks granules.

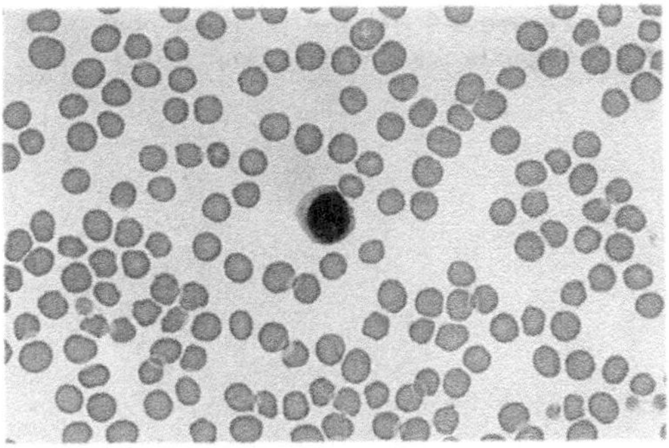

Figure 8-11 Small lymphocyte on canine blood smear. (Wright's stain; 65×.)

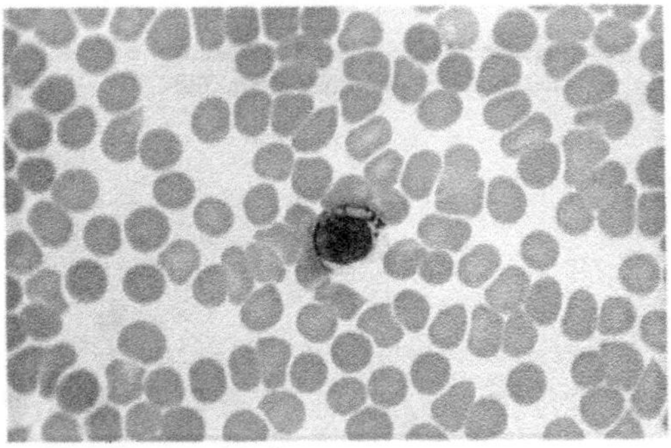

Figure 8-12 Canine granular lymphocyte. (Wright's stain; 330×.)

15. What are granular lymphocytes?

Granular lymphocytes vary in size from small to large and contain low numbers of small but prominent azurophilic granules (Figure 8-12). Often these cells are large and are referred to as "large granular lymphocytes" or "LGLs." The cytoplasmic granules are often loosely grouped together near a slight indentation of the nucleus. Granular lymphocytes occur in low numbers in healthy animals. Functionally, they correspond to either cytotoxic T lymphocytes or natural killer (NK) lymphocytes. Granular lymphocytes mediate cytotoxicity against neoplastic or microbe-infected cells by releasing proteins (e.g., perforin) that induce cell lysis.

16. What is a Kurloff body?

A Kurloff body is a single, large inclusion that occurs in a low percentage of the lymphocytes from South American rodents such as the guinea pig and capybara (Figure 8-13). This

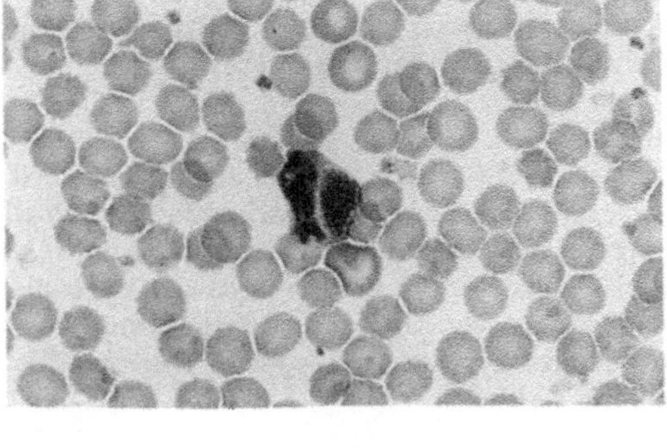

Figure 8-13 Lymphocyte with large inclusion (Kurloff body) in a guinea pig. (Wright's stain; 330×.)

inclusion is often as large as the nucleus and stains azurophilic. Lymphocytes containing a Kurloff body are considered a variant of granular lymphocytes.

17. Describe the function of lymphocytes.

Lymphocytes are involved in immune system functions, which are studied in depth by immunologists, not hematologists. Unlike other types of leukocytes, lymphocytes are a heterogeneous population of cells that have many different functions. In brief, B lymphocytes and plasma cells produce antibodies to specific antigens as part of the humoral response. Several types of T lymphocytes are involved in immunoregulation (*helper* or *suppressor* cells) of antibody-mediated and cell-mediated immune responses, as well as in cytotoxicity reactions against neoplastic, allogenic, or infected cells. The null lymphocytes (neither B nor T) include NK cells.

18. What types of lymphocytes occur in blood?

Identification of the different types of blood lymphocytes relies on species-specific antibodies against cluster differentiation (CD) antigens. For example, CD3 is a marker antigen of canine T lymphocytes, and CD79a is a marker antigen of canine B lymphocytes. Detection of these lymphoid antigen markers is not routinely performed, but the lymphocytes in blood of healthy animals consist of about 60% T cells and 30% B cells.

19. Describe the hematopoietic events that lead to production of neutrophils.

The marrow production of the granulocytic leukocytes and monocytes is linked to a common stem cell. The pluripotential stem cell proliferates in response to stem cell factor and interleukin-6 (IL-6), and differentiates to lineage-specific progenitor cells that can become neutrophils, monocytes, eosinophils, or basophils. These progenitor cells differentiate into the precursors that are recognizable on bone marrow smears (Figure 8-14). The early precursors of granulocytic leukocytes (myeloblasts, promyelocytes, and myelocytes) undergo up to five mitotic divisions. Differentiation of these precursors into mature granulocytes produces changes in nuclear shape (from round to indented to lobulated), progressive condensation of nuclear chromatin, and the appearance of cytoplasmic granules (azurophilic and specific). The replication and maturation of one myeloblast to 16 or 32 segmented neutrophils occur in 6 days during health. However, this maturation time is shortened during inflammation to increase the number of neutrophils available for tissue emigration.

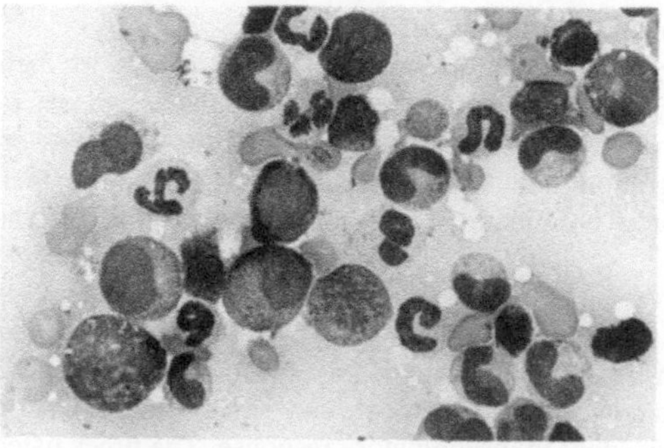

Figure 8-14 Canine bone marrow smear showing increased granulopoiesis and predominance of neutrophilic precursors. (Wright's stain; 330×.)

20. What are colony-stimulating factors?

Colony-stimulating factors (CSFs) are a class of glycoproteins that stimulate the marrow production of neutrophils and monocytes. CSFs have granulocyte (G-CSF), granulocyte-macrophage (GM-CSF), and macrophage (M-CSF) specificity and are produced by lymphocytes and macrophages at sites of inflammation. These factors act by preventing the apoptosis of neutrophilic and monocytic precursors, a process that normally limits the number of mature cells produced in marrow. The increased survival of precursors induced by CSFs leads to increased neutrophils and monocytes in blood. In addition, CSFs enhance the functional activity of mature neutrophils and monocytes.

21. Identify the different compartments in blood and marrow where neutrophils occur.

a. *Circulating pool.* Large numbers of segmented neutrophils occur in the flowing blood within blood vessels. The neutrophils in the circulating pool are those counted in the leukogram.

b. *Marginal pool.* In readiness to enter tissue, many segmented neutrophils are closely associated with the endothelial cells lining capillaries and postcapillary venules. These neutrophils are not in free-flowing blood and are not represented on the leukogram. The numbers of neutrophils in the circulating and the marginal pools are about equal, except in cats, whose marginal pool contains three times more neutrophils.

c. *Storage pool.* The storage pool consists of the nondividing neutrophils in marrow: segmented neutrophils, band neutrophils, and metamyelocytes. These precursors will continue to mature into segmented neutrophils and can provide several days' supply of segmented neutrophils in dogs. The storage pool is the largest source of neutrophils.

d. *Proliferative (mitotic) pool.* The proliferative pool consists of the actively dividing neutrophil precursors in bone marrow: myeloblasts, promyelocytes, and myelocytes.

22. Do marrow and blood compartments similar to those for neutrophils exist for other leukocytes?

Eosinophils and monocytes have circulating and marginal pools in blood that correspond to those for neutrophils, but these cells do not have marrow storage pools. Lymphocytes primarily reside in lymphoid tissues, not in marrow or blood.

23. Describe the marrow production of monocytes.

Interleukin-3 (IL-3) and M-CSF specifically induce the stem cell committed to the neutrophil and monocyte lineage (colony-forming unit [CFU]-GM) to differentiate into the monocytes. The progression of monoblast to promonocyte to monocyte occurs in only 2 days, and mature monocytes quickly leave the marrow to enter blood. Few monocytes and their precursors exist in the marrow, so they are seldom recognized or evaluated on bone marrow smears.

24. What is unique about the kinetics of blood lymphocytes?

Lymphocytes are continuously moving among the different lymphoid tissues in their surveillance and response to antigens. They travel in both blood and lymphatic vessels to reach the lymphoid tissues. In blood, lymphocytes recognize specific adhesion molecules on endothelial cells, which leads to their emigration into lymphoid tissues. Lymphocytes then enter the lymphatic vessels, which eventually culminate in the thoracic duct that returns ("recirculates") lymphocytes to blood.

25. Compare the circulating blood transit time and tissue life span of leukocytes.

Blood transit time refers to the length of time that leukocytes spend in blood before emigrating to tissues. *Tissue life span* refers to how long the leukocyte survives outside the blood in tissues before undergoing apoptosis or being spent in inflammatory response. The times listed in Table 8-1 are approximate and can vary depending on the species, measurement methodologies used, and presence of inflammation.

Table 8-1 ***Transit Time and Tissue Life of Leukocytes***

LEUKOCYTE TYPE	BLOOD TRANSIT TIME	TISSUE LIFE SPAN
Neutrophil	7-10 hours	1-2 days
Eosinophil	0.5-18 hours	1 week
Basophil	6 hours	2 weeks
Monocyte	24 hours	Weeks to months
Lymphocyte	(Recirculates)	Weeks to years

9. LABORATORY EVALUATION OF LEUKOCYTES

Stephen D. Gaunt

1. What laboratory test results are included in the leukogram?

The *leukogram* consists of the laboratory tests used in the routine evaluation of leukocytes on the complete blood count (CBC). The *total leukocyte concentration* is measured by a cell-counting instrument. The next step is to determine the relative *percentage* of each leukocyte type. The stained blood smear is examined with a microscope using high-power (50× or 100×) oil-objective lenses. A tally is recorded of the leukocyte types observed in the thin, monolayer portion of smear. The percentage of each leukocyte type is multiplied by the total leukocyte count to obtain their *absolute concentration*. The absolute concentration of each leukocyte type (*not* their percentages) is compared to appropriate reference intervals for that animal to detect any increases or decreases. In addition, microscopic changes in the *morphology of leukocytes* are noted on the stained blood smear, typically using the 100× oil-objective lens.

2. How is the total leukocyte concentration measured?

In the manual procedure, leukocytes in an aliquot prepared with a dilution kit (e.g., Unopette) are counted on a *hemacytometer* using a microscope. This method is very time consuming and is relatively inaccurate, with up to a 20% margin of error. *Automated cell counters*, which make precise dilutions and count the leukocytes in a larger volume of blood, provide more accurate results (<5% error). *Impedance* cell counters detect the voltage changes caused by the nonconducting leukocytes as they pass through an electrical field. Newer cell counters use *flow cytometric* methods to channel leukocytes through the path of a laser light beam. Laser optical detectors obtain both size and light scatter information ("interrogation") about each leukocyte to differentiate it from other types of leukocytes and blood cells.

3. How are leukocytes counted in avian and nonmammalian blood?

Automated cell counters are unable to differentiate the nucleated erythrocytes and thrombocytes from leukocytes in avian and nonmammalian species. The leukocyte count can be calculated using the leukocyte differential from the stained blood smear and a hemacytometer count of the granulocytic leukocytes. The stain most often used to obtain the granulocyte count is *phloxine B,* which is marketed as a blood dilution kit for counting human eosinophils. In birds and reptiles, phloxine B stains the heterophils and eosinophils, not the lymphocytes and monocytes.

The formula for calculating the total leukocyte count (cells/μl) follows:

$$(\#\text{ stained granulocytes} \times 1.1 \times 16) \div (\%\text{ heterophils} + \%\text{ eosinophils})$$

With number of (#) stained granulocytes obtained from hemacytometer count (sum of both chambers) and percentages (%) obtained from stained smear.

4. How many leukocytes should be counted in the manual differential count?

When the total leukocyte count is within the reference interval, a percentage distribution based on the differential counting of 100 leukocytes is typically performed. Although counting more cells could produce greater accuracy, other sources of error are present (e.g., uneven distribution of different leukocytes across the blood smear). When significant *leukocytosis* is present, more leukocytes must be counted to accurately reflect leukocytes present in low numbers. One rule of thumb is to count 100 leukocytes for each 20,000 cells/microliter (μl) increment of the total leukocyte count. For example, when the total leukocyte count is 40,000/μl, a 200-cell differential would be performed. If there is significant *leukopenia,* however, it can be difficult to find 100 leukocytes on the smear. Therefore a percentage distribution of leukocytes may be obtained from a differential count of 50 or even 25 leukocytes.

5. Can automated hematology analyzers provide differential leukocyte concentrations?

Some hematology analyzers (e.g., Vet ABC, IDEXX QBC) produce a three-part leukocyte differential (neutrophils, eosinophils, and combined lymphocyte/monocytes). The newer flow cytometric analyzers (e.g., Bayer Advia, Abbott Cell-Dyne, IDEXX LaserCyte) produce a five-part differential leukocyte counts. These instruments perform well with leukocytes from healthy animals. However, differential counts during abnormal conditions such as left shifts and leukemias are inaccurate. Therefore, despite its own limitations, microscopic examination of the stained blood smear currently remains the "gold standard" for obtaining the differential leukocyte concentrations in animals.

6. Which hematologic stains are used to evaluate leukocyte morphology?

The classic hematologic stains are Romanowsky stains, such as Wright's and Giemsa, which have eosinophilic and basophilic dyes dissolved in alcohol. Although they produce optimal staining of blood cells, these dye solutions are unstable, and the staining procedure requires several minutes. Modified Romanowsky stains (e.g., Diff-Quik) that use water-soluble dyes were developed. These dyes are more stable and rapidly stain the cells on blood smear (<1 minute). The only shortfall of the quick stains is failure to consistently stain the metachromatic granules in basophils (and mast cells) and the azurophilic granules in granular lymphocytes.

7. When should a differential leukocyte count *not* be performed?

If a significant number (>10%) of the leukocytes on the blood smear are smudged, pyknotic, or otherwise unidentifiable, the differential leukocyte count should be abandoned. The counting of only recognizable leukocytes would produce percentages that are skewed because of the "missing" leukocyte types and inaccurate calculation of the absolute leukocyte concentrations.

8. What precaution will prevent the adverse effect of sample storage on leukocytes?

Leukocytes, particularly neutrophils, begin to undergo apoptosis within hours after the blood sample is collected. In addition, exposure to the anticoagulant EDTA will induce cytoplasmic vacuolization and other morphologic changes in leukocytes. Refrigeration of the blood sample will not prevent these changes. If the blood sample will not be analyzed immediately or will be sent to an outside laboratory, a blood smear should be prepared, within minutes if possible. This step will minimize the morphologic changes that occur with aging or storage of leukocytes. The air-dried blood smear should be stored at room temperature and protected from vermin and humidity until staining by the laboratory.

9. How do nucleated erythrocytes affect the leukogram?

Most cell-counting methodologies include nucleated red blood cells (nRBCs) as leukocytes and report a falsely increased leukocyte concentration. Whenever a blood smear is examined for the differential leukocyte count, any nRBCs encountered should be recorded as a separate tally. When the tally of nRBCs exceeds 5 per 100 leukocytes, the initial "leukocyte" concentration must be adjusted downward to remove the counted nRBCs.

The following formula calculates the corrected leukocyte concentration (WBC conc.) when nRBCs are present:

$$\text{Corrected WBC conc.} = (\text{Initial WBC conc.} \times 100)/(100 + \#\ \text{nRBCs})$$

Most laboratories make this correction for nRBCs on their CBC report. However, not all do, so the clinician should be aware of whether this calculation is still needed.

10. Can other conditions falsely *increase* the leukocyte concentration reported by the hematology analyzer?

Cell-counting errors should be suspected when the total leukocyte concentration from an automated cell counter does not match the density of leukocytes on the stained blood smear. The leukocyte count should be confirmed with a different cell counter or a manual hemacytometer count. One or more of the following conditions can produce overcounting of leukocytes on certain hematology analyzers:

a. Heinz bodies in erythrocytes (most common in cats)
b. Clumped platelets or macroplatelets (most common in cats)
c. Incomplete lysis of erythrocytes, especially reticulocytes from certain nondomestic animals (e.g., prairie dogs)
d. Lipemia

11. What conditions will falsely *decrease* the total leukocyte concentration reported by the hematology analyzer?

Undercounting occurs when the leukocytes in blood sample are not detected by the cell counter. The most common cause is large platelet clumps that incorporate leukocytes and mask them from the cell counter. A rare condition is *leukergy,* when leukocytes occur in loose clusters or aggregates that are not counted as individual leukocytes (Figure 9-1). Leukergy is associated with collection of blood into EDTA (but not other calcium-chelating anticoagulants such as citrate). In both conditions, the undercounting error is confirmed by examining the leukocyte density on blood smear. The error is corrected by collecting another blood sample that avoids the inciting problem (platelet clumping or EDTA-induced leukergy).

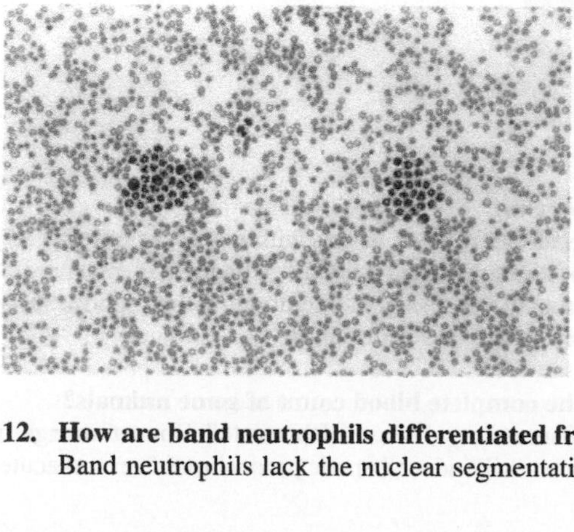

Figure 9-1 Low-magnification view of a canine blood smear with aggregates of leukocytes (leukergy) that produced an undercounting of leukocytes in the blood sample. (Wright's stain; 60×.)

12. How are band neutrophils differentiated from segmented neutrophils?

Band neutrophils lack the nuclear segmentation that occurs in segmented neutrophils. The classic appearance of the band neutrophil is a C- or S-shaped nucleus with smooth and parallel nuclear margins. The presence of a single constriction of any degree along the nuclear margin is sufficient to classify that cell as a *segmented,* not a band, neutrophil. Band and segmented neutrophils have a similar cytoplasmic and nuclear chromatin appearance (Figure 9-2).

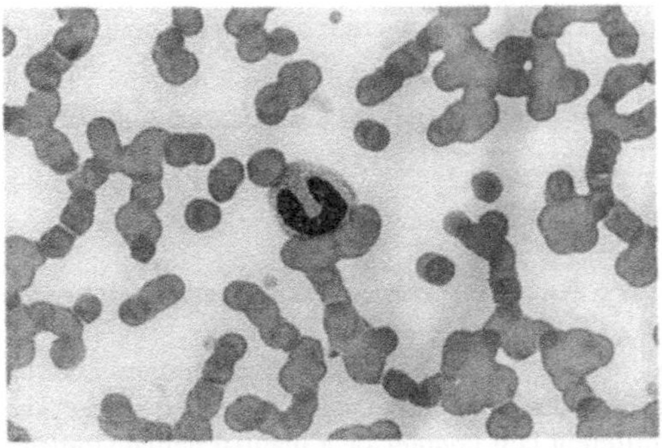

Figure 9-2 Band neutrophil from a horse. (Wright's stain; 330×.)

13. How are monocytes differentiated from band neutrophils?

Monocytes and band neutrophils are the leukocytes most likely to be mistaken for the other. Monocytes can have a band-shaped nucleus, especially in dogs, although the nuclear chromatin is less condensed compared with band neutrophils (Figure 9-3). A better distinguishing feature is the basophilic cytoplasm of monocytes, which can be quickly gauged by comparison to the less basophilic cytoplasm of segmented neutrophils on the smear. If present in monocytes, cytoplasmic vacuoles are discrete round vacuoles. Band neutrophils with toxic change can also have cytoplasmic basophilia and indistinct cytoplasmic vacuoles, which makes it more difficult to differentiate them from monocytes.

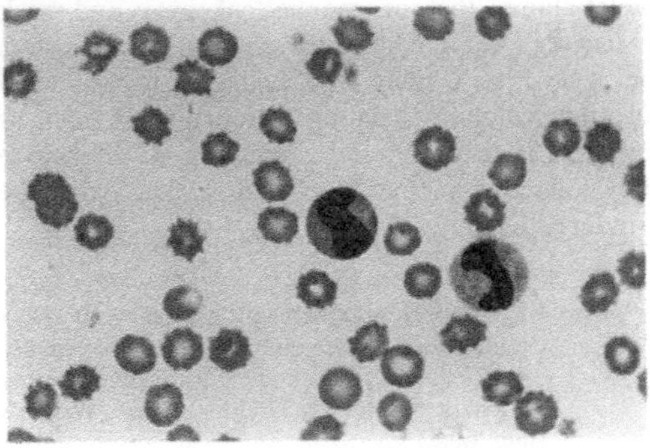

Figure 9-3 Band neutrophil and monocyte from a cat. The monocyte *(center)* has a more basophilic cytoplasm and less condensed nuclear chromatin. (Wright's stain; 330×.)

14. Describe the appearance of metamyelocytes.

Metamyelocytes are the granulocytic precursors of band neutrophils and occur infrequently in blood as part of a left shift. An indented or kidney-shaped nucleus distinguishes metamyelocytes from band neutrophils. The nuclear chromatin is less condensed and the cytoplasm more basophilic in metamyelocytes than in band and segmented neutrophils.

15. Why is a fibrinogen test included on the complete blood count of some animals?

Horses and ruminants often develop inflammatory disease without a significant change in the leukogram. However, inflammatory cytokines will induce hepatic production of several acute-phase reactant proteins. One of these proteins, fibrinogen, is relatively easy to measure, so it is included on large animal CBCs to augment the detection of inflammation. Although most often caused by inflammation, increased fibrinogen concentration can also result from dehydration.

16. How is plasma fibrinogen measured?

The fibrinogen laboratory test relies on the semiselective precipitation of fibrinogen when plasma is heated to 56° C for 3 minutes. The assay is simple to perform and is reasonably specific and sensitive for detection of increased fibrinogen concentrations in horses and ruminants. However, this methodology is not sufficiently sensitive to detect changes (increases or decreases) in the fibrinogen concentration of cats and dogs.

17. Can leukocytosis interfere with tests on the complete blood count or chemistry panel?

The presence of marked leukocytosis (>50,000 cells/μl), whether lymphocytic or granulocytic, can affect the following tests:

a. *Hemoglobin*. The nuclei from increased numbers of leukocytes increase the turbidity of lysed blood, which the hemoglobinometer incorrectly reads as increased hemoglobin. This artifactually increased hemoglobin leads to erroneous calculation of an increased mean corpuscular hemoglobin concentration (MCHC).

b. *Glucose*. When blood from an animal with leukocytosis is submitted for serum chemistries, the serum or plasma should be rapidly separated because leukocytes (particularly neutrophils) will catabolize glucose in vitro. The leukocytes may also contribute to increased in vivo utilization of blood glucose.

c. *Potassium*. The extremely increased numbers of leukocytes that occur with leukemia can release enough intracellular potassium into the serum or plasma in vitro to produce an artifactual increase in potassium (pseudohyperkalemia).

18. What are the indications for examining a "buffy coat" smear?

Smears with concentrated numbers of blood leukocytes are needed when the presence of certain nucleated cells or infectious agents are suspected but were not observed on a routine blood smear. Searches for microorganisms such as *Histoplasma* or *Hepatozoon americanum* within leukocytes or circulating neoplastic cells (e.g., mast cells) are more fruitful when buffy coat smears are examined.

19. How is a "buffy coat" smear prepared?

A buffy coat smear is made by centrifuging an EDTA-anticoagulated blood sample at high speed to sediment the blood cells from plasma. The visible white layer (unless the animal is leukopenic) containing packed leukocytes and platelets will be above the packed erythrocytes. Although a microcapillary (microhematocrit) tube filled with blood can be used to prepare this smear, a 2-ml blood sample is preferred because it produces a more accessible and larger buffy coat layer to prepare multiple hand-drawn smears.

20. When is a bone marrow evaluation indicated for evaluation of leukocytes?

When neutropenia is present, with decreased granulopoiesis suspected as the cause, a bone marrow aspirate (or marrow core biopsy if aspiration is unsuccessful) should be considered. Blood neutrophil concentrations can fluctuate dramatically and rapidly, so a leukogram collected just before the marrow sampling is recommended to confirm the neutropenia. Marrow evaluation will document changes in myeloid:erythroid (M/E) ratio, maturation sequences of neutrophilic precursors, morphologic abnormalities in neutrophilic precursors, and presence of abnormal cells in marrow. Obviously, if neutrophilia is present, granulopoiesis is clearly effective and bone marrow evaluation is not indicated.

10. INTERPRETATION OF THE LEUKOGRAM

Stephen D. Gaunt

1. What is the predominant blood leukocyte during health in the domestic animals?

In cats, dogs, and neonatal ruminants, neutrophils are the most abundant leukocyte, followed by lymphocytes. In mature ruminants, lymphocytes are the predominant leukocyte, with fewer neutrophils. In horses and pigs, numbers of neutrophils and lymphocytes are approximately equal. Eosinophils occur in very low numbers on blood smears from healthy animals, and basophils are almost never observed.

2. What is a left shift?

The term *left shift* indicates the presence of neutrophil precursors in blood, typically increased numbers of band neutrophils and rarely metamyelocytes and earlier precursors. A left shift occurs when the number of segmented neutrophils in the blood pools and marrow storage pools are depleted by excessive emigration to inflammatory sites. Band neutrophils (and earlier precursors) will prematurely leave the marrow at this point. Although often occurring with bacterial infections, left shifts also result from noninfectious causes of inflammation, such as tissue necrosis and immune-mediated disease.

3. How are left shifts categorized?

Leukograms with an increased concentration of band (or earlier) neutrophils are often categorized as "regenerative" or "degenerative" left shifts. Increased concentrations of both segmented and band neutrophils constitute a *regenerative left shift*. This is regarded as a somewhat favorable change, since the granulopoietic response of marrow is maintaining an appropriately increased concentration of segmented neutrophils during inflammation. No uniform definition exists for *degenerative left shift*. Some maintain it is the opposite of a regenerative left shift, with the segmented neutrophil concentration within or below its reference interval and with increased band (or earlier) neutrophils. Others restrict "degenerative" to leukograms with absolute concentrations of band neutrophils that exceed the segmented neutrophils, a rare event. Despite controversy over the definition, it is agreed that a degenerative left shift is of greater concern than a regenerative left shift. With degenerative left shift, marrow granulopoiesis is unable to maintain an appropriate segmented neutrophil concentration because of granulopoietic suppression and/or excessive demand for blood neutrophils at sites of inflammation.

4. Define mature neutrophilia.

The term *mature hemophilia* describes an increased concentration of segmented neutrophils and no band neutrophils (or earlier precursors) on the leukogram. It is observed in many different conditions, and without knowledge of the degree of neutrophilia, it can be a relatively nonspecific finding. However, mature neutrophilia is a convenient term to describe leukograms with neutrophilia and no left shift.

5. What is a right shift?

The term *right shift* describes increased numbers of hypersegmented neutrophils, with five or more nuclear lobes. Hypersegmented neutrophils are not specifically included in the leukocyte differential count, so right shifts are not quantitated like left shifts. Hypersegmentation of neutrophils usually occurs as an aging change, when neutrophils circulate in blood for a longer time. Right shifts occur most often in animals (especially dogs) on glucocorticoid therapy or with hyperadrenocorticism, since glucocorticoids inhibit the emigration of neutrophils from blood vessels and prolong their circulation. Rarer causes of hypersegmentation are developmental disorders of neutrophils, such as erythroid macrocytosis of poodles, vitamin B_{12} maladsorptive disorder in giant schnauzers, myelodysplasia in animals with myelogenous leukemia, and benign idiopathic neutrophil hypersegmentation in horses (Figure 10-1).

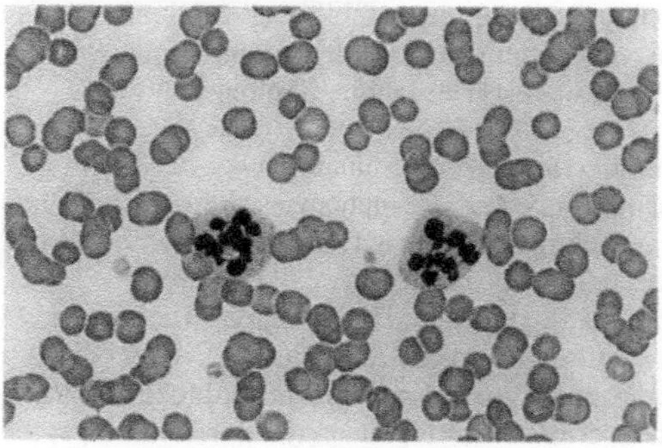

Figure 10-1 Hypersegmented neutrophils on blood smear from a horse with benign idiopathic hypersegmentation syndrome. (Wright's stain; 330×.)

6. What are the components of a glucocorticoid-induced ("stress") leukogram?

Stress leukograms occur in all animals but are most common and pronounced in dogs. Endogenous and exogenous glucocorticoids affect the concentration of most leukocytes. A prime feature of the stress leukogram is mature neutrophilia, resulting from increased release of segmented neutrophils from the marrow storage pool, as well as demargination of blood neutrophils to the circulating neutrophil pool. Monocytosis also occurs in dogs because monocytes shift from their marginal pool to the circulating monocyte pool. Another characteristic finding is lymphopenia, the result of diminished recirculation of lymphocytes from lymphoid tissues to venous blood. Chronic glucocorticoid administration also causes lysis of lymphocytes. Eosinopenia may be present, probably because eosinophils are sequestered in marrow or other tissues. The stress leukogram develops over several hours and peaks 6 to 8 hours after administration of exogenous glucocorticoids. These leukocyte changes persist up to several days, depending on the type and dose of glucocorticoid.

7. What is the maximal degree of neutrophilia expected in a stress leukogram?

The segmented neutrophil concentration typically increases two to three times the upper limit of its reference interval in stress leukograms. In dogs, for example, the segmented neutrophil concentration may be as high as 35,000 cells/microliter (µl) because of endogenous/exogenous glucocorticoids. Many inflammatory leukograms with a mature neutrophilia occur in the same range as stress leukograms, making differentiation of stress and inflammatory leukograms difficult without a clinical history and physical examination of the patient.

8. What disease should be suspected when a stress leukogram is absent in a clinically ill animal?

Unchanged or even increased concentrations of lymphocytes and eosinophils (instead of lymphopenia and eosinopenia) during illness suggest a "relaxed" leukogram. These changes are characteristic of dogs and cats with hypoadrenocorticism. The lack of mineralocorticoids produces distinctive electrolyte findings in animals with hypoadrenocorticism, but the lack of glucocorticoids produces the distinctive changes on the leukogram.

9. What is a physiologic leukogram?

The *physiologic leukogram* typically occurs in young (<12 months of age) animals, although it is least likely to occur in dogs. The leukocyte changes are mediated by epinephrine during the "fight or flight" response that occurs with excitement, fear, or anxiety or with physical exertion, including parturition or convulsions. The distinguishing feature of the physiologic leukogram is lymphocytosis. The lymphocytosis is attributed to increased entry of lymphocytes into blood, presumably from splenic contraction and muscular activity that enhance the lymphatic and thoracic duct flow of lymphocytes into blood. A mature neutrophilia is also present, caused by demargination of blood neutrophils. The increased cardiac output and blood flow apparently sweep neutrophils from the marginal pool into the circulating neutrophil pool. Minimal changes occur in monocyte, eosinophil, and basophil concentrations. The physiologic leukogram is observed infrequently, in part because this leukocytosis resolves within 30 minutes.

10. Describe the components of an inflammatory leukogram.

On the *inflammatory leukogram,* neutrophil concentrations may vary from decreased to increased during inflammation. The blood concentration depends on the balance between the rate of blood neutrophil emigration to tissues in response to increased chemoattractants, and the rate of marrow granulopoiesis that replaces the blood neutrophils. The monocyte concentration often parallels an increase in neutrophils, since they share a common stem cell (colony-forming unit [CFU]-GM) and respond to granulocyte-macrophage colony-stimulating factor (GM-CSF). Increased numbers of band neutrophils may be released from the marrow storage pool with depletion of segmented neutrophils. Lymphopenia and eosinopenia may also occur with inflammation. Although lymphopenia and eosinopenia are often attributed to concurrent glucocorticoid release, inflammatory mediators can induce these changes independent of glucocorticoids. Depending on the cause of inflammation, eosinophilia may actually occur.

11. Compare the changes in leukocyte concentration that occur in stress, physiologic, and inflammatory leukograms.

	LEUKOGRAM		
LEUKOCYTE PARAMETER	STRESS	PHYSIOLOGIC	INFLAMMATORY
Total leukocytes	Increased	Increased	Decreased to increased
Segmented neutrophils	Increased	Increased	Decreased or increased
Band neutrophils	Absent	Absent	Absent or increased
Lymphocytes	Decreased	Increased	Decreased to increased
Monocytes	Increased	Unchanged	Unchanged or increased
Eosinophils	Decreased	Unchanged	Unchanged or increased

12. Rank the domestic animals by their ability to develop maximal degrees of neutrophilia during inflammation.

(1) Dog
(2) Cat
(3) Horse
(4) Cattle

13. Are there "panic values" for changes on the leukogram?

Severe neutropenia (<500 or <1000 cells/μl) is the only leukocyte change that requires the immediate attention of the clinician. When caused by decreased marrow production, severe neutropenia is especially a concern because improvement of the neutrophil concentration is not likely in the short term. Animals with severe neutropenia are at risk to develop sepsis, so administration of prophylactic antibiotics should be considered to prevent bacterial infection.

14. What changes on serial leukograms would be considered favorable in animals with inflammatory disease?

a. Diminishment of prior neutrophilic leukocytosis
b. Diminishment or absence of prior left shift
c. Increase in segmented neutrophil concentration if previously neutropenic
d. Increase in lymphocyte concentration if previously lymphopenic
e. Decrease in elevated plasma fibrinogen concentration in horses and cattle

15. List the general mechanisms (with appropriate examples) that cause neutropenia.

a. Excessive emigration to tissues during inflammation (acute bacterial infection, sepsis, necrosis)
b. Endotoxin-induced margination (equine salmonellosis)
c. Decreased marrow granulopoiesis
   (1) Viruses (feline leukemia virus [FeLV], feline immunodeficiency virus [FIV], parvoviruses)
   (2) Cellular infiltration of marrow (myelophthistic conditions, e.g., lymphosarcoma, myelofibrosis, granulomatous disease)
   (3) Toxins (bracken fern in cattle, estrogen and sulfadiazine in dogs)
   (4) Familial (adult Belgian Tervuren, cyclic hematopoiesis in grey collie)
d. Increased destruction of neutrophils (immune-mediated neutropenia)

16. Why are cattle more likely to develop neutropenia with acute inflammation?

This common finding in cattle is attributed to a smaller storage pool of segmented neutrophils in marrow or slower replenishment of this storage pool with segmented neutrophils. In cattle with acute inflammation, particularly localized inflammation such as mastitis, neutropenia (often with a left shift) is initially present for 1 to 2 days. For this reason, degenerative left shifts are not unusual in cattle with acute inflammation and do not carry the same concern associated with this leukogram in other animals. Increased marrow granulopoiesis should quickly compensate and lead to "rebound" neutrophilic leukocytosis in the ensuing days.

17. Why does endotoxemia cause neutropenia?

One of the many systemic effects of endotoxin is to enhance the adhesion of blood neutrophils to the endothelial surface by activating adhesion molecules. Redistribution of blood neutrophils occurs as a shift from the circulating to marginal pool, manifested as a severe neutropenia. Because the neutrophils essentially remain in blood but are marginated and are not represented on the leukogram, the change is termed *pseudoneutropenia*. The neutropenia is an acute but transient change often followed by neutrophilia, since endotoxin causes release of neutrophils from the marrow storage pool.

18. Why does severe neutropenia occur with parvoviral infection?

Canine and feline parvoviruses target cells with a high mitotic rate, including hematopoietic precursors. The blood and marrow pools of segmented neutrophils are quickly depleted because of the short half-life of neutrophils and the lack of replenishment by impaired granulopoiesis. In addition, loss of villous enterocytes results from viral damage to the intestinal crypt cells. The resulting increased enteric absorption of endotoxin further aggravates the neutropenia in parvovirus-infected animals. Neutropenia without thrombocytopenia or anemia are the classic hematologic findings in parvoviral infections.

19. List two general mechanisms (with appropriate examples) that cause neutrophilia.

a. Demargination of blood neutrophils and/or marrow pool release
   (1) Glucocorticoids (administration, hyperadrenocorticism)
   (2) Epinephrine (anxiety, physical exertion)

b. Increased granulopoiesis and marrow storage pool release
   (1) Inflammatory diseases
      (a) Infectious (bacterial, fungal, feline infectious peritonitis [FIP])
      (b) Noninfectious (immune mediated, necrosis, hemolysis)
   (2) Paraneoplastic (production of CSFs by neoplasms)
   (3) Acute or chronic granulocytic leukemia

20. List specific diseases that cause extreme neutrophilia in the dog.

a. Pyometra
b. Other localized neutrophilic inflammatory diseases, such as prostatitis, pancreatitis, and peritonitis
c. *Hepatozoon americanum* infection
d. Immune-mediated hemolytic anemia
e. Early phase of estrogen toxicosis (rare)
f. Paraneoplastic neutrophilia (rare)
g. Leukocyte adhesion defect (rare)
h. Chronic granulocytic leukemia (rare)

Because dogs can develop a higher degree of neutrophilia than other animals, extremely high concentrations of neutrophils (>50,000/μl) are possible. The leukogram may include a mature neutrophilia or a regenerative left shift. Although studies have demonstrated a lower rate of survival in dogs (and cats) with extreme neutrophilia, the disease causing this leukocytosis is a likely determinant of survivability.

21. What is a leukemoid response?

The term *leukemoid response* was coined to describe leukograms with neutrophilic leukocytosis, marked left shift with bands and earlier precursors, and reactive lymphocytes. These leukograms were found to be inflammatory in origin, but the initial blood smear was more suggestive of myelogenous leukemia. Unfortunately, this term is incorrectly applied to leukograms with extreme neutrophilia (>50,000/μl) that lack a left shift or have a modest left shift (bands only). The inflammatory origin of these leukograms is quite evident, and myelogenous leukemia is not likely. These leukograms are correctly described as "marked" or "extreme" neutrophilia. The "leukemoid" terminology is intended for the rare leukogram with marked left shift, for which leukemia is a realistic differential diagnosis.

22. What acute change in neutrophil concentration is expected after surgical correction of pyometra in dogs?

Pyometra is a classic example of localized intense neutrophilic inflammation, which induces a significant increase in granulopoiesis. After hysterectomy, the chemotactic signals causing neutrophil emigration to the inflammatory site immediately disappear. However, the neutrophilic precursors in the expanded proliferative and storage pools in marrow continue to mature and release neutrophils, which causes an even greater degree of neutrophilia after surgery. Granulopoiesis will quickly down-regulate, and the neutrophilia will abate after a few days.

23. In which tissues is inflammation *not* likely to induce an inflammatory leukogram?

Neutrophilic inflammation in the urinary bladder, intestine, epidermis, and central nervous system typically causes minimal or no change in the leukogram. This is attributed to loss of inflammatory mediators (e.g., CSFs) or their seclusion in protected tissue spaces. Therefore, no systemic inflammatory response is reflected in granulopoiesis and the leukogram.

24. List conditions associated with eosinophilia.

a. Hypersensitivity ("allergic") reactions
   (1) Skin: eosinophilic granuloma complex

(2) Respiratory tract: eosinophilic bronchopneumopathy, asthma
(3) Intestinal tract: eosinophilic enteritis

b. Parasitism (ectoparasites, endoparasites)
(1) Skin
(2) Respiratory tract
(3) Intestinal tract

c. Mast cell tumor
d. Hypoadrenocorticism in dogs ("relaxed" leukogram)
e. Hypereosinophilic syndrome in cats (increased interleukin-5 [IL-5] production?)
f. Eosinophilic leukemia
g. Paraneoplastic (production of IL-5 by neoplasm)

25. List conditions associated with basophilia.

a. Hypersensitivity reactions to ectoparasites, endoparasites, and drugs
(1) Skin
(2) Respiratory tract
(3) Intestinal tract

b. Mast cell tumors
c. Eosinophilic granuloma
d. Myeloproliferative diseases
e. Basophilic leukemia

26. List conditions associated with lymphocytosis.

a. Inflammatory-induced antigenic stimulation
(1) Infectious (especially ehrlichiosis, rickettsiosis)
(2) Noninfectious

b. Vaccination (antigenic stimulation)
c. Physiologic leukogram (epinephrine-induced shift from lymphoid tissues)
d. Hypoadrenocorticism (lack of glucocorticoids)
e. Persistent lymphocytosis in cattle infected with bovine leukemia virus (BoLV)
f. Lymphoid leukemias

27. List conditions associated with lymphopenia.

a. Stress or hyperadrenocorticism (endogenous glucocorticoids)
b. Glucocorticoid therapy
c. Acute inflammation
d. Viral infection
e. Decreased recirculation of lymphocytes from lymphoid tissues:
Chylous effusions caused by anterior mediastinal mass, congestive heart failure, or thoracic duct leakage
f. Decreased recirculation of lymphocytes from intestinal lymphatics
(1) Lymphangiectasia
(2) Intestinal neoplasm
(3) Granulomatous inflammation

g. Congenital immunodeficiencies (e.g., severe combined immunodeficiency)

28. List conditions associated with monocytosis.

a. Acute or chronic inflammation
(1) Infectious (fungal, bacterial)
(2) Noninfectious (immune mediated, necrosis, hemolysis)

b. Glucocorticoids (endogenous or exogenous)
c. Monocytic or myelomonocytic leukemia

29. Why is monocytosis a favorable indicator for recovery from leukopenia?

After transient suppression of hematopoiesis and development of leukopenia, an increased blood concentration of monocytes typically precedes the recovery of neutrophils and other granulocytic leukocytes. Monocytes have a rapid marrow transit time (2 days for monoblasts to differentiate to monocytes), versus the longer marrow transit time (6 days) for differentiation of segmented neutrophils from myeloblasts. In addition, monocytes rapidly leave the marrow, whereas neutrophils enter a marrow storage pool, which can delay their entry into blood.

30. What is the significance of mast cells on blood smear?

Mastocytemia, or the presence of mast cells in blood, is often associated with disseminated mast cell neoplasms or mast cell leukemia in dogs and cats. However, low numbers of mast cells are also observed on blood or "buffy coat" smears in several inflammatory diseases of the dog, including immune-mediated hemolytic anemia, parvoviral infection, dermatitis, pleuritis, and peritonitis. The morphology of mast cells with inflammatory diseases may be similar to neoplastic mast cells, with varying degrees of metachromatic granulation evident in both disease types (Figure 10-2).

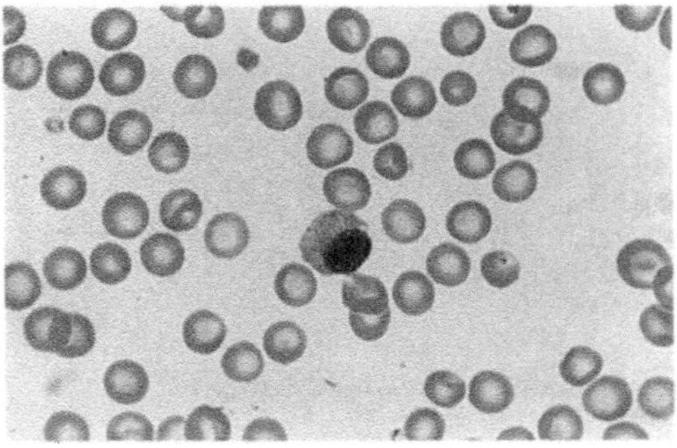

Figure 10-2 Mast cell on the blood smear of a dog. (Wright's stain; 330×.)

11. ALTERED LEUKOCYTE MORPHOLOGY AND FUNCTION

Stephen D. Gaunt

1. What are reactive lymphocytes, or immunocytes?

Immunocytes are large-sized lymphocytes with intensely basophilic cytoplasm and occasionally a prominent nucleolus that appear similar to lymphoblasts. These cells may be more similar to plasma cells, with a clear Golgi area in basophilic cytoplasm, an eccentric nucleus, and even cytoplasmic inclusions (Russell bodies). These cells occur in low numbers, with most of the lymphocytes appearing normal. These reactive lymphocytes are observed in animals undergoing immune response, typically during infectious inflammatory diseases or after vaccination. The low number of these cells and the clinical history provide the convincing evidence that these lymphocytes are antigenically stimulated, not neoplastic (Figure 11-1).

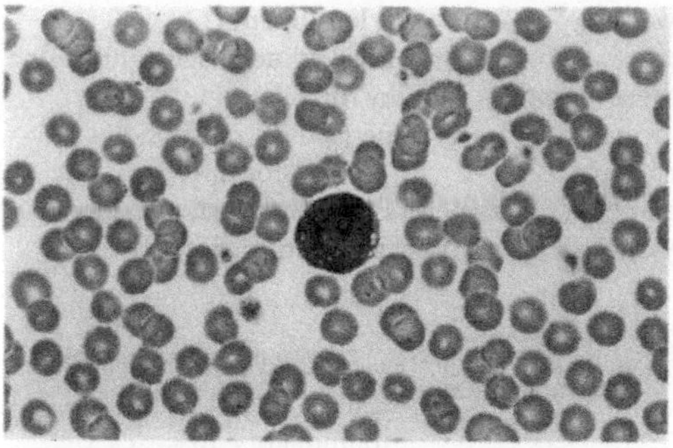

Figure 11-1 Reactive lymphocyte (immunocyte) from a cat. (Wright's stain; 330×.)

2. What are toxic changes in neutrophils?

Cytoplasmic changes occur in blood neutrophils during intense inflammation from many causes (infectious or noninfectious). The toxic changes observed in neutrophils include Döhle bodies, diffuse cytoplasmic basophilia, cytoplasmic ("foamy") vacuolization, and infrequently, toxic granulation (Figure 11-2). *Döhle bodies* are small (1-2 μ), lightly basophilic inclusions that occur in low numbers near the periphery of cytoplasm. Döhle bodies may also occur in low numbers of neutrophils in healthy cats.

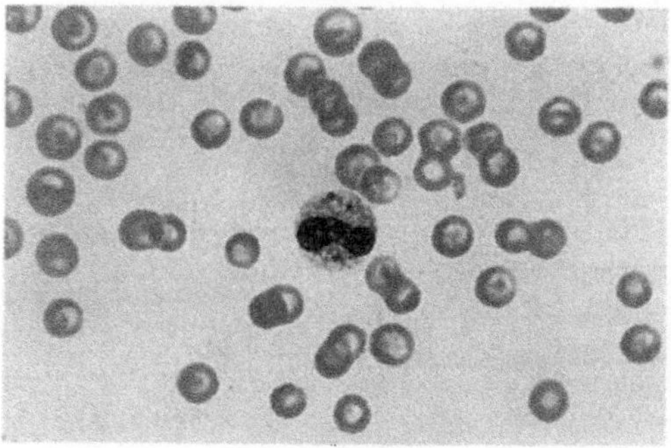

Figure 11-2 Band neutrophil with Döhle bodies, cytoplasmic basophilia, and cytoplasmic vacuolization. (Wright's stain; 330×.)

3. What causes the formation of toxic changes in neutrophils?

These changes first appear in early neutrophil precursors in the marrow as a developmental abnormality and are not induced in mature neutrophils by "toxins." For example, Döhle bodies and the cytoplasmic basophilia are rough endoplasmic reticulum and free ribosomes, respectively, that normally disappear in early neutrophil precursors. The cytoplasmic vacuolization results from disruption of cytoplasmic granules in neutrophilic precursors. Toxic changes apparently result from the heightened and quickened pace of granulopoiesis during particularly intense inflammatory responses.

4. How are toxic changes reported by laboratories?

Any toxic change(s) observed in blood neutrophils should be included in the "leukocyte morphology" comments on the complete blood count (CBC). Different toxic changes may occur individually, in various combinations, and in varying degrees between neutrophils. Because of this variability in occurrence and the lack of clinical correlation, grading systems for toxic changes are not used in most laboratories.

5. What causes abnormal granulation in neutrophils?

The rare reports of increased prominence of azurophilic granules in neutrophils and other granulocytes (especially basophils) and monocytes include the following:

a. Observed in some normal foals and Birman cats
b. Occur in inflammatory diseases as a toxic change
c. Chediak-Higashi syndrome in cattle and Persian cats (abnormal fusion of granules)
d. Lysosomal storage diseases (mucopolysaccharidosis in dogs and cats, Figure 11-3)

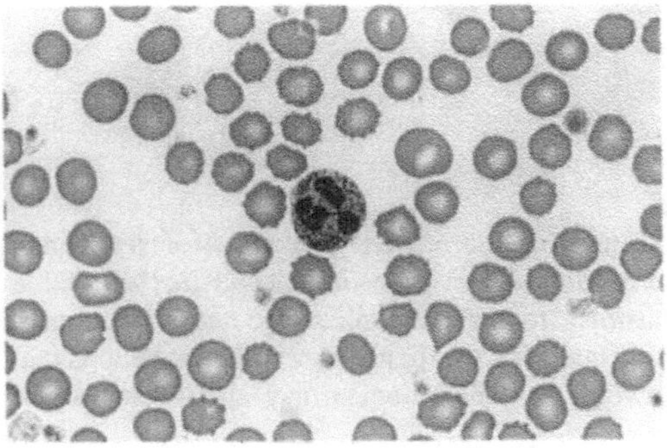

Figure 11-3 Neutrophils with prominent cytoplasmic granules in a young dog with mucopolysaccharidosis, MPS VII. (Wright's stain; 330×.)

6. What is the significance of giant neutrophils?

Segmented neutrophils that are up to twice the size of normal neutrophils, but with otherwise unremarkable morphology, are rarely observed on blood smears. This finding indicates *dysgranulopoiesis,* in which a mitotic cell division was likely skipped by an early precursor and larger neutrophils resulted. Giant neutrophils occur with inflammatory diseases and in cats with feline leukemia virus (FeLV) infection (Figure 11-4).

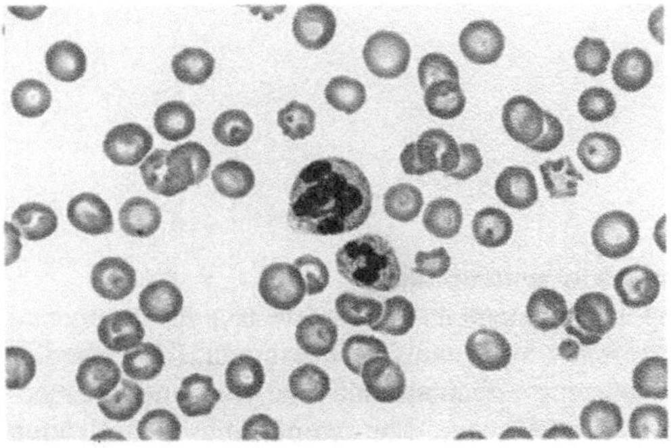

Figure 11-4 Blood smear from a dog with giant and normal-sized neutrophils. (Wright's stain; 330×.)

7. What are pyknotic cells?

Senescent leukocytes normally undergo apoptosis, with marked condensation and fragmentation of the nuclear chromatin. The resultant pyknotic cell has an intact cytoplasm and one or more round, variably sized dense inclusions. This change typically occurs in tissues once leukocytes leave blood. However, pyknotic cells are encountered on blood smears prepared hours after the sample collection (Figure 11-5). It is logical to assume that these cells were formerly neutrophils, because of their short life span, but the identity of pyknotic cells cannot be presumed.

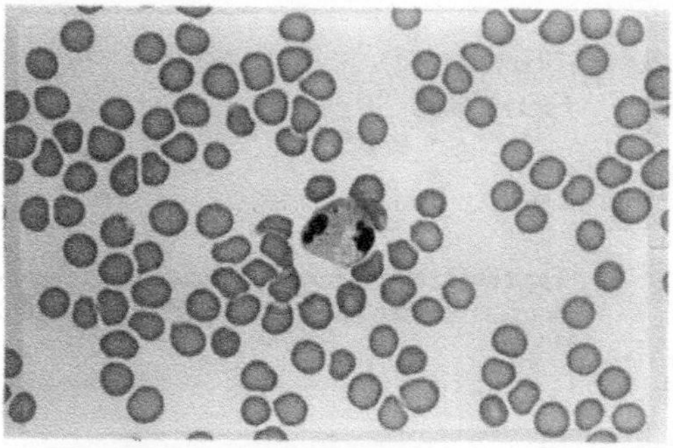

Figure 11-5 Pyknotic leukocyte on canine blood smear. (Wright's stain; 330×.)

8. What are "basket" cells?

The term *basket cell* describes nuclei without intact cytoplasm that appear as basophilic smudges. The smudged nucleus may have a crisscrossed linear pattern that resembles a woven "basket." These nuclei originate from fragile leukocytes that were lyzed during blood cell preparation. Increased numbers of smudged cells occur most often with leukemic cells (Figure 11-6), leukocytes from severely ill animals (particularly horses with endotoxemia), and avian blood cells. In these cases the blood sample can be spiked with an albumin solution or homologous serum before preparing the smear; this may decrease the number of smudged cells. Another cause of basket cells is autolysis from prolonged storage of blood sample.

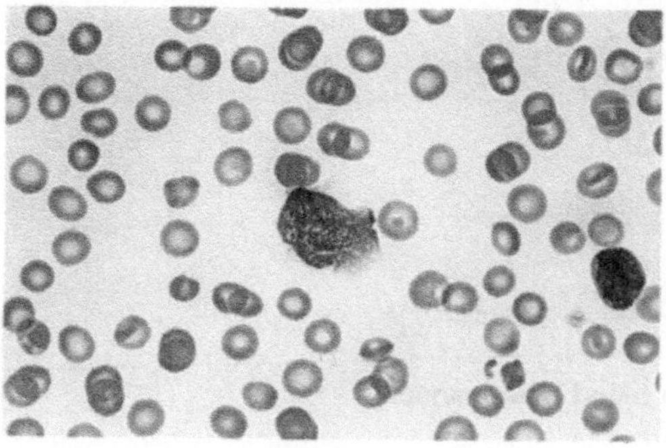

Figure 11-6 Smudged or "basket" cell on blood smear from a dog with lymphoblastic leukemia. (Wright's stain; 330×.)

9. List microorganisms that can occur in blood neutrophils or monocytes.

a. *Ehrlichia ewingii* in neutrophils of dogs, *Anaplasma phagocytophilia* (formerly *Ehrlichia equi*) in neutrophils of horses and other species (Figure 11-7)

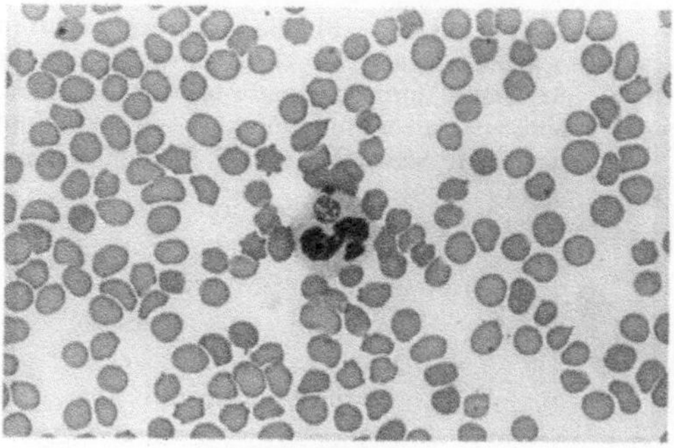

Figure 11-7 Morula of *Anaplasma phagocytophilia* (formerly *Ehrlichia equi*) in blood neutrophil of a horse. (Wright's stain; 330×.)

b. *Histoplasma* in dogs and cats (Figure 11-8)
c. *Hepatozoon americanum* or *H. canis* in dogs (Figure 11-9)
d. Canine distemper viral inclusions in dogs
e. *Cytauxzoon felis* schizonts in cats
f. Bacteria (e.g., *Mycobacterium,* enteric bacilli)

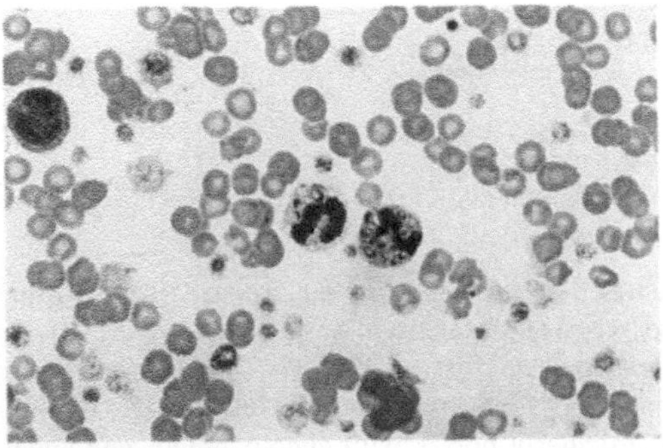

Figure 11-8 Multiple *Histoplasma* organisms in canine neutrophils. (Wright's stain; 330×.)

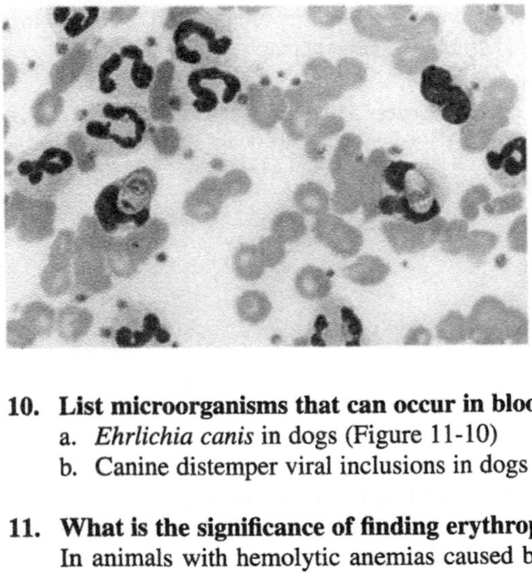

Figure 11-9 Gamont of *Hepatozoon americanum* in two leukocytes on buffy coat smear from a dog. (Wright's stain; 330×.)

10. List microorganisms that can occur in blood lymphocytes.

a. *Ehrlichia canis* in dogs (Figure 11-10)
b. Canine distemper viral inclusions in dogs (Figure 11-11)

11. What is the significance of finding erythrophagocytosis on a blood smear?

In animals with hemolytic anemias caused by immune-mediated removal of erythrocytes,

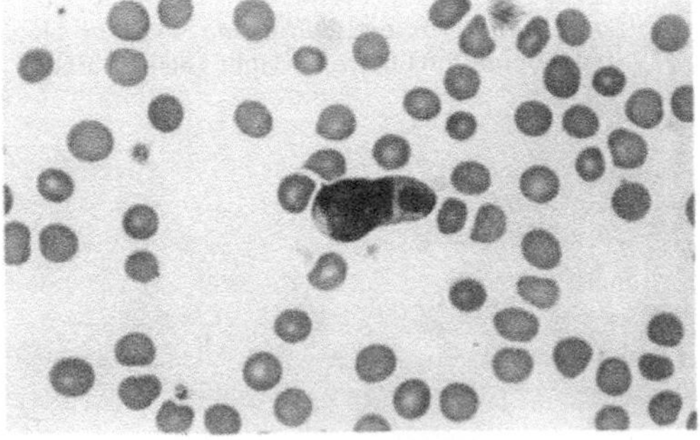

Figure 11-10 Morula of *Ehrlichia canis* in a canine lymphocyte. These inclusions occur transiently during the early phase of infection, and a search for this morula is not a fruitful method for detecting *E. canis.* (Wright's stain; 330×.)

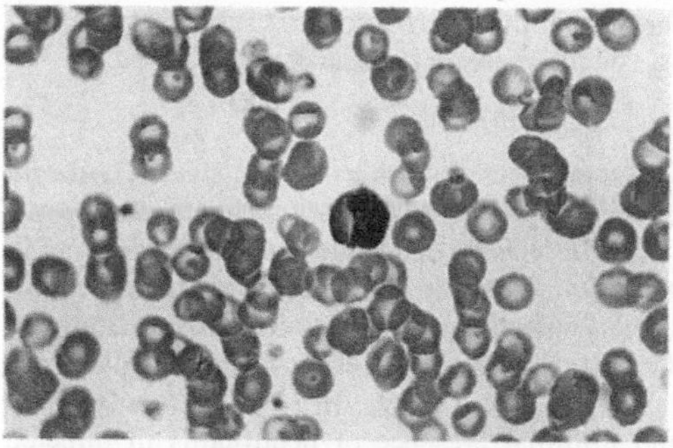

Figure 11-11 Viral inclusion in lymphocyte from a dog with canine distemper viral infection. Although many dogs develop this viral infection, the inclusions in blood cells are rarely observed. These viral inclusions often stain more prominently with the rapid Romanowsky stains, such as Diff-Quik. (Wright's stain; 330×.)

monocytes or macrophages with phagocytosed erythrocytes can be observed rarely on blood smears. *Erythrophagocytosis* occurs on blood smears of dogs with immune-mediated hemolytic anemia (Figure 11-12), cats with *Mycoplasma haemofelis* infection, foals with neonatal isoerythrolysis, and horses with equine infectious anemia viral infection. More rarely, erythrophagocytosis by circulating neoplastic cells (e.g., mast cell leukemia of dogs and cats, histiocytic sarcoma in dogs) has been observed on blood smears.

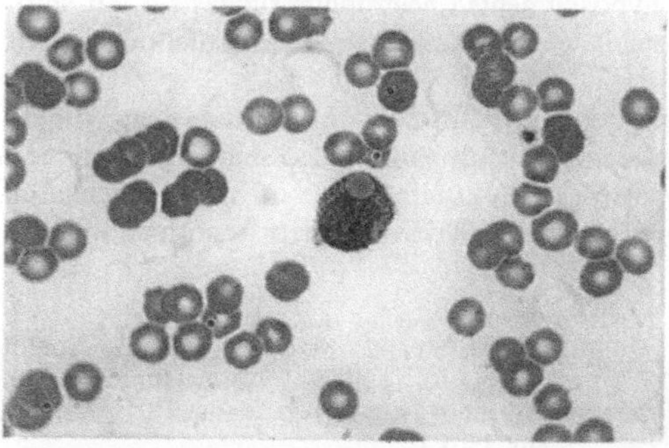

Figure 11-12 Erythrophagocytosis by monocyte in a dog with hemolytic anemia. (Wright's stain; 330×.)

12. What are sideroleukocytes?

Neutrophils or monocytes rarely contain variably sized golden-brown granules of hemosiderin. The iron content of these granules can be verified with an iron stain such as Prussian blue. *Sideroleukocytes* occur in animals with hemolytic anemias, particularly dogs with immune-mediated hemolytic anemia (Figure 11-13) and horses with acute equine infectious anemia viral

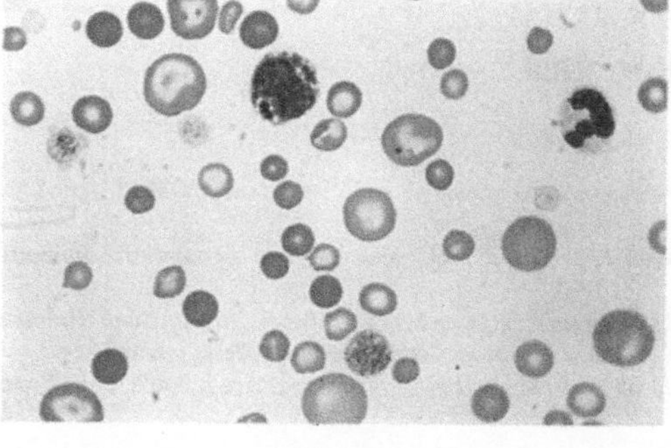

Figure 11-13 Monocyte with cytoplasmic hemosiderin granules in a dog with immune-mediated hemolytic anemia. (Wright's stain; 330×.)

infection. Rarely, horses with extensive metastases of malignant melanoma have blood neutrophils that contain black melanin granules, which resemble hemosiderin granules.

13. What are CLAD and BLAD?

Canine leukocyte adhesion defect (CLAD, reported in Irish setters) and *bovine leukocyte adhesion defect* (BLAD, reported in Holsteins) are rare congenital diseases in which neutrophils have normal morphology but are dysfunctional. The molecular defect is linked to the abnormality of a membrane adhesion protein in the integrin family, identified as CD18, that is necessary for adhesion of neutrophils to vascular endothelial cells. Affected neutrophils are unable to emigrate from blood vessels to sites of inflammation. The bactericidal activity of these neutrophils is also abnormal. Affected animals are observed at a few months of age, with marked neutrophilic leukocytosis, recurrent bacterial infections, and minimal presence of neutrophils in infected tissues. The diagnosis is confirmed by demonstrating decreased immunoreactivity for CD18 on neutrophils.

14. What is Pelger-Huet syndrome?

In Pelger-Huet syndrome, nuclear lobulation of neutrophils, eosinophils, and basophils decreases, but the function of these cells is not significantly altered. The nucleus of affected neutrophils is round, band, or peanut shaped, with a bilobed nucleus ("pince nez" cell) being the maximal segmentation observed. The "drumstick appendage" is lacking in neutrophils of affected females. Although the nuclear shape of these hyposegmented neutrophils suggests a left shift, the colorless cytoplasm and darkly condensed nuclear chromatin indicate the actual maturity of these cells.

Pelger-Huet syndrome occurs as a benign congenital disorder in dogs and cats (Figure 11-14). In cattle, horses, and pigs, hyposegmentation of neutrophils and eosinophils occurs as a transient disorder during severe inflammatory disease. In acquired cases of hyposegmentation ("psuedo–Pelger-Huet") the segmentation of granulocytic leukocytes reverts to normal once the inflammatory condition resolves.

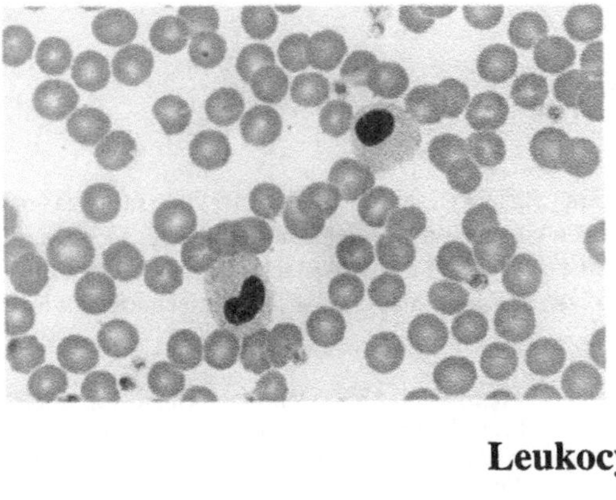

Figure 11-14 Myelocyte-like neutrophil and bandlike neutrophil in a healthy dog with congenital Pelger-Huet anomaly. (Wright's stain; 330×.)

Leukocytes

BIBLIOGRAPHY

Feldman BF, Zinkl JG, Jain NC, editors: *Schalm's veterinary hematology*, ed 5, Baltimore, 2000, Lippincott, Williams & Williams.

Harvey JW: Leukocytes. In *Atlas of veterinary hematology: blood and bone marrow of domestic animals*, Philadelphia, 2001, Saunders, pp 45-74.

Latimer KS, Prasse KW: Leukocytes. In Latimer KS, Mahaffey E, Prasse KW, editors: *Duncan and Prasse's veterinary laboratory medicine: clinical pathology*, Ames, 2003, Iowa State University Press, pp 46-79.

Stockham SL, Scott MA: Leukocytes. In *Fundamentals of veterinary clinical pathology*, Ames, 2002, Iowa State University Press, pp 49-83.

Plasma Proteins

12. DISORDERS AND LABORATORY EVALUATION

Ronald D. Tyler, Rick L. Cowell, and James H. Meinkoth

1. What is protein dyscrasia?

Protein dyscrasia refers to a protein with an abnormal structure, as in dysfibrinogenemia.

2. What is dysproteinemia?

Dysproteinemia is the presence of either normal plasma proteins at abnormal concentrations or abnormal proteins in the blood, e.g., hyper and hypoalbuminemia, hyper and hypoglobulinemia.

3. What are the two major categories of plasma proteins, and how are their concentrations usually determined?

The two major categories of plasma proteins are *albumin* and *globulin*. Their concentrations are determined by measuring total protein (TP) and albumin concentrations, then calculating the globulin concentration by subtracting the albumin concentration from the TP concentration.

4. Where are the major plasma proteins synthesized?

The liver synthesizes albumin and essentially all plasma globulins other than immunoglobulins and von Willebrand's factor. The lymphoid system synthesizes immunoglobulins, and endothelial cells (and megakaryocytes) synthesize von Willebrand's factor.

5. List two major functions of albumin.

a. Transport substances with low plasma solubility
b. Provide oncotic pressure

6. What are the general causes of severe hypoalbuminemia?

a. Hemorrhage
b. Glomerular disease (protein-losing nephropathies)
c. Gastrointestinal loss (protein-losing gastroenteropathies)
d. Decreased hepatic production of albumin

7. What are some supportive features of each of the four general causes of severe hypoalbuminemia?

a. *Hemorrhage:* concurrent anemia (usually a regenerative anemia unless iron deficiency anemia has developed), evidence of hemorrhage
b. *Glomerular disease:* moderate to marked proteinuria with benign urine sediment
c. *Gastrointestinal loss:* diarrhea (generally present but not always)
d. *Decreased hepatic production of albumin:* low blood glucose and urea nitrogen concentrations; elevated concentration of bile acids; hepatic transaminases and biliary enzymes may be elevated. Diarrhea is also present in some cases.

8. How does inflammation influence serum albumin and globulin concentrations?

During inflammation, albumin catabolism increases and albumin synthesis decreases, resulting in lower albumin concentrations. Concurrently, globulins increase due to increased production of inflammatory globulins, such as fibrinogen, alpha-2 macroglobulin, haptoglobin, ceruloplasmin, alpha-1 antitrypsin, and immunoglobulins. As a result, albumin concentration often decreases by about 1 gram per deciliter (g/dl) for each 3 to 4 g/dl increase in globulin concentration.

9. What are the advantages of measuring plasma or serum protein by refractometry?

Refractometry is a rapid, easy, and rather inexpensive method of measuring total protein and can be done at the clinic while the patient is in the examination room, if necessary.

10. Name two colormetric methods of measuring plasma or serum protein.

a. Biuret method
b. Lowry method

11. What is the chemical method most often used to measure plasma or serum protein in clinical laboratories?

Because of its simplicity, accuracy, and precision, the biuret method is the chemical method of choice for measuring TP concentration in serum or plasma in the clinical laboratory.

12. What is the basis of the biuret method of protein measurement?

The biuret method is based on the formation of a blue peptide–copper complex in alkaline solution and is the most widely used colorimetric method for TP concentration assay.

13. How sensitive is the biuret method for protein measurement?

The biuret method is accurate for assay of protein concentrations from 1 to 10 g/dl. Thus it is adequate for measurement of total plasma and serum protein concentrations, but not for the measurement of the very low levels of protein often found in body fluids, such as cerebrospinal fluid (CSF), urine, and transudates.

14. What is the basis of the phenol-Folin-Ciocalteau method for protein measurement?

The phenol-Folin-Ciocalteau method is based on the reaction of the reagent with the phenolic groups of tryptophan and tyrosine in proteins to form a blue color.

15. Which is better for measuring plasma or serum albumin concentration in domestic animals, the bromocresol green method or the 2-(4′-hydroxyazobenzene) benzoic acid method?

The bromocresol green (BCG) method is the dye-binding procedure that is most acceptable for determining serum albumin levels in domestic animals. Many human laboratories use a 2-(4′-hydroxyazobenzene) benzoic acid (HABA) procedure, which produces erratic results in domestic animals.

16. Can serum albumin concentration be measured by electrophoresis?

Serum protein electrophoresis is the most accurate method for measurement of albumin and is used as the reference method for the colorimetric procedures. However, serum protein electrophoresis is not routinely used to determine albumin levels because of its high cost and the time requirement for processing.

17. How is plasma or serum globulin concentration usually determined, and what are factors to consider when using it?

Serum globulin level is generally not measured but instead is determined mathematically by subtracting the albumin level from the TP level, with the difference being the globulin level. Therefore the globulin level represents all the nonalbumin protein measured in the TP level, and errors in measurement of TP or albumin level will erroneously alter the calculated globulin level.

The serum globulin level can be measured colorimetrically or by serum protein electrophoresis. However, these procedures are costly and time consuming and therefore are only used in rare instances.

18. What is the diagnostic value of the albumin/globulin ratio?

An increased albumin/globulin (A/G) ratio may occur with any factor that increases albumin or decreases globulin. A decreased A/G ratio may occur with any factor that decreases albumin or increases globulin. For best interpretation of the A/G ratio, absolute TP, albumin, and globulin values must also be considered.

19. Is serum or plasma preferred for protein electrophoresis?

Generally, serum is preferred for protein electrophoresis, and hemolysis should be avoided. Besides obscuring the patterns of other serum proteins, fibrinogen and hemoglobin produce monoclonal spikes and can be misdiagnosed as monoclonal gammopathies.

20. What factors influence protein migration during electrophoresis?

Direction and rate of migration of the different proteins are determined by the type of charge (positive or negative) of the protein, strength of the charge, size of the protein, intensity of the electrical field, and support medium through which the proteins are induced to migrate. To compare results of serum protein electrophoresis, the support medium, pH, buffer, and electric current should be known. Cellulose acetate is the most frequently used support medium.

21. Does serum electrophoresis identify changes in individual proteins?

Serum protein electrophoresis does not separate individual proteins, other than albumin, and therefore does not specifically identify changes in proteins other than albumin. Instead, electrophoresis separates proteins into groups of similarly charged and sized proteins. A change (increase or decrease) in the area of the electrophoretic pattern where a protein migrates indicates a change (increase or decrease) in that protein and/or another protein migrating in the same area. Therefore, serum protein electrophoresis generally provides only an estimate of which similarly charged and sized groups of proteins have increased or decreased. It usually does not indicate a specific diagnosis but instead indicates a general disease process, such as inflammation or immune response. An important exception is monoclonal spikes.

22. How are monoclonal peaks in electrophoretograms recognized?

Because of its homogeneity, albumin is used as a guide for differentiating sharp monoclonal globulin peaks (monoclonal spikes) from polyclonal peaks. Monoclonal peaks should be as sharp or sharper than the albumin peak.

23. What is the most common pathologic cause of monoclonal peaks in serum electrophoretograms?

Plasma cell myeloma is the most common cause of monoclonal spikes.

24. Besides plasma cell myeloma, what diseases may infrequently be associated with a monoclonal peak in serum protein electrophoretograms?

Monoclonal gammopathies resulting in peaks may be associated with the following:

a. Lymphosarcoma (occasionally)
b. Canine ehrlichiosis
c. Canine lieshmaniasis
d. Feline infectious peritonitis
e. Plasmacytic gastroenterocolitis
f. Chronic pyoderma
g. Idiopathic causes

25. What are two nonpathologic causes of monoclonal peaks in electrophoretograms?

a. Hemoglobin (subsequent to intravascular or in vitro hemolysis)
b. Fibrinogen (if plasma is used)

26. Can protein electrophoresis be performed on fluids other than serum and plasma?

Protein electrophoresis can also be performed on urine, CSF, abdominal fluid, and thoracic fluid.

27. How does the globulin fraction separate on electrophoresis?

There are three major globulin fractions: alpha (α) globulins, beta (β) globulins, and gamma (γ) globulins. The α-globulins are the most anodally migrating, and γ-globulins are the least anodally migrating. Depending on the species, one or more of the three major globulins may divide into subfractions during migration. Globulin subfractions are identified by numeric subscripts, such as α_1, α_2, β_1, β_2, γ_1, γ_2, and γ_3, with the smaller number representing the most anodal subfraction.

28. What are some components of the alpha-globulin fraction?

In most species other than the ruminant, α-globulin migrates as two fractions, α_1 (sometimes called "fast alpha") and α_2 (sometimes called "slow alpha"). The α_1-globulins tend to be smaller than α_2-globulins, but they are functionally indistinct. High-density lipoproteins (HDLs), sometimes called α-lipoproteins, migrate in the α_1 fraction. Important members of the α_2 fraction include very-low-density lipoproteins (VLDLs) or pre-β-lipoproteins, low-density lipoproteins (LDLs) or β-lipoproteins, α_2-macroglobulin, haptoglobin, and ceruloplasmin. LDLs were originally named β-lipoproteins because they migrate in the beta region on paper. On cellulose acetate, however, LDLs migrate in the α_2 region.

29. What are some diagnostic implications of changes in the alpha-globulin fraction?

Some causes of increases in the α_2 fraction are nephrotic syndrome, acute inflammation, glucocorticoids (prednisone), and haptoglobin-hemoglobin complexes. Increases in VLDL, LDL, and α_2-macroglobulin cause the increase in the α_2-globulin fraction that occurs with nephrotic syndrome. The α_2-macroglobulin haptoglobin and ceruloplasmin are sometimes called "acute inflammatory proteins" because their concentration increases during acute inflammation. Prednisone has been shown to induce increased haptoglobin levels in dogs. Also, hemolyzed samples can result in α_2-globulins being increased due to the presence of haptoglobin-hemoglobin complexes, and a monoclonal peak may be present.

30. What are some components of the beta-globulin fraction?

In most domestic species other than the ruminant, β-globulins migrate as β_1 (fast beta) and β_2 (slow beta) fractions. Hemopexin, transferrin, and complement C3 and C4 migrate in the beta region. Fibrinogen may migrate in the late β_2 region (the region closest to the gamma regions) but usually trails the β_2-globulins in the early gamma region. However, serum should be used for protein electrophoresis instead of plasma because fibrinogen interferes with the migration of other proteins and can form a monoclonal spike, leading to confusion in interpretation. Some highly charged immunoglobulins, usually IgM and IgA, migrate in the late β_2 region. IgM and IgA usually extend from the β_2 region to the γ_2 region. Therefore, immune stimulation, especially early when IgM is abundantly produced, or plasma cell malignancy can increase β-globulins, but more specifically, β_2-globulins as well as γ_1- and γ_2-globulins.

31. What are some diagnostic implications of changes in the beta-globulin fraction?

Increases in β-globulins alone occur infrequently but suggest active liver disease, suppurative dermatopathies, and occasionally the nephrotic syndrome. Transferrin appears to be primarily responsible for the increase in β-globulins seen with liver disease, although hemopexin and complement also increase. If antigenic stimulation occurs during liver disease, IgM may also increase in the β_2 region or fast gamma region. Antigenic stimulation with resultant IgM and complement increases is thought to be responsible for the increase in β-globulins associated with suppurative dermatopathies. The increase in β-globulin seen with the nephrotic syndrome results from increased transferrin. Monoclonal peaks in the beta region indicate plasma cell myeloma, Waldenström's macroglobulinemia, lymphosarcoma, and rarely, canine ehrlichiosis. Also, plasma samples and hemolyzed samples should be avoided, since fibrinogen and hemoglobin can form monoclonal peaks in the beta region and cause slurring of other peaks. Monoclonal peaks should be as sharp as the albumin peak. Monoclonal peaks in the beta region usually represent IgM or IgA.

Decreases in the late β-globulin fraction suggest decreased immunoglobulin concentration resulting from immune suppression or immunodeficiency syndrome.

32. What are some components of the gamma-globulin fraction?

The gamma fraction migrates as two fractions, γ_1 (fast) and γ_2 (slow). IgA, IgM, and IgE migrate primarily in the γ_1 region, and IgG migrates primarily in the γ_2 region. Immunoglobulin types, such as IgG versus IgM, cannot be determined by routine serum protein electrophoresis.

33. What are the diagnostic implications of changes in the gamma-globulin fraction?

Increases in the gamma region indicate immune stimulation and subsequent immunoglobulin production. During early immune stimulation (the first few weeks), the increase in γ-globulins may be more prominent in the β_2, γ_1, and γ_2 regions, reflecting the preponderance of IgM production. As the immune response matures, the IgM level and thus the β_2- and fast γ-globulins will decrease, whereas the IgG and thus the midrange and slow gamma regions will increase.

Decreases in the γ-globulin fraction suggest decreased immunoglobulin concentration resulting from immune suppression or immunodeficiency syndrome.

34. What is beta-gamma bridging?

Beta-gamma bridging refers to an electrophoretic pattern in which there is no clear separation between the β_2 and γ_1 fractions.

35. What causes beta-gamma bridging?

Beta-gamma bridging results from an increase in IgA and/or IgM and is purported to be almost pathognomonic of chronic active hepatitis, although it is also occasionally produced by low-grade gammopathy due to lymphosarcoma.

36. Can the heat precipitation method be used for measuring fibrinogen consumption, such as occurs during disseminated intravascular coagulation?

The heat precipitation method is not sufficiently sensitive at low plasma fibrinogen concentrations.

37. Why does subtracting total serum protein from total plasma protein *not* provide an accurate estimate of fibrinogen concentration?

Subtraction of total serum protein (TSP) concentration from total plasma protein (TPP) concentration to determine fibrinogen concentration is inaccurate because of the following:

a. Some coagulation factors remain in the clot along with fibrinogen.
b. Procedures used to assay TPP and TSP are not sufficiently precise.
c. Different procedures are often used to assay TPP and TSP. For example, TPP is often measured by the hematology unit using refractometry, and TSP is often measured in the chemistry unit using an automated chemistry analyzer.

38. What is the interpretive value of changes in fibrinogen?

Plasma fibrinogen levels are frequently determined in large animals as an indicator of inflammation (increased fibrinogen levels) and occasionally in small animals when evaluating certain coagulopathies, such as disseminated intravascular coagulation (DIC). During inflammation, both production and consumption of fibrinogen increase, and production of fibrinogen often increases more than consumption of fibrinogen, resulting in increased plasma fibrinogen concentration. Because dehydration causes a relative increase in plasma fibrinogen concentration, dehydration must be ruled out before accepting an increase in fibrinogen as evidence of inflammation. Because some inflammatory diseases do not result in more fibrinogen being produced than is being consumed, the absence of an increase in plasma fibrinogen concentration does not rule out inflammation.

39. When assessing dehydrated animals, how does one accommodate for the increase in fibrinogen concentration caused by dehydration?

To accommodate for dehydration, the percent of TPP that is fibrinogen is calculated by dividing the fibrinogen concentration (g/dl) by the TPP concentration (g/dl), then multiplying the result by 100. When fibrinogen represents 10% or more of the TPP concentration (a calculated value ≥ 10), inflammation is indicated. Because some inflammatory diseases do not result in more fibrinogen being produced than is being consumed, a fibrinogen concentration less than 10% of the total protein (calculated value <10) does not rule out inflammation.

40. What are Bence Jones proteins, and what is their diagnostic significance?

Bence Jones proteins are unpaired light chains produced by plasma cell myelomas. They are detected in approximately 50% of human and canine cases of plasma cell myeloma. Bence Jones proteins are filtered by the kidney and are present in the urine. Although Bence Jones proteins do not react (give a positive protein reaction) with the urine dipstick tests, they can be detected in urine samples by sulfosalicylic acid turbidometric test, by electrophoresis, or by a proteinaceous precipitate forming when heating the urine sample to 56° C for 15 minutes and the precipitate returning to solution with further heating to 100° C for 3 minutes. Documenting their presence aids in the diagnosis of plasma cell myeloma.

41. What are some causes of elevated total protein concentration?

Hyperproteinemia results from increased plasma globulins or decreased plasma water content (hemoconcentration). Therefore, causes of hyperproteinemia are dehydration, inflammation (infectious and noninfectious), and neoplastic conditions. These conditions may occur singly or in combination. Specific examples follow:

- a. Inflammation
  - (1) Infectious
    - (a) Bacterial
    - (b) Viral (e.g., feline infectious peritonitis, equine infectious anemia)
    - (c) Protozoal
    - (d) Fungal
    - (e) Rickettsial
  - (2) Noninfectious
    - (a) Neoplasia (especially if necrotic areas are present)
    - (b) Foreign body granuloma
    - (c) Antigenic response
- b. Neoplastic paraprotein production
  - (1) Plasma cell myeloma
  - (2) Some lymphomas
- c. Dehydration

42. What is panhyperproteinemia?

Panhyperproteinemia refers to elevated TP concentration caused by concurrently increased albumin and globulin concentrations.

43. What causes panhyperproteinemia?

Dehydration is the only condition that causes increased plasma albumin levels. Therefore, patients with panhyperproteinemia are dehydrated. If the increase in globulins is greater than the increase in albumin (i.e., A/G ratio is low), there is a previous or concurrent inflammatory response. However, absence of a low A/G ratio does not rule out concurrent inflammation.

44. What other hematologic changes occur during panhyperproteinemia?

Total protein (TP), hematocrit (Hct) or packed cell volume (PCV), hemoglobin (Hgb), and erythrocyte or red blood cell (RBC) count are elevated by dehydration. However, these values may not be elevated outside the normal range; that is, the values may simply range from low normal to high normal. Also, an anemic animal may have the anemia masked by dehydration. Because sequestration of white blood cells (WBCs) and platelets in small vessels (including splenic sinuses) tends to increase during dehydration, WBC and platelet values do not increase as greatly as TP, Hct, Hgb, and RBC values during dehydration alone.

45. What are causes of hyperproteinemia without concurrent hyperglobulinemia (an uncommon finding)?

Hyperproteinemia without hyperglobulinemia requires serum albumin to be greatly elevated. Because hyperalbuminemia is invariably associated with dehydration in the clinical setting, hyperalbuminemia without hyperglobulinemia indicates dehydration with concomitant hypoglobulinemia or low-normal globulin concentration. Possible causes include the following:

a. Failure of passive transfer in the neonate with concomitant dehydration
b. Combined immunodeficiency (CID) with concomitant dehydration
c. Age influence. Very young/old animal with low-normal globulin level may have globulin level in high-normal range with dehydration.
d. Low-normal globulin level with dehydration

46. What are causes of hyperproteinemia without concurrent hyperalbuminemia?

Hyperproteinemia without hyperalbuminemia requires serum globulin concentration to be elevated. This situation is usually produced by hypoalbuminemia with increased globulin production. Increased globulin production is often associated with a decrease in albumin concentration of about 1 g/dl for every 3 to 4 g/dl increase in globulin concentration. Causes of increased globulin production include the following:

a. Chronic systemic inflammation (usually requires an associated immune response for hyperglobulinemia to develop)
b. Immune stimulation
c. Plasma cell myeloma
d. Lymphosarcoma

47. Does a normal total protein concentration rule out abnormalities in albumin and globulin levels?

Abnormalities in the albumin and globulin levels can be present with a normal TP concentration. Common causes include the following:

a. Hypoalbuminemia with concomitant hyperglobulinemia
 (1) Hepatoinsufficiency
 (2) Inflammatory bowel disease causing a protein-losing enteropathy
b. Immediately after hemorrhage, before sufficient interstitial fluid has shifted into the blood to lower plasma protein concentration

c. Plasma loss with concomitant dehydration
   (1) Hemorrhage with dehydration
   (2) Exudation from large surface areas with dehydration
   (3) Protein-losing nephropathy with dehydration
   (4) Protein-losing enteropathy with dehydration

48. What are causes of low total protein values?

Low TP concentration, or *hypoproteinemia,* can be caused by increased plasma protein loss, decreased plasma protein production, decreased protein absorption, increased protein catabolism, age, or a combination of these causes. Increased protein metabolism may also contribute in some cases.

Plasma protein loss can be caused by the following:

a. Hemorrhage (both albumin and globulin lost in equal proportions)
b. Severe exudation from large surface areas, such as the pleural and peritoneal cavities, intestines, and skin
c. Lymphangiectasia caused by conditions such as congestive heart failure, intestinal diseases causing protein-losing enteropathies (if enteropathy is caused by inflammatory disease [e.g., histoplasmosis] and causes the globulin level to increase, the TP concentration may decrease, stay within the reference range, or even be mildly increased depending on the degree of globulin increase), and idiopathic lymphangiectasia (both albumin and globulin lost in approximately equal proportions)
d. Conditions in which albumin is predominantly lost (primarily protein-losing nephropathy caused by conditions such as renal amyloidosis, glomerulosclerosis, and glomerulonephritis)

Decreased plasma protein production can be caused by the following:

a. Hepatoinsufficiency
b. Severe malnutrition
c. Combined immunodeficiency

Increased protein catabolism can be caused by the following:

a. Cachexia of cancer
b. Severe malnutrition

Age influences TP concentration. Normal TP concentrations of very young or old animals are lower than those in normal adults.

49. What is the diagnostic value of albumin concentration?

Evaluation of albumin concentration is helpful in the diagnosis of patients with suspected dehydration, liver disease, renal disease, and gastrointestinal disease and with vague, nondescript signs.

a. Elevated albumin concentration almost invariably indicates dehydration (if the patient has not been transfused with plasma proteins recently).
b. Normal albumin concentration tends to make certain diseases less likely (e.g., severe protein losing nephropathy, severe protein losing enteropathy, severe hepatoinsufficiency).
c. Low albumin concentration can be caused by the following:
   (1) Hemorrhage
   (2) Severe exudation from large surface areas (e.g., pleural and peritoneal cavities, intestines, skin)
   (3) Lymphangiectasia caused by conditions such as congestive heart failure, intestinal diseases (inflammatory or neoplastic), and idiopathic lymphangiectasia
   (4) Protein-losing nephropathy
      (a) Renal amyloidosis
      (b) Glomerulosclerosis
      (c) Glomerulonephritis

(5) Decreased albumin production
  (a) Hepatic insufficiency
  (b) Severe malnutrition
(6) Increased albumin catabolism
  (a) Cachexia of cancer and chronic disease
  (b) Severe malnutrition

50. What is the diagnostic value of globulin concentration?

Because globulins are so highly varied, many conditions can cause increases or decreases in one or more components of the globulin fraction. However, change from normal in the total globulin value generally requires change in plasma immunoglobulin concentration because immunoglobulins make up the bulk of plasma globulins by weight.

a. Elevated globulin concentration *(hyperglobulinemia)* indicates immune stimulation or chronic inflammation with increased immunoglobulin production.
b. Normal globulin concentration tends to make chronic systemic immune stimulation unlikely because this usually results in an elevated globulin concentration. (*Note*: Chronic inflammation that is not systemic (cystitis) does not tend to elevate the globulin level.)
c. Low globulin concentration *(hypoglobulinemia)* indicates low immunoglobulin concentration and can be caused by conditions such as hemorrhage, protein-losing gastroenteropathy, immunosuppression, immunodeficiency syndromes, and severe malnutrition.

51. What are methods for determining immunoglobulin G concentration in foals and calves?

Several methods are available to measure IgG, and marked variation in results may occur between methods. Therefore, one must follow the interpretive guidelines for the specific method used. Methods for determining IgG in foals and calves include the following:

a. Serum protein electrophoresis
b. Single radial immunodiffusion assay (SRID): foals, calves
c. Glutaraldehyde coagulation test: foals, calves
d. Latex agglutination test (Foalcheck): foals
e. Zinc sulfate turbidity test: foals, calves
f. Sodium sulfate precipitation test: calves

52. Should serum, plasma, or whole blood be used for estimating immunoglobulin G concentration?

Serum should be used to estimate IgG because fibrinogen and other plasma and blood components may interfere with the assays.

53. Which method for estimating immunoglobulin G concentration in foals and calves is most accurate?

The most accurate method for estimating IgG in foals and calves is the single radial immunodiffusion assay.

54. What serum immunoglobulin G concentration indicates sufficient passive transfer in foals?

Although 400 mg/dl was long considered evidence of sufficient passive transfer in foals, concentrations of 800 mg/dl or greater are currently considered necessary. IgG concentrations less than 200 mg/dl are considered evidence of the failure of passive transfer. IgG concentrations of 200 to 800 mg/dl are considered evidence of partial passive transfer.

55. What serum immunoglobulin G concentration indicates sufficient passive transfer in calves?

At this time, no guidelines have been universally agreed on to indicate passive transfer in calves, although the following two guidelines are provided:

Guideline A
- Greater than 1000 mg/dl is evidence of passive transfer.
- Less than 500 mg/dl is evidence of failure of passive transfer.

Guideline B
- Greater than 1600 mg/dl is evidence of passive transfer.
- From 800 to 1600 mg/dl is evidence of partial passive transfer.
- Less than 800 mg/dl indicates failure of passive transfer.

Myeloproliferative Disorders

13. MYELOPROLIFERATIVE DISORDERS

Tarja Juopperi and Heather Leigh DeHeer

1. Define the term leukemia.

The term *leukemia* literally means "white blood." This term was initially used to describe disorders characterized by the abnormal finding of large numbers of leukocytes present in the peripheral blood. *Leukemias* are neoplastic disorders that result from the uncontrolled and excessive proliferation of hematopoietic cells within the bone marrow. As the malignant cells increase in number, they replace the normal bone marrow and are frequently observed in abundance in the peripheral blood ("white blood"). Occasionally, leukemic cells may not circulate in the peripheral blood and remain in the bone marrow (*aleukemic* leukemias), or rarely, low numbers of leukemic cells may be seen (*subleukemic* leukemias). With these disorders the blood would not appear "white," although leukemia is present. In addition to finding leukemic cells circulating in the peripheral blood, the cells may infiltrate other organs (e.g., spleen, liver).

2. What are myeloproliferative disorders?

The term *myeloproliferative disorder* encompasses an assortment of diseases, including acute myeloid leukemias, chronic myeloproliferative disorders, and myelodysplastic syndromes. This category of neoplastic disorders is used to describe a group of clonal malignancies arising from neoplastic myeloid cells (all hematopoietic cells other than lymphocytes) that originate in the bone marrow.

3. How are myeloproliferative disorders classified?

Myeloproliferative disorders can initially be classified as acute or chronic based on the degree of differentiation and maturity of the neoplastic cells. In *acute* myeloproliferative disorders, the neoplastic cells are immature and they do not progress beyond the "blast" stage (myeloid precursors). In contrast, *chronic* myeloproliferative disorders are characterized primarily by the proliferation of excessive numbers of mature and well-differentiated hematopoietic cells. In addition, this terminology was previously used to reflect the biologic behavior of the neoplasm and the life expectancy of the patient; with acute disorders having a rapid onset and a poor prognosis and chronic disorders exhibiting a prolonged and progressive clinical course.

Myeloproliferative disorders can be further classified based on the cell type as erythroid, granulocytic, monocytic, megakaryocytic, or a combination of these.

4. How common are myeloproliferative disorders?

Myeloid leukemias are uncommon in veterinary medicine and are seen less frequently than lymphoproliferative diseases. Although documented in several domestic species, myeloproliferative disorders are observed more often in the dog and cat (approximately 5% and 10%-15% of hematopoietic neoplasms, respectively).

5. Briefly discuss the etiology of myeloproliferative disorders.

The etiology of spontaneously occurring myeloproliferative disorders has not yet been determined for the majority of species in which these diseases have been documented (including dogs). Cats are an exception, as feline leukemia virus (FeLV) and feline immunodeficiency virus (FIV) are frequently associated with myeloproliferative disorders in this species.

6. What tests are used to diagnose a myeloproliferative disorder?

Myeloproliferative disorders result in the production of excessive numbers of abnormal hematopoietic cells that interfere with normal hematopoiesis. The clinical signs and laboratory findings exhibited by a patient with a myeloproliferative disorder will reflect the hematopoietic cell lines that have been affected as a result of impaired or disturbed hematopoiesis. The results of diagnostic tests will also vary depending on the type of myeloproliferative disorder (acute leukemia, chronic leukemia, or myelodysplastic syndrome). Box 13-1 lists tests that may be used to diagnose a myeloproliferative disorder (in conjunction with a complete history and physical examination).

Box 13-1 ***Diagnostic Tests for Myeloproliferative Disorders***

Complete blood count (cell counts and microscopic evaluation) ± cytochemical stains
Bone marrow aspirate and cytological evaluation ± cytochemical stains
Bone marrow core biopsy + histochemical stains
Flow cytometry and immunophenotyping (blood or bone marrow specimen)
Feline leukemia virus (FeLV) and feline immunodeficiency virus (FIV) testing*

*Cats suspected of having a myeloproliferative disorder should be tested.

7. Can special techniques be used in the identification and classification of myeloproliferative disorders?

Numerous specialized techniques can be used to evaluate myeloproliferative disorders, including the use of cytochemical stains, immunophenotyping (by flow cytometry or immunohistochemical staining), cytogenetics, and molecular analyses. These techniques can be employed to provide supplemental information that may enable further classification of the neoplasm. Definitive classification may be critical to patient management because the prognosis and treatment of the disorders may differ.

Cytochemical Stains

Because it can be difficult to determine cell lineage definitively based solely on morphology, several cytochemical stains are available to aid in the classification of myeloid leukemias. Table 13-1 lists cytochemical stains that may be used to help identify various cell types.

Table 13-1 *Cytochemical Stains Used to Identify Cells of Myeloid Lineage*

CELL TYPE	CYTOCHEMICAL STAIN
Granulocytes	Myeloperoxidase
	Sudan black B
	Chloroacetate esterase
	Leukocyte alkaline phosphatase*
Monocytes	Nonspecific esterase
Myelomonocytic	Myeloperoxidase
	Sudan black B
	Chloroacetate esterase
	Nonspecific esterase
Megakaryocytic	Nonspecific esterase
	Acetylcholinesterase

*Normally absent in canine and feline neutrophils.

Immunophenotyping

Flow cytometric immunophenotyping is an additional diagnostic test that can assist in identifying cell lineage. Cells are differentiated based on the expression of surface antigens. In veterinary medicine, flow cytometry is more useful in the diagnosis of lymphoid neoplasms because a number of antibodies are available for the identification of various subtypes of lymphocytes. However, a few antibodies also are available to aid in the diagnosis of monocytic myeloid disorders. CD14 surface antigen expression is currently used to identify cells of monocytic origin.

Cytogenetics and Molecular Analyses

These supplementary techniques are used primarily in human medicine; limited veterinary studies have been performed.

14. ACUTE MYELOID LEUKEMIAS

Tarja Juopperi and Heather Leigh DeHeer

1. What are acute myeloid leukemias?

Acute myeloid leukemias (AMLs) are disorders that result from the uninhibited proliferation of a clone of malignant myeloid cells. The neoplastic cell is derived from a hematopoietic stem cell that has the ability to produce cells of the myeloid lineage (erythroid, granulocytic, monocytic, and megakaryocytic). Because lymphocytes are not usually involved in these disorders, AML has also been referred to as *acute nonlymphocytic leukemia* (ANLL). AMLs are characterized by increased numbers of immature myeloid cells (blasts) in the bone marrow and frequently in the peripheral blood. As the blast cells accumulate within the bone marrow, they replace the normal cellular constituents and often result in peripheral cytopenias (severe anemia, thrombocytopenia).

2. List the clinical signs and physical examination findings that can be seen with AML. What are the related hematologic/cytologic findings?

Animals with AML typically present with a history of nonspecific illness, such as anorexia, weight loss, vomiting, or diarrhea of short duration (days to weeks). Specific clinical signs and physical examination findings may also be seen as a consequence of bone marrow infiltration by leukemic cells (resulting in cytopenias). Abnormal findings may be directly attributable to the hematopoietic cell line that is affected. Table 14-1 lists the clinical signs and physical examination findings frequently seen with animals that have AML and the associated hematologic or cytologic findings.

Table 14-1 *Clinical Signs and Physical Examination Findings Attributable to AML*

CLINICAL SIGNS/ PHYSICAL EXAMINATION	HEMATOLOGIC/ CYTOLOGIC	PATHOPHYSIOLOGY/ POSSIBLE CAUSE
Pallor Lethargy Weakness Icterus*	Anemia	Myelophthisis (decreased production) Immune-mediated destruction (secondary to neoplasia) Maturation arrest of precursors Hemorrhage (if thrombocytopenia also present)
Persistent/recurrent fever Infections	Neutropenia	Myelophthisis Functional defects in neutrophils
Epistaxis Petechiae/ecchymoses Hemorrhage Lameness, hemarthrosis	Thrombocytopenia	Disseminated intravascular coagulation Splenic sequestration Myelophthisis Platelet dysfunction
Splenomegaly Hepatomegaly Lymphadenopathy (mild) Bone pain (lameness) Icterus†	Increased numbers of blasts (cytology)	Infiltration by leukemic cells

*As a result of hemolysis.
†As a result of hepatic infiltration.

3. What are the potential peripheral blood findings in an animal with AML?

The hematologic features of AML are diverse, and animals may exhibit a wide range of peripheral blood findings. Hematologic abnormalities vary depending on the subtype of AML present, but cytopenias (anemia and thrombocytopenia) are the most frequent findings. Total leukocyte and blast cell counts are unpredictable, ranging from decreased to within normal range to greatly elevated (leukocytosis is more common). Table 14-2 lists potential peripheral blood findings in an animal with AML.

4. How is AML diagnosed?

The initial test needed to diagnose AML is a complete blood count (CBC) in conjunction with morphologic examination of a blood smear. A tentative diagnosis of AML can be made if large numbers of myeloblasts are noted in the circulation. Cytochemistry or flow cytometry is usually necessary for confirmation. Occasionally, low numbers or rare circulating leukemic cells are observed in the peripheral blood, necessitating bone marrow examination for a definitive diagnosis (also needed for subtyping).

Table 14-2 *Possible Peripheral Blood Findings in Animal with AML*

CELL TYPE	PERIPHERAL BLOOD FINDINGS
Erythrocytes	Anemia* (severe, nonregenerative)
	Dyserythropoiesis (megaloblastic rubricytes, macrocytosis)
	Normoblastemia (circulating nucleated red blood cells)
Leukocytes	Leukocytosis* (marked)
	Leukopenia (neutropenia)
	Dysgranulopoiesis (giant forms, hypersegmentation)
	Monocytosis
	Circulating blasts* (variable numbers)
Platelets	Thrombocytopenia*
	Thrombocytosis (rare)
	Abnormal platelets (giant, vacuolated, or containing large granules)
	Circulating megakaryocytes (micromegakaryocytes)

*Most frequent findings.

On bone marrow examination, the key finding needed to diagnose AML is a 30%* or greater presence of blasts (myeloblasts, erythroblasts, monoblasts, or megakaryoblasts) in the bone marrow. This can be accomplished by cytologic examination of the bone marrow, consisting of performing a differential count (minimum 200 nucleated cells) and determining the percentage of nonlymphoid blasts in the bone marrow. AML must be distinguished from lymphoid neoplasms because the prognosis varies considerably. Morphologic examination may allow for identification of the leukemic cells as myeloid. However, additional diagnostic tests (e.g., cytochemical stains, immunophenotyping) may be necessary to determine cell lineage definitively.

Once AML is diagnosed, the neoplasm is typically classified into a particular subtype. The classification is based on the degree of differentiation of the neoplastic cells, predominant cell lineage involved, and number of blast cells present.

5. Is histologic examination of the bone marrow necessary for a diagnosis of AML?

Examination of a blood smear and bone marrow cytology are frequently the only diagnostic tests that are required to diagnose AML. Histopathologic examination may be essential if cytologic examination is not possible or is nondiagnostic (dry tap, hypocellular specimen). The biopsy may also provide additional information regarding the overall cellularity, presence of myelofibrosis, and infiltration pattern of the tumor. A core biopsy is less useful for examination of cellular morphology, since it is difficult to appreciate the fine cellular detail readily observed by cytology.

6. List the various types of AML. How are these types classified?

The current system used to classify AML in animals was derived from the French-American-British (FAB) classification system used in human medicine. This system helped to standardize the classification of myeloproliferative disorders. According to this classification scheme, various subtypes of AML exist in animals. These subtypes are defined primarily by cellular morphology (noting degree of differentiation) and the cell lineage. The specifics regarding the morphologic identification of myeloid hematopoietic precursors and the classification of AML are beyond the scope of this chapter; interested readers are referred to articles pertaining to

*Note: In human medicine the blast percentage to diagnose AML has been reduced to 20% by the World Health Organization. Several veterinary pathologists have suggested the use of a similar cutoff point.

Table 14-3 *Veterinary Classification of Acute Myeloid Leukemias*

SUBTYPE	FAB*	CELL ORIGIN
Acute undifferentiated leukemia	AUL	Undifferentiated/unidentifiable
Myeloblastic leukemia without maturation	M1	Minimal granulocytic differentiation
Myeloblastic leukemia with maturation	M2	Granulocytic
Promyelocytic leukemia	M3	Promyelocytes (granulocytic)
Acute myelomonocytic leukemia	M4	Granuolcytic and monocytic
Monoblastic leukemia	M5a	Monocytic
Monocytic leukemia	M5b	Monocytic
Erythroleukemia	M6	Erythroid and granulocytic
Erythremic myelosis	M6-Er	Erythroid
Megakaryoblastic leukemia	M7	Megakaryocytic

*French-American-British classification.

Table 14-4 *Frequency of AML in Certain Domestic Species*

SPECIES	SUBTYPE
Cat	M1 and M2 (myeloblastic): most common
	M6 and M6Er (erythroid): second most common (reported primarily in cats)
	M7 (megakaryocytic): rare
Dog	M1 and M2 (myeloblastic): most frequent
	M5a and M5b (monocytic): second most common
	M6 and M6-Er (erythroid): rare
	M7: rare
Horse	M4 (myelomonocytic): most frequently reported

AML. Table 14-3 lists the subtypes of AML according to the FAB classification system, as well as the cell of origin.

7. Which of the AML subtypes occur more frequently?

AMLs are rare in domestic species. Although most of the subtypes have been documented in animals, certain subtypes are reported more often than others. Table 14-4 lists the most frequent subtypes of AML reported in the cat, dog, and horse.

8. What differential diagnoses should be considered before making a diagnosis of AML?

a. *Lymphoma and acute lymphoblastic leukemia*. It is important to rule out an acute lymphoblastic leukemia or the hematogeneous phase of lymphoma before diagnosing AML (as the response to treatment and prognosis differ). When morphologic examination of the cells is not definitive, additional tests (e.g., cytochemical stains, immunophenotyping, histopathology, electron microscopy) can be used to determine cell lineage.

b. *Hyperplastic responses*. A defining characteristic of AML is the excessive numbers of blasts present in the bone marrow. However, other conditions may have a similar appearance and must be ruled out before diagnosing AML. Increased numbers of immature cells may be seen in association with diseases that cause a hyperplastic response (e.g., immune-mediated disorders). Additionally, a bone marrow that is attempting to recover from an insult (e.g., panleukopenia/parvovirus infection, chemotherapy treatment) that has greatly disrupted hematopoiesis may appear similar (as the marrow attempts to regenerate, increased numbers of blasts are seen). History and physical examination findings aid in differentiating these causes. Monitoring the peripheral blood and bone marrow can provide evidence that the findings are compatible with regeneration and recovery of the bone marrow.

c. *Other myeloproliferative disorders*. Myelodysplastic syndromes and chronic myeloproliferative disorders can transition into AML. Specific criteria have been established to aid in differentiating these disorders (see previous questions).

9. What is the prognosis and current treatment for AML?

Currently, the prognosis for all subtypes of AML in animals is poor. Animals typically have a short survival time, seldom more than 3 months. The mainstay of AML treatment is the use of cytoreductive chemotherapeutics. Because the cytotoxic drugs currently available fail to induce or maintain remission, treatment of AML has been disappointing. These disorders are not as responsive to chemotherapy as lymphoid tumors. Furthermore, chemotherapeutic agents frequently cause substantial suppression of hematopoiesis (potentially resulting in significant cytopenias), necessitating supportive care.

15. CHRONIC MYELOPROLIFERATIVE DISORDERS

Tarja Juopperi and Heather Leigh DeHeer

1. What are chronic myeloproliferative disorders?

Chronic myeloproliferative disorders (CMPDs) are clonal bone marrow disorders that result in the production of excessive numbers of mature, morphologically unremarkable, hematopoietic cells of the myeloid lineage (erythrocytes, granulocytes, and platelets). These neoplastic conditions arise from the proliferation of an abnormal hematopoietic stem cell that retains its ability to differentiate and mature. Although the term encompasses a variety of diseases and each disorder is unique, there is considerable overlap of clinical and laboratory features among the CMPDs. In contrast to acute leukemias, CMPDs tend to have a protracted clinical course.

2. Identify the diseases classified as CMPDs and the primary cell line affected.

The CMPDs are classified primarily based on the hematopoietic cell line that predominates. However, it is important to recognize that all the myeloid lineages (granulocytic, megakaryocytic, erythroid) may be involved in each of the diseases. In addition, the presence or absence of marrow fibrosis is an important diagnostic criterion for classification of CMPDs. Table 15-1 lists the CMPDs and the predominant hematopoietic cell lines affected.

Note: Traditionally this category encompassed the following four disorders: polycythemia vera, essential thrombocythemia, idiopathic myelofibrosis, and chronic myelogenous leukemia.

3. What clinical or laboratory features do the CMPDs have in common?

The similarities among the CMPDs are the result of a marked proliferation of leukemic cells. Table 15-2 lists common features of CMPDs provided by physical examination, peripheral blood, and bone marrow findings.

Table 15-1 ***Classification of Chronic Myeloproliferative Disorders***

DISORDER	PREDOMINANT CELL LINE
Polycythemia vera*	Erythroid (erythrocytes)
Essential thrombocythemia*	Megakaryocytic (platelets)
Chronic idiopathic myelofibrosis*	Megakaryocytic and myeloid (platelets and granulocytes)
Chronic Myeloid Leukemias	
Chronic myelogenous leukemia*	Myeloid (granulocytes)
Chronic neutrophilic leukemia*	Neutrophils
Chronic eosinophilic leukemia*	Eosinophils
Chronic basophilic leukemia	Basophils
Chronic monocytic leukemia	Monocytes
Chronic myelomonocytic leukemia	Granulocytes and monocytes
Mast cell leukemia	Mast cells

*Recognized as CMPDs by the World Health Organization classification system.

Table 15-2 ***Common Features of Chronic Myeloproliferative Disorders***

DIAGNOSTIC TEST	FINDING	PATHOPHYSIOLOGY/ POSSIBLE CAUSE
Physical examination	Organomegaly (splenomegaly, hepatomegaly)	Infiltration and proliferation of leukemic cells resulting in organ enlargement
Peripheral blood examination	High cell counts* (leukocytosis, polycythemia, thrombocytosis)	Effective hematopoiesis resulting in large numbers of mature cells being released into peripheral blood
Bone marrow examination	Hypercellular marrow* Orderly maturation	Proliferation of neoplastic hematopoietic cells

*Most often seen. However, bone marrow failure (ineffective hematopoiesis) may be observed in the late stages of CMPDs.

4. Can CMPDs transform into acute leukemias?

All the CMPDs have the potential to progress into acute myeloid leukemias. In veterinary medicine, little is known about the transformation rate of each disorder.

5. What tests are used to diagnose CMPDs?

The diagnosis of a CMPD is challenging. Critical diagnostic tests include complete blood count (CBC) and peripheral blood smear examination, bone marrow aspirate cytology, and bone marrow core biopsy with histopathology. In human medicine, genetic testing such as cytogenetics and molecular analyses are important criteria in the diagnostic workup. To diagnose a CMPD, it is essential to correlate the history and physical examination findings with the results of laboratory testing. Although diagnostic criteria exist for each disorder, a major component of the diagnostic workup is the exclusion of reactive processes.

6. What is polycythemia vera?

The term *polycythemia* or *erythrocytosis* is used to describe an abnormally elevated red blood cell (RBC) mass, as measured by hemoglobin or hematocrit. *Polycythemia vera* (PV) is a neoplastic hematopoietic stem cell disorder typified by excessive erythropoiesis. The neoplastic clone proliferates uncontrollably and independent of the mechanisms that regulate RBC production, resulting in increased numbers of mature RBCs in circulation. Although the erythroid cell line is predominantly affected, other hematopoietic cells of myeloid origin may also be involved. PV has been documented primarily in the dog and the cat.

7. List the major history and clinical findings associated with polycythemia vera.
The history and clinical findings in an animal with PV are related to the marked increase in RBC mass that accompanies this disease. The excessive proliferation of mature erythrocytes often increases blood viscosity, causing reduced blood flow within vessels and suboptimal delivery of oxygen to tissues (tissue hypoxia). Box 15-1 lists clinical findings associated with PV.

Box 15-1 *History and Clinical Findings Associated with Polycythemia Vera*

- Hyperemic mucous membranes
- Dilated retinal vessels
- Splenomegaly (mild)
- Neurologic manifestations
  - Behavior changes
  - Ataxia
  - Blindness
  - Seizures
- Increased bleeding tendencies
  - Hematemesis
  - Hematochezia
- Nonspecific findings
  - Anorexia
  - Lethargy
  - Polyuria, polydipsia

8. List the major peripheral blood and bone marrow findings associated with polycythemia vera.
Table 15-3 lists peripheral blood and bone marrow findings associated with PV.

9. How is polycythemia vera diagnosed?
A diagnosis of PV requires documentation of an absolute increase in RBC mass and exclusion of other causes of polycythemia. To diagnose an absolute polycythemia, the possibility of a relative polycythemia should initially be eliminated. A relative increase in RBC mass may result

Table 15-3 *Peripheral Blood and Bone Marrow Findings Associated with Polycythemia Vera*

SITE	MAJOR FINDINGS
Peripheral blood	Elevated red cell mass (typical range 65%-81%)
	Morphologically unremarkable erythrocytes
	Red cell indices can vary (normocytic normochromic to microcytic hypochromic)
	Neutrophilia* (mild)
	Thrombocytosis*
Bone marrow	Myeloid:erythroid ratio <1
	Marked erythroid hyperplasia with orderly maturation
	Granulocytic and megakaryocytic hyperplasia
	Fibrosis possible

*Not typical in animals (seen in humans with PV).

from decreased plasma volume caused by dehydration. Splenic contraction (caused by catecholamine release) can also increase RBC mass by releasing mature erythrocytes into circulation, resulting in an increased RBC count. With both these situations (hemoconcentration or redistribution), the true or total body RBC mass is not increased; these are transient conditions.

Once an absolute polycythemia is confirmed, the elevation in RBC mass should be classified as primary or secondary based on erythropoietin production and concentration. *Erythropoietin* is a glycoprotein produced by the renal interstitial cells that stimulates erythrocyte production. With *primary polycythemia* (PV) the neoplastic cells proliferate independently of normal regulatory mechanisms (autonomous of erythropoietin levels), and animals with PV tend to have normal to low erythropoietin levels.

Secondary polycythemia arises from increased secretion of erythropoietin. This category can be further divided into *appropriate* or *inappropriate* with respect to tissue oxygenation. Increased serum erythropoietin levels and the resultant polycythemia are appropriate in situations when tissue hypoxia is present. Inappropriate increases in erythropoietin also occur, regardless of tissue oxygenation status (independent of tissue hypoxia). The increase in serum erythropoietin and RBC mass that occurs with inappropriate polycythemia is unwarranted and unnecessary.

Table 15-4 lists conditions associated with relative, primary, and secondary appropriate and inappropriate polycythemia.

Table 15-4 ***Conditions Associated with Polycythemia and Diagnostic Tests***

TYPE	CAUSE	DIAGNOSTIC TESTS
Relative	Dehydration Splenic contraction (epinephrine)	Physical examination: assess hydration status Confirm elevation (repeat PCV) Fluid therapy (rehydrate)
Absolute: Primary	Myeloproliferative disorder (polycythemia vera)	Minimum database* Bone marrow evaluation Erythropoietin levels Endogenous erythroid colony formation (in vitro) Rule out other causes
Absolute: Secondary (appropriate)	High altitude Methemoglobinemia Pulmonary disease Cardiac disease: right-left cardiovascular shunting	Minimum database* Cardiac evaluation Arterial blood gas analysis Erythropoietin levels
Absolute: Secondary (inappropriate)	Renal lesions: neoplasia (benign or malignant), cysts, hydronephrosis Other tumors: uterine myoma, hepatoma	Minimum database* Abdominal ultrasound/radiographs Erythropoietin levels

PCV, Packed cell volume.
*Complete blood count (CBC), chemistry panel, and urinalysis.

10. What is the current treatment for polycythemia vera?

Current therapy for PV centers on decreasing the RBC mass to reduce the risk of hyperviscosity and the associated complications of thrombosis and hemorrhage. Phlebotomy is a noninvasive method to lower the number of circulating erythrocytes. Although this procedure results in a temporary reduction in erythrocyte numbers, it can be difficult to control or manage a patient with PV using only this method. Myelosuppressive therapy (e.g., hydroxyurea) can be used if excessive phlebotomy is required.

11. What is essential thrombocythemia?

Essential thrombocythemia (ET) is a hematopoietic stem cell disorder that results in the clonal expansion of cells of the megakaryocytic lineage. In ET, numerous platelets are detected in the peripheral blood (marked thrombocytosis) because of the continual proliferation of mature, well-differentiated megakaryocytes. ET is a rare myeloproliferative disorder, although it has been reported in the dog and cat.

12. List the major history and clinical findings associated with essential thrombocythemia?

As there are few documented clinical cases of ET in animals, Box 15-2 lists history and clinical findings associated with ET in humans. Patients may be asymptomatic or exhibit clinical signs related to the marked increase in platelets that accompanies ET (signs of hemorrhage or thrombosis).

Box 15-2 ***History and Clinical Findings Associated with Essential Thrombocythemia (Humans)***

Nonspecific findings*
Inappetence
Lethargy
Weight loss
Signs related to disorders of primary hemostasis (platelet-type bleeding)
Petechiae, ecchymoses
Bleeding from mucosal surfaces
Signs related to thrombosis
Dyspnea (pulmonary)
Arterial or venous thrombosis
May also be asymptomatic

*Most consistent findings in animals with essential thrombocythemia.

13. List the major peripheral blood and bone marrow findings associated with essential thrombocythemia.

Table 15-5 lists peripheral blood and bone marrow findings associated with ET.

14. How is essential thrombocythemia diagnosed?

A diagnosis of ET is made by exclusion of all other possible causes of a severe thrombocytosis (e.g., reactive thrombocytosis, other neoplastic conditions). No single pathognomonic laboratory finding differentiates ET from other disorders. Documentation of a persistent and greatly elevated platelet count should be followed by diagnostic tests that help to exclude disease processes that can appear similar to ET. Common causes of an extreme thrombocytosis (e.g., inflammatory disease, iron deficiency) should be considered before a rare disorder such as ET is diagnosed. Box 15-3 lists differential diagnoses for ET.

In human medicine, exclusion of secondary causes of an extreme thrombocytosis is also critical to the diagnosis of ET. The Polycythemia Vera Study Group (PVSG) has established criteria to aid in the diagnosis of ET (Box 15-4). Similar criteria may be used in veterinary patients to help rule out reactive processes.

Table 15-5 *Peripheral Blood and Bone Marrow Findings Associated with Essential Thrombocythemia*

SITE	MAJOR FINDINGS
Peripheral blood	Persistent and marked thrombocytosis* (1-5 million) Variable platelet size (anisocytosis) Elevated platelet distribution width (PDW) Bizarre platelet shapes, agranular cytoplasm Megakaryocyte fragments White cell count: normal to slightly elevated Normal red cell mass or anemia (if bleeding)
Bone marrow	Normocellular to moderately hypercellular Normal myeloid:erythroid ratio Marked megakaryocytic hyperplasia* (usually normal morphology) Megakaryoblasts less than 30% of population Myelofibrosis (not typical)

*Key findings.

Box 15-3 *Differential Diagnosis of Essential Thrombocythemia*

Causes of Thrombocytosis

- Physiologic thrombocytosis
  - Exercise, epinephrine
- Reactive thrombocytosis*
  - Neoplasia
  - Iron deficiency
  - Postsplenectomy
  - Chronic hemorrhage
  - Chronic infectious disease
  - Rebound from thrombocytopenia
  - Acute/chronic inflammatory disorders
- Drug therapy
  - Vincristine
  - Corticosteroids
- Other chronic myeloproliferative disorders
  - Polycythemia vera
  - Idiopathic myelofibrosis
  - Chronic myelogeneous leukemia
- Megakaryocytic leukemia

*Common causes of a persistent thrombocytosis.

15. What is the current treatment for essential thrombocythemia?

The paucity of reported cases of ET precludes definitive information regarding the prognosis and treatment of the disease in animals. In humans, ET is an indolent disorder, and patients frequently have a good prognosis (long-term survival). Treatment is considered for patients suspected of having an increased risk of hemorrhagic or thromboembolic complications (marked thrombocytosis). Protocols may include cytoreductive therapy (hydroxurea) to control cell counts or antiaggregant agents (aspirin).

16. What is chronic idiopathic myelofibrosis?

Chronic idiopathic myelofibrosis (CIM), also known as "agnogenic myeloid metaplasia" and "myelosclerosis with myeloid metaplasia," is a condition resulting from the clonal proliferation of hematopoietic cells (primarily megakaryocytes and granulocytes), which is accompanied by myelofibrosis (deposition of excess collagen/reticulin in the bone marrow). Myelofibrosis results from the proliferation of fibroblasts due to cytokine stimulation (a reactive process) rather than from the propagation of neoplastic mesenchymal cells. *Extramedullary hematopoiesis* (EMH),

Box 15-4 *PVSG Criteria for Diagnosis of Essential Thrombocythemia (Humans)*

Platelet count >600,000 cells/μl
Normal red cell mass (normal hemoglobin)
Normal serum iron concentration, presence of stainable iron (bone marrow)
Absence of Philadelphia chromosome*
No evidence of bone marrow fibrosis
No known cause for reactive thrombocytosis

PVSG, Polycythemia Vera Study Group.
*Has not been detected in animals.

the production of hematopoietic cells at a site other than the bone marrow, is a characteristic feature of CIM. Neoplastic hematopoietic cells leave the bone marrow and lodge in other locations (typically the liver and spleen) and proliferate, causing enlargement of affected organs. CIM has been induced experimentally in animals; reports of naturally occurring disease are rare. The majority of cases of myelofibrosis occur secondary to disease processes such as bone marrow necrosis, irradiation, hemolytic anemias, or other neoplasias (leukemia/lymphoma).

17. Describe the major peripheral blood and bone marrow findings associated with chronic idiopathic myelofibrosis.

The morphologic findings in CIM vary depending on the degree of bone marrow fibrosis present (hypercellular vs. hypocellular marrow). Cytopenias and ineffective hematopoiesis result from increased deposition of collagen within the bone marrow replacing the normal cellular elements. Because CIM is uncommon in animals, Table 15-6 lists characteristic peripheral blood and bone marrow findings in humans with CIM.

Table 15-6 *Peripheral Blood and Bone Marrow Findings Associated with Chronic Idiopathic Myelofibrosis (Humans, Fibrotic Stage)*

SITE	MAJOR FINDINGS
Peripheral blood	Leukoerythroblastosis (immature granuolcytes and nucleated red blood cells)
	Dacrocytes (teardrop-shaped erythrocytes)
	Anemia
	Leukopenia or leukocytosis
	Dysgranulopoiesis
	Bizarre platelet shapes
Bone marrow	Variable fibrosis
	Decreased cellularity (can also be normocellular or hypercellular)
	Dysplastic megakaryocytes
	Megakaryocytic hyperplasia
	Osteosclerosis

18. How is chronic idiopathic myelofibrosis diagnosed?

The diagnosis of CIM requires documentation of the characteristic features of the disorder and the exclusion of all other causes of myelofibrosis. EMH may be initially suspected based on physical examination findings such as splenomegaly or hepatomegaly. Confirmation of EMH is made by cytologic or histologic examination of the organ. Peripheral blood and bone marrow examinations (cytology and histopathology) are necessary for the diagnosis of CIM. Peripheral blood findings such as leukoerythroblastosis and the presence of dacrocytes support CIM. Bone marrow evaluation is mandatory to document fibrosis. It is important to note that laboratory findings will vary depending on stage of disease. To diagnose CIM, it is crucial to rule out other potential causes of myelofibrosis, such as malignant diseases (e.g., leukemias, metastatic carcinomas), other CMPDs (e.g., PV, ET, CML), immune-mediated disease, and radiation therapy. In human medicine, chromosomal analysis is also performed, although a specific genetic abnormality has not been identified.

19. What is chronic myelogenous leukemia?

Chronic myelogenous leukemia (CML) is a neoplastic clonal disorder arising from a hematopoietic stem cell. Although all the cells of the myeloid lineage can be affected, CML is characterized by the marked proliferation of granulocytic cells. The severe leukocytosis detected with this disorder consists primarily of neutrophils and their precursors, although increases in eosinophils and basophils may also be seen. CML often has an indolent clinical course, but it can terminate in an acute blast crisis. CML is a rare disorder that has been documented in the dog.

20. What are the major history and clinical findings associated with chronic myelogenous leukemia?

Animals with CML present for nonspecific signs, such as anorexia, lethargy, or weight loss. Occasionally, animals may be asymptomatic, and evidence for CML is found on routine laboratory testing. Splenomegaly and hepatomegaly have also been reported.

21. List the major peripheral blood and bone marrow findings associated with chronic myelogenous leukemia.

Table 15-7 lists peripheral blood and bone marrow findings associated with CML.

Table 15-7 ***Peripheral Blood and Bone Marrow Findings Associated with Chronic Myelogenous Leukemia***

SITE	MAJOR FINDINGS
Peripheral blood	Marked leukocytosis (usually >100,000 cells/μl) Neutrophilia with left shift Myeloblasts (may be present in circulation in low numbers) Eosinophilia Basophilia Mild-moderate anemia Thrombocytopenia
Bone marrow	Myeloid:erythroid ratio >1 (increased) Hypercellular bone marrow Myeloid hyperplasia Orderly maturation (mature cells predominant)

22. How is chronic myelogenous leukemia diagnosed?

In human medicine the diagnosis of CML is based on the detection of the Philadelphia chromosome. The chromosomal defect in CML is a reciprocal translocation between chromosomes 9 and 22, resulting in the creation of the fusion protein BCR-ABL. This protein can transform hematopoietic cells in such a manner that their growth and survival are independent of cytokines (protects cells from apoptosis). The Philadelphia chromosome has not yet been identified in animals, so the diagnosis of CML relies heavily on the exclusion or elimination of other diseases that can stimulate a marked leukocytosis (e.g., inflammation, immune-mediated disease).

23. What differential diagnoses should be considered before making a diagnosis of chronic myelogenous leukemia?

The major differential diagnoses that need to be considered before making a diagnosis of CML are any conditions that can incite a marked leukocytosis. It is important to rule out the following processes:

a. Inflammation (e.g., pyometra, pyothorax)
b. Immune-mediated diseases (e.g., hemolytic anemia)
c. Infectious diseases (e.g., *Hepatozoon canis*) or other tumors (paraneoplastic response)
d. Other chronic myeloproliferative disorders

24. What is the current treatment for chronic myelogenous leukemia?

Chemotherapeutic agents such as hydroxyurea have been used for the treatment of CML in animals. Survival times in treated dogs are variable, ranging from 41 days to more than 690 days. Transformation from CML to an acute leukemia has been documented in both untreated and treated animals.

16. MYELODYSPLASTIC SYNDROMES

Tarja Juopperi and Heather Leigh DeHeer

1. Define the term myelodysplastic syndrome.

The term *myelodysplastic syndrome* (MDS) refers to a heterogeneous group of hematologic disorders characterized clinically by ineffective and disorderly hematopoiesis. Despite the name, myelodysplastic disorders are not "dysplastic" disorders; rather, MD disorders are neoplastic conditions that result from the clonal expansion of an abnormal hematopoietic stem cell and manifest as peripheral blood cytopenias and dysplastic changes seen in blood and bone marrow.

2. Briefly discuss the etiology of MDS.

In the human literature, MDS can be divided into two major categories based on the etiology: primary or secondary. *Primary* MD syndromes are spontaneously occurring disorders; the etiology and the initiating cause are unknown. *Secondary* MD syndromes result from exposure to ionizing radiation, environmental toxins, and chemotherapy treatment. Secondary conditions are seen less frequently than primary disorders, and the majority of secondary MDS cases are therapy related, particularly after treatment with alkylating agents or topoisomerase II inhibitors.

Myelodysplastic syndromes are rare in veterinary medicine and have been reported in the cat (most frequently), dog, and horse (uncommon). In cats, MDS is suspected to be associated with feline leukemia virus (FeLV) infection because about 80% of cats with MDS are FeLV positive. Predisposing events or underlying etiologies have not yet been identified in other species.

3. Explain the pathogenesis of MDS.

The exact pathogenesis of MDS is unknown. However, the development of MDS is thought to arise from deoxyribonucleic acid (DNA) damage in a hematopoietic stem cell that induces a malignant phenotype. The clonal expansion of the malignant pluripotential stem cell can result in the abnormal production of a variety of myeloid cells, including neutrophils, monocytes, erythrocytes, and platelets. In rare human cases of MDS, lymphoid cells may also be clonally derived. The proliferation of the abnormal stem cell results in the accumulation of progenitors in the bone marrow (a hypercellular marrow) with simultaneous peripheral cytopenias. This paradoxical finding may result from the failure of the stem cells to differentiate or from an increased rate of apoptosis in the bone marrow (with many hematopoietic cells undergoing programmed cell death in the marrow, low numbers of mature hematopoietic cells are in the peripheral blood). Defective maturation, dysplastic changes, and functional abnormalities are also noted in many of the progeny of the neoplastic hematopoietic stem cells.

4. List possible functional abnormalities detected in patients with MDS.

In human patients, functional abnormalities have been demonstrated in the hematopoietic cells produced by the abnormal stem cell. Recurrent infections or bleeding tendencies may be seen as a result of abnormal neutrophil or platelet function, respectively. Similar clinical findings have been documented in animals with MDS, although further investigation is necessary to document functional defects. Table 16-1 lists functional abnormalities detected in humans with MDS.

Table 16-1 ***Functional Abnormalities Documented in Humans with MDS***

CELL TYPE	FUNCTIONAL ABNORMALITY
Red cells	Enzyme defects, reduced enzyme levels
	Cell surface antigen changes
	Abnormal iron metabolism
Neutrophils	Abnormal adhesion, chemotaxis, and phagocytosis
	Reduced microbial killing
	Reduced myeloperoxidase activity
	Can result in recurrent infections
Platelets	Abnormal adhesion and aggregation (dense granule storage pool and microtubule defect)
	Can result in bleeding tendencies

5. Are any chromosomal abnormalities or genetic changes associated with MDS?

In human medicine, clonality has been confirmed using cytogenetic and molecular techniques. However, the genetic changes responsible for the neoplastic transformation of the hematopoietic stem cell have not yet been elucidated. Point mutations in Ras genes (a family of proto-oncogenes) have been found to occur in about 3% to 33% of human patients with MDS. Chromosomal gains, losses, and translocations have also been described in human patients, with chromosomes 5, 7, 8, and Y reported most. None of the chromosomal abnormalities is specific for MDS, but some are highly associated with certain subtypes and have prognostic significance. For example, MDS patients with deletion of long arm of chromosome 5 have a relatively favorable prognosis, longer survival time, and a low rate of transformation to acute leukemia. The use of cytogenetic analysis or molecular techniques as a diagnostic tool has not been thoroughly investigated for veterinary cases of MDS.

6. How is MDS diagnosed?

The diagnosis of MDS is based on the history, clinical signs, and morphologic examination of the peripheral blood and bone marrow. Cytogenetic analysis is an important diagnostic tool in human medicine. Because MDS encompasses a heterogeneous group of disorders, the presenting signs and laboratory abnormalities may vary. The key to diagnosis of MDS is the presence of persistent cytopenias, despite a hypercellular bone marrow (ineffective hematopoiesis), in conjunction with dysplastic changes in one or more hematopoietic cell lines. It is essential to note that transient dysplastic changes may be seen in the bone marrow with other conditions, and these diseases must be excluded before making a diagnosis of MDS.

7. What differential diagnoses should one consider before making a diagnosis of MDS?

Several diseases can be similar in appearance to MDS, and these disorders should be ruled out before MDS is diagnosed. Dysplastic changes in hematopoietic cells may be seen with nutritional deficiencies (e.g., vitamin B_{12}, folate), may be drug induced (e.g., vincristine, chloramphenicol), may be congenital (e.g., poodle macrocytosis, congenital dyserythropoiesis), and may result from lead toxicity or immune-mediated hematologic disorders. Dysplastic changes seen with these disorders are polyclonal (unlike MDS, which is a clonal disorder) and should be excluded first before making a diagnosis of MDS.

8. What are the major history and clinical findings associated with MDS?

The history, clinical signs, and physical examination findings in an animal with MDS may be variable. Clinical signs are frequently attributable to the type and severity of the cytopenias present. Animals may present for nonspecific signs, such as lethargy, anorexia, and weight loss. Because anemia is frequently present, animals may show evidence of pallor and weakness. Less often, animals display clinical signs due to thrombocytopenia, such as petechiae or ecchymoses. Animals with neutropenia may have recurrent bacterial infections. MDS may also be an incidental finding on routine screening tests.

9. Describe the major peripheral blood findings associated with MDS.

The main peripheral blood findings associated with MDS are a persistent cytopenia or cytopenias (bicytopenia or pancytopenia are common). Animals are usually anemic (may be severe), and the anemia is frequently nonregenerative. Thrombocytopenia is a common finding. Neutropenia may also be seen. Dysplastic changes may be observed in the peripheral blood, and various cell lines can be affected. Possible dysplastic changes for the erythroid lineage may include macrocytosis (common finding in cats), poikilocytosis, and normoblastemia (presence of nucleated red blood cells) without polychromasia. Dysplastic myeloid changes may include abnormal cell size (gigantism), hypo/hypersegmentation, and hypo/hypergranulation. Platelets may be seen that are giant, bizarre in shape, or abnormally granulated. In addition, circulating blast cells may be seen in the peripheral blood, although they do not exceed 5% of blood leukocytes.

10. Discuss the findings expected on cytologic examination of the bone marrow with MDS.

Cytologic examination of the bone marrow in MDS usually reveals a hypercellular to normocellular marrow (although a hypocellular marrow may be noted). One of the key findings with MDS is persistent peripheral cytopenias in the presence of a hyperplastic bone marrow. An increase in blast cell number is typically seen, but the percentage of blasts does not exceed 30%. The hallmark is the observation of dysplastic changes in one or more cell lines. Maturation defects are also observed, such as left shifts and asynchrony of maturation.

11. List the possible dysplastic changes and features in the blood or bone marrow with MDS.

Box 16-1 lists morphologic abnormalities associated with MDS.

Box 16-1 ***Morphologic Abnormalities Associated with MDS***

Erythroid Lineage (Dyserythropoiesis)	Granulocytic Lineage (Dysgranulopoiesis)	Megakaryocytic Lineage (Dysmegakaryopoiesis)
Megaloblastic changes (large amounts of cytoplasm, immature nucleus)	Cell gigantism	Micromegakaryocytes
Nuclear-cytoplasmic asynchrony	Ring forms of neutrophils	Large mononuclear megakaryocytes
Multinucleate erythroblasts	Nuclear-cytoplasmic asynchrony	Megakaryocytes with multiple small and separated nuclei
Abnormal nuclear shapes and fragmentation	Multinucleation	Giant platelets
Ringed sideroblasts and siderocytes	Nuclear blebs	Agranular, or hypergranular platelets
Excess rubriblasts (left shifts)	Hyposegmentation and abnormal chromatin condensation (Pelger-Huet–like syndrome)	Bizarre-shaped platelets
Abnormal red cell morphology (anisocytosis, poikilocytosis, macrocytosis)	Hypersegmentation	
Normoblastemia (circulating nucleated red blood cells)	Hypogranulation, abnormal granulation	
	Increased myeloblasts (left shifts)	

12. If MDS is suspected, why would a bone marrow core biopsy be performed, and what information would this procedure provide?

The diagnosis of MDS can be made based on peripheral blood and bone marrow aspirate examination. However, a bone marrow core biopsy can provide useful information and may be necessary when aspiration is unsuccessful. Marrow biopsy is the most accurate method of determining bone marrow cellularity and can demonstrate disruption of the marrow architecture. *Myelofibrosis,* the deposition of excess collagen and increased fibroblasts in the bone marrow, may be seen in patients with MDS and can be detected on examination of a core biopsy. This procedure is diagnostically useful because dysplastic changes can also be identified, as well as abnormal localization of immature hematopoietic precursors.

13. How is MDS distinguished from chronic myeloproliferative disorders?

One of the main characteristics that aids in differentiating a chronic myeloproliferative disorder (CMPD) from MDS is that CMPDs generally result in effective hematopoiesis. Bone marrow examination of CMPDs usually reveals a hypercellular marrow (as with MDS), but typically with increased numbers of one or more hematopoietic cell lines in the peripheral blood (leukocytosis). In contrast, MDS results in ineffective hematopoiesis and peripheral blood cytopenias. In addition, dysplastic changes in hematopoietic cells are not a frequent finding with CMPDs (morphology of the cells is typically unremarkable), unlike MDS. Occasionally it can be difficult to distinguish between these two disorders because they can have similar or overlapping features if CMPDs transform into a more aggressive disorder that mimics MDS.

14. How is MDS differentiated from acute myeloid leukemia?

The major criterion in differentiating MDS from acute myeloid leukemia (AML) is the percentage of blast cells in the bone marrow. MDS patients have less than 30% blasts present in the marrow, whereas 30% or greater is indicative of an acute leukemia. Recently the World Health Organization (WHO) reduced the blast percentage from 30% to 20% to diagnose AML in humans. A number of veterinary pathologists have modified the classification of MDS/AML in animals to correspond with this change.

15. What is meant by leukemic transformation or progression?

If additional DNA damage occurs in the abnormal hematopoietic stem cell, MDS may transform or progress into an acute leukemia, most often AML. In humans the transformation rate (range 10%-60%) depends on the subtype of MDS involved. Lower transformation rates typically occur with subtypes that have low numbers of blasts present in the bone marrow. Leukemic transformation has been demonstrated in veterinary patients with MDS, but data are inadequate to determine the transformation rate accurately.

16. How are myelodysplastic syndromes classified?

Classification systems for MDS have been designed to allow for consistency and uniformity in reporting. These systems are based on morphologic evaluation of blood and bone marrow. The French-American-British (FAB) cooperative group developed a classification system that outlines five subtypes of MDS. FAB differentiates the subtypes on the basis of the percentage of blast cells in the peripheral blood and bone marrow, percentage of ringed sideroblasts in the bone marrow, presence of monocytosis in the peripheral blood, and number of cell lines showing dysplastic changes. The five subtypes are as follows:

(1) Refractory anemia (RA)
(2) Refractory anemia with ringed sideroblasts (RARS)
(3) Refractory anemia with excess blasts (RAEB)
(4) Refractory anemia with excess blasts in transformation (RAEB-t)
(5) Chronic myelomonocytic leukemia (CMML)

Not all patients can be classified in the FAB scheme, and other classification systems have been created. More recently, WHO has reclassified many of the human malignant hematologic disorders and has removed CMML from the MDS category and placed it in a new separate group known as the "myeloproliferative/myelodysplastic diseases." In veterinary medicine the FAB classification system has been used to classify MDS and has been modified to better reflect the disease in animals. The three main subtypes in this system are as follows:

(1) MDS erythroid predominant
(2) MDS refractory cytopenia
(3) MDS excess blasts

Table 16-2 lists the criteria for each subtype.

Table 16-2 *Myelodysplastic Syndrome Subtypes: Modified FAB Classification (Veterinary)*

MDS SUBTYPE	BLAST % IN BONE MARROW	MYELOID/ERYTHROID RATIO
Erythroid predominant (MDS-Er)	<30% of all nucleated cells (ANCs)	<1
Refractory cytopenia (MDS-RC)	<6% of ANCs (excluding rubriblasts)	>1
Excess blasts (MDS-EB)	6%-29% of ANCs (excluding rubriblasts)	>1

FAB, French-American-British system.

17. What is the prognosis for MDS?

MDS carries a poor prognosis; animals typically survive only days to months. However, prognosis can depend on the MDS subtype and the severity of the cytopenias present, with low blast cell counts and mild-moderate cytopenias associated with longer survival. In some cases, MDS can transition into an acute leukemia. In humans, prognosis is based on the percentage of bone marrow blasts and the number and type of cytogenetic abnormalities. The presence and severity of cytopenias are also important. An international prognostic scoring system has been devised in human medicine that considers these factors and provides a prognostic score for an individual patient that is highly predictive of survival. A similar prognostic scoring system has not yet been created for veterinary patients.

18. What is the current treatment for MDS?

The treatment of MDS has been disappointing because therapies are not well established. Supportive therapy is the basis of treatment and, depending on the cytopenias present, typically consists of blood transfusions as necessary and antibiotics. Additional therapeutics investigated for the treatment of MDS include hematopoietic growth factors (e.g., erythropoietin, granulocyte colony-stimulating factor) and differentiating agents (e.g., retinoic acid analogs). It is thought that differentiating agents will cause terminal differentiation of the abnormal clone, resulting in maturation of the cell and loss of its ability to proliferate (has been successful in vitro). Chemotherapy has also been used, particularly when excessive numbers of blasts are present in bone marrow and/or peripheral blood.

Lymphoproliferative/Myeloproliferative Disorders

BIBLIOGRAPHY

Bass MC, Schultze AE: Essential thrombocythemia in a dog: case report and literature review, *J Am Animal Hosp Assoc* 34:197-203, 1998.

Blue JT: Myelodysplastic syndromes and myelofibrosis. In Feldman BF, Zinkl JG, Jain NC, editors: *Schalm's veterinary hematology,* ed 5, 2000, Philadelphia, Lippincott, Williams & Wilkins, pp 682-688.

Dorfman M, Dimski DS: Paraproteinemias in small animal medicine, *Compend Cont Educ Pract Vet* 14:621-631, 1992.

Greenberg PL: Myelodysplastic syndromes. In Hoffman R, Benz EJ, Shattil SJ, et al, editors: *Hematology: basic principles and practice,* ed 3, New York, 2000, Churchill Livingstone, pp 1106-1127.

Grindem CB: Classification of myeloproliferative diseases. In August JR, editor: *Consultations in feline internal medicine,* ed 3, Philadelphia, 1997, Saunders, pp 499-508.

Grindem CB: Acute myeloid leukemia. In Feldman BF, Zinkl JG, Jain NC, editors: *Schalm's veterinary hematology,* ed 5, Philadelphia, 2000, Lippincott, Williams & Wilkins, pp 717-726.

Harvey JW, West CL: Prednisone-induced increases in serum alpha-2-globulin and haptoglobin concentrations in dogs, *Vet Pathol* 24:90-92, 1987.

Heaney ML, Golde DW: Myelodysplasia, *N Engl J Med* 340:1649-1660, 1999.

Jacobs RM, Messick JB, Valli VE: Tumors of the hemolymphatic system. In Meuten DJ, editor: *Tumors in domestic animals,* ed 4, Ames, 2002, Iowa State University Press, pp 180-198.

Jain NC, Blue JT, Grindem CB, et al: Proposed criteria for classification of acute myeloid leukemia in dogs and cats, *Vet Clin Pathol* 20:63-82, 1991.

Kaneko JJ: Serum proteins and the dysproteinemias. In Kaneko JJ, Harvey JW, Bruss ML, editors: *Clinical biochemistry of domestic animals,* ed 5, New York, 1997, Academic Press, pp 117-137.

Lowenberg B, Downing JR, Burnett A: Acute myeloid leukemia, *N Engl J Med* 341:1051-1059, 1999.

Perkins P: Hematologic abnormalities accompanying leukemia. In Feldman BF, Zinkl JG, Jain NC, editors: *Schalm's veterinary hematology,* ed 5, Philadelphia, 2000, Lippincott, Williams & Wilkins, pp 740-746.

Raskin RE, Valenciano A: Cytochemical tests for diagnosis of leukemia. In Feldman BF, Zinkl JG, Jain NC, editors: *Schalm's veterinary hematology,* ed 5, Philadelphia, 2000, Lippincott, Williams & Wilkins, pp 755-763.

Rogers KS, Forrester SD: Monoclonal gammopathy. In Feldman BF, Zinkl JG, Jain NC, editors: *Schalm's veterinary hematology,* ed 5, Philadelphia, 2000, Lippincott, Williams & Wilkins, pp 932-936.

Stockham SL, Scott MA: Proteins. In *Fundamentals of veterinary clinical pathology,* Ames, 2002, Iowa State University Press, pp 251-276.

Tefferi A: Myelofibrosis with myeloid metaplasia, *N Engl J Med* 342:1255-1265, 2000.
Thomas JS: Overview of plasma proteins. In Feldman BF, Zinkl JG, Jain NC, editors: *Schalm's veterinary hematology*, ed 5, Philadelphia, 2000, Lippincott, Williams & Wilkins, pp 891-898.
Thomas JS: Protein electrophoresis. In Feldman BF, Zinkl JG, Jain NC, editors: *Schalm's veterinary hematology*, ed 5, Philadelphia, 2000, Lippincott, Williams & Wilkins, pp 899-903.
Vardiman JW, Harris NL, Brunning RD: The World Health Organization (WHO) classification of the myeloid neoplasms, *Blood* 100:2292-2302, 2002.
Watson ADJ: Erythrocytosis and polycythemia. In Feldman BF, Zinkl JG, Jain NC, editors: *Schalm's veterinary hematology*, ed 5, Philadelphia, 2000, Lippincott, Williams & Wilkins, pp 216-222.
Weiss DJ, Smith SA: A retrospective study of 19 cases of canine myelofibrosis, *J Vet Intern Med* 16:174-178, 2002.
Willard MD: Hypoalbuminemia. In Feldman BF, Zinkl JG, Jain NC, editors: *Schalm's veterinary hematology*, ed 5, Philadelphia, 2000, Lippincott, Williams & Wilkins, pp 937-940.
Zoran D: Immunodeficiency disorders. In Feldman BF, Zinkl JG, Jain NC, editors: *Schalm's veterinary hematology*, ed 5, Philadelphia, 2000, Lippincott, Williams & Wilkins, pp 941-946.

Section II
Lymphoproliferative Disorders

Heather Leigh DeHeer and Tarja Juopperi

17. OVERVIEW AND LYMPHOMA/ LYMPHOSARCOMA

1. Which disorders are included in the category of lymphoproliferative diseases?

Lymphoproliferative disorders include any neoplastic expansion of lymphoid cells. Three broad categories of lymphoproliferative disorders are traditionally recognized: lymphomas, leukemias, and plasma cell neoplasms, as discussed separately in this chapter and the other two chapters of this section. In general, lymphoid proliferations arising from neoplastic transformation of lymphoid cells in the bone marrow are termed *leukemias,* and those arising outside marrow tissues are termed *lymphomas*. Proliferations of plasma cells are conventionally considered separately from other lymphoid neoplasms and are subdivided similarly according to site of origin. Plasma cell neoplasms arising in or involving bone marrow are called *myelomas* and those arising outside marrow tissues are called *plasmacytomas*.

Neoplastic transformation can occur at any stage of lymphoid cell maturation, from early progenitor to fully differentiated, mature cell. Neoplastic proliferations of poorly differentiated lymphoid cells include acute lymphoblastic leukemia (ALL) and lymphoblastic lymphomas. Proliferations involving more mature, differentiated lymphoid cells include small cell and intermediate-sized cell lymphomas and chronic lymphocytic leukemia (CLL).

2. Is there a difference between lymphoma and lymphosarcoma?

A common contraction of the term "malignant lymphoma," *lymphoma* is the conventional human nomenclature for lymphoid neoplasms arising as solid tissue masses in organs outside the bone marrow.[1] The term "lymphoma" is a misnomer in that the suffix *oma* typically denotes a benign neoplasm. However, a benign form of this lymphoid neoplasm does not occur in either human or veterinary medicine. For this reason, the "malignant" portion of malignant lymphoma is understood, and the abbreviated *lymphoma* is often used alone. *Lymphosarcoma* is a term used in veterinary literature to denote malignant lymphoma. Therefore the terms lymphoma, malignant lymphoma, and lymphosarcoma are synonymous. Because of its acceptance within human literature, the term *lymphoma* is be used throughout this text.

3. What is the incidence rate of lymphoma in different veterinary species?

Lymphoma is by far the most common hematopoietic tumor in the dog, accounting for 80% to 90% of these tumors[2] and approximately 5% to 7% (up to 24% reported)[3] of all canine neoplasms. Incidence rate is estimated to be 13 to 24 per 100,000 dogs at risk annually.[3]

As in the dog, lymphoma is generally thought to be the most common of the feline hematopoietic tumors, accounting for 50% to 90% of these tumors in the cat.[2] Some authors question the current validity of these statistics, however, because they were generated in studies conducted before widespread availability and use of feline leukemia virus (FeLV) vaccination and testing. Indeed, the change in incidence of FeLV infection has greatly changed both the age and the site distribution of lymphoma in cats. More recent surveys indicate a 25% incidence of FeLV infection in cats with lymphoma, in contrast to 60% to 70% reported in earlier studies.[4]

Although occurring much less frequently in the horse than in either dogs or cats, lymphoma is still among the most common malignant neoplasms of horses, accounting for 1% to 3% of equine malignancies.[5] Lymphoma was the fifth most common malignancy diagnosed in equine patients in a University of California survey.[6]

In the cow the occurrence of lymphoma varies with age and husbandry practices. Although the most frequent malignant neoplasm of dairy cattle, lymphoma is second in frequency to ocular squamous cell carcinoma if production type is not considered.[6] Prevalence has been reported at 18 per 100,000 slaughtered cattle in the United States, although incidence rates vary dramatically in age-stratified studies.[6] Lymphoma is reported to occur infrequently in the absence of bovine leukemia virus (BLV) infection.[7]

4. Does age play a role in the incidence of lymphoma?

In general, occurrence of lymphoma increases with increasing patient age. Middle-aged to older animals are most often affected. In dogs the average age at diagnosis is 6 to 9 years.[3] Lymphoma may develop in younger animals, however, and has been reported to occur in dogs as young as 4 months and in the bovine[6] and equine[5] fetus. Unfortunately, lymphoma in younger animals is often a high-grade, aggressive type.[4]

A bimodal age distribution is seen in the development of lymphoma in cats and in cattle.[2,6] This is largely attributable to the incidence of a retroviral etiology in these species. In cats, lymphoma incidence increases at 2 to 3 years age, then again at 6 to 12 years.[6] These peaks represent very different manifestations of lymphoma. Lymphoma occurring in younger cats is more often thymic in origin, is more frequently associated with FeLV infection, and is more often the T cell phenotype.[8] In contrast, lymphoma in older cats is more frequently alimentary in origin, is of B cell phenotype, and is less often associated with FeLV infection.

As with cats, cattle may develop lymphoma subsequent to retroviral-induced mutagenesis. The causative agent in cattle is BLV. In contrast to cats, however, viral-associated lymphoma is more prevalent in older cattle. Spontaneous lymphomas are more common in younger cattle.

5. Are breed predispositions seen with lymphoma?

In the dog a number of breed predispositions in the development of lymphoma have been documented. Scottish terriers, boxers, basset hounds, bulldogs, Labrador retrievers, bullmastiffs, Airedale terriers, and Saint Bernards are all reported to be overrepresented.[2,3,6] In contrast, other breeds may be at decreased risk for development of lymphoma. Dachshunds and Pomeranians have been reported as underrepresented. A genetic predisposition has been suggested in the dog as a result of familial incidence of lymphoma in Rottweilers, otter hounds, and bullmastiffs.[3,6]

Cats also exhibit breed predispositions. The oriental breeds, in particular the Siamese, have been reported to be overrepresented in development of lymphoma.[6,8]

In cattle, breed predispositions are not actually seen, but dairy breeds do exhibit an increased incidence of lymphoma relative to that seen in beef cattle.[6] This is thought to be attributable the differences in average age and management practices.

No breed predispositions are recognized in the horse.[6]

6. What is the importance of classifying lymphoma, and which features are used in classification?

The goal of any classification scheme is to enable the accurate prediction of prognosis from the disease diagnosis. This is achieved by dividing a single disorder into various subdisorders having similar manifestations, rates of progression, responses to treatment, and clinical outcomes. With a more precise diagnosis, veterinarians can more specifically tailor therapy, more accurately predict survival, and more reliably advise pet owners throughout the course of disease.

A variety of criteria may be useful to subclassify lymphomas further, including anatomic location, cell morphology, histologic tumor appearance, and cell immunophenotype. Distinct variations in tumor behavior are seen among the various anatomic sites of lymphoma. Age is also important, particularly in the feline and bovine, in which anatomic site, age, and viral infection are closely linked. Anatomic features such as mitotic index (reflecting tumor cell proliferation rate) may predict response to therapy. Lymphomas may be subcategorized into *low grade* (0-1 mitotic figures per high-power field [HPF]), *intermediate grade* (2-4 mitotic figures/HPF), and *high grade* (>5 mitotic figures/HPF).[6] Disease progression and response to therapy both increase with increasing tumor grade.

7. Discuss the anatomic categorization of lymphoma in veterinary species.

Anatomic classification of lymphoma is common mode of tumor categorization in veterinary medicine. Anatomic forms include mediastinal (thymic), alimentary (gastrointestinal), cutaneous (and subcutaneous), multicentric (generalized), and extranodal (solitary or regional) forms, based on site of primary tumor involvement. The incidence of various anatomic forms varies among species (Table 17-1).[3,9]

Table 17-1 ***Incidence of Various Anatomic Forms of Lymphoma in Common Domestic Animals***

SPECIES	MULTICENTRIC	ALIMENTARY	MEDIASTINAL	CUTANEOUS	EXTRANODAL
Canine	>80%	5-7%	5%Rare	Rare	
Feline	Third most common	Most common	Almost as common as alimentary	Rare Most are nonepitheliotropic	Fourth most common*
Bovine	Most common overall	—	Most common form in calves	Second most common adult form	—
Equine	Most common	Second most common	Rare	Rare	Rare Ocular and respiratory most common sites

*Kidney is the most common extranodal site. Incidence of nervous system involvement is 12% and is most common in feline leukemia virus–positive young adults. Both nasopharyngeal and ocular forms are more common in the cat than the dog.

Multicentric lymphoma is the predominant form in most animals and frequently involves peripheral lymph nodes, liver, spleen, kidneys, heart, and bowel. *Alimentary* forms involve the gastrointestinal wall, mesenteric lymph nodes, and abdominal viscera. *Mediastinal* lymphoma involves thymus and mediastinal lymph nodes and may extend into adjacent tissues. *Cutaneous* lymphoma may be primary or may occur with metastasis of lymphoma from other sites. Primary cutaneous lymphoma includes epitheliotropic (mycosis fungoides), and nonepitheliotropic (dermal) forms. A unique subcutaneous form is seen in the horse. *Extranodal* lymphoma refers to tumors arising in anatomic sites not encompassed in the other categories, including primary renal, nasopharyngeal, ocular, and neural lymphomas. As with cutaneous lymphoma, secondary involvement of kidney, nasopharynx, eye, and nervous system may occur with lymphoma arising elsewhere, particularly in the multicentric form.

Cat

Mediastinal and alimentary forms are most common in the cat. The alimentary type occurs most often in older, FeLV-negative cats and may be diffuse or may occur as solitary lesions. Solitary alimentary lymphomas occur more often in the cat than the dog.[3] B lymphocyte phenotype is most common. Among alimentary lymphomas in the cat, 50% to 80% arise within small intestine, with the remaining 25% in the stomach, ileocecocolic junction, and colon (in decreasing order of frequency). Lymphoplasmacytic enteritis may be a predisposing factor and may progress to alimentary lymphoma.[4] The mediastinal form occurs in younger, FeLV-positive cats and involves the thymus and the mediastinal and sternal lymph nodes.[4,6] T lymphocyte phenotype is most common in this form. Pleural effusion frequently occurs and may occasionally contain neoplastic cells. Hypercalcemia, a frequent manifestation of thymic lymphoma in dogs, is uncommon in cats.[4] Prevalent sites of extranodal lymphoma in cats include the kidneys, eyes and retrobulbar space, central nervous system (CNS), nasal cavity, and skin. Renal involvement may also be seen, with extension of lymphoma arising in the alimentary tract. One quarter to one half of cats with renal lymphoma are FeLV positive.[8] CNS extension occurs in 40% to 50% of feline renal lymphoma cases. Primary CNS lymphoma is primarily extradural and associated with the spinal canal. A strong association with FeLV infection is seen; 85% to 90% of cats with primary CNS lymphoma are infected. Lymphoma is second only to meningioma in frequency among feline CNS tumors. Extranodal primary nasal lymphoma is usually localized, although systemic involvement occasionally occurs. It is usually of B lymphocyte phenotype, and affected cats are most often FeLV negative. Primary ocular lymphoma is more common in cats than in dogs. Cutaneous lymphoma, either primary or less frequently secondary to metastasis of multicentric lymphoma, is seen most often in older, FeLV-negative cats and may be focal or diffuse. Two forms are seen: epitheliotropic, most often of T lymphocyte phenotype, and nonepitheliotropic, most often of B lymphocyte phenotype.[4]

Dog

Multicentric lymphoma, accounting for 80% to 85% of canine lymphoma cases, is the most common anatomic form seen in the dog. Alimentary lymphoma is the second most frequent and accounts for 5% to 7% of canine cases.[3,6] As in the cat, alimentary lymphoma may occur either multifocally or diffusely throughout the submucosa and lamina propria of the small intestine in the dog. Lymphocytic plasmacytic inflammation may be associated with alimentary lymphoma, which some consider a potentially prelymphomatous change. Thymic lymphoma is seen in 5% of dogs and is most often of T lymphocyte phenotype.[3] Cutaneous lymphoma in the dog may be solitary or generalized, and epitheliotropic and nonepitheliotropic forms are described. As in the cat, epitheliotropic lymphoma in the dog is most often of T lymphocyte phenotype.[6] This form may involve oral mucosa and extracutaneous sites as well.[3] A rare form of cutaneous T cell lymphoma, Sézary syndrome, has been reported in the dog, cat, and horse and is associated with circulating atypical lymphoid cells that have convoluted nuclei.[3,4,10] Nonepitheliotropic cutaneous lymphoma in the dog may be of either B or T lymphocyte phenotype. The B lymphocyte type characteristically spares the epidermis and is concentrated in the middle to deep dermis.[3]

Horse and Cattle

In the horse, as in the dog, the multicentric form is most prevalent. Alimentary is the second most common, followed by thymic, extranodal cutaneous, ocular, and respiratory forms, which are rarely reported.[6,8]

As in the cat, prevalence of the various anatomic forms of lymphoma in cattle varies with age and viral status. In younger, BLV-uninfected cattle, thymic lymphoma is most often seen. In older cattle, BLV lymphomagenesis is associated with development of multicentric lymphoma. Because affected animals in either group are often presented late in the course of disease, lesions are frequently widespread and multicentric. Cutaneous lymphoma is a distinct entity in adult cattle that manifests as waxing and waning, raised, hairless, sometimes ulcerated lesions concentrated over the neck, shoulders, and perineum. Development of multicentric lymphoma eventually occurs.[6]

8. What is immunophenotype, and what is the role of immunophenotyping in characterizing lymphoma?

Each cell type within the body carries on its surface a combination of membrane-associated surface proteins that are unique to its lineage or origin, the *immunophenotype*. The process by which these surface proteins are identified using protein-specific antibody labeling is called *immunophenotyping*. This process has enabled more specific and reproducible cell identification among cells that are not reliably distinguished morphologically.

Undifferentiated lymphoid origin cells may be reliably distinguished from other discrete cells (hematopoietic cells, as well as anaplastic epithelial and mesenchymal cells) through immunophenotypic detection of combinations of surface proteins unique to their lymphoid lineage. Immunophenotyping has also permitted the identification of subsets of lymphocytes that behave uniquely both in health and in disease. Three broad categories of lymphocytes are described: B lymphocytes, T lymphocytes, and null cells. The B and T subsets are by far the largest and can be further subdivided by specialty function or stage of maturation using this same technology. This has permitted extremely specific identification of the neoplastic lymphocyte cell type in lymphomas, which in many cases is predictive of disease progression, response to therapy, and ultimate outcome.

In the dog, lymphoma phenotype is linked with tumor behavior and prognosis. For example, incidence of hypercalcemia in canine lymphoma patients overall is approximately 10%. A much greater incidence of hypercalcemia (40%-50%) is seen in dogs with thymic T cell lymphoma,[8,6] illustrating a difference in behavior among this subset of neoplastic lymphocytes. Compared with B cell lymphomas, T cell tumors exhibit a poorer remission rate with chemotherapy, a shorter disease-free interval, and reduced survival. Among B cell tumors, those exhibiting decreased B5 surface antigens are characterized by shorter remission and survival times.[3]

The majority of lymphoma in the cat, the dog, the horse, and in adult cattle is of B cell phenotype.[2,6] B cell tumors may be infiltrated with large numbers of nonneoplastic T lymphocytes, an entity commonly referred to as "T cell–rich B cell lymphomas." This variant has been reported most often in the horse, but also in the cat, dog, and pig.[11] Anatomic distribution and phenotype are often associated. T lymphocyte phenotype predominates in mediastinal forms in the dog, cat, and calf[6] and in the CNS form in the cat.[4]

9. Which human lymphoma classification schemes have been used in veterinary medicine?

A number of human lymphoma classification schemes have evolved over the years that attempt to correlate the neoplastic cell type and tumor histologic features with tumor behavior to predict clinical prognosis more accurately. Veterinary hematopathologists have applied these models to lymphoma in domestic animals with varying degrees of success. Subsets of lymphoma in domestic animals have been found to behave similarly to their human counterparts. Human lymphoma classification schemes used in veterinary medicine in recent decades include the Rappaport classification system, the Kiel classification scheme, the National Cancer Institute (NCI) Working Formulation, and the World Health Organization (WHO) classification.

The *Rappaport system* is the oldest classification followed in veterinary medicine. It was accepted as a classification for human non-Hodgkin's lymphomas (NHLs) in 1956.[12] This system considers pattern of growth (follicular or diffuse) and cytologic features of the neoplastic lymphoid cells (well differentiated, poorly differentiated, or "histiocytic") in classification of tumor type. In contrast to human medicine, veterinary follicular lymphomas are uncommon. Also, advances in biotechnology and cell identification have all but eliminated use of the confusing term "histiocytic" to describe lymphomas. Ultimately, such a classification system based on morphology alone has been found to be an inadequate predictor of biologic behavior and prognosis of lymphoma in animals.

The *Kiel system* added immunophenotype to cell morphology in classifying lymphoma, resulting in improved prognostic value compared with the Rappaport system.[2]

The *NCI Working Formulation* represented an attempt to unify the existing human lymphoma classification schemes by developing a consensus report among the leading authors on lymphoma classification during the late 1970s,[13] in the hope of permitting more meaningful comparison of data from human clinical trials.[3] This classification correlated patient survival data with neoplastic cell morphology (large, small, cleaved, or blastic) and histologic pattern (follicular or diffuse).[12] Neoplastic cell immunophenotype was not considered.

The most current classification scheme is the *WHO system,* revised in 2001. This system incorporates neoplastic cell morphology, immunophenotype, as well as clinical and survival information to classify lymphoma more meaningfully into subtypes with genuine clinical differences in behavior and prognosis.

Common among these systems is the division of lymphoma types by *grade*. Low, high, and sometimes intermediate grades are described (Table 17-2).[3,6] Features typical of low-grade lymphomas include small cell size, low mitotic rate, slow progression, long survival, and poor response to therapy. Features typical of high-grade lymphomas include high mitotic rate, rapid progression, and better response to therapy.

Table 17-2 ***Comparison of Lymphoid Neoplasms by Grade for Classification Schemes***

TUMOR GRADE	UPDATED KIEL FORMULATION	NCI-WF
Low	Lymphocytic Lymphoplasmacytic Lymphoplasmacytoid Centrocytic, follicular Centroblastic/centrocytic, follicular small cells	Diffuse small lymphocytic • Plasmacytoid • Intermediate Follicular small cleaved Follicular mixed
Intermediate	Centroblastic/centrocytic, follicular large cells Centrocytic, diffuse Centroblastic/centrocytic, diffuse small cells Centrocytic, diffuse large cells	Follicular large Diffuse small cleaved Diffuse mixed Diffuse large cleaved Diffuse large noncleaved
High	Centroblastic, monomorphic Centroblastic, polymorphous Immunoblastic Lymphoblastic Lymphoblastic	Immunoblastic Small noncleaved Small noncleaved, Burkitt type

NCI-WF, National Cancer Institute Working Formulation.

In applying human classification schemes to lymphoma in domestic species, several differences are observed. In contrast to humans, follicular lymphoma in dogs occurs rarely.[6,12] In addition, few canine lymphomas are classified as low-grade tumors (5%-29%).[3] Similar to the dog, most feline tumors are also intermediate to high grade (85%-90%).[4] In dogs the majority of small cell tumors are T lymphocyte derived, and the majority of high-grade lymphomas are B lymphocyte derived.[12] Using the Kiel classification scheme, high-grade lymphomas exhibit less complete remission and a shorter disease-free interval.[6,12] Lymphomas classified as high grade by the NCI Working Formulation exhibit shorter survival time.[6]

10. Has an etiology been identified in any species to explain the development of lymphoma?

No clear etiology for the development of lymphoma has been identified in the dog. A genetic component is suggested by the familial occurrence of lymphoma in related bullmastiffs,[3] otter hounds, and Rottweilers.[6] Unlike cats and cattle, no retroviral etiology has been confirmed in dogs, although viral particles have been isolated from canine lymphoma tissue cultures.[3] Immune dysfunction may play a role. An increased incidence of lymphoma has been reported in dogs diagnosed with immune-mediated thrombocytopenia.[14] In humans, exposure to certain herbicides, including 2,4-dichlorophenoxyacetic acid (2,4-D), has been implicated as a risk factor for lymphoma. A similar trend has observed in dogs; owners of dogs with lymphoma applied 2,4-D to their lawns or employed commercial lawn care companies more frequently than owners of dogs without lymphoma, but findings have been questioned elsewhere. Some association has also been found between exposure to magnetic fields and development of lymphoma in dogs.[3]

FeLV retroviral infection was the major cause of hematopoietic neoplasia in the cat before the widespread availability of testing and vaccination, associated with 60% to 70% of reported cases. More recent surveys suggest the role of FeLV has diminished, accounting for approximately 25% of recent feline hematopoietic neoplasias. Paralleling the shift in the viral status of cats, a shift in the anatomic distribution, patient signalment, and phenotype of lymphoma in cats has been observed.[4] FeLV-associated forms of lymphoma (young cats, thymic and CNS location, T cell phenotype) now constitute a relatively smaller proportion of all feline lymphomas. Feline immunodeficiency virus (FIV) infection has also been indirectly linked with development of B cell lymphoma, perhaps secondary to defective immune surveillance.[2] Common FeLV diagnostic modalities include enzyme-linked immunosorbent assay (ELISA; CITE test) for p27 viral antigen, immunofluorescent antibody (IFA) testing for p27 in blood or bone marrow, and virus isolation. FIV diagnostic modalities include the CITE test for serum antibodies, Western blot, or IFA testing.

In cattle, BLV infection is the major etiology of lymphoma in adult animals. BLV is a member of the retrovirus family and is transmitted horizontally, most often through blood or colostrum. Once inoculated, animals develop subclinical infection, during which BLV replicates in B lymphocytes. Approximately one third of infected animals with BLV develop a persistent polyclonal B cell lymphocytosis over the ensuing 3 to 5 years. This persistent lymphocytosis is considered a preneoplastic condition. Of these animals, another third will ultimately progress to develop malignant B cell lymphoma or lymphoid leukemia.

11. Describe the typical presenting signs in animals with lymphoma.

Presenting signs are highly variable, depending on the anatomic location and degree of disease progression at presentation. In dogs the multicentric form is most common, accounting for more than 80% of cases, and these dogs typically present with solitary or generalized lymphadenopathy, with or without splenomegaly, hepatomegaly, bone marrow involvement, or other organ involvement. From 20% to 40% of these dogs have additional clinical signs of illness, including weight loss, lethargy, anorexia, and fever.[3] Unlike the dog, peripheral lymphadenopathy alone is uncommon in the cat.

In cats the most common forms of lymphoma are alimentary and mediastinal, with nodal involvement possible in both forms.[4] Cats with the gastrointestinal form typically present with 1 to 3 months of weight loss, anorexia, panhypoproteinemia, and malabsorption.[3] Vomiting, diarrhea, dyschezia/tenesmus, and peritonitis secondary to bowel rupture have also been reported.[2] In 75% to 80% of cases a focal intestinal mass or diffusely thickened bowel loops are palpable.[4] Mesenteric lymphadenopathy, splenomegaly, or hepatomegaly may be present.[4]

Cats with the mediastinal form typically present with coughing, regurgitation, or dyspnea. A noncompressible anterior mediastinum, as well as dull heart and lung sounds, may be evident. Pleural effusion is common, is often chylous, and may contain atypical lymphoid cells.[4] Horner's syndrome may be seen.[2] An estimated 10% to 40% of dogs with mediastinal lymphoma are hypercalcemic and often present with polyuria and polydipsia.[2,3] Precaval syndrome (edema of head, neck, and forelimbs) may be seen in dogs with compression or invasion of cranial vena cava.[3,8]

Extranodal lymphoma signs vary with site of involvement. Cutaneous lymphoma may be generalized or multifocal. Alopecia, erythema, pruritus, nodules, plaques, and ulcers may be seen with or without peripheral lymphadenopathy.[15] CNS lymphoma may be solitary or diffuse and may cause seizures, paresis, paralysis, lameness, or muscle atrophy.[2] Tail flaccidity and upper motor neuron paralysis of the bladder have also been reported.[4] Patients with ocular lymphoma may have uveitis, glaucoma, thickening of the iris, hyphema, retinal detachment, or sudden blindness. Nasal lymphoma may be associated with chronic serosanguineous nasal discharge or facial deformity.[8] Renal lymphoma results in irregularly enlarged kidneys, often bilaterally, and clinical signs of renal failure.[2]

12. Which hematologic or biochemical abnormalities are most often seen with lymphoma?

In animals with lymphoma, complete blood count (CBC) may be normal, or in the presence of bone marrow involvement, cytopenias or atypical circulating cells may be present.[2] The majority of dogs and cattle with lymphoma are hematologically normal, whereas one half of horses and two thirds of cats exhibit some hematologic abnormality.[6] Anemia is the most common hematologic abnormality and is typically normocytic, normochromic and nonregenerative (anemia of chronic disease).[3,8] Hemolytic anemia may also occur, as reported in the dog and horse.[3,6]

Neutrophilia is present in approximately 25% to 40% of canine cases[3] but is less common in the other species.[6] Lymphopenia occurs in 20% of dogs and 50% of cats.[6] Lymphocytosis is seen with equal frequency as lymphopenia in the dog (20%)[3,6] and is occasionally seen in cattle.[6] The presence of atypical circulating lymphoid cells may signify progression to a leukemic phase and is more often found in the later stages of disease.[6] As many as one quarter of cats have a leukemic blood profile at diagnosis.[4] Leukemia is a common manifestation of lymphoma in calves.[6] Thrombocytopenia is seen in 30% to 50% of canine cases[3] but is infrequently associated with clinical signs of hemorrhage.[6] Of horses with lymphoma, 20% exhibit thrombocytopenia, although in the presence of concurrent immune-mediated hemolytic anemia, thrombocytopenia is invariably present.[6]

Biochemical abnormalities depend on organ involvement. Increased hepatic leakage of the enzymes alanine aminotransferase (ALT) and aspartate aminotransferase (AST) may signal hepatic infiltration. Patients with renal lymphoma are often azotemic, attributable to renal insufficiency or failure. Hypercalcemia is seen in 10% to 15% of dogs with all forms of lymphoma[6] but in as many as 40% of dogs with thymic lymphoma.[3,8] Hypercalcemia is rare in the cat.[4] Clinical signs associated with hypercalcemia include anorexia, weight loss, muscle weakness, lethargy, polyuria, polydipsia, and rarely, CNS depression.[3] Hypoproteinemia and hypoalbuminemia may be seen with alimentary or renal lymphoma resulting from chronic protein loss.[8] Rare lymphomas may be associated with monoclonal hyperglobulinemia.[6]

13. What is a paraneoplastic syndrome, and how are these syndromes associated with lymphoma?

The term *paraneoplastic syndrome* refers to an indirect clinical manifestation of neoplasia in the body. Tumors other than lymphoma may be associated with paraneoplastic syndromes, and any given syndrome may be seen accompanying more than a single tumor type.

A number of these syndromes have been described in association with lymphoma and tend to manifest more often in the dog than the cat.[2] *Anemia of chronic disease* is the most common paraneoplastic disorder of lymphoma seen domestic animals. Hemolytic anemia may also occur, as reported in the dog and horse.[3,6]

Other hematologic paraneoplastic syndromes in animals with lymphoma may include eosinophilia, which is proposed to occur in response to tumor cell interleukin-5 (IL-5) production. This rarely reported finding is usually found in association with T cell neoplasms in ferrets, horses, cats, and dogs.[1,16-18] The paraneoplastic manifestation of eosinophilia, particularly when seen in association with lung disease, is sometimes referred to as "Loeffler-like syndrome."[19]

Hypercalcemia is among the more common paraneoplastic syndromes seen in lymphoma and is thought to result from neoplastic cell liberation of parathyroid hormone–related protein (PTHrp).[3] Of dogs with mediastinal T cell lymphoma, 10% to 40% are hypercalcemic and typically present with polyuria and polydipsia.[2,3] If persistent, hypercalcemia may result in irreversible renal damage.[2,8] Hypercalcemia is a rare finding in the cat.[4]

Hypergammaglobulinemia (monoclonal gammopathy) is reported in dogs with lymphoma[3] without plasmacytoid differentiation.[6] When hypergammaglobulinemia is present in sufficient amount, hyperviscosity syndrome may be evident[6] (see Chapter 19, Plasma Cell Neoplasia).

Occurrence of paraneoplastic disorders may complicate or delay treatment for lymphoma.[2] Intravenous (IV) fluid diuretic therapy, and in extreme cases pharmacologic agents (e.g., calcitonin), to control ionized serum calcium levels may be indicated with severe hypercalcemia. Veterinary patients with renal failure may require IV fluid support as well. In those with cardiac or circulatory complications from hypergammaglobulinemia or hyperviscosity syndrome, plasmaphoresis may be useful.[20]

14. What additional testing is useful in confirming the diagnosis of lymphoma?

In veterinary patients with generalized lymphadenopathy or cutaneous lesions, fine-needle aspiration cytology may be a useful, easy, rapid, and inexpensive method to confirm infiltration by neoplastic lymphoid cells. In clinical settings where more invasive procedures are feasible, bone marrow biopsy, ultrasound-guided aspiration cytology of visceral organs, and evaluation of cavitary effusions may also prove beneficial. Other diagnostic modalities vary with the suspected form of lymphoma. Nasal flushing may be diagnostic in animals with nasal lymphoma. Cerebrospinal fluid (CSF) evaluation may be useful in suspected neural lymphomas.

Neoplastic lymphocyte morphology may vary from well-differentiated and mature-appearing to poorly differentiated, immature, or anaplastic cells (Figures 17-1 to 17-4) Well-

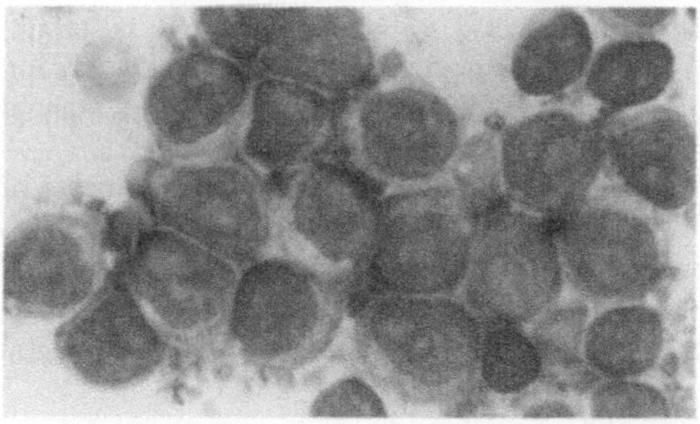

Figure 17-1 Lymphoma, small intestinal mass lesion, canine (300×). Neoplastic cells are 15 to 18 μm in diameter, with eccentrically located, irregularly ovoid nuclei having lightly clumped chromatin and one or more large, moderately indistinct nucleoli. Cytoplasmic fragments (lymphoglandular bodies) are plentiful in the background. A single erythrocyte is present in the upper-left corner for size reference.

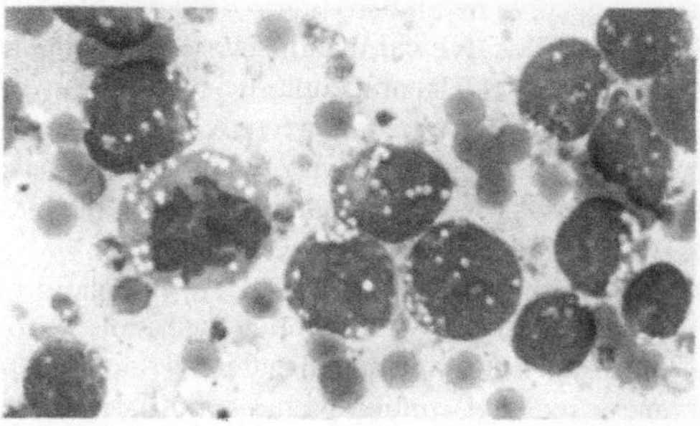

Figure 17-2 Lymphoma, kidney, feline (300×). Neoplastic cells are 12 to 16 μm in diameter, with eccentrically located, irregularly round to ovoid nuclei having lightly clumped chromatin and multiple small, indistinct nucleoli. Cytoplasm is scanty and exhibits prominent punctate vacuolation. This morphologic variation is seen more often with renal, intestinal, and thymic lymphomas. A single mitotic figure is present at center left.

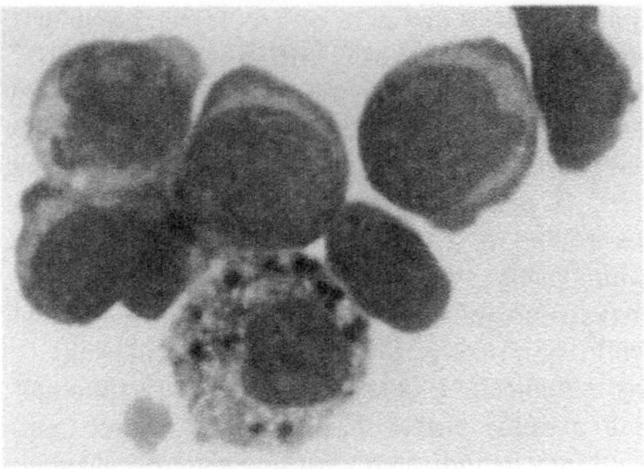

Figure 17-3 Lymphoma, pleural effusion, feline (375×). Neoplastic cells are 10 to 20 μm in diameter, with eccentrically located, irregularly ovoid to cerebriform nuclei having lightly clumped chromatin and one or more variably sized, moderately indistinct nucleoli. Cytoplasm may extend in blunt pseudopodia, a relatively common feature in fluid specimens. A single hemosiderin-laden macrophage is present at center bottom.

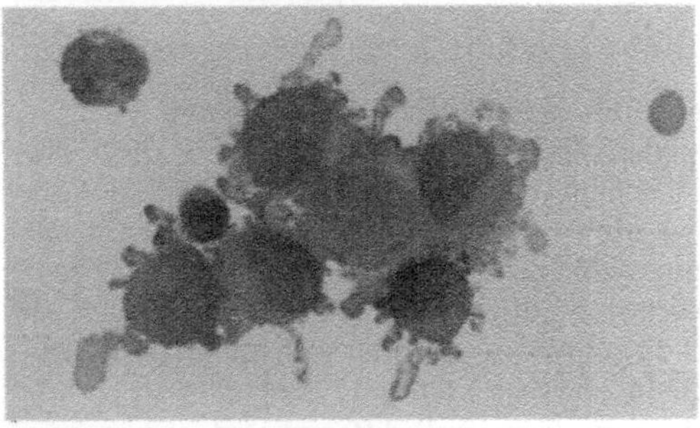

Figure 17-4 Lymphoma, cerebrospinal fluid, canine (300×). Neoplastic cells are very large, 15 to 25 μm in diameter, with eccentrically located, round to ovoid nuclei having lightly clumped chromatin and multiple small, indistinct nucleoli. Cytoplasm is abundant and extends in numerous elongate pseudopodia. A single small lymphocyte, an erythrocyte, and a mononuclear cell are also present. (Courtesy Carol B. Grindem, MD, North Carolina State University.)

differentiated small cell lymphomas may be difficult to distinguish from normal lymphocytes by aspiration cytology alone. Likewise, poorly differentiated or anaplastic lymphomas may lack sufficient morphologic features to distinguish them reliably as being lymphoid in origin. Additional testing modalities, such as cytochemical stains, immunophenotypic analysis, clonality assessment, and biopsy with histopathology, may be needed to confirm a suspicion of lymphoid neoplasia.

Whole–lymph node excision and biopsy is useful in small cell lymphomas when loss of normal architecture is critical to diagnosis. In T cell–rich B cell lymphoma and Hodgkin's lymphoma, the relatively small numbers of neoplastic cells and the relatively large numbers of nonneoplastic inflammatory cells greatly complicate diagnosis.[21] Cytology alone is of limited use. In addition, biopsy may be needed to distinguish lymphoma from nonneoplastic peripheral lymph node hyperplasia of young cats.[6]

Cytochemical staining to differentiate lymphoid from nonlymphoid tumors relies mainly on the ability of these stains to identify nonlymphoid cells specifically, because lymphoid cells fail to stain with most cytochemical stains. For example, positive myeloperoxidase or Sudan black B staining suggests granulocytic or monocytic cell origin.[22] Positive nonspecific esterase staining is seen in monocytic, lymphocytic, and occasionally other cell types, although the pattern of staining differs; lymphocytic cells tend to stain focally, whereas monocytic cells stain diffusely with nonspecific esterase. Failure of a neoplastic cell population to stain in a characteristic manner with cytochemical stains does not automatically suggest a lymphoid origin. Abnormalities in maturation, function, or structure of neoplastic cells may alter staining properties.

Immunophenotyping is useful to confirm that poorly differentiated cells are lymphoid in origin, to ascertain stage of maturation, and to distinguish B cell from T cell phenotype for prognostic purposes. Immunophenotypic analysis may use flow cytometry and fluorescent-labeled antibodies directed against cell membrane-associated surface proteins.[23] Alternatively, immunohistochemical stains may be applied to formalin-fixed or frozen tissues, or immunocytochemical staining can be performed on blood smears or cytologic preparations.[24]

Clonality assessment may be of benefit in distinguishing nonneoplastic from neoplastic lymphocyte proliferations, particularly when lymphocyte morphology is mature.[25] Detection of a uniform T cell receptor or an immunoglobulin gene rearrangement using polymerase chain reaction (PCR) fragment analysis in a population of T cell or B cell lymphocytes, respectively, suggests a clonal lymphocyte proliferation most compatible with a neoplastic process.

15. What staging system is used for lymphoma, and what purpose does staging serve?

The WHO staging system is most often used in staging lymphoma in domestic animals. This system divides lymphoma into stages based on the extent of organ involvement and the presence or absence of systemic signs (Table 17-3).[3]

Table 17-3 ***WHO Clinical Staging System for Lymphoma in Domestic Animals***

STAGE	EXTENT OF ORGAN INVOLVEMENT
I	Involvement of a single lymph node or organ (except bone marrow)
II	Involvement of multiple lymph nodes in a regional area
III	Generalized lymph node involvement
IV	Liver and/or splenic involvement (with/without stage III)
V	Bone marrow and/or peripheral blood involvement (with/without stages III/IV)
A*	Without systemic signs
B*	With systemic signs

WHO, World Health Organization.
*Each stage is subclassified.

Complete staging involves assessment of any peripheral lymphadenopathy to verify tumor involvement; thoracic radiography to assess mediastinal or pulmonary involvement; abdominal ultrasound evaluation of mesenteric lymph nodes, liver, spleen, and other abdominal viscera; and bone marrow biopsy. Bone marrow biopsy is important, even in the absence of atypical circulating cells, because the incidence of bone marrow involvement (57%) is double that of peripheral blood effects (28%) in dogs. Using this staging system, more than 80% of dogs present in stage III to V (advanced) lymphoma.[3]

Because of the frequency of visceral involvement in the cat, an alternate feline-specific staging system has been proposed (Table 17-4).[4]

The value of staging lymphoma is in permitting selection of appropriate therapy, enabling accurate assessment of response to therapy, allowing for improved detection of relapse, and determining accurate prognosis.

16. What treatment options exist for veterinary patients with lymphoma?

Because of the diversity possible in manifestation of lymphoma, no single treatment protocol would be suitable for all animals. Treatment decisions are governed by disease stage/substage, presence or absence of paraneoplastic disease, overall patient health, owner finances, time and commitment level, and occurrence of treatment-related side effects.[3] Overall, current treatment modalities for lymphoma in cats and dogs achieve high initial response rates (70% and 90%, respectively), making pursuit of treatment rewarding for both the veterinarian and the pet owner. Because current therapeutic regimens are usually not curative, eventual relapse of multidrug-resistant disease should be anticipated.[26]

Lymphoma is considered a systemic disease, requiring a systemic approach to therapy. Chemotherapeutic drugs, alone or in combination protocols, are the standard mode of treatment.

Table 17-4 *Clinical Staging System for Feline Lymphoma*

STAGE	EXTENT OF ORGAN INVOLVEMENT
I	Single tumor (extranodal) or single anatomic area (nodal) Includes primary intrathoracic tumors
II	Single tumor (extranodal) with regional lymph node involvement Two or more nodal areas on same side of diaphragm Two single (extranodal) tumors with/without regional lymph node involvement on same side of diaphragm Resectable primary gastrointestinal tract tumor with/without involvement of associated mesenteric lymph nodes only
III	Two single tumors (extranodal) on opposite sides of diaphragm Two or more nodal areas above and below diaphragm All extensive primary unresectable intraabdominal tumors All paraspinal or epidural tumors, regardless of other tumor sites
IV	Stages I-III with liver and/or spleen involvement.
V	Stages I-IV with initial involvement of central nervous system and/or bone marrow.

Combination protocols typically yield higher success rates (response rates) than single-agent protocols.[3] As mentioned, initial response rates are very good. Conventional chemotherapy protocols typically achieve complete remission in 60% to 90% of affected dogs, with a median survival of 6 to 12 months. Chemotherapy is typically well tolerated by dogs, with only a minority exhibiting dose-limiting toxicity. Major dose-limiting toxicities include neutropenia and thrombocytopenia, necessitating routine assessment of CBC throughout treatment. In patients with fewer than $2.0 \times 10^3/\mu l$ neutrophils and $50 \times 10^3/\mu l$ platelets in circulation, therapy should be withheld.[3] One exception to this general rule would apply to patients with myelophthisis prior to treatment.

Once remission has been achieved, the question arises, "Is maintenance therapy appropriate or desirable?" Inferences from human and canine lymphoma studies suggest that maintenance therapy is not only unnecessary but may even be detrimental.[3] Animals maintained on chemotherapeutic agents once remission was achieved demonstrated no prolongation of disease-free interval or survival.[3] Findings suggest that these dogs are at greater risk of development of drug resistance, further jeopardizing the success of any rescue protocol.[3] The added cost and risks of maintenance therapy cannot be justified.

In the uncommon cases of lymphoma, surgery or radiation therapy may play a role in treatment. Surgery is indicated in many solitary tumors, necrotic lesions, or obstructive masses. Radiation therapy is most useful with stage I or II lymphoma (localized or regionalized disease), for palliation of pain, or experimentally, with whole-body irradiation and bone marrow transplantation.

Alternative modalities in treatment of lymphoma include use of retinoids, such as isotretinoin (Accutane) and etretinate (Tegison), or photodynamic therapy in cutaneous lymphomas, which often have poor response to traditional chemotherapy.[3] Monoclonal antibody therapy (e.g., CL/Mab 231) is sometimes used in combination with nonimmunosuppressive chemotherapy. The principle behind this strategy is to induce complement-mediated or antibody-dependent pathways of cell cytotoxicity to destroy tumor cells.[2] Topical therapy has also been attempted in cutaneous forms of lymphoma, although only rarely in veterinary medicine due to practicality. Topical mechlorethamine (Mustargen) has been used, but response is variable and often only palliative.[3] Nutritional support is an important consideration as well, particularly in the cat, because of the frequency of anorexia as a side effect.[4]

Two main treatment options exist for relapse of lymphoma: reinduction or rescue therapy. *Reinduction therapy* involves administration of the same chemotherapy protocol that initially induced remission. The likelihood of response and the duration of response are typically half that encountered in initial therapy.[4] *Rescue therapy* involves the use of an alternate drug or a drug protocol withheld for a drug-resistant case. Such agents include mitoxantrone, doxorubicin, lomustine, and MOPP (mechorethamine, Oncovin [vincristine], procarbazine, prednisone).[26]

17. What does a diagnosis of lymphoma mean for patient survival, and what factors assist in determining prognosis?

Most lymphomas in domestic species are considered high grade, and most animals present in advanced stages of disease. Therefore longevity after diagnosis in untreated cases is brief; survival of only 4 to 6 weeks without treatment can be expected in both dogs and cats.[26]

Complete cure is rare, reported in only 10% of canine cases.[3]

Life expectancy is improved with chemotherapeutic intervention. Steroid therapy alone can double longevity to 3 months[26] and is an option when financial constraints exist. The best results are achieved using combination chemotherapy. Complete remission is achieved in 60% to 90% of affected dogs, with a median survival of 6 to 12 months.[3] Remission rates and durability in general are poorer in the cat. Complete remission is seen in 50% to 70% of feline patients, with a median survival of 6 months.[4] With relapse of lymphoma, prognosis is poorer due to development of drug resistance.

Factors influencing success of treatment include location of disease, clinical stage, presence or absence of clinical signs, histologic tumor grade, immunophenotype, exposure to previous chemotherapeutic agent or steroids (affecting likelihood of multidrug resistance), patient health status, presence of paraneoplastic syndromes, and development of dose-limiting side effects.[3]

In cats, FeLV status is also influential in prognosis.[4]

Some generalizations concerning determination of prognosis can be made. The higher clinical stages of lymphoma are associated with a shorter disease-free interval and decreased patient survival. Likewise, substage B of any stage carries a worse prognosis than substage A of the same stage. Although low-grade lymphomas exhibit a worse response to chemotherapy than intermediate-grade or high-grade forms, the slower progression of these disorders often translates into longer patient survival. In the dog, lymphomas of T cell phenotype carry a worse prognosis than those of B cell type, regardless of tumor histologic grade.[3] This same association has not been confirmed in the cat.[4] Lymphoma patients with hypercalcemia also have a worse prognosis, thought to be an indirect effect of the association of hypercalcemia with T cell phenotype.[2]

Prognosis of lymphoma among the various anatomic forms also differs. Cutaneous, diffuse alimentary, and CNS lymphomas tend to be associated with poor prognosis (less so if disease is localized).[3] Treatment of diffuse alimentary lymphoma tends not to be as successful as with localized gastrointestinal disease amenable to surgical resection. Localized CNS lymphoma is amenable to treatment using radiation, which outperforms chemotherapeutic options for lymphomas in this location. CNS lymphoma chemotherapy response rates are typically low and of short duration. Also, cases with diffuse marrow involvement (which are often impossible to distinguish reliably from lymphoid leukemia) tend to have a poor prognosis.[3]

Improved molecular testing modalities have led to investigations into the utility of tumor cell proliferation markers to predict prognosis. Early studies suggest argyrophilic nucleolar organizer region (AgNOR) enumeration may be of prognostic value (higher AgNOR counts correlate with shorter patient survival).[3] Bromodeoxyuridine (BrdU) labeling, which is used to assess tumor doubling time, may also be useful.[3]

18. What is Hodgkin's lymphoma, and has this entity been described in veterinary medicine?

Hodgkin's lymphoma is a lymphoid neoplasm of humans unique in both its behavior and morphology.[21] Unlike the non-Hodgkin's forms, Hodgkin's lymphoma is a slowly progressive and often curable tumor that arises in a single node and spreads through contiguous nodes. Histologically, it consists of low numbers of neoplastic Reed-Sternberg cells (or their variants) interspersed amid numerous lymphocytic and inflammatory cells. For this reason, diagnosis may be challenging without whole–lymph node excisional biopsy and histopathology. Cytology is frequently unrewarding. Establishing a specific diagnosis of Hodgkin's lymphoma is vital given the marked difference in its rate of progression and prognosis from other forms of lymphoma.

A veterinary counterpart to Hodgkin's lymphoma has been described infrequently in ferrets, skunks, killer whales, rats, mice, horses, dogs, and cats.[16,21]

19. What is large granular lymphoma, and how is it detected in veterinary species?

Large granular lymphoma, also called "lymphoma of large granular lymphocytes," is a morphologically unique variant of alimentary lymphoma in which the neoplastic cells contain magenta cytoplasmic granules best visualized with Wright-Giemsa stain.[4,27,28] The name of this disorder can be misleading in that neither the neoplastic cells nor the granules they contain are consistently "large." Phenotypic analysis has demonstrated a T cell or natural killer (NK) cell phenotype. T cell phenotype is most common and typically exhibits the following pattern of immunoreactivity: CD3 positive, CD8 positive or negative, CD-57–like perforin positive, CD20 negative, with T cell receptor gene rearrangement.[4,28]

This lymphoma variant has been reported in a number of veterinary species, including cats, dogs, horses, rats, ferrets, birds, guinea pigs, and mice.[28,29] Incidence of large granular lymphoma is thought to be low, although diagnosis by histopathology alone may be misleading because neoplastic cell granules fail to stain consistently with routine hematoxylin-eosin (H&E).[27] Middle-aged to older animals are most often affected and present with clinical signs referable to disease of the gastrointestinal tract, including anorexia, weight loss, chronic or intermittent vomiting, hypoalbuminemia, and diarrhea.[27,28] Tumors typically arise as mass lesions in jejunum or mesenteric lymph nodes that are palpable on physical examination. Splenic involvement is relatively common.[27] A leukemic blood profile is also possible[27,28] (Figure 17-5). Treatment and response rates are comparable to other forms of alimentary lymphoma. An association with FeLV infection has not been demonstrated.[27]

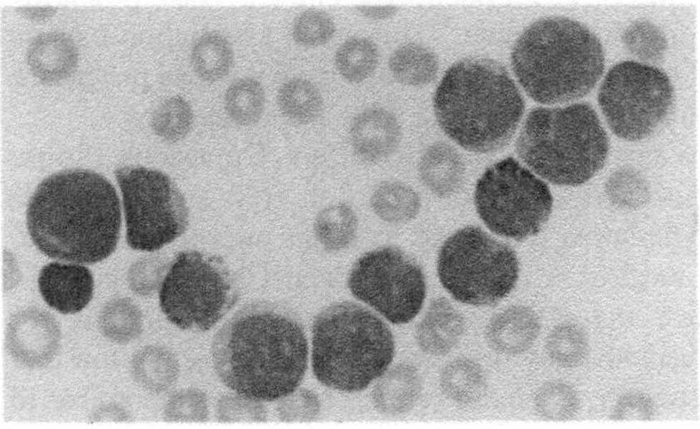

Figure 17-5 Acute lymphoblastic leukemia (ALL) of granular lymphocytes (LGL leukemia), peripheral blood, canine (300×). Circulating neoplastic lymphoid cell count exceeded $100 \times 10^3/\mu l$. These cells measured 10 to 16 μm in diameter, with eccentrically located, irregularly round nuclei having lightly clumped chromatin and multiple small, prominent nucleoli. Cytoplasm occasionally contains few to moderate numbers of variably coarse, magenta-staining granules. In this case, neither the neoplastic cells nor the granules within them are particularly "large," illustrating the confusion sometimes surrounding the term "large granular lymphocyte."

REFERENCES

1. Duncan JR, Prasse KW, Mahaffey EA: Hematopoietic neoplasms. In *Veterinary laboratory medicine: clinical pathology,* ed 3, Ames, 1994, Iowa State University Press, pp 63-74.
2. Morris J, Dobson J: Haematopoietic system. In *Small animal clinical oncology,* Philadelphia, 2001, Saunders, pp 228-250.
3. Vail DM, MacEwan EG, Young KM: Canine lymphoma and lymphoid leukemias. In Withrow SJ, MacEwen EG, editors: *Small animal clinical oncology,* ed 3, Philadelphia, 2001, Saunders, pp 558-586.

4. Vail DM, MacEwen EG: Feline lymphoma and leukemias. In Withrow SJ, MacEwen EG, editors: *Small animal clinical oncology,* ed 3, Philadelphia, Saunders, 2001, pp 590-608.
5. Savage CJ: Lymphoproliferative and myeloproliferative disorders, *Vet Clin North Am Equine Pract* 14(3):563-578, 1998.
6. Jacobs RM, Messick JB, Valli VE: Tumors of the hemolymphatic system. In Meuten DJ, editor: *Tumors in domestic animals,* ed 4, Ames, 2002, Iowa State University Press, pp 119-180.
7. Cockerell GL, Reyes RA: Bovine leukemia virus-associated lymphoproliferative disorders. In Feldman BF, Zinkl JG, Jain NC, editors: *Schalm's veterinary hematology,* ed 5, Philadelphia, 2001, Lippincott, Williams & Wilkins, pp 614-619.
8. Vail DM: Lymphoma. In Feldman BF, Zinkl JG, Jain NC, editors: *Schalm's veterinary hematology,* ed 5, Philadelphia, 2001, Lippincott, Williams & Wilkins, pp 620-625.
9. Gabor LJ, Malik R, Canfield PJ: Clinical and anatomical features of lymphosarcoma in 118 cats, *Aust Vet J* 76(11):725-733, 1998.
10. Polkes AC et al: B-cell lymphoma in a horse with associated Sezary-like cells in the peripheral blood, *J Vet Intern Med* 13:620-624, 1999.
11. Aquino SM et al: Progression of an orbital T-cell rich B-cell lymphoma to a B-cell lymphoma in a dog, *Vet Pathol* 37:465-469, 2000.
12. Messick JB, Calderwood Mays MB: Classification of lymphomas. In Feldman BF, Zinkl JG, Jain NC, editors: *Schalm's veterinary hematology,* ed 5, Philadelphia, 2001, Lippincott, Williams & Wilkins, pp 604-613.
13. Valli VE et al: The histologic classification of 602 cases of feline lymphoproliferative disease using the National Cancer Institute Working Formulation, *J Vet Diagn Invest* 12:295-306, 2000.
14. Keller ET: Immune-mediated disease as a risk factor for canine lymphoma, *Cancer* 70:2334-2337, 1992.
15. Moriello KA: Cutaneous lymphoma and variants. In Feldman BF, Zinkl JG, Jain NC, editors: *Schalm's veterinary hematology,* ed 5, Philadelphia, 2001, Lippincott, Williams & Wilkins, pp 648-659.
16. Blomme EAG, Foy SH, Chappell KH, LaPerle KMD: Hypereosinophilic syndrome with Hodgkin's-like lymphoma in a ferret, *J Comp Pathol* 120:211-217, 1999.
17. Barrs VR, Beatty JA, McCandlish IA, Kiper A: Hypereosinophilic paraneoplastic syndrome in a cat with intestinal T-cell lymphosarcoma, *J Small Anim Pract* 43(9):401-405, 2002.
18. Duckett WM, Matthews HK: Hypereosinophilia in a horse with intestinal lymphosarcoma, *Can Vet J* 38:719-720, 1997.
19. Valli VE, Jacobs RM, Parodi AL, et al: Histological classification of hematopoietic tumors in domestic animals, Second series, vol VIII. Armed Forces Institute of Pathology and World Health Organization Collaborating Center for Worldwide Reference of Comparative Oncology, Washington, DC, 2002.
20. Vail DM: Plasma cell neoplasias. In Withrow SJ, MacEwen EG, editors: *Small animal clinical oncology,* ed 3, Philadelphia, 2001, WB Saunders, pp 654-659.
21. Walton RM, Hendrick MJ: Feline Hodgkin's-like lymphoma: 20 cases (1992-1999), *Vet Pathol* 38:504-511, 2001.
22. Raskin RE, Nipper MN: Cytochemical staining characteristics of lymph nodes from normal and lymphoma-affected dogs, *Vet Clin Pathol* 61(2):62-67, 1992.
23. Weiss DJ: Application of flow cytometric techniques to veterinary clinical hematology, *Vet Clin Pathol* 31(2):72-82, 2002.
24. Moore PF, Affolter VK, Vernau W: Immunophenotyping in the dog. In Bonagura JD, editor: *Kirk's current veterinary therapy.* XIII. Small animal practice, Philadelphia, 2000, Saunders, pp 505-509.
25. Dreitz MJ, Ogilvie G, Sim GK: Rearranged T lymphocyte antigen receptor genes as markers of malignant T cells, *Vet Immunol Immunopathol* 69:113-119, 1999.
26. Vail DM: Lymphoma: principles of management. In Feldman BF, Zinkl JG, Jain NC, editors: *Schalm's veterinary hematology,* ed 5, Philadelphia, 2001, Lippincott, Williams & Wilkins, pp 626-630.
27. Moore AS, Ogilvie GK: Lymphoma. In Ogilvie GK, editor: *Feline oncology: a comprehensive guide to compassionate care,* Trenton, NJ, 2001, Veterinary Learning Systems, pp 199-200.
28. Wellman ML: Lymphoproliferative disorders of large granular lymphocytes. In Feldman BF, Zinkl JG, Jain NC, editors: *Schalm's veterinary hematology,* ed 5, Philadelphia, 2001, Lippincott, Williams & Wilkins, pp 642-647.
29. Kariya K, Konno A, Ishida T: Perforin-like immunoreactivity in four cases of lymphoma of large granular lymphocytes in the cat, *Vet Pathol* 34(2):156-159, 1997.

18. LYMPHOID LEUKEMIAS

1. What is the hallmark of lymphoid leukemia, and how is this disorder distinguished from lymphoma?

Lymphoid leukemia is primarily a disease of bone marrow, peripheral blood, and in later stages, tissues outside the marrow. In most cases, lymphoid leukemia is thought to arise within bone marrow, but it may infrequently arise within the thymus or spleen and subsequently colonize the bone marrow.[1] Classically, lymphoid leukemia is distinguished by the presence of high numbers of circulating neoplastic lymphoid cells in peripheral blood. *Aleukemic* and *subleukemic* forms do occur, in which neoplastic cells are absent or are not visualized in significant numbers in peripheral blood, respectively, necessitating evaluation of bone marrow for definitive diagnosis.

Lymphoid leukemia and lymphoma may both involve tumors of B cell, T cell, or null cell phenotype.[2,3] In addition, both may involve mature-appearing or undifferentiated cells. The only means by which lymphoid leukemias can be routinely distinguished from lymphomas is with appropriate disease staging to determine sites of tumor involvement. Bone marrow involvement must be documented to diagnose leukemia. Lymphoid leukemia cannot be distinguished from stage V lymphomas characterized by extensive bone marrow involvement.

2. How are lymphoid leukemias classified?

Leukemias are classified into acute or chronic categories according to the degree of maturity or differentiation of the neoplastic lymphoid cell involved. *Acute lymphoid leukemia* (ALL) arises from proliferation of early, undifferentiated, immature progenitor cells, resulting in the arrest of lineage development (Figure 18-1). In contrast, *chronic lymphoid leukemia* (CLL) arises from late-stage precursors, resulting in proliferation of fairly well-differentiated cells[4] (Figure 18-2). In animals the acute form of lymphocytic leukemia is more common than the chronic form.[1]

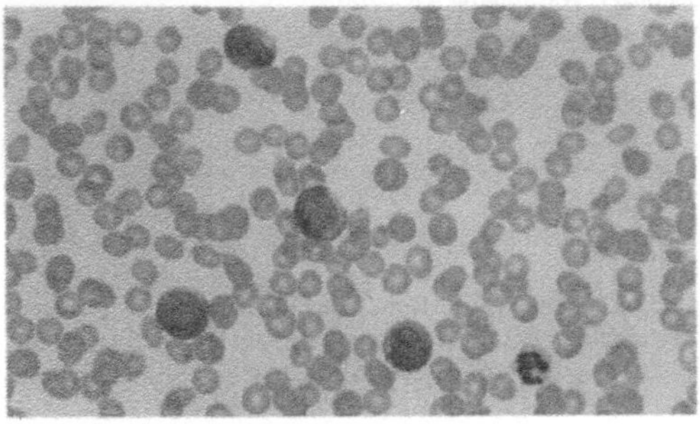

Figure 18-1 Acute lymphoid leukemia (ALL), peripheral blood, canine (150×). Circulating neoplastic lymphoid cell count was $18 \times 10^3/\mu l$. Moderate to marked anemia, marked thrombocytopenia, and marked neutropenia were also present. Neoplastic cells are blastic in morphology, measuring 15 to 18 µm in diameter, with eccentrically located, irregularly round nuclei having lightly clumped chromatin and multiple small, indistinct nucleoli. A single neutrophil is present in the lower-right aspect for size reference.

The French-American-British (FAB) Cooperative Group has defined a classification scheme that further subdivides ALL by patient age and neoplastic cell morphology into three subdisorders termed *L1, L2,* and *L3*. This system may be applied to ALL in veterinary patients, but prognostic usefulness is questionable.[1,2] Alternatively, lymphoid leukemia may be classified by neoplastic cell phenotype into B cell, T cell, or natural killer (NK) cell phenotype. Prognostic utility of leukemia phenotyping in veterinary species remains to be seen.[2]

3. How do acute and chronic leukemias differ in behavior?

Behavior of acute and chronic lymphoid leukemia is distinct. Acute leukemias tend to exhibit more aggressive behavior and rapid progression than chronic leukemias. In acute forms,

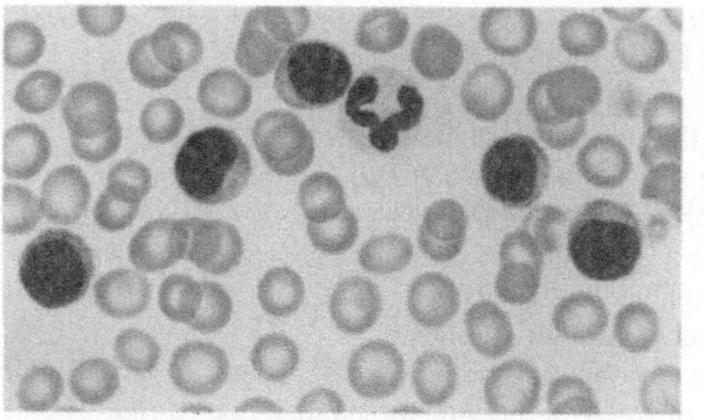

Figure 18-2 Chronic lymphoid leukemia (CLL), peripheral blood, canine, 300×. Circulating neoplastic lymphoid cell count exceeded $200 \times 10^3/\mu l$. Mild to moderate anemia and moderate thrombocytopenia were also present. Neoplastic cells measured 8 to 10 μm in diameter, with eccentrically located, round nuclei having dense, coarsely clumped chromatin and no visible nucleoli. Morphology is typical of mature small lymphocytes.

neoplastic cells exhibit a greater tendency to proliferate at the expense of bone marrow hematopoietic cells, ultimately resulting in myelophthisis. This manifests clinically as variable cytopenias and increased vulnerability to infection (usually secondary to neutropenia). As neoplastic cells spill into peripheral blood in increasing numbers, increased blood viscosity and thrombosis, as well as organ infiltration (particularly of liver, spleen, and lymph nodes), are possible.[4]

Chronic lymphoid leukemias typically exhibit a slower pattern of progression; a prodromal phase of months to years is thought to occur.[1] Clinical signs are also relatively mild, and lethargy may be the only outward sign of illness.[1,4] In many cases, chronic lymphocytic leukemia is diagnosed incidentally on routine hematologic evaluation. Bone marrow involvement is generally significantly less extensive, at least in the early phases of disease, than in the acute form. When present, cytopenias tend to be milder in severity.[1]

4. What is the incidence of lymphoid leukemia in veterinary species?

Compared with lymphoma, both ALL and CLL occur less often. Among lymphoid leukemias, ALL is more common than CLL. The reported proportion of all canine leukemias that are lymphoid in origin varies. Leukemias of lymphoid origin were recently reported to represent one third of all leukemias diagnosed in the dog.[1] Another report suggests that lymphoid leukemias are the predominant type in the dog.[5] Certainly among the chronic leukemias, CLL is most common in all species.[4]

In the cat, lymphoid leukemias make up the majority of all leukemias diagnosed. Leukemias occur more frequently in the cat overall, accounting for approximately one third of all hematopoietic neoplasia in this species,[6] likely as a result of the effects of feline leukemia virus (FeLV) infection.[4]

ALL typically affects young to middle-aged dogs and cats, with a median reported age of 5.5 and 5 years, respectively.[1] Among dogs, affected males outnumber females about three to two.[5]

CLL is primarily a disorder of middle-aged and older dogs, cattle, and cats.[1] Median reported age in the dog is 10.5 years.[1] As with ALL, male dogs have a higher rate of incidence, outnumbering affected females about two to one.[5] CLL is reported only rarely in the cat and does not appear to be related to FeLV infection.[6]

5. Has an etiology been determined in the development of lymphoid leukemia?

Viral infection is probably the best-defined etiology associated with leukemia development in cats and cattle. Of cats diagnosed with ALL, 60% to 80% will test positive for FeLV infection.[6] FeLV infection has been reported in as many as 90% of all leukemias in cats.[4] Other, as yet unknown factors (possibly genetic) must act in concert with FeLV in development of leukemia, however, because tumor rates with experimental infection are much lower.[4] Bovine leukemia virus (BLV) infection in cattle is associated with development of lymphocytic leukemia, although the incidence is lower than that of BLV-associated lymphoma.[7]

In dogs, no specific etiology in the development of lymphoid leukemia has been identified. Unlike cats and cattle, no retroviral cause has been implicated.[5]

6. How is immunophenotyping useful in the diagnosis of lymphoid leukemia?

As with lymphoma, immunophenotyping may be useful to confirm a lymphoid lineage when insufficient or ambiguous neoplastic cell morphologic features exist to distinguish these cells reliably from either myeloid or anaplastic epithelial or mesenchymal tumors. Immunophenotyping is also used to subclassify lymphoid leukemias into T cell, B cell, or null cell phenotypes, which may influence treatment decisions and prognosis.

In the dog, ALL is of varied phenotype. In one case series, T cell, B cell, and null cell phenotypes each constituted about one third of cases described.[8] In another case series, B cell phenotype was seen in half of cases, with the other half consisting of an equal mix of T cell and null cell phenotypes of large granular lymphocyte leukemia.[9] Another series documented 40% T cell, 40% null cell, and 20% B cell phenotype in canine ALL.[10] A higher proportion of canine CLL is reported to be of T cell phenotype (two thirds to three quarters of cases).[1,5]

7. What are the typical presenting signs in veterinary patients with lymphoid leukemia?

As many as 50% of patients diagnosed with CLL are asymptomatic. In these animals, diagnosis is frequently made incidental to routine hematologic evaluation. In other patients, mild or vague signs of progressive disease may be present, including vomiting, diarrhea, fever, pallor, lethargy, polyuria, polydipsia, weight loss, and mild lymphadenopathy and hepatosplenomegaly.[4]

In contrast, acute leukemias tend to be associated with a greater frequency of nonspecific signs, including weakness, anorexia, vomiting, diarrhea, fever, pale mucous membranes, mild lymphadenopathy (although less dramatic than in lymphoma), and hepatosplenomegaly.[1,4] Infrequently in advanced disease, myelophthisis may result in thrombocytopenia and clinical signs of hemorrhage. Neurologic manifestations, including neuropathies, paresis, and ocular complications (e.g., retinal detachment, hyphema, glaucoma), may occur rarely.[4] Calves may present severely cachectic with marked, symmetric lymphadenopathy.[1]

8. What hematologic or biochemical abnormalities are typically seen in leukemic animals at presentation?

In ALL, extensive bone marrow infiltration leads to varying degrees of anemia, neutropenia, and thrombocytopenia, and thus hematologic abnormalities are common. Many dogs have normocytic, normochromic and nonregenerative anemia, which may be severe. Leukocytosis, neutropenia, and high numbers of circulating neoplastic cells are also common.[5] In aleukemic or subleukemic cases, leukopenia is more typical. Cats most often have normal to decreased leukocyte numbers, and a moderate to marked nonregenerative anemia. Circulating neoplastic cells are less common than in the dog.[6]

Bone marrow involvement in CLL is often less extensive than in ALL, at least early in the course of disease, and thus hematologic abnormalities are often less severe. Both dogs and cats with CLL may have mild nonregenerative anemia and thrombocytopenia. Leukocyte numbers are variable because of fluctuations in the number of circulating neoplastic cells, but leukocyte count is typically the most striking hematologic feature.[5] Most dogs have leukocyte counts greater than $30 \times 10^3/\mu l$ and most cats greater than $50 \times 10^3/\mu l$. In either species, counts may exceed $100 \times 10^3/\mu l$, attributable to abundant circulating neoplastic cells. These cells often have sufficiently mature morphology as to be indistinguishable from nonneoplastic mature small lymphocytes. Ruling out other causes for persistent small lymphocytosis is essential. Neutrophil numbers usually are adequate.

Hypergammaglobulinemia and monoclonal gammopathies have been reported to occur in 30% and 68% of canine CLL cases, respectively. Monoclonal gammopathies are most often of the immunoglobulin M (IgM) type.[3] As with lymphoma, other biochemical abnormalities depend on extent of organ involvement. Increased hepatic leakage enzymes, alanine aminotransferase (ALT) and aspartate aminotransferase (AST), may signal hepatic infiltration. Veterinary patients with extensive renal involvement may be azotemic, attributable to renal insufficiency or failure.

9. Are paraneoplastic syndromes a concern in lymphoid leukemia?

Hypergammaglobulinemia has been reported as a fairly frequent occurrence in dogs with CLL (as many as 68% of dogs in one study).[3] IgM was the most frequent immunoglobulin type detected in these cases. Because of its larger size and polymerizing capabilities, IgM is more frequently associated with hyperviscosity syndrome than the other immunoglobulin types. Consequently, this paraneoplastic syndrome has been reported occasionally in the dog.[1] The presence of concurrent CLL and IgM monoclonal gammopathy is termed *Waldenström's macroglobulinemia*.[5] In 10% of canine CLL cases, reduced immunoglobulin levels are present and may increase the risk of infection.[4]

The occurrence of severe hyperviscosity syndrome may necessitate intervention before diagnostic testing or treatment is instituted. Plasmaphoresis is one therapeutic option.

10. How is a diagnosis of lymphoid leukemia established?

Diagnosis of any leukemia, lymphoid or nonlymphoid, requires bone marrow examination. In ALL or CLL, lymphoid cells should constitute greater than 30% of nucleated cells within the marrow.[1,2] In more recent publications, this threshold has been reduced to 20%.[11] In ALL and in the late stages of CLL, neoplastic cells may efface the marrow. Neoplastic cell morphology and clinical history help in determining acute or chronic classification. Lymphoid leukemia cannot be distinguished from stage V lymphomas characterized by extensive bone marrow involvement.

Bone marrow examination is also vital to assess the extent of normal hematopoiesis for prognostic purposes and therapeutic considerations.[4]

11. What additional testing is available to confirm the diagnosis of lymphoid leukemia?

In ALL, neoplastic cell morphology alone may be insufficient or misleading to confirm a lymphoid cell lineage. Cytochemical staining or immunophenotyping may be necessary to verify the diagnosis. The diagnostic value of cytochemical staining relies mainly on the ability of these stains to identify nonlymphoid cells specifically, because lymphoid cells fail to stain with most cytochemical stains. For example, positive myeloperoxidase or Sudan black B staining suggests granulocytic or monocytic cell origin.[12] Positive nonspecific esterase staining is seen in both monocytic and lymphocytic and occasionally other cell types, although the pattern of staining differs; lymphocytic cells tend to stain focally, whereas monocytic cells stain diffusely with nonspecific esterase. Failure of a neoplastic cell population to stain in a characteristic manner with cytochemical stains does not automatically suggest a lymphoid origin. Abnormalities in maturation, function, or structure of neoplastic cells may alter staining properties.

Neoplastic lymphocytosis in CLL, particularly during the early phase of disease, may be difficult or impossible to distinguish reliably from a nonneoplastic, reactive lymphocytosis. By establishing that a population of lymphocytes is expressing an identical constellation of surface proteins through immunophenotypic analysis, a clonal proliferation is supported. Detection of a uniform T cell receptor or immunoglobulin gene rearrangement using polymerase chain reaction (PCR) fragment analysis within a population of T cell or B cell lymphocytes, respectively, suggests a clonal lymphocyte proliferation most compatible with a neoplastic process.[9,13]

12. Are patients with lymphoid leukemia "staged" in a manner similar to patients with lymphoma?

Staging of lymphoid leukemias is not routinely performed in veterinary medicine. Currently, ALL and advanced cases of CLL are classified and approached therapeutically in a manner equivalent to stage V lymphoma. The staging system in Table 18-1 has proven valuable prognostically in human CLL.[5]

Table 18-1 *Clinical Staging System for Human Chronic Lymphocytic Leukemia*

STAGE	EXTENT OF ORGAN INVOLVEMENT
0	Lymphocytosis only Absolute lymphocyte count $\geq 15 \times 10^3/\mu l$ Proportion of lymphocytes in bone marrow $\leq 40\%$ in normocellular or hypercellular marrow
I	Lymphocytosis plus enlarged lymph nodes
II	Lymphocytosis plus hepatomegaly and/or splenomegaly
III	Lymphocytosis plus anemia (hemoglobin ≤ 7.0 g/dl)
IV	Lymphocytosis plus thrombocytopenia (platelets $\leq 100 \times 10^3/\mu l$), with or without lymph node enlargement, hepatomegaly, and splenomegaly

13. What treatment options exist for veterinary patients with lymphoid leukemia?

Of immediate and vital concern in the treatment of lymphoid leukemia is the prompt restoration of normal hematopoiesis.[5] This is primarily achieved with the use of chemotherapeutic drugs. In the interim, supportive therapy may be needed and may include red cell or platelet transfusions, antibiotic protection, and fluid therapy. The neoplastic cells of acute leukemias are more vulnerable to the effects of chemotherapy due to their more rapid rate of cell division. However, the occurrence of side effects (particularly life-threatening neutropenia) and organ failure (due to extensive neoplastic cell infiltration) may limit success of treatment.

Combination protocols are most often used in the treatment of ALL. Chemotherapeutic agents used are essentially those used in lymphoma, including vincristine, prednisone, L-asparaginase, and doxyrubicin. Response rate is frequently disappointing. In dogs, complete remission is expected in only 20% of those treated with vincristine and prednisone, with partial remission in another 20%.[5] Success rates are even lower in cats.[6] Complete remission is defined as the absence of detectable neoplastic cells in either bone marrow or peripheral blood. Maintenance therapy is continued weekly (or at 2- to 3-week intervals if doxyrubicin is used) during remission.[5] Recombinant erythropoietin and granulocyte-macrophage colony-stimulating factor (GM-CSF) may be useful to support hematopoiesis in patients with severe myelosuppression caused by myelophthisis or chemotherapy.[2,4]

Treatment of CLL is more controversial because of the indolent nature of the disease. In the absence of clinical signs or hematologic abnormalities other than lymphocytosis, treatment may be withheld. Most agree that treatment is indicated in patients with anemia, thrombocytopenia, lymphadenopathy, hepatosplenomegaly, or lymphocytosis in excess of $60 \times 10^3/\mu l$. Chlorambucil, with or without prednisone, is the most effective therapeutic regimen to date. In humans, chlorambucil in conjunction with prednisone has been proven superior to chlorambucil alone, possibly due to lymphocytolytic properties of prednisone. Cyclophosphamide is sometimes used in patients with advanced bone marrow infiltration. Aggressive combination chemotherapy protocols used in treatment of lymphoma are occasionally employed as last resort. Goals of treatment are primarily palliative, with complete remission only rarely achieved. Despite this, survival of 1 to 3 years with good quality of life can be expected because of the slow progression rate of CLL.[3,5]

Occasionally, animals with CLL will develop an aggressive, rapidly progressive ALL-like phase. This is recognized clinically as an alteration in neoplastic cell phenotype from a mature small cell to a large blast cell appearance. This transformation is also seen in humans with CLL (Richter's syndrome) and is associated with a poor prognosis.[1,5]

14. What does a diagnosis of lymphoid leukemia mean to survival? Also, what rate of treatment success can be expected, and what factors assist in determining prognosis?

Prognosis for patients with ALL is poor. Only 20% to 40% of dogs diagnosed with ALL achieve complete or partial remission, with survival of only 1 to 3 months.[4] A subtype of ALL in dogs with a more intermediate cell morphology has been described and may be associated with a better prognosis.[5] Fewer cats with ALL (one third) respond to chemotherapy than cats with lymphoma (two thirds). Survival may be longer in cats (1 to 7 months) than in dogs.[4]

In CLL the prognosis is better for patient survival. Bone marrow involvement is typically less extensive, sparing hematopoiesis, and disease progression is more gradual due to slower neoplastic cell proliferation rates. Survival longer than 1 year is seen in both the dog[4] and the cat.[6] T cell phenotype CLL, as with its lymphoma counterpart, may be associated with a poorer prognosis.[3]

REFERENCES

1. Jacobs RM, Messick JB, Valli VE: Tumors of the hemolymphatic system. In Meuten DJ, editor: *Tumors in domestic animals,* ed 4, Ames, 2002, Iowa State University Press, pp 119-180.
2. Modiano JF, Helfand SC: Acute lymphocytic leukemia. In Feldman BF, Zinkl JG, Jain NC, editors: *Schlam's veterinary hematology,* ed 5, Philadelphia, 2001, Lippincott, Williams & Wilkins, pp 631-637.
3. Helfand SC, Modiano JF: Chronic lymphocytic leukemia. In Feldman BF, Zinkl JG, Jain NC, editors: *Schlam's veterinary hematology,* ed 5, Philadelphia, 2001, Lippincott, Williams & Wilkins, pp 638-641.
4. Morris J, Dobson J: Haematopoietic system. In *Small animal clinical oncology,* Philadelphia, 2001, WB Saunders, pp 228-250.
5. Vail DM, MacEwan EG, Young KM: Canine lymphoma and lymphoid leukemias. In Withrow SJ, MacEwen EG, editors: *Small animal clinical oncology,* ed 3, Philadelphia, 2001, Saunders, pp 558-586.
6. Vail DM, MacEwen EG: Feline lymphoma and leukemias. In Withrow SJ, MacEwen EG, editors: *Small animal clinical oncology,* ed 3, Philadelphia, Saunders, 2001, pp 590-608.
7. Cockerell GL, Reyes RA: Bovine leukemia virus-associated lymphoproliferative disorders. In Feldman BF, Zinkl JG, Jain NC, editors: *Schalm's veterinary hematology,* ed 5, Philadelphia, 2001, Lippincott, Williams & Wilkins, pp 614-619.
8. Ruslander DA, Gebhard DH, Tompkins MB, et al: Immunophenotypic characteristics of canine lymphoproliferative disorders, *In Vivo* 11(2):169-72, 1997.
9. Vernau W, Moore PF: An immunophenotypic study of canine leukemias and preliminary assessment of clonality by polymerase chain reaction, *Vet Immunol Immunopathol* 69:145-64, 1999.
10. Weiss DJ: From cytometric and immunophenotypic evaluation of acute lymphocytic leukemia in dog bone marrow, *J Vet Intern Med* 15:589-594, 2001.
11. Valli VE, Jacobs RM, Parodi AL, et al: Histological classification of hematopoietic tumors in domestic animals, Second series, vol VIII. Armed Forces Institute of Pathology and World Health Organization Collaborating Center for Worldwide Reference of Comparative Oncology, Washington, DC, 2002.
12. Raskin RE, Nipper MN: Cytochemical staining characteristics of lymph nodes from normal and lymphoma-affected dogs, *Vet Clin Pathol* 61(2), 62-67, 1992.
13. Dreitz MJ, Ogilvie G, Sim GK: Rearranged T lymphocyte antigen receptor genes as markers of malignant T cells, *Vet Immunol Immunopathol* 69:113-119, 1999.

19. PLASMA CELL NEOPLASIA

1. Which disorders are included in the plasma cell neoplasia group?

Plasma cell neoplasms include multiple myeloma, Waldenström's macroglobulinemia, solitary osseous plasmacytomas, and extramedullary plasmacytomas. Multiple myeloma is the most important based on incidence and severity[1,2] and has been reported in the dog, cat, horse, cow, and pig.[3]

Each of these disorders is thought to arise from a single neoplastic B lymphocyte (monoclonal proliferation), although biclonal and polyclonal tumors have been described. *Extramedullary plasmacytomas* arise outside the bone marrow, and their behavior varies with site of origin. Cutaneous and oral extramedullary plasmacytomas are relatively common in older dogs and generally benign in behavior.[4] In contrast, noncutaneous extramedullary plasmacytomas, especially those arising within the gastrointestinal (GI) tract, are much more aggressive in behavior and often spread to regional lymph nodes. *Solitary osseous plasmacytomas* arise as a focal skeletal lesion and frequently progress to systemic multiple myeloma.[2]

Multiple myeloma involves neoplastic proliferation of B lymphocytes in bone marrow and in extramedullary tissues. Frequently these B lymphocytes retain their secretory function and produce complete immunoglobulin proteins or protein subunits, resulting in an increased plasma protein concentration. *Waldenström's macroglobulinemia* is a subtype of multiple myeloma in which the neoplastic B lymphocytes produce immunoglobulin M (IgM).

2. How common is multiple myeloma in veterinary species?

In the dog, multiple myeloma is relatively uncommon, accounting for less than 1% of all malignant neoplasms, approximately 8% of all hematopoietic tumors, and 4% of all bone tumors.[1,5] Older dogs are typically affected, with a reported age distribution of 8 to 10 years.[1,3] No gender or breed predisposition is consistently reported.[2]

In other domestic species, occurrence of multiple myeloma is very rare. In the cat, multiple myeloma accounts for less than 1% of all hematopoietic tumors.[5] As with dogs, older cats are most often affected, and no gender predisposition has been reported.[2,5]

3. Has an etiology been found to explain the development of multiple myeloma?

No specific etiology has been determined to cause multiple myeloma in domestic species. Genetic predispositions, viral infection, chronic immune stimulation, and carcinogen exposure may all play a role in tumor development.[1] In one large case series of canine multiple myeloma, German Shepherds were overrepresented.[1,3] Cocker spaniels may be overrepresented in development of extramedullary plasmacytomas, accounting for 24% of affected dogs in one study.[3] Multiple myeloma has not been associated with feline leukemia virus (FeLV) or feline immunodeficiency virus (FIV) infection in the cat.[1]

4. What is the M-component?

The *M-component*, also called *myeloma protein* or *M protein,* refers to the immunoglobulin proteins or protein fragments produced by secretory neoplastic B lymphocytes. It includes the various immunoglobulin types (IgG, IgA, IgM), light chains (Bence Jones proteins), and heavy chains. The production of M-component by neoplastic B lymphocytes is termed *paraproteinemia*. Although this is a more common manifestation of multiple myeloma, it may also occur rarely in association with other plasma cell neoplasms.[2,3,6]

IgG and IgA paraproteinemia have an almost equal rate of occurrence in the dog.[3] IgG is most frequently reported in the cat.[1,7] IgM paraproteinemia occurs less frequently and is termed (Waldenström's) macroglobulinemia. All typically manifest as a monoclonal protein spike (monoclonal gammopathy) on serum protein electrophoresis, although biclonal gammopathies have also been reported.[3,6,8] Nonsecretory multiple myeloma is rarely reported in the dog.[3]

Other diseases may infrequently be associated with a monoclonal gammopathy and must be distinguished from multiple myeloma. Monoclonal gammopathy has been associated with lymphoma, ehrlichiosis, leishmaniasis, plasmacytic gastroenterocolitis, chronic pyoderma, feline infectious peritonitis (FIP), and idiopathic causes.[3,6]

Because of their small molecular weight, Bence Jones proteins (light chains) are readily filtered through the glomerulus and are passed in urine.[1] This is referred to as *Bence Jones proteinuria* (BJP) and is seen in 25% to 40% of dogs and 60% of cats with multiple myeloma.[3] Traditional urine protein dipstick methodology does not detect BJP, necessitating use of more specialized testing, such as immunoelectrophoresis. With significant proteinuria, the sulfasalcytic acid (SSA) test will be positive with BJP.

Cryoglobulins are paraproteins that are insoluble at temperatures less than 37° C.[7] Failure to detect cryoglobulins may occur if blood collection and clotting are not performed at body temperature to avoid precipitation and loss of these proteins. Clinical manifestations of *cryoglobulinemia* result from sludging of blood and obstruction of small vessels, particularly in the extremities, where blood may cool sufficiently to allow precipitation of cryoprotiens.[6] Affected animals may present with cyanosis and necrosis of the skin of the distal extremities. Cryoglobulinemia has been reported in association with multiple myeloma in the dog, cat, and horse.[7]

Concentration of M-component is often proportional to tumor burden and therefore may be useful in monitoring response to therapy as well as tumor recurrence.

5. What presenting signs are common in animals with multiple myeloma?

Clinical signs are usually nonspecific but may include fever, pale mucous membranes, lethargy, mild lymphadenopathy, and hepatic or splenic enlargement. Pathology may be attributable to neoplastic cell infiltration of various organs and paraproteinemia. Other common clinical signs may be related to skeletal involvement, bleeding disorders, hyperviscosity, immune dysfunction, and renal disease.

Skeletal involvement may be focal or diffuse. Focal osteolytic lesions are primarily seen in the dog[2] and may result in lameness or pathologic fracture.[1,3] An estimated 25% to 66% of dogs with IgG- and IgA-secreting tumors will develop osteolytic lesions. In contrast, dogs with IgM-secreting tumors only rarely present with osteolytic lesions.[3] Sites most frequently involved are those of active hematopoiesis, including vertebra, pelvis, ribs, skull, and metaphysis of long bones.[1,3] Diffuse skeletal lesions include osteopenia and osteoporosis, which may result from secretion of osteolytic factors, including osteoclast activating factor and parathyroid hormone–related protein (PTHrp), by neoplastic cells.[1] Hormonal effects of osteolytic factors may contribute to the development of hypercalcemia. Hypercalcemia is rarely seen in the cat but may affect 15% to 20% of dogs with multiple myeloma.[2]

Bleeding disorders are a frequent complication, affecting approximately one third of dogs with multiple myeloma. Clinical manifestations of hemorrhage may include epistaxis, petechiae, ecchymoses, bruising, gingival bleeding, and GI bleeding. A number of mechanisms may contribute to the development of hemostatic abnormalities. Thrombocytopenia may result from myelophthisis of the bone marrow. Platelet function may be impaired as a result of paraprotein-coating of platelets interfering with platelet aggregation. Paraproteins may also adsorb minor coagulation factors, causing a functional factor decrease of sufficient magnitude to prolong activated partial thromboplastin time (aPTT) and prothrombin time (PT).[1] Paraprotein binding of ionized calcium may likewise contribute to functional hypocalcemia, further impacting the coagulation cascade.[2]

Hyperviscosity syndrome is a possible consequence of paraprotein secretion by neoplastic cells. Although it may develop with any type of paraproteinemia, hyperviscosity syndrome most often is a complication of IgM- and IgA-secreting myelomas, attributable to the higher molecular weight of these proteins and their ability to polymerize. Hyperviscous blood may sludge in small vessels, impairing delivery of oxygen and nutrients to tissues and predisposing to thrombus formation. Common manifestations include cerebral disease (seizures, ataxia, dementia), cardiac disease (cardiomyopathy, exercise intolerance, syncope, cyanosis), and ocular disease (sudden blindness, retinal detachment, tortuous retinal vessels, retinal hemorrhage). Hyperviscosity syndrome has been reported in 20% of dogs with multiple myeloma and less often in cats.[1] Enhanced rouleaux formation, evident on peripheral blood smears, may signal the presence of hyperviscosity syndrome[2] (see Figure 19-1).

Animals with multiple myeloma are at increased risk of infection as a result of immune dysfunction. Susceptibility to infection is a leading cause of death in affected animals. Contributing to immunocompromise is a marked decrease in production of normal immunoglobulins as a consequence of paraproteinemia.[1] In addition, leukopenia resulting from myelophthisis, particularly neutropenia, potentiates vulnerability to infection.[2] Diminished immune surveillance may increase the risk of additional tumor development. Veterinary patients with multiple myeloma have a higher prevalence of concurrent tumors.[6]

Renal disease ("myeloma kidney") is another common presenting feature of multiple myeloma, occurring one third to one half of affected dogs.[1-3] Pathogenesis is multifactorial.[1] Protein deposition in the glomeruli (Bence Jones proteins, amyloid, or intact immunoglobulin) and protein cast formation in tubules may occur. Renal tumor metastasis is also possible. Impaired perfusion from anemia of chronic disease and hyperviscosity syndrome may contribute. Hypercalcemia impairs tubular concentrating ability and may lead to dystrophic mineralization. Immune dysfunction may increase the risk of urinary tract infection and pyelonephritis. Any or all of these conditions may contribute concurrently to development of renal failure in veterinary patients with multiple myeloma.

6. What hematologic or biochemical abnormalities are expected in veterinary patients with multiple myeloma?

A variety of hematologic abnormalities may be evident in veterinary patients with multiple myeloma. Cytopenias are seen frequently. A normocytic, normochromic and nonregenerative anemia (anemia of chronic disease) is present in 60% to 70% of affected dogs.[1,5] Development of anemia may result from myelosuppression and myelophthisis. Blood loss secondary to impaired hemostasis, as well as reduced red cell life span due to coating by paraproteins, and hyperviscosity syndrome may also contribute in some cases.[1] Thrombocytopenia and leukopenia may occur through similar mechanisms, although less often than anemia, and are seen in only 16% to 30% and 25% of dogs, respectively.[1,5] Leukocytosis attributable to neutrophilia or circulating neoplastic B lymphocytes has been reported in 16% and 10% of dogs, respectively.[5,6]

Biochemical abnormalities are highly variable as a result of the wide array of clinical syndromes possible. Paraproteinemia may result in increased serum globulins, decreased albumin/globulin (A/G) ratio, and decreased synthesis of albumin. Azotemia, hyperphosphatemia, and hypoalbuminemia may be evident in patients with renal disease. Evidence of hepatocellular injury and cholestasis may be present in patients with liver involvement.

7. How is a diagnosis of multiple myeloma established?

Diagnosis of multiple myeloma is based on demonstration of at least two of the following features:

a. *Monoclonal* (or less frequently, biclonal) *gammopathy*. Confirm with serum protein electrophoresis or immunoelectrophoresis.
b. *Bone marrow plasmacytosis* (ideally >20%-30%, but often 10%-15%). Detection of atypical plasma cell morphology or occurrence of plasma cells in dense aggregates or sheets may increase suspicion.
c. *Bence Jones proteinuria*. Confirm with urine immunoelectrophoresis.
d. *Osteolytic skeletal lesions,* particularly of the pelvis, vertebral column, and metaphyseal region of long bones. These lesions may manifest as either punctate radiopacities or generalized osteoporosis.

8. What additional testing may be valuable in confirming a diagnosis of multiple myeloma?

In the presence of lymphadenopathy, hepatomegaly, splenomegaly, or other organomegaly, fine-needle aspiration cytology may be useful to confirm tissue infiltration by neoplastic plasma cells. Morphology may vary from well-differentiated, mature-appearing plasma cells to poorly differentiated, immature lymphoid cells or pleomorphic atypical plasmacytoid cells (Figures 19-1 to 19-3). Biopsy with histopathology may be similarly useful, with the added benefit of permitting special staining for amyloid (Congo red) as well as immunohistochemistry for immunoglobulin and B cell lymphocyte markers.

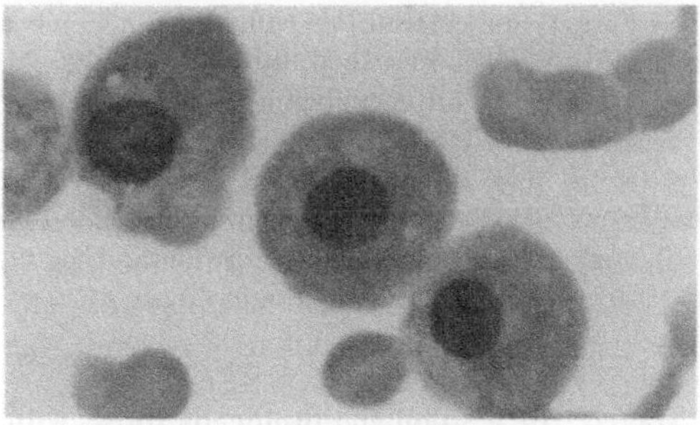

Figure 19-1 Multiple myeloma, bone marrow, canine (375×). Normal hematopoietic elements are effaced by a monomorphic population of atypical plasma cells with round nuclei having coarsely clumped chromatin and rare small, indistinct nucleoli. Cytoplasm is abundant, lightly granular, and contains a glassy amorphous fringe of immunoglobulin at the periphery. Note the prominent rouleaux formation in the upper-right corner, suggesting increased plasma protein concentration typical of multiple myeloma.

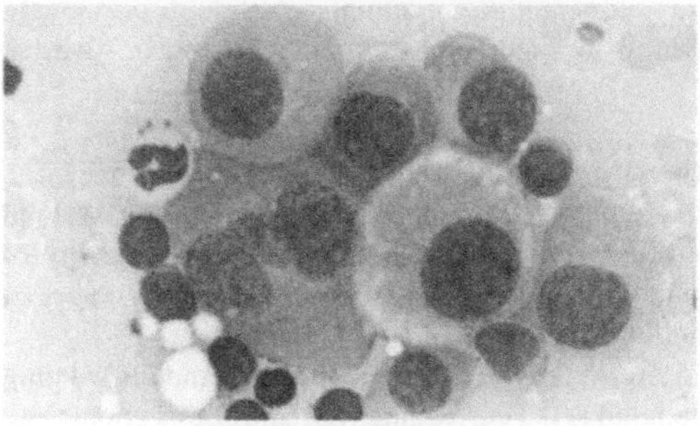

Figure 19-2 Malignant plasmacytoma, lymph node, feline (300×). Neoplastic cells are large to extremely large and contain eccentrically located, round nuclei with coarsely stippled chromatin and occasional small nucleoli. Cytoplasm is moderate to abundant in volume and occasionally contains a faint perinuclear halo. A single multinucleated cell is present. Several mature small lymphocytes and a single neutrophil are present to the left of the neoplastic plasma cells for size reference.

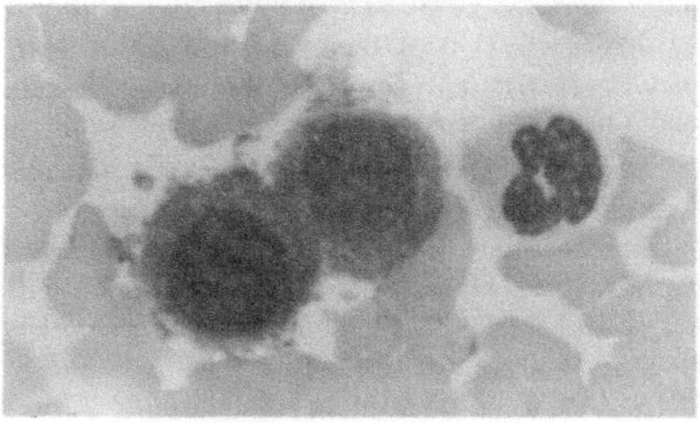

Figure 19-3 Multiple myeloma, leukemic phase; peripheral blood; feline (375×). This peripheral blood smear is from the same patient depicted in Figure 19-2, who ultimately developed multiple myeloma, hyperviscosity syndrome, and circulating neoplastic cells. The circulating cells were smaller, measuring 12 to 15 μ in diameter, with eccentrically located, round nuclei having coarsely clumped chromatin and a moderate volume of deeply basophilic cytoplasm. Occasionally, these cells were fringed with eosinophilic-staining, amorphous, glassy material compatible with immunoglobulin. Rouleaux formation was prominent. A single neutrophil is on the right for size reference.

9. Are paraneoplastic syndromes a concern in multiple myeloma?

Paraneoplastic syndromes are a major concern in veterinary patients with multiple myeloma and contribute greatly to the clinical manifestations of the disease. Paraproteinemia is present in the majority of cases, although nonsecretory myelomas have been reported rarely.[3] Hyperviscosity syndrome, hemolytic anemia, bleeding diatheses, renal disease, and immune dysfunction are all potential consequences of paraproteinemia.

Hypercalcemia is seen in 15% to 20% of canine cases[2,3,5] and is thought to result from secretion of osteoclast-stimulating factor, PTHrp, and other osteolytic factors.[2] It has been reported only rarely in the cat.[1] Hypercalcemia can contribute to impaired urine concentrating ability and development of renal failure. Polyneuropathy is another rare paraneoplastic syndrome reported in multiple myeloma patients.[5]

Paraneoplastic disorders may complicate or delay treatment for multiple myeloma. Intravenous (IV) fluid diuretic therapy, and in extreme cases pharmacologic agents (e.g., calcitonin), to control serum ionized calcium levels may be indicated with severe hypercalcemia.[1] Renal failure patients may also require IV fluid support. Bisphosphonate or mithramycin therapy has been used to reduce osteoclast activity, thus decreasing the incidence and severity of bone lesions and hypercalcemia.[5] In patients with cardiac or circulatory complications from hyperviscosity syndrome, plasmaphoresis may be useful. In severe thrombocytopenia resulting in hemorrhage, platelet or platelet-rich plasma transfusions may be necessary. Antibiotic protection, using nonnephrotoxic agents, is frequently indicated to safeguard against increased risk of infection in the presence of immunocompromise. Orthopedic stabilization of pathologic fractures is essential.[1]

10. Are patients with multiple myeloma "staged" in a manner similar to those with lymphoma?

No clinical staging system is currently in use for multiple myeloma.[5] Although previously described, staging systems did not prove useful in predicting tumor behavior or disease prognosis.[1]

11. What treatment options exist for animals with multiple myeloma?

Currently available chemotherapy can effectively reduce tumor burden, alleviate skeletal lesions and bone pain, reduce serum paraprotein concentration, and improve patient quality of life. More than 90% of patients exhibit complete or partial remission.[2] Despite this success, current therapeutic regimens are not curative, and tumor relapse should be expected.[1]

Chemotherapeutic agents currently used in multiple myeloma treatment include alkylating agents, sometimes combined with steroids. Melphalan is the current alkylating drug of choice and is generally well tolerated. Routine monitoring of complete blood count (CBC) is necessary to detect dose-limiting myelosuppression, particularly thrombocytopenia or neutropenia. This side effect is more problematic in the feline patient. Treatment is continued until relapse or dose-limiting myelosuppression occurs. Prednisone is often combined with melphalan and is thought to enhance its efficacy.[1] Cyclophosphamide and chlorambucil may be used instead of or in combination with melphalan or as rescue agents in relapse. Doxyrubicin, vincristine, and dexamethasone sodium phosphate may also be used in combination for rescue therapy.[1,2]

Response to therapy is monitored through assessment of clinical signs, biochemical parameters, resolution of skeletal lesions, and degree of bone marrow plasmacytosis. With successful therapy, reduction or resolution of anorexia, lethargy, and lameness should be evident in 3 to 4 weeks. Reduction of serum paraprotein concentration may take longer but should be expected within 3 to 6 weeks of institution of therapy. Because paraprotein concentration is often proportional to tumor burden, it is often useful in monitoring response to therapy as well as tumor recurrence. Resolution of skeletal lesions, ocular complications, and neuropathies may be slower to show improvement and may fail to resolve completely.[1]

12. What does a diagnosis of multiple myeloma mean in terms of survival? Also, what rate of treatment success can be expected, and what factors assist in determining prognosis?

Short-term prognosis of multiple myeloma is generally good with treatment. With chemotherapy, 75% to 90% of dogs exhibit a favorable response (either complete or partial remission), with survival of 12 to 18 months.[2,5] In animals presenting with one or more paraneoplastic syndromes, including hypercalcemia, Bence Jones proteinuria, renal failure, and extensive bone lesions, survival is reduced.[3] A good initial response to chemotherapy is considered a favorable prognostic indicator. No correlation has been documented between immunoglobulin type and disease prognosis.[5]

In cats, prognosis is less favorable because of their poorer response to chemotherapy. Dose-limiting myelosuppression is frequently problematic in cats.[1] If achieved, remission tends not to be durable, with survival of usually 2 to 3 months.[2]

In the dog, long-term prognosis of multiple myeloma is poor because current therapeutic regimens are not curative and eventual tumor relapse is inevitable. Death may result from progression of renal failure, development of infection, or owner-elected euthanasia for intractable bone pain.[2]

REFERENCES

1. Vail DM: Plasma cell neoplasms. In Withrow SJ, MacEwen EG, editors: *Small animal clinical oncology,* ed 3, Philadelphia, 2001, Saunders, pp 626-638.
2. Vail DM: Plasma cell tumors and macroglobulinemia. In Feldman BF, Zinkl JG, Jain NC, editors: *Schalm's veterinary hematology,* ed 5, Philadelphia, 2001, Lippincott, Williams & Wilkins, pp 654-659.
3. Jacobs RM, Messick JB, Valli VE: Tumors of the hemolymphatic system. In Meuten DJ, editor: *Tumors in domestic animals*, ed 4, Ames, 2002, Iowa State University Press, pp 119-180.
4. Cangul IT et al: Clinico-pathological aspects of canine cutaneous and mucocutaneous plasmacytomas, *J Vet Med A Physiol Pathol Clin Med* 49:307-312, 2002.
5. Morris J, Dobson J: Haematopoietic system. In *Small animal clinical oncology,* Ames, Iowa, 2001, Blackwell Science, pp 228-250.
6. Giraudel JM, Pages JP, Guelfi JF: Monoclonal gammopathies in the dog: a retrospective study of 18 cases (1986-1999) and literature review, *J Am Anim Hosp Assoc* 38:135-147, 2002.
7. Hickford FH et al: Monoclonal immunoglobulin G cryoglobulinemia and multiple myeloma in a domestic shorthair cat, *J Am Vet Med Assoc* 217(7):1029-1033, 2000.
8. Bienzle D, Silverstein DC, Chaffin K: Multiple myeloma in cats: variable presentation with different immunoglobulin isotypes in two cats, *Vet Pathol* 37:364-369, 2000.

Section III
Hemostasis

Bernard F. Feldman

20. OVERVIEW: HEMOSTATIC COMPONENTS AND DISORDERS

1. What is hemostasis?

Hemostasis is the maintenance of vascular integrity and blood fluidity necessary for the normal function of blood. The term *hemostasis* implies a balance between the extremes of hemostatic dysfunction: too little hemostasis resulting in hemorrhage and too much hemostasis resulting in thrombosis. When a blood vessel is injured, blood loss must be minimized by the rapid formation of a clot localized at the injury site. Hemostasis is involved in the healing process. When hemostasis is in balance, rapid clotting at the injury and appropriate healing occur. Imbalance resulting in too little hemostasis results in some component of significant blood loss due to hypocoagulation at the injury site. Imbalance resulting in too much hemostasis results in hypercoagulation or thrombosis, obstruction of vascular blood flow, and distal organ hypoxia and injury.

2. When is a hemostatic disorder suspected?

Lengthy or unabated hemorrhage after venipuncture suggests a hemostatic disorder. A hemostatic disorder also is suspected with petechiae, purpura, ecchymoses, body cavity hemorrhage, or the presence of excessive hematoma formation. A family history of bleeding or if the patient has experienced previous bleeding diatheses recently or as a young animal suggests a hemostatic disorder as well. Any evidence of excessive bleeding or bleeding in excess of the anticipated amount of hemorrhage from trauma should increase suspicion for a hemostatic disorder. Sudden onset of dyspnea or acute organopathy suggests a thrombotic process.

3. List the components of hemostasis in sequence.

The process of hemostasis is a diverse interplay among the vascular wall or endothelial cells, circulating platelets, coagulation proteins or factors, and the factors confining hemostasis to the appropriate area—the fibrinolytic system. Once endothelial damage has occurred and there is subendothelial collagen exposure, the sequence of appropriate hemostasis is initiated.

The endothelial response, *vascular constriction,* occurs first, followed quickly by the attachment of platelets to exposed subendothelial collagen, called *platelet adhesion.* Platelet adhesion is followed by recruitment of additional platelets to the area, or *platelet aggregation.* Stabilization of the platelet plug then occurs through the activation of the coagulation proteins or factors, resulting in *coagulation* or *fibrin formation.* Fibrin encompasses the platelet plug and provides the superstructure on which healing occurs. To keep the clot localized once fibrin formation has occurred, the backup fibrinolytic system is activated. *Fibrinolysis* ultimately prevents extension of the fibrin clot and breaks down fibrin to produce fibrin degradation products (FDPs) and fibrin split products (FSPs).

4. List activities of the endothelial cells.

Endothelial cells are among the most metabolically active cells in the mammalian body. Endothelial cells are involved with the material transfer of metabolic substances of varied size between blood and tissues. They also provide a relative barrier to blood cells, plasma, macromolecules, and particulate matter. Endothelial cells synthesize or metabolize numerous mediators, including von Willebrand factor, fibronectin, proteoglycans, and serotonin. These cells maintain thromboresistance, mediate vascular repair, and mediate cell migration and proliferation as well as thrombolysis. Endothelial cells also process antigen in cellular immunity.

5. Which clinical problems are associated with endothelial cells?

Potential problems with endothelial cells include ineffective vascular constriction and the lack of surrounding tissue support that occurs in older individuals as muscle mass decreases. Hyperadrenocorticism due to glucocorticoid increase also diminishes muscle mass, resulting in endothelial damage. Immune and septic activity against endothelial cells will cause vasculitis. Heatstroke is a common cause of severe vasculitis.

6. Why is platelet adhesion clinically important?

Platelet adhesion is required for primary hemostasis. Platelets do not adhere to healthy endothelium. Ligands such as collagen and von Willebrand factor are involved with platelet adhesion and are sequestered in the subendothelium. Intact endothelial cells secrete antithrombotic substances such as *prostacyclin* (PGI_2), a prostaglandin, vasodilator, and platelet inhibitor. Platelets are also repelled by the negatively charged surface of intact endothelium. Most canine cases involving poor platelet adhesion are associated with hereditary von Willebrand factor decrease or dysfunction.

7. What is von Willebrand factor, and why is it a clinical concern?

Von Willebrand factor is a large protein synthesized by megakaryocytes and endothelial cells. It is necessary for platelet adhesion and is the carrier protein for coagulation factor VIII—hemophilia A factor. The von Willebrand molecule is made of a series of subunits. Larger subunits, stored in endothelial cells, are most effective binding platelets. These subunits are released in response to various stimuli. Deficiency of von Willebrand factor results in lack of platelet adhesion, resulting in primary hemostatic dysfunction.

8. Why is platelet aggregation clinically important?

When a blood vessel is damaged, vascular constriction and platelet adhesion begin to reduce the rate of blood flow through that vessel. As platelets adhere, they begin to change physically, promoting platelet-to-platelet aggregation. Platelets also begin to produce and secrete platelet chemotactic substances, effectively recruiting other platelets to the injured area. The most important of these is thromboxane A_2 (TXA_2), a product of arachidonic acid metabolism. Prostacyclin is a platelet antiaggregant. When primary hemostasis is in balance, PGI_2 and TXA_2 allow platelet aggregation to occur at the injury site but prevent platelet aggregation distal to the site. The clinical use of most nonsteroidal antiinflammatory drugs (NSAIDs) interferes with the production of these two substances, resulting in inbalance and lack of primary hemostasis.

9. What are the potential clinical problems associated with platelets in primary hemostasis?

The potential problems with platelets are twofold, quantitative and qualitative. Quantitative problems include thrombocytopenia and thrombocytosis. Severe thrombocytopenia, less than 30,000 platelets per microliter (μl), will result in primary hemostatic problems manifest by bleeding. Clinically significant thrombocytosis, greater than 1 million platelets/μl, is less predictable. Bleeding occurs at least as often as thrombotic disorders. Qualitative platelet disorders, or thrombocytopathia, result in dysfunctional platelets. Although these disorders are found in myeloproliferative disorders and in rare congenital problems, the most common cause of thrombocytopathia is the inappropriate use of NSAIDs.

10. What are the clinical manifestations of a primary hemostatic disorder?

Specific types of bleeding are the most common clinical manifestations of a primary hemostatic dysfunction. These include small reddish spots, *petechiae,* found in mucosal areas or in friction areas such as in the axilla or inguinal regions. Multiple coalescing petechiae are called *purpura.* Bruising or ecchymosis is another clinical manifestation of primary hemostatic dysfunction. Petechiae, mucosal bleeding, purpura, and ecchymoses are the most common manifestations of primary hemostatic dysfunction, that is, endothelial problems or platelet qualitative/quantitative disorders.

11. What is secondary hemostasis?

Secondary hemostasis is the process of blood coagulation. For convenience, the coagulation pathways, or "cascades," have been divided into the extrinsic, intrinsic, and common pathways. It is clinically useful to think of secondary hemostasis in terms of these three pathways, although much more interaction actually occurs between the pathways than is implied. All the enzymatic coagulation proteins (factors) circulate in inactive forms in plasma and become activated, sequentially, by numerous and diverse events, ultimately producing fibrin.

12. What are the essential components of secondary hemostasis?

a. Negatively charged phospholipid surface, most often provided by the inner bilayer of the platelet cytoplasmic membrane
b. Ionized calcium
c. Tissue factor (factor III), a glycoprotein that is part of the cytoplasmic membrane of most cells, including endothelial cells
d. Contact activation factors, including factors XII, XI, and the bradykinin precursors prekallikrein and high-molecular-weight kininogen
e. The remaining factors of the intrinsic pathway (factors IX and VIII), the extrinsic pathway (factor VII), and the common pathway (factors X, V, II, and fibrinogen)

13. What is the extrinsic pathway?

The *extrinsic pathway,* the most important of the three pathways in vivo, consists of factor VII activated by tissue factor (rarely called factor III) in the presence of ionized calcium (which is the elusive factor IV, but is never called that). Since tissue factor or tissue thromboplastin is extrinsic to the immediate area in and around blood vessels, the pathway has been named the "extrinsic" pathway. Activated factor VII in turn activates factor X in the common pathway. The remainder of the factors in the common pathway (after factor X is activated) include factors V, II (prothrombin), and I (fibrinogen), which are sequentially activated, producing fibrin. Fibrin stabilizes the platelet plug. Actually, activated prothrombin becomes thrombin, which among many other activities, cleaves fibrinogen to form fibrin.

14. What is the intrinsic pathway?

The *intrinsic pathway* consists of factors XII, XI, IX, and VIII. Factors XII and XI are called the *contact factors* because they are activated by contact with numerous other factors intrinsic to the vasculature. The additional contact factors are portions of the kinin system and include prekallikrein (PK) and high-molecular-weight kininogen (HMWK). Activation of the intrinsic pathway results in activation of the common pathway and, again, production of fibrin. It is interesting to note that deficiencies of factor XII, PK, and HMWK do not cause bleeding.

15. What is the common pathway?

The *common pathway* includes factors X, V, prothrombin (II) and fibrinogen (I).

Factor X, activated with ionized calcium, and activated factor V are bound to platelet membranes. This combination results in activation of prothrombin to thrombin that is bound to the site of injury. Thrombin is an active enzyme amplifying the coagulation pathways and forming fibrin from cleaved fibrinogen.

16. What anticoagulant is used when collecting blood for tests of secondary hemostasis (coagulation)?

The anticoagulant of choice is sodium citrate. It is important to add the correct amount of blood to anticoagulant: 9 parts blood to 1 part anticoagulant. Deviation from this ratio will significantly change the results (given in seconds), resulting in erroneous interpretation of results. Sodium citrate and ethylenediaminetetraacetic acid (EDTA) inhibit coagulation through calcium chelation. Sodium citrate is a relatively poor chelator of calcium. EDTA is an excellent chelator of calcium. Use of EDTA-anticoagulated blood in coagulation testing will cause unpredictable results. Heparin works as an anticoagulant by activating antithrombin III (ATIII), a natural inhibitor of many coagulation factors (all the proenzymes, except the nonenzymatic factors VIII, V, and fibrinogen). Heparin and EDTA are never used as anticoagulants when collecting blood for hemostasis testing.

17. What coagulation test examines the extrinsic and common pathways?

One-stage prothrombin time (OSPT), usually referred to as the *prothrombin time* (PT), examines the extrinsic and common pathways. PT examines factors VII (extrinsic pathway) and factors X, V, prothrombin (II) and fibrinogen (I) (common pathway). The basics of the test are the addition of calcium (factor IV) and tissue factor (TF; factor III) to warmed citrated plasma. If all the factors in the extrinsic and common pathways are quantitatively and qualitatively adequate, PT will be within the reference limits.

18. What coagulation test examines the intrinsic and common pathways?

The *activated partial thromboplastin time* (aPTT) examines the intrinsic and common pathways. The aPTT examines factors XII, XI, IX, and VIII (intrinsic pathway) and factors X, V, II, and I (common pathway). The basics of the test require the addition of an "activating substance," a phospholipid-based material (the "partial thromboplastin"), and calcium to warmed citrated plasma. If all the factors in the intrinsic and common pathways are quantitatively and qualitatively adequate, aPTT will be "normal."

The *activated coagulation time* (aCT) also examines the intrinsic and common pathways and is a useful "in-house" screening test for these pathways. Compared with aPTT, the aCT is insensitive to intrinsic and common pathway problems. If aCT is prolonged, aPTT will be prolonged. Also, aCT may be "normal" and aPTT prolonged. If a hemostatic problem is suspected and aCT is "normal," aPTT should be performed. In rare patients with prolonged thrombocytopenia, aCT may be prolonged and aPTT within reference limits.

19. Will platelet problems (thrombocytopenia, thrombocytosis, thrombocytopathia) affect prothrombin time or activated partial thromboplastin time?

No, because both tests use a platelet substitute in the testing process. PT and aPTT are not affected by platelet problems. The platelet substitute in the PT is tissue thromboplastin. The platelet substitute in the aPTT is the "partial thromboplastin."

20. What is thrombin time, or thrombin clotting time?

Thrombin time (TT), also called *thrombin clotting time* (TCT), is both a qualitative and a quantitative test of fibrinogen. If there is a low concentration of fibrinogen or if fibrinogen is dysfunctional, the TT will be prolonged. The basics of the test require the addition of thrombin (activated prothrombin; factor IIa) to warmed citrated plasma.

21. What is antithrombin III?

Antithrombin III (AT-III) is a natural inhibitor of some of the coagulation factors (all the proenzymes). The nonenzymatic factors VIII, V, and fibrinogen are not affected by AT-III. When the proenzymes are activated, AT-III, especially in the presence of heparin compounds, will effectively inhibit the activated factors that become enzymes. AT-III bound to endothelial cells participates in controlling the coagulation process at the periphery of the vascular injury site.

22. What are proteins C and S?

Proteins C and S are vitamin K–dependent anticoagulant factors that, in the presence of ionized calcium and negatively charged phospholipid, are potent inactivators of activated factors V and VIII. The activated protein C–protein S complex also initiates fibrinolysis.

23. What is tertiary hemostasis or fibrinolysis?

The final stage of hemostasis is repair of vascular damage, lysis of the fibrin clot, and reestablishment of vascular patency and normal blood flow. Fibrinolysis is mediated by *plasmin,* a potent proteolytic enzyme. Plasmin circulates as an inactive precursor, *plasminogen*. Once activated to plasmin, plasminogen degrades cross-linked fibrin within clots to release FDPs, including the cross-linked fragment known as D-dimer. Activators of plasminogen include *tissue plasminogen activator* (tPA) and *urokinase plasminogen activator* (uPA). Vascular endothelial cells synthesize and release tPA in response to many stimuli, including bradykinin. uPA is synthesized by the kidneys.

Excessive fibrinolysis, the main dysfunctional state of tertiary hemostasis, is an uncommon disease, with testing abnormalities similar to those of secondary hemostasis.

21. PLATELETOPATHIES

1. What is the clinical presentation of thrombocytopenia in dogs and cats?

The clinical impression of thrombocytopenia, thrombocytopathia, and endothelial cell problems cannot easily be differentiated based on clinical presentation. The only somewhat specific clinical signs are petechiae, purpura, and ecchymosis. This type of bleeding is often associated with mucous membranes or friction areas such as the axilla or inguinal areas. Other, nonspecific signs may include hematuria, epistaxis, hematochezia, and hemoptysis. Fever is often present in an actively bleeding animal. If the buccal mucosal bleeding time is prolonged in a dog or cat with appropriate platelet numbers, the prolongation is probably caused by thrombocytopathia or endothelial problems. Remember that thrombocytosis causes unpredictable clinical signs.

2. What is the buccal mucosal bleeding time?

The buccal mucosal bleeding time (BMBT) is used when platelet dysfunction (thrombocytopathia, von Willebrand's disease) or endothelial cell dysfunction is suspected. In dogs or cats with platelet counts less than 70,000/μl, the BMBT is often prolonged. If petechiae are present, a BMBT will add no additional information and need not be performed because petechiae are specific for a primary system dysfunction. Therefore, in effect, the use of the BMBT is reserved for nonthrombocytopenic patients with evidence of primary hemostatic disorders. The patient is placed in lateral recumbency, and a firm (not tight) gauze tie is used to fold back and expose the buccal mucosa. Hand movement tends to affect the test, so a gauze tie is used. A nonvascular area is selected. A guillotine-like "bleeding time device" (e.g., Simplate II) is placed *lightly* on this area and triggered. A stopwatch is started. At 30-second intervals and without touching the wound, blood leaking from the wound is soaked up. The time from the creation of the minor incision(s) until blood stops flowing from the wound is the BMBT. In dogs and cats, the BMBT reference interval in my practice is 1.7 to 4.2 seconds. Most results are near the low end of the reference interval.

3. Can a "guarded" scalpel or the "toenail" bleeding time be used?

These "scalpel" and "toenail" tests should *not* be used. Although all these tests, including the BMBT, are somewhat crude, at least the BMBT has built-in controls; the other tests do not. The BMBT has withstood scientific scrutiny in the form of published articles in the veterinary literature.

4. Which etiologies should be considered with a thrombocytopenic patient?

Thrombocytopenia is seldom "idiopathic." Not uncovering an etiology simply underlines limited diagnostic abilities as regards this common clinical presentation. Although platelet numbers can be affected by severe hemorrhage, thrombocytopenia is seldom severe and is usually >70,000 cells/µl. A careful history with specific questions regarding anticoagulant rodenticides, other drugs, recent vaccinations, and tick infestations is essential. An infectious or immune-mediated etiology is the most likely cause of thrombocytopenia. Serology for the common tick-borne diseases only examines the "tip of the iceberg." In fact, unless a specific etiology is uncovered, 3 to 4 weeks of appropriate antimicrobial therapy is indicated in conjunction with other forms of therapy.

5. What do hemogram reports indicating the platelet count is "adequate" really mean?

The numbers of platelets associated with "adequate" platelet numbers do differ somewhat between laboratories, but this is a moot point. It is essential to obtain an actual platelet count by estimation, manual counts, or instrument counts obtained in the production of the hemogram. Ideally, the platelet count determined by the instrument should be corroborated by the technologist's or clinical pathologist's visual estimation; these should be in close agreement. This is somewhat problematic in feline hematology because more than 60% of feline blood specimens contain platelet clumps despite numerous efforts to stop clumping. The word "adequate" in relation to platelet counts in a patient without observable hemorrhage or suspected occult hemorrhage is usually satisfactory. All instrument-produced hemograms include a direct platelet count that may or may not actually be reported.

6. What does mean platelet volume mean?

The *mean platelet volume* (MPV) is the platelet equivalent of the red blood cell mean cell volume (MCV). An increased MPV indicates that mean platelet size is increased—the presence of macroplatelets. Macroplatelets are usually an indication of young or reactive platelets responding to increased thrombopoiesis—increased concentrations of thrombopoietin. (Apparently, macroplatelets are observed along with reduced platelet counts in Cavalier King Charles Spaniels.) A decreased MPV indicates decreased mean platelet size or presence of microplatelets. Microplatelets may be the only early indication of complement-mediated, immune-mediated attack against platelets.

7. Can bone marrow examination be accomplished when thrombocytopenia is severe?

Bone marrow aspiration or biopsy is necessary if the cause of the thrombocytopenia has not been ascertained. Any questionable cytopenias or multiple cell line cytopenias necessitate marrow examination to aid in determining etiology. Hemorrhage, if present at all with severely thrombocytopenic patients, is usually modest and easily controlled by pressure. Hemorrhage is uncommon or modest in thrombocytopenic patients in general. When platelet-related hemorrhage is observed and considered significant, both reduced platelet numbers and platelet dysfunctional states (a combination) are probable.

8. Should a hemostasis profile be performed on a thrombocytopenic patient?

Tests may be clinically useful and include prothrombin time (PT), activated partial thromboplastin time (aPTT), thrombin time (TT), examination of blood for schistocytes, and determination of fibrin-fibrinogen degradation products (FDPs). None of these tests should be prolonged or positive with isolated thrombocytopenia. Abnormal tests would suggest the potential of a more involved process or other etiologies. One consideration would be disseminated intravascular coagulation (DIC) inducing thrombocytopenia. BMBT will be prolonged with severe thrombocytopenia and will not be useful. Activated coagulation time (aCT) may be prolonged if thrombocytopenia is severe (fewer than 10,000 platelets/μl).

9. Identify general categories or processes that cause thrombocytopenia.

Infectious disease is statistically the most common etiology of thrombocytopenia in dogs and cats. Infections may include rickettsial diseases and systemic mycoses in dogs and retroviral diseases in cats. Toxoplasmosis and hemobartonellosis can also cause thrombocytopenia in cats. Immune-mediated disease is also an important category. Neoplasia, especially lymphoproliferative neoplasia, has been associated with both immune-mediated hemolytic disease and thrombocytopenia.

10. What is (are) the best test(s) to help determine the etiology of thrombocytopenia?

In a clinical setting the etiology of thrombocytopenia is often determined by exclusion. Flow cytometric tests for detection of platelet antibodies in serum have largely preempted the older platelet factor 3 (PF3) test and bone marrow megakaryocyte immunofluorescence. None of these tests can consistently differentiate a primary immune-mediated cause from a secondary cause (e.g., infectious etiology), and time and availability of such testing are major considerations. Antinuclear antibody titers, if significantly elevated and with other considerations, may indicate an immune etiology such as systemic lupus erythematosus (SLE).

11. What are the common infectious etiologies that cause thrombocytopenia?

Geographic considerations often affect which infectious etiologies are common and therefore which tests are selected. A good historical examination considers travel. Testing for infection includes serology for *Rickettsia* and *Ehrlichia* (including *Ehrlichia platys* where appropriate). Testing for *E. canis, E. equi,* and *Rickettsia rickettsii* must be considered. Heartworm disease and leptospirosis are additional considerations. Retroviral examination in cats is recommended (FeLV, FIV, FIP). Ehrlichial infections have been reported in cats. Babesiosis must be considered in dogs.

12. Are fresh whole blood or platelet transfusions effective?

In most thrombocytopenic patients, hemorrhage is not significant and use of blood products is not necessary. Blood products should be considered if intracranial, intraocular, or periadrenal hemorrhage is occurring or suspected. The effect of fresh blood or platelet-rich plasma on the total patient platelet count is problematic in the long term. Transfused platelets are rapidly destroyed. Unless multiple units of blood products are used, whole blood or platelet concentrates will not result in a notable sustained increase in platelet counts. Typed and matched red cell concentrates are encouraged if anemia is present.

13. What causes thrombocytosis?

Three general categories should be considered when platelet counts consistently exceed 1 million platelets/μl:

a. Bone marrow disorders
b. Disorders secondary to disease states
c. Physiologic thrombocytosis

14. What is essential thrombocythemia?

Essential thrombocythemia is a rare myeloproliferative disorder characterized by persistent and often extreme thrombocytosis. This disease is also referred to as "idiopathic thrombocythemia" and "primary hemorrhagic thrombocythemia." Both hemorrhage and thrombosis have been described in dogs. Nonregenerative and regenerative anemia, hypogranular macroplatelets, basophilia, and spurious hyperkalemia have been observed in animals ultimately diagnosed as having essential thrombocythemia.

15. What is reactive thrombocytosis?

Reactive thrombocytosis, or secondary thrombocytosis, is characterized by transiently increased platelet counts in conditions other than myeloproliferative disorders. These conditions include neoplasia, gastrointestinal inflammatory disorders (e.g., pancreatitis, inflammatory bowel disease, hepatitis, colitis), immune-mediated disease, blood loss or hemorrhage causing iron deficiency, trauma (e.g., fractures), drug therapy (e.g., glucocorticoids), and postsplenectomy status in dogs.

16. What is physiologic thrombocytosis?

Physiologic thrombocytosis results from increased mobilization of platelets from splenic and nonsplenic (perhaps pulmonary) pools. Physiologic thrombocytosis may also result from stress and prolonged exercise.

17. What is thrombocytopathia?

Thrombocytopathia is a term used to describe platelet qualitative or functional disorders. Dysfunctional platelets are suspected when there is clinical hemorrhage (petechiae, purpura, ecchymosis) despite appropriate or mildly decreased platelet numbers. BMBT is often prolonged.

18. Identify causes of acquired platelet dysfunction associated with hemorrhage.

Acquired platelet dysfunction is suspected when hemorrhage associated with primary hemostatic disorders is observed and thrombocytopenia and vascular disorders have been ruled out. Causes include uremia, dysproteinemia, infectious agents, envenomation by insects or snakes, hepatic disease, neoplasia, and numerous drugs, including those also suspected of causing thrombocytopenia. The most common acquired platelet dysfunction in cats and dogs is drug-induced platelet dysfunction.

19. Identify causes of acquired platelet dysfunction associated with hypercoagulation or thrombosis.

This disorder is also called "platelet hyperresponsiveness" and "prothrombotic state." Cause are disparate and include diabetes mellitus, hyperadrenocorticism, protein-losing diseases (e.g., protein-losing gastrointestinal and renal diseases), neoplasia (e.g., sarcoma, carcinoma), and infectious processes (e.g., heartworm disease, feline infectious peritonitis).

20. What is the most common inherited platelet dysfunctional disease?

Von Willebrand's disease (vWd) is the most common canine hereditary bleeding disorder. Qualitative or quantitative problems with the large plasma glycoprotein known as *von Willebrand factor* (vWf) cause vWd. Other inherited platelet dysfunctional states include canine thromasthenic thrombopathia (observed in Great Pyrenees and otter hounds), bassethound thrombopathia, Spitz thrombopathia, and storage pool deficiency or cocker spaniel bleeding disorder.

Chédiak-Higashi syndrome in cats and canine cyclic hematopoiesis in grey collies are also platelet dysfunctional diseases.

21. How does von Willebrand's disease affect platelets?

Von Willebrand factor is produced by bone marrow megakaryocytes and by vascular endothelial cells. vWf is found adsorbed to platelet surfaces and adsorbed to subendothelial collagen. vWf is essential for platelet adhesion to subendothelial collagen and is also involved in platelet aggregation. The clinical signs of vWd are similar to those of other thrombopathias and most often manifest as mucous membrane hemorrhage (hematuria, gastrointestinal bleeding, epistaxis) or, in severe disease states, as significant hemorrhage.

22. How is von Willebrand's disease best diagnosed?

Routine universal tests of secondary hemostasis, including PT and aPTT, are unaffected by vWd. The disease can be diagnosed using laboratory tests for direct evaluation of the vWf gene. Genetic testing using molecular technology is accomplished in specialized laboratories. Quantitation is done through rocket immunoelectrophoresis or enzyme-linked immunosorbent assay (ELISA) technology. Collection and handling can affect these tests. It is not advisable to obtain blood from a stressed, ill, or recently exercised animal. Females in heat should not be tested. A clean venipuncture is required. Blood is carefully placed (to prevent hemolysis) into a tube with sodium citrate as an anticoagulant, with strict attention placed on the essential ratio of 9 parts blood to 1 part sodium citrate. Ideally, nonhemolyzed plasma (hemolysis causes unpredictable results in vWf quantitation) should be removed using plastic pipettes, and the plasma should be placed in plastic tubes with plastic stoppers. The plasma should be transported to the laboratory on ice or frozen until examination.

23. Is buccal mucosal bleeding time useful as a screening test for von Willebrand's disease?

BMBT is best used as a crude presurgical assessment of the status of primary hemostasis and as such will be prolonged in most veterinary patients with moderate to severe decreases in vWf. A prolonged BMBT requires prophylactic treatment. An appropriate BMBT does not necessarily ensure appropriate surgical hemostasis, since anesthetics and drugs may affect platelet function in patients with modestly reduced vWf.

22. DISORDERS OF SECONDARY HEMOSTASIS (COAGULATION DEFECTS)

1. What is secondary hemostasis, and what are associated tests?

Secondary hemostasis is the sequential activation of coagulation proteins (factors) resulting in conversion of soluble fibrinogen to insoluble fibrin. For convenience, the coagulation proteins are grouped into the intrinsic, extrinsic, and common coagulation pathways.

Prothrombin time (PT) tests for quantitative and qualitative adequacy of proteins in the extrinsic and common coagulation pathways. *Activated partial thromboplastin time* (aPTT) tests for qualitative and quantitative adequacy of proteins in the intrinsic and common pathways. *Thrombin time* (TT) tests for quantitative and qualitative aspects of fibrinogen. Depending on the affected pathway, the appropriate test will be prolonged if a single factor or factors are inadequate quantitatively or qualitatively.

2. What are the clinical signs of secondary (coagulation) defects?

Bleeding into tissues or body cavities is most characteristic of coagulation defects. Coagulation defects often result in hematoma formation; pleural, peritoneal, or retroperitoneal hemorrhage; hemarthrosis; and hemorrhage between the planes of large muscle groups. Delayed bleeding or rebleeding is also characteristic. Usually, venipuncture is uncomplicated. Mucosal or frictional area bleeding is uncommon.

3. How are acquired coagulation defects differentiated from inherited defects?

Inherited coagulation defects often occur in animals at a young age and with a history of previous hemorrhage. Siblings (especially male) and other relatives probably will also have bleeding defects. Inherited coagulation defects usually are associated with a single coagulation protein. Acquired coagulation defects occur at any age, and there is no history of previous bleeding or affected relatives. Acquired coagulation defects often affect multiple coagulation proteins.

4. What is the most common acquired coagulopathy?

Toxicosis with anticoagulant rodenticides is the most common acquired secondary hemostatic disorder. This toxicosis is sometimes difficult to diagnose because bleeding is often occult, occurring in body cavities or between planes of large muscle groups. No specific and relatively easy laboratory test can corroborate this diagnosis, although tests can strongly suggest rodenticide toxicosis. The most common clinical treatment errors are inadequate dosages of vitamin K_1 and inadequate duration of treatment.

5. What are the vitamin K–dependent coagulation proteins?

The four major vitamin K–dependent coagulation proteins involved in functional clotting activity are factor II (also known as prothrombin), factor VII, factor IX, and factor X. Proteins C and S are also vitamin K–dependent proteins but have anticoagulant activity.

6. What does vitamin K dependence mean?

Factors II, VII, IX, and X are produced by hepatocytes in an inactive or precursor form. To become functional, glutamic acid in the precursor protein must be carboxylated. This is called gamma-carboxyglutamic acid. The carboxylation process requires the presence of vitamin K. In the absence of vitamin K, these proteins are only present in nonfunctional forms.

7. How do anticoagulant rodenticides affect coagulation?

The active hydroquinone form of vitamin K is necessary for the carboxylation and epoxidation required to change the precursor proteins into the functional forms of factors II, VII, IX, and X. Hydroquinone is converted into the inactive epoxide form of vitamin K as these factors are activated. The active form, hydroquinone, must be regenerated by enzymatic reductions. Anticoagulant rodenticides act by inhibiting the reduction reaction. This quickly reduces the concentration of the hydroquinone form of vitamin K and thus the concentration of functional vitamin K–dependent proteins.

8. How can vitamin K be inhibited without involving rodenticides?

Because vitamin K is fat soluble and is taken up by the intestinal tract with fatty acids, conditions that lead to maldigestion or malabsorption of fats in the diet can also cause reduction in vitamin K concentration. Conditions to rule out include infiltrative bowel disease, lymphangiectasia, exocrine pancreatic deficiency, and biliary obstruction. Bile acids facilitate intestinal absorption of fat. Prolonged oral antibiotic therapy with second-generation and third-generation cephalosporins may lead to mild vitamin K deficiency as the result of decreased bacterial synthesis. These conditions should be considered clinically for completeness but are infrequent causes of severe vitamin K depletion.

9. Identify first- and second-generation rodenticides causing toxicosis and the resulting clinical considerations.

The first-generation hydroxycoumarins included warfarin and dicoumarin. Second-generation hydroxycoumarins are brodifacoum, bromadiolone, and difenacoum. The first-generation indanediones include diphacinone, chlorphacinone, pindone, and valone. The second-generation hydroxycoumarins and first-generation indanediones are highly potent compared with first-generation hydroxycoumarins.

Toxicity with these potent coumarins may last for several weeks or even, in worst-case scenarios, several months. Therefore, therapy should be continued for at least 3 weeks, followed by 1 week of testing to ensure relapse does not occur.

10. How soon after rodenticide ingestion will clinical signs of toxicosis manifest?

Manifestation of clinical signs largely depends on ingested dosage of the intoxicant and activity of the patient. The more potent coumarins may result in hemorrhagic tendency within hours. Intoxication may take as long as 2 days to 1 week. More active patients tend to hemorrhage earlier than more sedentary patients.

11. What is the best approach to diagnosis of vitamin K inhibition?

Coagulation factor VII in the extrinsic pathway is vitamin K dependent, has the shortest half-life, and therefore the shortest inactivation time; thus tests that examine factor VII, among others, should be performed. PT examines factors VII, X, V, II, and I, and the PIVKA test examines factors VII, X, and II (the proteins produced but not activated by vitamin K are called the "proteins induced by vitamin K absence," or PIVKA proteins). Either test probably will become prolonged hours before the patient manifests clinical signs. Eventually, as the inactive form of other vitamin K–dependent proteins predominate, the other universal tests of coagulation, activated coagulation time (aCT) and aPTT will also become prolonged. It is important to note that if PT or the PIVKA test is not prolonged and aPTT is prolonged, for example, vitamin K inhibition is highly unlikely.

12. What is the appropriate therapeutic approach to vitamin K inhibition?

If ingestion of the toxicant is recent, emesis or gastric lavage may prevent toxicosis. Once hemorrhage is manifest or suspected, emesis and gastric lavage are contraindicated because of the risk of inducing further hemorrhage. If the amount and sites of patient hemorrhage are not considered clinically significant, vitamin K_1 therapy (phytonadione, phylloquinone, or phytomenadione) should be administered. Since vitamin K is fat soluble, vitamin K_1 therapy is best administered by subcutaneous (SC) or oral routes. Intramuscular (IM) injection does not result in appropriate blood concentrations of vitamin K more quickly than using oral and SC routes, and intramuscular hematoma formation is probable. Intravenous (IV) vitamin K also does not result in appropriate blood concentrations of vitamin K more quickly than using oral or SC routes, and anaphylaxis may occur. If the toxicant is one of the first-generation hydroxycoumarins and the animal no longer is exposed to this rodenticide, 5 days of appropriate therapy will suffice. If the toxicant is an indanedione or second-generation hydroxycoumarin, 3 weeks of therapy will usually suffice, as long as testing for an additional week is negative.

13. Can other forms of vitamin K be used to treat vitamin K inhibition in small animals?

Vitamin K_3 (menadione or menophthone) is the only other form of vitamin K that should or could be used. Although cheaper, K_3 is much less effective, and appropriate blood concentrations are often not achieved for several days. Vitamin K_3 therapy should never substitute for vitamin K_1 therapy.

14. What is the appropriate therapeutic approach to a patient hemorrhaging from vitamin K inhibition?

A minimum of several hours is required after administration of vitamin K_1 to initiate vitamin K–dependent factor activation. Therefore, supplying activated vitamin K coagulation proteins through administration of typed and (minor) crossmatched fresh or fresh frozen plasma is indicated. Of course, vitamin K_1 therapy should be administered concurrently with the blood product. Only if the patient's red cell mass appears reduced should a typed and (major and minor) crossmatched red cell product (whole blood; packed red cells) be considered.

15. What type of testing is recommended once vitamin K1 therapy is stopped?

Approximately 3 hours after the last dosage of vitamin K_1, PT or PIVKA testing is performed and the results considered as baseline data. At 48 hours and again at 96 hours after baseline testing, these tests should be repeated. Any prolongation in either of these tests, at either time, requires reinstating vitamin K_1 therapy for a minimum of several weeks, with additional retesting. During the initial 96-hour postbaseline testing period, any evidence of fever or lack of appetite requires examination because rebleeding is likely.

16. Describe secondary hemostatic disorders other than rodenticide toxicosis.

Hepatic disease, disseminated intravascular coagulation (DIC), and circulating antibodies to coagulation proteins all can induce clinical signs similar to those of toxicosis, including hematoma formation, hemorrhage into body cavities or between large muscle groups, and hemarthrosis. Because PT and aPTT are often prolonged, it is clinically difficult to differentiate between hepatic disease and DIC, especially DIC secondary to hepatic disease. History, clinical impression, platelet counts, fibrin and fibrinogen degradation product concentrations, and hepatic biochemical and ultrasonographic examination may be helpful. Circulating antibodies to coagulation proteins have been rarely reported in the veterinary literature. A lupus anticoagulant resulting in thrombotic disease has been reported in one dog. Factor VIII inhibitors resulting in hemorrhage have been described in hemophilic dogs.

17. Can mast cell neoplasia result in systemic, multisite hemorrhage?

Heparin is a physiologic inhibitor of coagulation. Mast cell tumors contain significant concentrations of heparin, so a hemorrhagic tendency may result. Heparin works with antithrombin III, inhibiting many activated coagulation proteins and resulting in prolongation of PT and aPTT.

18. What are the inherited coagulopathies?

Single coagulation protein (factor) deficiencies of virtually all known factors have been described. Usually these factor deficiencies manifest in young animals. The classic hemophilias inherited in a sex-linked recessive pattern are factor VIII deficiency and factor IX deficiency. These diseases have prolonged aPTT and appropriate PT. Interestingly, although aPTT is prolonged in factor XII deficiency, there is no bleeding tendency. The inheritance pattern of the other coagulation proteins is autosomal dominant. Factor I (fibrinogen) deficiency has both autosomal dominant and recessive patterns of inheritance. Factor X deficiency is autosomal recessive. In the Devon Rex cat, vitamin K–dependent protein deficiency is currently considered to have an autosomal recessive inheritance pattern.

19. What are the genetic expectations of the sex-linked (X-linked) hemophilias: hemophilia A (VIII deficiency) and hemophilia B (IX deficiency)?

Unless the male is a modest hemophiliac, it is improbable that he will grow to breeding age. Typically, hemophilia is a male disease with female carriers. If a carrier female is bred to a normal male, the possibilities include 25% normal females, 25% carrier females, 25% normal males, and 25% affected males. Differentiating the males will depend on the presence of hemorrhage in the affected male and prolonged aPTT. With hemophilia A, factor VIII concentration will be low. Both the carrier female and the normal female will have appropriate aPTTs. However, the carrier female will have much lower factor VIII concentration than her normal female sibling.

If a hemophilic male is bred to a normal female, all the females of this breeding will be obligate carriers, and all the males will be normal.

23. DISSEMINATED INTRAVASCULAR COAGULATION AND THROMBOSIS

1. What is disseminated intravascular coagulation (DIC)?

Disseminated intravascular coagulation is the result of a primary inflammatory or tissue-damaging process. DIC is a complex syndrome involving a transition between accelerated activation of platelets, coagulation proteins, and plasmin evolving into consumption of coagulation proteins, platelets, and inhibitors of fibrinolysis. Coagulation is accelerated systemically when the following occur:

a. Blood comes into contact with tissues containing tissue thromboplastin or subendothelial collagen.
b. Significant quantities of circulating white blood cells, inflammatory mediators, or cytokines are present.
c. Significant contact occurs between coagulation proteins and phospholipids from platelets or red blood cells (RBCs).
d. Circulating tissue debris is present from RBCs, tissue necrosis, tumor tissue, or heartworms.

Uncontrolled coagulation leads to rapid consumption of platelets, consumption or degradation of coagulation proteins, and consumption or degradation of natural anticoagulants—DIC.

2. How is DIC diagnosed?

The diagnosis of DIC is based on clinical suspicion, knowledge of the pathophysiologic mechanisms responsible in associated diseases, and abnormal serial tests of hemostasis indicative of this secondary process. The clinical signs of DIC depend on the phase the patient is experiencing. The phase of DIC depends on the intensity of the underlying disease, concentration and variety of inhibitors present, and length of time the coagulation mechanisms are exposed to the initiators. An ideal hemostasis laboratory profile includes the prothrombin time (PT), activated partial thromboplastin time (aPTT), platelet count, fibrinogen concentration, fibrin-fibrinogen degradation product (FDP) concentration, and antithrombin III (AT-III) concentration. These tests should be serially evaluated to determine trends in any patient thought to have a primary disease likely to initiate DIC but with nondiagnostic test results.

3. Describe the phases of DIC.

a. *Peracute* (hypercoagulable) *phase,* characterized by no or few overt clinical signs
b. *Acute* (consumptive) *phase,* characterized by venipuncture oozing or modest hemorrhage
c. *Chronic phase,* characterized by no clinical signs of oozing blood

4. What are the laboratory test expectations in the peracute or hypercoagulable phase of DIC?

The PT and aPTT are within reference limits or have a shortened time (below reference limits) in the peracute phase. Platelet numbers are normal, which should increase clinical suspicion because platelet counts in most systemic inflammatory disorders are at the upper end of the reference interval or above the reference interval. Fibrinogen concentration is appropriate or modestly declining, which should also increase clinical suspicion because fibrinogen concentration in most systemic inflammatory disorders is at the upper end of the reference interval or above the reference interval. FDP and AT-III concentrations are within the reference range.

5. What are the laboratory test expectations in the acute or consumptive phase of DIC?

The laboratory findings in the acute phase are most characteristic of DIC. This includes prolongation of the PT and aPPT, decreasing platelet numbers, decreasing fibrinogen concentrations, increasing FDP concentrations, and decreasing concentrations of AT-III.

6. What are the laboratory test expectations in the chronic phase of DIC?

The PT and aPTT remain prolonged in the chronic phase. Platelet numbers remain decreased. Fibrinogen concentration is most unpredictable and may be within reference limits or severely decreased. The concentration of FDPs depends on the adequacy of the mononuclear phagocytic system (MPS). If the MPS in the liver and spleen is not overwhelmed by tissue and hemostatic debris, FDPs will remain appropriate or mildly elevated. If the MPS is fully saturated with tissue and hemostatic debris, FDPs will be notably elevated. The concentrations of AT-III may remain decreased in more fulminant clinical situations or return toward baseline or the reference interval in less fulminant situations.

7. Is the activated coagulation (aCT) time useful in the laboratory diagnosis of DIC?

Activated coagulation time (aCT) examines the intrinsic and common coagulation pathways. Therefore aCT identifies the same coagulation protein problems as aPTT. Accomplished serially, aCT will help define trends. It is much less sensitive than the aPTT; aCT requires marked deficiencies in coagulation proteins before becoming prolonged. If a process associated with DIC is suspected and the aCT result is within reference limits, aPTT should be performed. If the aCT result is prolonged, however, there is no need to perform aPTT because it also will be prolonged. Remember that there is potential for prolongation of aCT if the platelet count is greatly decreased. Marked thrombocytopenia will not cause prolongation of aPTT.

8. List clinical diseases and their initiators in DIC.

a. Systemic inflammatory response syndrome (SIRS) initiates DIC by exposure of subendothelial collagen, accelerating the immune response, release of inflammatory mediators, and in pancreatitis, release of trypsin. Uncontrolled immune-mediated cellular destruction results from circulating RBC membrane phospholipid, cellular debris, and cytokine release.

b. Trauma and burns can initiate DIC by similar mechanisms to SIRS and immune-mediated disease.

c. Metabolic acidosis and severe shock result in exposure of subendothelial collagen. Shock also accelerates the immune response and prevents clearance of activated coagulation proteins and delivery of coagulation protein inhibitors.

c. Neoplasia exposes subendothelial collagen and results in increased concentrations of intravascular tissue debris.

d. Hepatosplenic disease results in inadequate production of coagulation proteins and inadequate clearance of activated coagulation proteins and tissue debris.

e. Heartworm disease results in increased circulation of tissue thromboplastin.

f. Envenomation activates coagulation factor X.

g. Heatstroke exposes subendothelial collagen.

h. Endotoxemia can cause activation of coagulation proteins.

9. What is the logical treatment approach to DIC?

Successful therapy in DIC depends on early suspicion and detection in critically ill animals. Ameliorating or mitigating the primary instigating process is an essential component of DIC therapy. A logical approach to DIC treatment includes promotion of capillary flow, support of target organs where microthrombi may cause ischemia or hemorrhage, coagulation factor replacement therapy, and administration of heparin as needed.

10. How is therapy in DIC monitored?

Plasma antithrombin activity is the key test for both diagnosis and monitoring of DIC. The activity of AT-III declines in early DIC as this endogenous anticoagulant is consumed. Activity less than 80% (the plasma pool AT-III concentration is considered 100%) is considered diagnostic for DIC in humans. When AT-III concentration falls below 60% in critically ill humans, a 96% mortality rate is described. Concentrations less than 90% should be continuously monitored. Clinical experience in dogs suggests that AT-III concentrations less than 80% are indicative of DIC. Concentrations less than 60% indicate risk for thrombosis or DIC and require heparin therapy and AT-III replacement. Concentrations less than 30% are critical, with immediate risk for thrombosis, DIC, and death. These patients require heparin and aggressive and immediate AT-III replacement therapy.

11. What is thrombophilia?

A coordinated interaction and regulation between endothelium, platelets, coagulation factors, and fibrinolysis are necessary for appropriate hemostasis. Alterations in Virchow's triad (changes in blood flow, alteration of coagulation factors, and endothelial damage) provide the baseline of thromboembolic disease. Hypercoagulability or prothombotic state, or *thrombophilia,* denotes a predisposition to increased thrombotic risk. Thrombophilia comprises several congenital, familial, and acquired disorders of the hemostatic system that predispose a patient to thromboembolic events. Deficiencies in inhibitors of coagulation (AT-III, protein C) are known to potentiate thrombosis. Impaired fibrinolysis also potentiates thrombosis.

12. Identify disorders predisposing to thrombus formation and thromboembolization.

Immune-mediated disease (hemolysis or thrombocytopenia, vasculitis, amyloidosis, phlebitis), infection, parasitism, neoplasia (e.g., hemangiosarcoma), protein-losing nephropathy or gastroenteropathy (loss of AT-III), and trauma (intravenous catheters, irritating or hyperosmolar substances) are factors that predispose to thrombus formation and thromboembolization.

13. Identify alterations in blood flow that predispose to thrombus formation and thromboembolization.

Hypovolemia caused by shock, trauma, burns, or organic disease increases thrombotic risk. Cardiac disease, including vegetative endocarditis, valvular insufficiency, and vascular abnormalities, may also predispose to thromboembolization. Congestive heart failure (CHF) and other hemodynamic disorders are also other risk factors.

14. What are the clinical manifestations of thrombosis?

Thrombosis can occur in veins, arteries, capillaries, and heart chambers. Localized vascular obstruction and embolization of the thrombi result in the clinical manifestations of thrombosis, which are variable in nature and severity depending on location and size of the thrombus. Acute dyspnea is often associated with pulmonary thrombosis. Some patients develop hemoptysis. Those with infarction or embolization in the genitourinary system can present with hematuria, abdominal pain, and abdominal splinting. Embolization of viscera may cause vomiting and fecal or urinary incontinence. Distal aortic emboli in cats results in marked pain in the affected limb, which lacks a pulse and is cool on palpation. The affected limb may be pale.

15. How is thrombosis diagnosed?

Diagnosis of thrombosis usually requires sophisticated diagnostic techniques, including digital subtraction angiography, contrast venography and arteriography, radioactive fibrinogen scanning, impedance plethysmography, and Doppler ultrasonography. Abnormal scintigraphic ventilation or perfusion scans increase the index of suspicion for thrombotic disease.

16. Without the availability of specialized studies, how can the clinical laboratory help in the diagnosis of prothrombotic or thrombotic states?

Routine universal tests of hemostasis such as PT and aPTT are useful in detecting hypercoagulable DIC states. In fact, the ability of the laboratory to perform hemostasis screening beyond the routine PT and aPTT is the secret for effective prothrombotic state screening. For example, decreasing concentration of AT-III or protein C increases the probability of thrombotic risk or actual thrombosis. Photometric assays of platelet aggregation may assist in monitoring antiplatelet therapy by helping to determine pharmacologic or pathologic alterations in platelet function.

17. What does the presence of fibrin-fibrinogen degradation products mean?

Fibrin-fibrinogen degradation products (FDPs), also known as fibrin-fibrinogen split products (FSPs), are the result of the conversion of plasminogen to plasmin and the resultant digestion of both cross-linked and non-cross-linked fibrin and fibrinogen. The presence of these products, without supporting historical, clinical, or laboratory aberrations, is difficult to interpret. In patients with modest compromise of the mononuclear phagocytic system (MPS), FDPs are often present if there has been trauma and significant hematoma formation or intracavity hemorrhage. In patients at risk for DIC or thrombosis with an effective MPS, FDPs will usually not be present until the process is fulminant. However, it is important to realize that the presence or absence of FDPs does not confirm or rule out diagnosis of DIC or thrombosis.

When plasmin directs enzymatic activity to cross-linked fibrin monomers, in the presence of fibronectin, D-dimers are produced. Although the presence of D-dimers plays an important role in the diagnosis of DIC in human medicine, their presence in nonhuman animal species is currently difficult to interpret. In my experience with numerous D-dimer test systems, there are excessive numbers of false-positive tests.

Hemostasis

BIBLIOGRAPHY

Bateman SW, Mathews KA, Abrams-Ogg ACG: Disseminated intravascular coagulation in dogs: review of the literature, *J Vet Emerg Crit Care* 8:29-44, 1998.

Bell WR: The physiology of disseminated intravascular coagulation, *Semin Hematol* 31:19-25, 1994.

Boudreaux MK: Acquired platelet dysfunction. In Feldman BF, Zinkl JG, Jain NC, editors: *Schalm's veterinary hematology,* ed 5, Baltimore, 2000, Lippincott, pp 496-500.

Brooks M: Von Willebrand disease. In Feldman BF, Zinkl JG, Jain NC, editors: *Schalm's veterinary hematology,* ed 5, Baltimore, 2000, Lippincott, pp 509-515.

Darien BJ: Acquired coagulopathy. V. Thrombosis. In Feldman BF, Zinkl JG, Jain NC, editors: *Schalm's veterinary hematology,* ed 5, Lippincott, Baltimore, 2000, pp 574-580.

Darien BJ: Fibrinolytic system. In Feldman BF, Zinkl JG, Jain NC, editors: *Schalm's veterinary hematology,* ed 5, Baltimore, 2000, Lippincott, pp 544-555.

Holloway SA: Disseminated intravascular coagulation. In Day M, Mackin A, Littlewood J, editors: *Manual of canine and feline haematology and transfusion medicine,* Gloucester, UK, 2000, British Small Animal Veterinary Association, pp 253-262.

Jergens AE, Turrentine MA, Krause AH, Johnson GS: Buccal mucosal bleeding time of healthy dogs and of dogs in various pathological states, including thrombocytopenia, uremia, and von Willebrand's disease, *Am J Vet Res* 48:1337-1342, 1987.

Johnstone IB: Coagulation inhibitors. In Feldman BF, Zinkl JG, Jain NC, editors: *Schalm's veterinary hematology,* ed 5, Baltimore, 2000, Lippincott, pp 538-543.

Kirby B, Rudloff E: Acquired coagulopathy. VI. Disseminated intravascular coagulation. In Feldman BF, Zinkl JG, Jain NC, editors: *Schalm's veterinary hematology,* ed 5, Baltimore, 2000, Lippincott, pp 581-587.

LaRue MJ, Murtaugh RJ: Pulmonary thromboembolism in the dog: 47 cases (1986-1987), *J Am Vet Med Assoc* 197:1368-1372, 1990.

Lewis DC: Disorders of platelet number. In Day M, Mackin A, Littlewood J, editors: *Manual of canine and feline haematology and transfusion medicine,* Gloucester, UK, 2000, British Small Animal Veterinary Association, pp 183-196.

Lewis DC: Immune-mediated thrombocytopenia. In Day M, Mackin A, Littlewood J, editors: *Manual of canine and feline haematology and transfusion medicine,* Gloucester, UK, 2000, British Small Animal Veterinary Association, pp 219-228.

Littlewood JD: Differential diagnosis of haemorrhagic disorders in dogs, *J Small Anim Pract* 14:172-180, 1992.

Littlewood JD: Disorders of secondary haemostasis. In Day M, Mackin A, Littlewood J, editors: *Manual of canine and feline haematology and transfusion medicine,* Gloucester, UK, 2000, British Small Animal Veterinary Association, pp 209-218.

Littlewood JD: Haemophilia A. In Day M, Mackin A, Littlewood J, editors: *Manual of canine and feline haematology and transfusion medicine,* Gloucester, UK, 2000, British Small Animal Veterinary Association, pp 237-242.

Mackin A: Anticoagulant rodenticides. In Day M, Mackin A, Littlewood J, editors: *Manual of canine and feline haematology and transfusion medicine,* Gloucester, UK, 2000, British Small Animal Veterinary Association, pp 243-252.

Mandell CP: Essential thrombocythemia and reactive thrombocytosis. In Feldman BF, Zinkl JG, Jain NC, editors: *Schalm's veterinary hematology,* ed 5, Baltimore, 2000, Lippincott, pp 501-508.

Mischke R, Nolte JA: Hemostasis: introduction, overview, laboratory techniques. In Feldman BF, Zinkl JG, Jain NC, editors: *Schalm's veterinary hematology,* ed 5, Baltimore, 2000, Lippincott, pp 519-525.

McConnell MF: Haemostatic diagnostic techniques. In Day M, Mackin A, Littlewood J, editors: *Manual of canine and feline haematology and transfusion medicine,* Gloucester, UK, 2000, British Small Animal Veterinary Association, pp 173-182.

McConnell MF: Overview of haemostasis. In Day M, Mackin A, Littlewood J, editors: *Manual of canine and feline haematology and transfusion medicine,* Gloucester, United Kingdom, 2000, British Small Animal Veterinary Association, pp 165-172.

Prater MR: Acquired coagulopathy. I. Avitaminosis K. In Feldman BF, Zinkl JG, Jain NC, editors: *Schalm's veterinary hematology,* ed 5, Baltimore, 2000, Lippincott, pp 544-555.

Ruiz de Gopegui R, Navarro T: Vascular wall: endothelial cell. In Feldman BF, Zinkl JG, Jain NC, editors: *Schalm's veterinary hematology,* ed 5, Baltimore, 2000, Lippincott, pp 526-527.

Russell KE, Grindem CB: Secondary thrombocytopenia. In Feldman BF, Zinkl JG, Jain NC, editors: *Schalm's veterinary hematology,* ed 5, Baltimore, 2000, Lippincott, pp 487-495.

Scott MA: Immune-mediated thrombocytopenia. In Feldman BF, Zinkl JG, Jain NC, editors: *Schalm's veterinary hematology,* ed 5, Baltimore, 2000, Lippincott, pp 478-486.

Stokol T: Disorders of platelet function. In Day M, Mackin A, Littlewood J, editors: *Manual of canine and feline haematology and transfusion medicine,* Gloucester, UK, 2000, British Small Animal Veterinary Association, pp 197-208.

Tablin F: Platelet structure and function. In Feldman BF, Zinkl JG, Jain NC, editors: *Schalm's veterinary hematology,* ed 5, Baltimore, 2000, Lippincott, pp 448-452.

Weiss DJ: Platelet production defects. In Feldman BF, Zinkl JG, Jain NC, editors: *Schalm's veterinary hematology,* ed 5, Baltimore, 2000, Lippincott, pp 448-452.

Williamson LH: Antithrobin III: a natural anticoagulant, *Comp Cont Educ Pract Vet* 13:100-107, 1991.

Zimmerman KL: Drug-induced thrombocytopenias. In Feldman BF, Zinkl JG, Jain NC, editors: *Schalm's veterinary hematology,* ed 5, Baltimore, 2000, Lippincott, pp 472-477.

Section IV
Acid-Base Disorders

24. INTRODUCTION TO ACID-BASE ABNORMALITIES

James H. Meinkoth and Rick L. Cowell

1. What four basic parameters are typically measured on a routine blood gas analysis?

a. pH: a measure of the acidity of the blood
b. PO_2: partial pressure (tension) of oxygen, the amount of O_2 dissolved in the blood
c. PCO_2: partial pressure (tension) of carbon dioxide, the amount of gaseous CO_2 dissolved in the blood; used as a measure of the respiratory component of acid-base disturbances
d. $[HCO_3^-]$: concentration of bicarbonate in the blood; used as a measure of the metabolic component of acid-base disturbances

2. How are the four basic parameters determined?

The pH, PaO_2, and PCO_2 are all directly measured using electrodes specific for the desired parameter. $[HCO_3^-]$ is calculated based on the relationship between pH and PCO_2. Many other calculated values might be reported, depending on the laboratory and the instrument used.

3. Is arterial or venous blood preferred for blood gas analysis?

Analyzing arterial or venous blood depends on the information the clinician is seeking. Arterial blood is needed for a meaningful interpretation of PO_2. The arterial PO_2 (PaO_2) allows evaluation of the oxygenation of arterial blood, dependent only on respiratory function. Venous PO_2 is affected by tissue utilization of oxygen as well as respiratory function. Thus, if an animal is in shock and has slow tissue perfusion, venous PO_2 may be greatly decreased despite a normal PaO_2. Similarly, an animal that is severely anemic has decreased oxygen-carrying capacity. This animal has a normal PaO_2, but as blood passes through the tissue, oxygen is depleted and venous PO_2 may be greatly reduced.

Venous blood is more easily collected and is acceptable for evaluation of pH, bicarbonate, and PCO_2 concentrations. Because of changes similar to those described for PO_2, measurement of pH, PCO_2, and bicarbonate in venous blood may give a more accurate reflection of the acid base status of the tissues than do arterial samples. This is particularly true in situations such as cardiac arrest.

4. What is the proper method for collecting and handling samples for blood gas analysis?

Samples are collected in heparinized syringes. Heparin (1000 units/ml) is drawn into a 3-cc syringe and then expelled back into the bottle. This leaves a small amount of heparin coating the syringe barrel and in the dead space of the syringe. This small amount of heparin is sufficient to anticoagulate a 3-ml whole-blood sample. Heparin solution is acidic and will falsely lower pH and HCO_3^- if too much heparin is left in the syringe before collecting the sample.

Once the sample (arterial or venous) is drawn into the syringe, any air bubbles are removed, and the syringe is capped by sticking the needle into a rubber stopper to prevent equilibration with room air. The sample should be immediately analyzed or delivered to the laboratory for analysis. If the sample cannot be analyzed within about 15 minutes, it should be placed in an ice bath, and accurate results can be obtained for up to about 3 hours and possibly longer.

5. What changes would be expected from delayed analysis of a sample?

If the sample is not analyzed in a timely fashion, artifacts are induced, the result of metabolism by the cells in the blood. Cellular metabolism will utilize oxygen, thus lowering Po_2, and will produce lactic acid, thus lowering both pH and bicarbonate.

6. What changes would be expected from excessive exposure to room air?

Exposure to room air may result from failure to cap the syringe in which the sample is collected or from the presence of large air bubbles in the sample that are not removed. Room air has a Po_2 higher than and a Pco_2 lower than blood. Thus an artificial increase in Po_2 and an artificial decrease in Pco_2 may be seen.

7. What is pH?

pH is a measurement of the hydrogen ion concentration $[H^+]$. The notation of a lowercase *p* means the "power of," so pH is the power of $[H^+]$.

By definition, pH = –log $[H^+]$. Because of the negative log, there is an inverse relationship between pH and hydrogen ion concentration, which sometimes leads to confusion. As $[H^+]$ *increases,* the pH *decreases* (becomes more acidic), and as $[H^+]$ *decreases*, the pH *increases* (becomes more alkaline). The normal hydrogen ion concentration in biologic fluid is measured in nanoequivalents per liter (nEq/L), about one-millionth the concentration of most other electrolytes (e.g., Na^+, Cl^-, K^+).

8. Why is $[H^+]$ measured as pH rather than as concentration?

The concept of pH was designed to "simplify" the representation of the wide range of H^+ ions found in chemical systems. The range of $[H^+]$ in biologic systems that is compatible with life is much narrower, and the concept of pH is probably not needed. It would undoubtedly be simpler to refer to $[H^+]$ in nEq/L, but pH is now used because of tradition. Keep in mind that a change in pH of 1 unit (e.g., 7.4 to 6.4) represents a 10-fold change in $[H^+]$. Similarly, a change of 0.3 pH units represents a twofold change in $[H^+]$.

9. If hydrogen ions are present in such low concentrations compared with other electrolytes, why are changes in pH so important?

Hydrogen ions are extremely reactive molecules. The proteins of the body, including enzymes, have many dissociable groups that can either bind or release hydrogen ions. Gain or loss of hydrogen ions can change the structure and function of these proteins. Therefore, changes in $[H^+]$ can have profound effects on the body.

10. What normal physiologic factors potentially alter pH?

Protein metabolism results in the daily generation of fixed acids. Carbohydrate metabolism results in the generation of CO_2, a volatile acid. CO_2 is a potential acid because in the presence of carbonic anhydrase, it can bind with water to form carbonic acid (H_2CO_3).

11. What are the definitions of an "acid" and a "base"?

An *acid* is a substance that can donate a hydrogen ion, whereas a *base* is an H^+ acceptor. A general equation would be:

$$\underset{\text{(acid)}}{HA} \leftrightarrow H^+ + \underset{\text{(base)}}{A^-} \qquad \text{(Equation 1)}$$

In which A^- acts as a base because it can bind to free H^+ ion.

12. What are the normal body defenses that serve to protect against changes in pH?

The body contains many buffers, which blunt changes in pH. A *buffer* is a substance that can gain or lose hydrogen ions and thus minimize changes in pH. A buffer pair consists of a weak acid (HA) and its conjugate base (A^-). If a large amount of hydrogen ions are added to a system, the buffer pair binds some of the H^+ ion, thus minimizing the change in pH.

13. What are some of the important buffers in the body?

In the *extracellular fluid* the main buffer is the bicarbonate (HCO_3^-)/carbonic acid (H_2CO_3) system. Hemoglobin is the most significant nonbicarbonate buffer of the extracellular fluid, with other plasma proteins contributing to a lesser degree. In *cells* the primary buffers are proteins, organic phosphates, and inorganic phosphates. The bicarbonate buffer system is the buffer system measured for diagnostic purposes.

14. What are the components of the bicarbonate buffer system?

Bicarbonate binds to H^+ ion to form carbonic acid (H_2CO_3). Under the influence of carbonic anhydrase, carbonic acid can break down to carbon dioxide and water. These reactions are reversible. Thus the bicarbonate system can be represented as:

$$H_2O + CO_2 \leftrightarrow H_2CO_3 \leftrightarrow HCO_3^- + H^+ \qquad \text{(Equation 2)}$$

The equilibrium of this reaction is such that the concentration of H_2CO_3 is insignificant compared with the concentrations of HCO_3^- and CO_2. Thus the reaction can be simplified and considered as:

$$H_2O + CO_2 \leftrightarrow HCO_3^- + H^+ \qquad \text{(Equation 3)}$$

An increase in CO_2 would shift the equilibrium of Equation 3 to the right, resulting in production of increased free H^+ ions *(acidosis)*. A decrease in CO_2 would shift the equilibrium to the left, thus decreasing free H^+ ions *(alkalosis)*. Thus, CO_2 acts as an acid. An increase in CO_2 is an *acidic* change, and a decrease in CO_2 is an *alkaline* change.

An increase in bicarbonate would shift the equilibrium of Equation 3 to the left, resulting in decreased H^+ ions (*alkalosis*). A decrease in HCO_3^- would shift the equilibrium to the right, generating free H^+ ions (*acidosis*). Thus, bicarbonate acts as a base. An increase in bicarbonate is an *alkaline* change, and a decrease in bicarbonate is an *acidic* change.

15. If there are numerous buffer pairs in the body, why is bicarbonate the only buffer system measured?

It is only necessary to measure one buffer system to evaluate acid-base status. Numerous buffer systems exist in the body, but all are in equilibrium. Following an acute acid load, all the buffers will share in buffering the H^+ ion change, dependent on their concentration and pK_a (see Question 16). Thus, if the relative concentrations of one buffer pair have changed, there will be a similar change in all other buffer pairs.

Of all the buffers, the bicarbonate/carbonic acid pair is the one that can easily be measured. Carbonic acid concentration is directly proportional to P_{CO_2}, which can easily be measured. Bicarbonate concentration can be directly measured or, more often, calculated using the P_{CO_2} and pH.

16. What is the pK_a of a buffer, and what is its significance?

The pK_a of a buffer pair is the pH at which the buffer is half dissociated, so that half the buffer exists as an acid (HA) and half exists as the base (A^-) or salt.

The significance is that a buffer is most effective at a pH within one unit of it pK_a. Thus, for a buffer to be most effective in plasma, it should have a pK_a within one unit of 7.4.

17. The pK_a of the bicarbonate buffer system is *not* within one pH unit of 7.4. If a buffer is normally most effective within one pH unit of its pK_a, what accounts for the effectiveness of this buffer system in maintaining normal plasma pH?

Most buffers are not under active physiologic control. They bind or release H^+ ions, depending on the relative concentration of all reactants, until they reach equilibrium. The bicarbonate system is unique in that it is an "open" system; the various components of the reaction can be added to or removed from system (e.g., CO_2 can be expired from the body). Also, the components of this system are under active control by the body, so the pH can be actively adjusted to a point different than would be reached by simply allowing the components to reach equilibrium passively.

With the bicarbonate system:

$$H_2O + CO_2 \leftrightarrow HCO_3^- + H^+$$

The concentration of CO_2 can be varied minute by minute through respiration. If this were a closed system as are the other buffers, the addition of an acute acid load (H^+) would shift the equilibrium of the equation to the left until a new equilibrium was reestablished. This would minimize the increase in [H^+] to some degree and would also result in a significant increase in Pco_2. However, the lungs can blow off the excess CO_2 generated by this reaction, which will allow more H^+ ions to be buffered, thus further minimizing the increase in [H^+]. Thus, by altering respiration to increase or decrease CO_2 concentration, the body can actively control pH.

In addition to controlling CO_2 concentrations, the kidney can regulate bicarbonate levels, although this response is much slower and requires days for full effect.

18. What is the difference between acidemia and acidosis and between alkalemia and alkalosis?

Acidemia and *alkalemia* refer to blood pH that is below or above reference range, respectively. *Acidosis* and *alkalosis* are processes that would tend to either lower or increase pH, whether or not a significant change in blood pH has actually occurred. Thus an animal may have an acidosis, but blood pH may still be in the normal range, either because the magnitude of the acidosis was not sufficient to change blood pH outside the normal range or because a concurrent alkalosis was negating the effect of the acidosis on blood pH.

19. What are the primary acid-base abnormalities that can be identified on a blood gas profile?

Four primary acid-base abnormalities can be identified, as follows:

a. ***Respiratory acidosis*** is an increase in Pco_2 resulting from hypoventilation. The increased CO_2 concentration shifts the equilibrium of the bicarbonate reaction (Equation 3) to the right and results in generation of free H^+ and thus a tendency to lower pH.
b. ***Respiratory alkalosis*** is a decrease in Pco_2 resulting from hyperventilation, the opposite of respiratory acidosis. The reduced CO_2 concentration shifts the equilibrium of the bicarbonate reaction to the left, thus reducing the free [H^+] and increasing pH.
c. *Metabolic acidosis* is a process that results in a decreased [HCO_3^-]. This can be the result of either loss of bicarbonate from the body or generation of excessive amounts of fixed acids. Either process results in an increased [H^+] and a tendency to decrease pH.
d. *Metabolic alkalosis* is characterized by increased [HCO_3^-] and increased pH, usually resulting from loss of stomach contents (and thus H^+ ions) or disproportionate loss of Cl^- ions from the body.

20. What are the compensatory responses expected for each of the primary acid-base disorders?

Compensatory (also called secondary or adaptive) changes are physiologic alterations that occur in an attempt to minimize the change in pH. The compensatory change occurs in the opposite system from the primary disorder (respiratory vs. metabolic) and occurs in the opposite pH direction. Thus the expected response to a metabolic acidosis (change of bicarbonate in the acid direction) would be a respiratory change in the alkaline direction (decreased Pco_2). The expected response to a metabolic alkalosis would be a respiratory change in the acid direction (increased Pco_2).

Similarly, the compensatory response to a respiratory acidosis would be an increase in bicarbonate (metabolic change in the alkaline direction), and the response to a respiratory alkalosis would be a decrease in bicarbonate.

21. Can the magnitude of the expected compensatory changes be estimated more specifically than simply looking for a change in the appropriate direction?

Formulas exist to calculate the expected response to the various primary acid-base disorders in humans. Although probably not accurate across species, these formulas are often applied to animals. Formulas for expected compensatory responses in dogs have been published and differ from typical human findings (Table 24-1). Formulas for other species have not been published.

It is important to remember that these formulas represent the *average* response seen in animals. Any given animal may have a greater or lesser response. Therefore the expected response cannot be interpreted too strictly, but rather should be used as a guideline.

Table 24-1 ***Compensatory Responses in Dogs with Primary Acid-Base Disorders***

PRIMARY DISORDER	EXPECTED COMPENSATORY RESPONSE
Metabolic acidosis	0.7 mm Hg decrease in Pco_2 for each 1.0 mEq/L decrease in $[HCO_3^-]$
Metabolic alkalosis	0.7 mm Hg increase in Pco_2 for each 1.0 mEq/L increase in $[HCO_3^-]$
Acute respiratory acidosis	0.15 mEq/L increase in $[HCO_3^-]$ for each 1.0 mm Hg increase in Pco_2
Chronic respiratory acidosis	0.35 mEq/L increase in $[HCO_3^-]$ for each 1.0 mm Hg increase in Pco_2
Acute respiratory alkalosis	0.25 mEq/L decrease in $[HCO_3^-]$ for each 1.0 mm Hg decrease in Pco_2
Chronic respiratory alkalosis	0.55 mEq/L decrease in $[HCO_3^-]$ for each 1.0 mm Hg decrease in Pco_2

Pco_2, Partial pressure of carbon dioxide; *$[HCO_3^-]$*, bicarbonate concentration.

22. What is the definition of a mixed acid-base disorder?

A *mixed* acid-base disorder is the occurrence of more than one of the four primary abnormalities in a patient. This may be the combination of a metabolic and a respiratory problem or the presence of both metabolic acidosis and alkalosis. The expected compensatory response to a primary abnormality is not considered a mixed acid-base disorder because this is a normal protective response.

23. What are the basic steps to interpreting data from a blood gas analysis?

a. The first step is evaluation of blood pH to determine whether an *acidemia* or *alkalemia* is present.

b. The next step is to determine if the change in pH is the result of a metabolic abnormality, respiratory abnormality, or both. To do this, evaluate Pco_2 (respiratory parameter) and $[HCO_3^-]$ (metabolic parameter). Usually, one of these parameters will have changed in the same direction as the pH change (acid or alkaline), and the other will have changed in the opposite direction. Whichever system has changed in the same direction as the pH change is the system that contains the underlying abnormality (the system changing in the opposite direction probably represents a compensatory response). If *both* systems have changed in the same direction as the pH change, both systems have an underlying abnormality, and a mixed acid-base abnormality is present.

c. The final step is to evaluate whether an appropriate compensatory response is present. Did the opposite system shift in the appropriate direction? In dogs the appropriate formula can be used to quantify the magnitude of the response.

24. What is the purpose of evaluating the magnitude of the compensatory response?

If the compensatory response has not occurred (no shift) or if the magnitude of the response is significantly less than or greater than expected, a mixed acid-base abnormality should be suspected. The patient should be evaluated for a second problem in the system in which the compensatory response should have occurred. If no problem can be found in this system, the "exaggerated" or "inadequate" compensatory response may simply represent normal variation for that individual.

25. How is it possible to have acid-base disturbances with a normal blood pH?

Although innumerable different disturbances can affect acid-base status, each can manifest itself in only one of two ways with regard to $[H^+]$: a tendency to increase $[H^+]$ or a tendency to decrease $[H^+]$. Two (or more) significant abnormalities can occur that have opposite effects on $[H^+]$ and thus negate each other, resulting in pH within the reference range. Such mixed acid-base disturbances should be considered when pH is normal but $[HCO_3^-]$ and P_{CO_2} are outside the reference ranges.

26. What is TCO_2?

TCO_2 stands for *total carbon dioxide* and is a measurement of the total amount of CO_2 (in different forms) in the blood. The majority of CO_2 in the blood is in the form of bicarbonate, so TCO_2 is an estimation of serum $[HCO_3^-]$. TCO_2 is provided on many serum chemistry profiles and can be used to screen for the presence of acid-base abnormalities. A small amount of the TCO_2 represents soluble CO_2 in the blood. Thus, the TCO_2 concentration is typically 1 to 2 mEq/L greater than the $[HCO_3^-]$.

27. What is base excess?

Base excess, another calculated value, is the amount of strong acid that would need to be added to the sample to bring the pH to 7.4 if the sample was maintained at a standard temperature and P_{CO_2} concentration. The purpose of the calculation, and normalization to a standard P_{CO_2}, is to try to separate the portion of a given change in total $[HCO_3^-]$ that is caused by metabolic disturbances from that caused by changes in P_{CO_2} (which will secondarily alter $[HCO_3^-]$ by shifting the equilibrium of Equation 3). If the base excess is positive, a metabolic alkalosis is present. If the base excess is negative (also called a *base deficit*), a metabolic acidosis is present. Base excess values are sometimes used to calculate the dose of bicarbonate to be given to an animal.

25. METABOLIC ACID-BASE ABNORMALITIES

James H. Meinkoth, Rick L. Cowell, and Karen Dorsey

1. What is a metabolic acidosis?

A metabolic acidosis is an acid-base disorder that results from either the loss of bicarbonate-rich fluids from the body or the accumulation of fixed acids. Accumulation of acids can be the result of increased metabolic production of acids (e.g., ketoacidosis) or decreased excretion of acids (e.g., renal failure).

2. How is metabolic acidosis identified on a blood gas profile?

As discussed in Chapter 24, metabolic acidosis is usually recognized when a patient has a decreased blood pH (acidosis) along with a concurrent decreased plasma bicarbonate concentration ([HCO_3^-], metabolic component). Metabolic acidosis may also be identified as part of a mixed acid-base abnormality in a patient with respiratory alkalosis, if the patient's [HCO_3^-] is lower than would be expected as part of a compensatory response to the alkalosis.

3. How common is metabolic acidosis?

Metabolic acidosis is probably the most common acid-base disorder seen in companion animals. Many common clinical conditions may produce this abnormality.

4. What are two general mechanisms by which metabolic acidosis may develop?

Metabolic acidosis develops by one of two main mechanisms:

a. Overproduction or overadministration of fixed acids that overwhelm the normal buffering capacity of the body, consuming bicarbonate; also termed a *titrational acidosis* because the buffers are being titrated by the excess acid
b. Loss of bicarbonate from the body in excessive amounts, as in animals with severe diarrhea.

5. Are there clinical signs that would suggest a patient has a metabolic acidosis?

Generally, the clinical signs present would reflect the underlying disease process rather than the metabolic acidosis itself. Humans have a deep, rhythmic respiratory pattern called Kussmaul's respiration, but this has not been described in veterinary species.

6. In the absence of a blood gas analysis, what findings on a routine chemistry profile might suggest the presence of a metabolic acidosis?

The most specific indicator of a metabolic acidosis on a routine chemistry profile would be a reduced *total carbon dioxide* (TCO_2). TCO_2 is a measurement of all forms of CO_2 in the blood. Dissolved CO_2 (which is the PCO_2 from a blood gas profile) is a minor portion of the total CO_2 content of the blood. The majority (~95%) of the CO_2 in the blood is in the form of bicarbonate, so TCO_2 is a reflection of [HCO_3^-].

Hyperchloremia with a normal serum sodium concentration would also suggest the presence of metabolic acidosis. Normally, changes in chloride concentration parallel changes in sodium concentration. However, when an animal has a metabolic acidosis caused by loss of bicarbonate (a negatively charge ion) from the body, an independent rise in chloride concentration will occur to maintain electroneutrality.

7. Define cation and anion.

A *cation* is a positively charged electrolyte, such as sodium, potassium, calcium, or magnesium. An *anion* is a negatively charged electrolyte, such as chloride, bicarbonate, or phosphate.

8. What is meant by electroneutrality?

In any body fluid, there must be an equal number of cations and anions. To maintain *electroneutrality,* if a cation is removed from a particular fluid component, either an anion must be removed along with it or a different cation must be added back to replace it. This is an important concept in understanding renal handling of ions and understanding electrolyte imbalances.

9. What is the anion gap, and what is the formula used for its calculation?

The *anion gap* is the difference between the amount of the commonly measured cations (e.g., sodium, potassium) and the commonly measured anions (e.g., chloride, bicarbonate) in the blood. Although many of these electrolytes are measured, the most common formula used is:

$$\text{Anion gap} = (Na^+ + K^+) - (Cl^- + HCO_3^-)$$

This calculation yields a positive number, usually between 15 and 25 in dogs and cats, indicating that there are fewer *measured* anions in the blood than there are *measured* cations.

10. What does the anion gap represent?

According to the concept of electroneutrality, there are equal numbers of total anions and total cations in the blood. The fact that there are less measured anions in the blood than measured cations indicates that there are more *unmeasured* anions in the blood than *unmeasured* cations (and the amount of this excess is identical to the amount of the excess *measured* cations). Therefore the magnitude of the difference between the measured cations and anions in the blood provides an indication of the *relative amounts* of *unmeasured* anions and cations in the blood.

If the measured anion gap increases to greater than normal, it means that the difference between unmeasured anions and unmeasured cations has also increased. This indicates either an increase in unmeasured anions or a decrease in unmeasured cations. In reality, the number of unmeasured cations is small and relatively constant. Therefore, increases in anion gap reflect an increase in unmeasured anions, most often organic acids of some type.

11. What is the clinical use of calculating an anion gap?

In a patient with a metabolic acidosis, calculating the anion gap can differentiate those conditions caused by excess production of organic acids (these have an increased anion gap) from those caused by other mechanisms (these have a normal anion gap).

12. What are some common causes of a metabolic acidosis with increased anion gap?

a. Lactic acidosis
b. Uremic acidosis
c. Ketoacidosis
d. Exogenous toxins that produce acidic metabolites

13. What exogenous toxins cause a high anion gap acidosis?

The most common endogenous toxin in veterinary medicine is ethylene glycol. In humans, salicylate intoxication and methanol poisoning also cause a high anion gap acidosis, but these toxins are not typically seen in companion animals.

14. What is the mechanism of acidosis in ethylene glycol poisoning?

In the liver, ethylene glycol is metabolized by the enzyme alcohol dehydrogenase. The initial metabolite is glycoaldehyde. Subsequent metabolism produces glycolic acid and glyoxylic acid. Glycolic acid is the metabolite responsible for the severe metabolic acidosis.

15. What symptoms associated with ethylene glycol poisoning would suggest this toxicity?

There are three clinical phases of ethylene glycol toxicity, caused by the different metabolites, as follows:

a. *Neurologic.* The initial signs are neurologic in nature. The animals may appear drunk or stuporous or may be comatose. This phase is seen within 12 hours of ingestion.
b. *Cardiorespiratory.* Tachypnea and tachycardia develop 12 to 24 hours after ingestion, although these are not obvious symptoms and may not be detected in many clinical cases.
c. *Renal.* Acute renal failure develops within 24 to 72 hours after ingestion, if a sufficient amount of ethylene glycol was ingested.

16. What are the typical laboratory findings in ethylene glycol toxicity?

Laboratory findings depend on the stage of intoxication when the animal is presented. Most animals are not presented until they are in renal failure. These animals have increased blood urea nitrogen (BUN), creatinine, and inorganic phosphate, typical of renal failure. Urine specific gravity is inadequately concentrated, or the animal may be anuric. The animal often has a profound metabolic acidosis, resulting in a low TCO_2 and a high anion gap. Early in the disease course the ethylene glycol metabolites may be the major contributor to the increased anion gap. Later in the disease the concentration of these metabolites decreases, and retained organic acids resulting from renal failure are the major contributors.

Hypocalcemia is present in many cases of ethylene glycol toxicity, a result of calcium being bound and precipitated in the form of calcium oxalate crystals.

Early after ingestion (<24 hours), a dramatic hyperosmolality is present, a result of the osmotic activity of the ethylene glycol and its metabolites, which are small molecules present in large amounts. The osmolarity reported on many chemistry profiles is a calculated estimate of the true osmolality and is based on the concentrations of the major osmotic particles normally found in the blood: electrolytes, urea, and glucose. The presence of an unmeasured osmotic substance such as ethylene glycol will not affect this calculation. This produces a discrepancy between calculated osmolarity and measured osmolality, which is termed an *osmole gap.*

17. How can a diagnosis of ethylene glycol toxicity be confirmed?

A history of ingestion is important, if this information is available. Kits are available to test for the presence of ethylene glycol, and results will be positive until the toxin is metabolized. Calcium oxalate monohydrate crystals are a characteristic finding in ethylene glycol toxicity and strongly support a diagnosis in animals with appropriate clinical signs.

18. How early can calcium oxalate crystals be found in the urine after ingestion?

Calcium oxalate crystals can be found in the urine less than 6 hours after ingestion, well before renal failure is present. This makes accurate evaluation of urine sediment critical in suspected cases.

19. What is ketoacidosis?

Ketoacidosis is a metabolic acidosis that results from the overproduction of ketone bodies, intermediate metabolites of fat metabolism that reflect a shift from carbohydrate metabolism to fat metabolism. Ketoacidosis can occur anytime that energy demands cannot be met by carbohydrate metabolism, such as starvation and in bovine ketosis. In small animals, ketoacidosis is most frequently the result of diabetes mellitus.

20. What are the ketone bodies produced in ketoacidosis?

a. Acetone
b. Acetoacetic acid
c. β-Hydroxybutyric acid

21. Do all ketones contribute to acidosis?

Acetone does not ionize and therefore does not contribute to acidosis. Both acetoacetic acid and β-hydroxybutyric acid are nearly completely dissociated at normal plasma pH and contribute to acidosis.

22. What laboratory findings suggest ketoacidosis as a cause of a high anion gap acidosis?

Ketoacidosis is suggested by the presence of increased concentrations of ketones in the urine. Ketones are easily excreted in the urine, and ketonuria occurs before significantly increased levels of ketones are present in the blood (hyperketonemia). Therefore, animals with sufficient ketones in the blood to cause acidosis should have greatly increased concentrations of ketones in the urine (3^+ to 4^+). Hyperketonemia can be directly confirmed by measuring β-hydroxybutyrate levels in the blood.

Because ketoacidosis in dogs and cats is usually the result of uncontrolled diabetes mellitus, hyperglycemia and glucosuria are also usually present.

23. What ketones are detected by the nitroprusside reaction?

Nitroprusside is the reagent used to detect ketones in urine, primarily acetoacetic acid; it reacts somewhat with acetone. Nitroprusside does not react with β-hydroxybutyrate, which is the predominant ketone produced in diabetes mellitus. Therefore, urine dipstick tests will typically underestimate the degree of ketonuria present.

24. What is the pathophysiology of acidosis associated with uremia?

The acidosis of renal failure results from reduced renal excretion of phosphates, sulfates, and organic acids normally excreted by the kidney. In chronic renal failure, compensatory responses of the kidney maintain acid-base status in the normal range until glomerular filtration rate (GFR) has been severely reduced (<20% of normal), and then the acidosis is generally mild to moderate. In acute renal failure the acidosis may be more severe because of insufficient time for the kidney to compensate.

25. When should uremia be suspected as the cause of a high anion gap acidosis?

Acid-base status is maintained until GFR is greatly decreased. Therefore a high anion gap resulting from renal failure is always associated with classic laboratory findings of renal failure: azotemia, inadequately concentrated urine, and usually hyperphosphatemia.

26. Under what situations does lactic acidosis develop?

Lactate production is the result of anaerobic metabolism. Tissue hypoxia over sufficient time will result in anaerobic metabolism and generation of lactic acidosis. Less often, lactic acidosis may occur in the absence of hypoxia, with defects in mitochondrial function.

27. What are some of the common causes of hypoxic lactic acidosis?

a. Reduced oxygen-carrying capacity of blood
   (1) Severe hypoxia (e.g., pulmonary disease)
   (2) Severe anemia
b. Poor tissue perfusion
   (1) Cardiovascular disease/arrest
   (2) Hypovolemia
   (3) Septic shock
c. Increased oxygen demand, exceeding normal capacity
   (1) Vigorous activity (e.g., racing Greyhounds)
   (2) Convulsions

28. When should lactic acidosis be suspected?

Lactic acidosis is suspected in a patient when a high anion gap acidosis is present, along with an appropriate clinical situation (e.g., poor tissue perfusion) and no evidence of other causes of high anion gap (no ketonuria, no uremia, no evidence of ethylene glycol toxicity).

29. How can lactic acidosis be definitively diagnosed?

Definitive diagnosis of lactic acidosis can be accomplished by determination of blood lactate concentration. However, this is frequently not available.

30. What are the most common causes of metabolic acidosis associated with a normal anion gap?

a. Diarrhea
b. Hypoadrenocorticism

c. Dilutional acidosis
d. Ammonium chloride administration
e. Renal tubular acidosis

31. How does diarrhea result in a normal anion gap acidosis?

The bicarbonate concentration [HCO_3^-] of intestinal fluids is greater than that of plasma, largely because of alkaline secretions from the pancreas and biliary tract. Excessive loss of HCO_3^- results in acidosis. The anion gap is normal because there is no unmeasured anion being produced. Instead, serum chloride concentration [Cl^-] is typically increased to compensate for the loss of HCO_3^- and maintain electroneutrality. However, if severe diarrhea leads to poor tissue perfusion, lactic acidosis may be superimposed on the bicarbonate loss and may increase the anion gap.

32. What is dilutional acidosis?

Dilutional acidosis occurs when plasma volume is expanded with large amounts of fluids (e.g., normal saline) that do not contain bicarbonate or other alkali. In addition to having no bicarbonate, normal saline contains a higher chloride concentration than plasma. Because Cl^- is reabsorbed in the kidney in competition with other anions such as HCO_3^-, this can promote bicarbonate loss in the urine.

33. What is renal tubular acidosis?

Renal tubular acidosis (RTA) is a group of diseases that result in metabolic acidosis because of either defective renal reabsorption of bicarbonate (type II RTA) or defective distal renal secretion of H^+ (type I RTA). These are uncommon diseases that are considered when a patient has a persistent normal anion gap metabolic acidosis with no identifiable cause.

34. What is the mechanism of metabolic acidosis in hypoadrenocorticism?

The metabolic acidosis in hypoadrenocorticism results from the aldosterone deficiency. Aldosterone promotes distal tubular secretion of H^+ as well as potassium ions (K^+). This occurs through both direct (H^+/ATPase pump) and indirect mechanisms. Aldosterone deficiency leads to reduced renal H^+ secretion and therefore acidosis. Because the acidosis results from defects in renal H^+ excretion, aldosterone deficiency is classified as a form of renal tubular acidosis (type IV RTA).

35. What changes on a blood gas profile characterize metabolic alkalosis?

Metabolic acidosis is identified by increases in both pH and bicarbonate. There is usually an adaptive increase in partial pressure of carbon dioxide (P_{CO_2}) as well.

36. Are there any physiologic limitations to the respiratory response to a metabolic alkalosis?

The respiratory response to metabolic alkalosis is an adaptive hypoventilation. Hypoventilation results in an increase in P_{CO_2}, which will shift the equilibrium of the bicarbonate equation to the right:

$$H_2O + CO_2 \leftrightarrow HCO_3^- + H^+$$

Oxygen is less diffusible across alveolar membranes than CO_2. Therefore, hypoventilation sufficient to raise P_{CO_2} will also decrease arterial oxygen partial pressure (P_{aO_2}), resulting in some degree of hypoxemia. However, hypoxemia will not override the pH-induced hypoventilation unless P_{aO_2} drops below 50 to 60 mm Hg, so this is usually not a significant impediment.

37. Are there clinical signs related to metabolic alkalosis?

Clinical signs generally relate to the underlying disease process causing the metabolic alkalosis rather than resulting from the alkalosis itself.

38. What findings on a routine chemistry profile would suggest the presence of a metabolic alkalosis?

Elevated TCO_2, a reflection of [HCO_3^-], would be the most direct support for the presence of a metabolic alkalosis. Metabolic alkalosis should also be considered when there is a low serum [Cl^-], in the absence of a similar reduction in serum sodium concentration [Na^+].

39. What are the major causes of metabolic alkalosis?

Vomiting of stomach contents and diuretic administration, both resulting in relative H^+ and Cl^- loss, are the most common causes of metabolic alkalosis. These are termed *chloride-responsive* causes. Chloride-resistant causes, unrelated to the loss of chloride-rich fluids, are much less common but may occur with primary hyperaldosteronism.

40. How does vomiting of stomach contents lead to metabolic alkalosis?

Stomach contents are high in H^+ and Cl^- ions, resulting in loss of these electrolytes along with fluid volume. Hydrogen ions are generated by the parietal cells in the stomach from the dissociation of carbonic acid ($H_2CO_3 \leftrightarrow H^+ + HCO_3^-$). For every H^+ ion secreted into the lumen of the stomach, an HCO_3^- ion is generated in the extracellular fluid (ECF). In the normal animal, pancreatic secretion of HCO_3^- balances the gastric H^+ secretion. In the animal vomiting stomach contents, the loss of gastric H^+ ions essentially results in generation of free HCO_3^- ions on a 1:1 basis. This leads to an increased ECF bicarbonate and thus alkalosis.

41. What factors are responsible for maintaining alkalosis?

The two main factors that prevent the correction of alkalosis by the body are the *volume deficit* and *chloride deficiency* that accompany gastric fluid loss. The fluid loss and resultant hypovolemia create a situation in which the body needs to maximally reabsorb sodium from the urine to maintain vascular volume. To maintain electroneutrality, the body needs either to reabsorb an anion along with sodium or to secrete another cation in exchange for it. Normally, most sodium is reabsorbed along with chloride in the proximal tubule. The chloride deficiency that occurs in animals with metabolic alkalosis results in increased delivery of free sodium to the distal tubules, where it is reabsorbed in exchange for H^+ and K^+ ions. This perpetuates the alkalosis and results in the development of hypokalemia.

42. How does administration of diuretics result in development of metabolic alkalosis?

Multiple mechanisms are involved in diuretic administration and development of metabolic alkalosis and relate to the following

a. Relative loss of Cl^- ions
b. Increased delivery of Na^+ to the distal tubules
c. Release of aldosterone from the resultant fluid volume loss

These factors lead to increased reabsorption of sodium in exchange for H^+ and K^+ in the distal tubules, as previously described.

Diuretics such as the loop diuretics inhibit sodium chloride (NaCl) transport in the loop of Henle. Although there is equal loss of both Na^+ and Cl^-, the plasma [Cl^-] is less than [Na^+]. Thus, loss of equal concentrations of these electrolytes represents a proportionately greater loss of chloride.

The resultant loss of fluid and the relative chloride loss are similar to the situation that occurs with loss of stomach contents. The inhibition of NaCl transport in the loop of Henle results in increased delivery of sodium to the distal tubules, where it is reabsorbed in exchange for H^+ and K^+ ions, resulting in alkalosis and hypokalemia.

26. RESPIRATORY ACID-BASE ABNORMALITIES

James H. Meinkoth, Rick L. Cowell, and Karen Dorsey

1. Define hypercapnia and hypocapnia.

Hypercapnia is an increase in the partial pressure of carbon dioxide (P_{CO_2}) of the blood. *Hypocapnia* is a decrease in P_{CO_2} of the blood. P_{CO_2} reflects alveolar ventilation. Increasing ventilation will decrease P_{CO_2}.

2. What is the difference between hypoxia and hypoxemia?

Hypoxia denotes decreased oxygen delivery to tissues, whereas *hypoxemia* denotes a reduction in the amount of oxygen dissolved in the blood (decreased Pa_{O_2}). Partial pressure of arterial oxygen (Pa_{O_2}) reflects the ability of the pulmonary system to oxygenate the blood. Hypoxemia often leads to hypoxia, depending on the severity of the hypoxemia.

3. Is it possible to have hypoxia without having hypoxemia?

Hypoxia can occur without hypoxemia. With severe anemia (but normal pulmonary function), there is a marked decrease in the total amount of oxygen dissolved in the blood, but Pa_{O_2} and the percent saturation of hemoglobin will be normal. As the blood perfuses the tissues and the dissolved oxygen is used, there will be insufficient oxygen "reserves" because of the reduced amount of hemoglobin available to carry oxygen. Poor tissue perfusion can also lead to tissue hypoxia with a normal Pa_{O_2}.

4. How is it possible to have hypoxemia without an increase in P_{CO_2}, since both hypoxemia and hypercapnia result from inadequate gas exchange?

First, oxygen does not diffuse across alveolar membranes as easily as does carbon dioxide. Therefore, during the development of pulmonary disease that interferes with gas exchange, O_2 diffusion may be impaired while CO_2 diffusion is normal. This will lead to hypoxemia with a normal P_{CO_2}. Also, respiration is normally controlled by P_{CO_2}-induced changes in hydrogen ion concentration [H^+]. Therefore, in the case of mild hypoxemia with a normal P_{CO_2}, there is no stimulus to increase respiration, and the hypoxemia is allowed to remain.

5. What is a respiratory acidosis?

A respiratory acidosis is a blood gas abnormality caused by a primary hypercapnia.

6. What changes on a blood gas analysis characterize a respiratory acidosis?

Respiratory acidosis is characterized by a decreased pH along with an increased P_{CO_2}. Pa_{O_2} is also decreased (hypoxemia). There is usually a compensatory increase in bicarbonate concentration [HCO_3^-].

7. What general mechanisms result in respiratory acidosis?

Respiratory acidosis is ultimately the result of decreased alveolar ventilation (gas exchange across the alveolar wall). Decreased alveolar ventilation may result from the following:

a. Any factor that interferes with neurologic control of respiration (e.g., drugs, central nervous system disease)
b. Mechanical obstruction (e.g., foreign body)
c. Restrictive pulmonary disease (e.g., pneumothorax, pleural effusion, masses)
d. Decreased gas exchange across the alveolar membrane (e.g., pneumonia, pulmonary edema)

8. Is Pa_{O_2} always decreased in respiratory acidosis?

Pa_{O_2} is *almost* always decreased in respiratory acidosis. Carbon dioxide diffuses across the alveolar spaces more easily than oxygen. Therefore any disease severe enough to limit CO_2 exchange will usually limit O_2 exchange as well, and hypoxemia will have developed before hypercapnia.

The one notable exception is an animal breathing supplemental oxygen. Animals on supplemental oxygen may not be hypoxemic, although the Pa_{O_2} would be lower than in a normal animal breathing a similar concentration of oxygen.

9. What Pa_{O_2} is expected in an animal breathing supplemental oxygen?

It is estimated that the Pa_{O_2} should be approximately five times the fractional concentration of oxygen in the inspired air (Fi_{O_2}). Thus an animal breathing room air (Fi_{O_2} ~21%) has a Pa_{O_2} near 100 mm Hg, whereas an animal breathing 100% oxygen has a Pa_{O_2} of about 500 mm Hg.

10. What is the expected degree of compensatory increase in bicarbonate in an animal with respiratory acidosis?

In an acute respiratory acidosis, HCO_3^- is increased approximately 1.5 mEq/L for each 10 mm Hg increase in P_{CO_2}. In a chronic situation, HCO_3^- increases approximately 3.5 mEq/L for each 10 mm Hg increase in P_{CO_2}.

11. Why is the expected compensatory response different in acute and chronic situations?

In a metabolic acid-base disorder, respiratory compensation occurs very quickly (minutes to hours). Therefore the compensatory response is typically maximal at the initial evaluation. In contrast, the renal compensatory response to respiratory acidosis takes several days to develop fully. After an acute increase in P_{CO_2}, the hydrogen ions generated are titrated by nonbicarbonate buffers, resulting in an initial increase in bicarbonate, which occurs within a few hours. This represents the expected compensatory response in an acute situation. The greater increase in bicarbonate expected in a chronic situation reflects this plus renal adaptive response.

12. What is a respiratory alkalosis?

A respiratory alkalosis is an acid-base disorder caused by a primary decrease in P_{CO_2}. Respiratory alkalosis is the result of alveolar hyperventilation.

13. Which changes on a blood gas profile signify a respiratory alkalosis?

An alkaline pH in conjunction with a decreased P_{CO_2} signifies a respiratory alkalosis. The bicarbonate is usually also decreased as a compensatory response. Pa_{O_2} is variable and may be normal or decreased, depending on the underlying cause of the disorder.

14. What is the magnitude of change in bicarbonate that is expected as part of the compensatory response?

As with the compensatory response to a *respiratory acidosis,* the magnitude of response expected for a *respiratory alkalosis* depends on whether the primary disorder is an acute or chronic situation. For acute respiratory alkalosis, HCO_3^- decreases approximately 2.5 mEq/L for every 10 mm Hg decrease in P_{CO_2}. For a chronic respiratory alkalosis, HCO_3^- decreases approximately 5.5 mEq/L for every 10 mm Hg decrease in P_{CO_2}. This is the expected response in dogs and may not be valid for other species.

15. What are the major mechanisms by which respiratory alkalosis develops?

Respiratory alkalosis results from increases in alveolar ventilation, although the stimulus for increased ventilation can vary. These mechanisms for respiratory alkalosis can be classified into one of three major groups:

a. Disorders that cause hypoxemia

b. Disorders that directly stimulate respiratory centers in the brain
c. Disorders that stimulate stretch and nociceptive receptors in the lungs in the absence of hypoxemia

16. How can hyperventilation lead to low P_{CO_2} when pulmonary disease is severe enough to result in hypoxemia due to poor diffusion of oxygen?

Again, since carbon dioxide is significantly more diffusible than oxygen, pulmonary disease may limit O_2 exchange before limiting CO_2 exchange. In such a case, hypoxemia-induced hyperventilation can result in excessive amounts of CO_2 being blown off from the lungs, resulting in hypocapnia and respiratory alkalosis.

17. How severe must hypoxemia become to induce respiratory alkalosis?

Respiration is normally controlled by CO_2-induced changes in $[H^+]$. Thus, P_{CO_2} is typically maintained at the expense of Pa_{O_2}. However, when Pa_{O_2} decreases to below 50 to 60 mm Hg, hypoxemia may stimulate peripheral chemoreceptors and override control of respiration. Hypoxemia-induced hyperventilation will not return P_{O_2} to normal; when the Pa_{O_2} returns to greater than 50 to 60 mm Hg, the hypoxemia drive is lost, and ventilation will be inhibited by the alkalosis. Therefore, animals with hypoxemia-induced respiratory alkalosis should have a Pa_{O_2} less than about 60 mm Hg. Respiratory alkalosis with a Pa_{O_2} greater than 60 mm Hg would suggest direct stimulation respiratory centers or stimulation of stretch receptors in the lungs.

18. What are common causes of respiratory alkalosis due to hypoxemia?

Any disease that increases the diffusion barrier across the alveoli can cause respiratory alkalosis through hypoxemia. Pneumonia, pulmonary edema, and pulmonary embolism can all result in decreased oxygenation. In addition, severe anemia can result in sufficient tissue hypoxia to stimulate hyperventilation, although the *arterial* P_{O_2} will be normal.

19. Which diseases cause respiratory alkalosis by direct stimulation of the respiratory center?

Hyperthermia, central nervous system diseases (e.g., trauma, infection), pain, anxiety, gram-negative sepsis, and certain drugs (e.g., salicylate intoxication) can result in direct stimulation of the respiratory center. In these cases, Pa_{O_2} will be normal.

Acid-Base Disorders

BIBLIOGRAPHY

DiBartola SP: *Fluid therapy in small animal practice,* ed 2, Philadelphia, 2000, Saunders, pp 189-210.

Rose BD: *Clinical physiology of acid-base and electrolyte disorders,* ed 4, New York, 1994, McGraw-Hill, pp 274-345, 500-514, 604-637.

Section V
Renal Function and Urinalysis

Heather L. Wamsley and A. Rick Alleman

27. EVALUATION OF RENAL FUNCTION

1. Briefly describe how urine is formed.

Urine represents the net effect of glomerular ultrafiltration of plasma and renal tubular excretion and reabsorption of substances into and out of the glomerular filtrate.

2. What is glomerular filtration rate (GFR)?

GFR is the rate at which the glomerulus forms the ultrafiltrate of plasma within Bowman's space.

3. What drives GFR?

The formation of the plasma ultrafiltrate within Bowman's space is a passive process that is driven primarily by glomerular hydrostatic pressure. The glomerular hydrostatic pressure directly reflects the hydraulic pressure generated by cardiac output and local renal vascular tone. Therefore, extrarenal factors that alter renal perfusion can affect GFR and elimination of nitrogenous wastes from the body.

4. What is the purpose of the glomerulus?

The glomerulus acts as a molecular sieve to form an acellular, low-protein ultrafiltrate of plasma that will eventually become urine.

5. Describe how the glomerulus functions as a molecular sieve.

The properly functioning glomerulus acts to exclude molecules from the ultrafiltrate based on their size, shape, and charge. Substances smaller than 68 kilodaltons (kD) may freely enter the filtrate. The concentrations of these substances within the filtrate may be modified later by renal tubular reabsorption or secretion. The glomerulus has a net negative charge that serves to repel negatively charged molecules from entering the filtrate, such as albumin. Its molecular mass (69 kD) and net negative charge prevent albumin from accumulating in the glomerular filtrate, as long as the glomeruli are functioning within normal limits.

6. How do the renal tubules participate in formation of urine?

The renal tubules function under the combinatorial regulation of multiple hormonal inputs to alter the initial glomerular filtrate in a way that maintains homeostasis and responds to the body's needs. For example, conserved substances are reabsorbed by the renal tubules, (e.g., glucose, amino acids, water-soluble vitamins), and wastes are secreted by the tubules (e.g., protons, ammonia).

7. How does the kidney function in total body water balance?

Under the control of antidiuretic hormone (ADH), aldosterone, and other hormones, the renal tubules modify the glomerular filtrate either by retention of water, which results in a concentrated urine, or by water excretion, which results in a dilute urine.

8. Define renal threshold.

Certain molecules (e.g., glucose) that readily enter the glomerular filtrate are almost entirely reabsorbed by the renal tubules, as long as the concentration within the filtrate is not excessive. *Renal threshold* refers to the maximal concentration of a given substance that the renal tubules can reabsorb. The substance will begin to appear in the urine when its concentration in the plasma, and therefore in the glomerular filtrate, exceeds this threshold reabsorptive capacity.

9. What is urea?

Urea is used as a serum biochemical marker of nitrogenous waste retention by the kidneys. Urea represents the endpoint of protein catabolism. During the process of protein catabolism, ammonium is generated. Within the liver, two molecules of ammonium are combined to form *urea* during the urea cycle in an energy-dependent reaction.

10. How does urea enter the blood?

The major source of blood urea comes from endogenous synthesis, primarily by the liver. A small portion of the urea that is filtered through the glomerulus is reabsorbed by the kidney and may reenter the general circulation. Additionally, a small amount of urea is found in the gut due to pancreatic secretions and movement of urea-containing water into the gut. However, little of this urea is directly absorbed as urea. Instead, it is converted to ammonia by enteric bacteria, which, in nonruminants, can then be absorbed and reenter the urea cycle.

11. How does protein catabolism affect blood urea nitrogen concentration?

Because urea is produced as the end product of protein metabolism, the blood urea nitrogen (BUN) concentration is directly proportional to the rate of protein catabolism. Therefore, diseases or physiologic states that alter the rate of protein catabolism can affect BUN.

12. List diseases or physiologic states that increase the rate of protein catabolism, and therefore may increase BUN concentration, in the absence of renal dysfunction.

a. Consumption of high-protein diet
b. Gastrointestinal (GI) hemorrhage
c. Prolonged strenuous exercise
d. Fever
e. Seizures
f. Acidosis
g. Hyperadrenocorticism/corticosteroid administration
h. Infection
i. Burns
j. Starvation
k. Possibly tetracycline administration

13. What happens to urea once it enters the bloodstream?

Once produced by the liver, urea enters the bloodstream and distributes throughout the total body water. Most urea is excreted from the body by the kidneys. A portion (at least 25% in humans) is removed from the bloodstream and metabolized to ammonia and carbon dioxide by the action of urease-producing enteric bacteria. The ammonia generated by enteric bacteria may then be absorbed and reenter the urea cycle. This results in a futile cycling of urea between the gut and the liver in nonruminants. (Controlling this generation of ammonia by enteric bacteria is especially important when managing hepatoencephalopathy.) In ruminants the ammonia generated by enteric bacteria is used as a substrate for amino acid synthesis by enteric organisms.

14. What is the fate of urea once it is presented to the glomerulus?

Because of the filtration pressure at the glomerulus, urea is passively moved across the glomerular basement membrane during the formation of the glomerular filtrate. The concentration of urea within the initial glomerular filtrate passively equilibrates with the concentration of urea in the blood. Therefore the blood urea concentration is equal to that contained within the initial glomerular filtrate. The filtrate's urea concentration is modified during its movement through distal portions of the nephron, such that the final concentration of urea within the urine is different than that in the initial glomerular filtrate.

15. Where do the renal tubules modify the concentration of urea in the initial glomerular filtrate?

As the filtrate moves through the tubules, the urea concentration is passively modified at the following three locations in the nephron:

a. Proximal tubule: urea passively reabsorbed from the filtrate
b. Descending limb of Henle's loop: urea passively secreted into the filtrate
c. Thin ascending limb of Henle's loop: urea passively reabsorbed from the filtrate

16. Is BUN concentration affected by the rate of renal tubular fluid flow?

The rate of renal tubular fluid flow does affect BUN. The movement of urea into and out of the filtrate occurs by passive diffusion, which depends on the fluid flow rate through the renal tubules. A more rapid flow rate through the tubules allows less time for passive reabsorption of urea and therefore more excretion of urea in the urine. Dehydrated patients have decreased renal tubular fluid flow rates, which allows greater reabsorption of urea and therefore less excretion of urea in the urine.

17. What is the fate of urea that is reabsorbed by the kidney?

Reabsorbed urea enters the renal interstitium, where it may remain as a component of the medullary solute concentration gradient. A portion of the reabsorbed urea may also reenter the general circulation and contribute to the BUN concentration.

18. What is creatinine?

Creatinine is used as a serum biochemical marker of nitrogenous waste retention by the kidneys. *Creatinine* is a product of decomposition of phosphocreatine, which is an energy storage molecule found in muscle. Creatinine is formed by a nonenzymatic, spontaneous, irreversible cyclization of phosphocreatine, which generates creatinine and free inorganic phosphate. Phosphocreatine is the sole precursor of creatinine.

19. How is phosphocreatine formed?

Creatine is formed in the liver using methionine and a precursor (guanidoacetate), which is generated by the pancreas, kidneys, and small intestines. Creatine leaves the liver, enters the general circulation, and is then taken up by muscle. Once within the muscle, a phosphate group is added to creatine by the action of creatine kinase to produce *phosphocreatine,* which is the sole precursor of creatinine.

20. How does creatinine enter the blood?

The serum creatinine concentration primarily represents the rate of phosphocreatine degradation by the muscle. However, small quantities of creatinine are supplied by intestinal absorption from animal-based feeds.

21. What factors influence the generation of serum creatinine?

The amount of creatinine formed each day depends on the total body content of its precursor, phosphocreatine. Total body phosphocreatine content depends on dietary intake of creatine and phosphocreatine from meat-based feeds, the rate of hepatic creatine synthesis, and the animal's muscle mass.

22. How is serum creatinine concentration affected by muscle mass?

Muscle mass is directly proportional to serum creatinine. Diseases that greatly decrease muscle mass, such as cachexia, can cause decreased serum creatinine. This explains why cachectic animals that are in renal failure may have an increased BUN concentration but a normal creatinine concentration. Conversely, increased muscle mass due to physical training can lead to mildly increased serum creatinine.

23. What happens to creatinine after it enters the blood?

After entering the blood stream, creatinine distributes throughout the total body water. It is removed from the bloodstream primarily by passive movement into the glomerular filtrate where it equilibrates with the plasma creatinine concentration. Colonic bacteria metabolize a significant portion of creatinine in humans. Unlike the situation with urea, these metabolites are reabsorbed to a limited degree.

24. Do the renal tubules alter the concentration of creatinine from that present in the initial glomerular filtrate?

For practical purposes in veterinary species, the concentration of creatinine in the glomerular filtrate is considered to undergo no modification during its passage through the tubules. However, there are exceptions to this generalization. In male dogs, very minimal tubular excretion of creatinine occurs. Tubular excretion of creatinine has also been documented in goats. When present, tubular excretion of creatinine occurs through an active process in the proximal tubules.

25. Is the serum creatinine concentration affected by the rate of renal tubular fluid flow?

Rate of renal tubular fluid flow does *not* affect serum creatinine. Creatinine is freely filtered at the glomerulus and in most veterinary species passes through the tubules unmodified. Therefore the rate of renal tubular fluid flow does not affect how much creatinine is removed from the serum and excreted by the kidneys. In those species that do excrete creatinine, excretion occurs by an active process rather than a passive one. As an active process, tubular excretion of creatinine is unaffected by the renal tubular fluid flow rate; therefore the renal clearance of creatinine can be used as an estimate of GFR.

26. Identify routine methods used to estimate glomerular function.

Measurement of serum levels of BUN and creatinine is usually performed to estimate glomerular function. BUN is a less reliable estimate of renal function than is creatinine, since levels in the blood are more easily affected by diet, gastrointestinal hemorrhage (increases BUN), and concurrent liver disease (decreases BUN). This is particularly important in ruminants and other gut fermenters, such as horses. The enteric flora of these animals can metabolize a significant portion of BUN to support amino acid biosynthesis. In these animals, creatinine is generally a more reliable indicator of glomerular function.

With renal disease, elevations in BUN and creatinine will generally parallel each other, although neither is a very sensitive indicator of renal disease. Elevations in BUN may not occur until 75% of the nephron mass is nonfunctional. BUN will then double each time the remaining functional mass is halved.

Creatinine clearance is a more accurate and sensitive method of measuring GFR. In some cases, creatinine clearance can detect as little as a 20% deficit in renal function. Additionally, measurement of urine albumin and creatinine (urine protein/creatinine ratio) is an easy and convenient way to detect glomerular damage.

27. How does the creatinine clearance test work?

Creatinine clearance measures the renal capacity to remove nitrogenous wastes from circulation. This test is commonly used in animals that have suspected renal disease but that are not yet azotemic (75% functional deficit is required for renal azotemia to be apparent). Creatinine clearance may also be used to monitor the progression of renal disease and response to therapy. The urine creatinine concentration is compared to the serum concentration over a specific period, during which the urine volume, serum creatinine, and urine creatinine are measured. The creatinine clearance test may be performed by measuring the clearance of endogenous creatinine, which requires a 24-hour urine collection period, or by measuring the clearance of subcutaneously administered, exogenous creatinine, which requires bladder lavage and two 20-minute collection periods separated by 60 minutes. In addition to a shorter collection period, the exogenous creatinine clearance test limits the interference of noncreatinine chromagens normally present in serum, which can falsely decrease results of the endogenous creatinine clearance test and lead to underestimation of renal function. Using the following calculation, the result is expressed as ml/min/kg:

$$\text{Urine volume (ml)} \times \text{Urine creatinine (mg/dl)}$$
$$\div \text{Time (min)} \times \text{Serum creatinine (mg/dl)} \times \text{Body weight (kg)}$$

28. Define azotemia.

Azotemia refers to the accumulation of nitrogenous wastes in the blood. BUN and creatinine are used as serum markers of nitrogenous waste accumulation. The term *azotemia* is used when urea and/or creatinine concentrations in the blood, serum, or plasma are increased above reference ranges. Azotemia may result from decreased delivery of urea and creatinine to the kidney, increased endogenous production of urea/creatinine, decreased renal clearance and excretion of urea/creatinine, or a combination of these mechanisms.

29. What are the possible anatomic localizations of disease processes that result in azotemia?

Azotemia may be localized to prerenal, renal, and postrenal causes. These causes are not mutually exclusive and may occur in various combinations. For example, a veterinary patient that is vomiting and that has acute renal failure may have a combination of both prerenal azotemia caused by dehydration (with renal hypoperfusion) and renal azotemia caused by the primary renal disease.

30. Define uremia.

Uremia specifically refers to azotemia along with clinical signs of the polysystemic consequences of renal failure, such as lethargy, depression, hyporexia, vomiting, weight loss, gastric ulceration, uremic encephalopathy, acidosis, osteopathy, and hypertension. An individual may be azotemic without being uremic. If uremic, however, an individual is also azotemic.

31. Why does gastrointestinal hemorrhage increase BUN, but not creatinine?

Urea is produced as the end product of protein metabolism, whereas the body's muscle mass serves as the source for serum creatinine. Therefore, BUN concentration is sensitive to dietary protein intake, whereas creatinine concentration is not. The blood lost into the GI tract during GI hemorrhage is a rich source of protein, which is digested and enters the urea cycle the same way as dietary protein.

32. What is meant by renal clearance of a substance?

Renal clearance of a substance is calculated by comparing the concentration of a substance in urine to concentration of the substance in serum. *Renal clearance* is a measure of the cumulative effects of glomerular filtration, tubular excretion, and tubular reabsorption of the substance. Renal clearance is calculated by dividing the urine concentration of the substance by the serum concentration of the substance: U_x/S_x.

33. Which endogenous substance has a renal clearance that can be used to approximate glomerular filtration rate?

Renal clearance of creatinine can approximate GFR. Creatinine is freely filtered at the glomerulus, but it is neither excreted nor reabsorbed by the renal tubules.

34. What is meant by fractional clearance or fractional excretion of a substance?

The *fractional clearance* or *fractional excretion* compares the concentration of a substance in urine to its concentration in the initial glomerular filtrate. The final concentration of a substance in urine reflects the actions of both the glomerulus and the renal tubules. It represents how much of the substance was initially filtered into the urine by the glomerulus and how much of the substance was then either removed from the filtrate (reabsorbed) or added to the filtrate (excreted) by the renal tubules. The fractional clearance of a substance is a calculation that compares the final urine concentration of the substance with its theoretic concentration in the initial glomerular filtrate. Fractional clearance is therefore an estimate of renal tubular function and the hormonal effects on renal tubular function (e.g., aldosterone).

35. How is fractional clearance calculated?

The fractional clearance of a substance is the ratio of the renal clearance of the substance and the renal clearance of creatinine. In normal patients, electrolytes are typically conserved by the renal tubules, such that the urine concentration is relatively low compared with plasma. Electrolytes are generally conserved, so their renal clearance is less than that of creatinine, which is excreted in urine at a high concentration compared with plasma. Therefore the fractional clearance (FC) of electrolytes in normal animals is typically much less than one.

$$FC_x = (U_x/S_x) \div (U_{Cr}/S_{Cr})$$

where
U_x = Urine concentration of the substance
S_x = Serum concentration of the substance
U_{Cr} = Urine concentration of creatinine
S_{Cr} = Serum concentration of creatinine

36. What is the normal 24-hour urine volume in dogs and cats, and which factors influence urine volume?

Normal 24-hour urine volume is variable and ranges from 20 to 45 ml/kg body weight for dogs and cats.

Urine production reflects the balance between water intake and water loss. Total water intake is represented by how much the patient drinks, the moisture contained in their diet, and any fluids administered. Water is lost both in the kidneys as a component of urine and through insensible losses, such as fecal moisture and evaporation from the upper respiratory tract. The amount of water excreted in urine reflects a balance between hormonal inputs, particularly ADH and aldosterone. The activity of these hormones and the renal tubular response to them can be influenced by the presence of endogenous or exogenous substances that alter renal tubular concentrating capacity (e.g., diuretics, other hormones, dietary components).

Insensible fluid loss is variable. In a normal patient, it is approximately equal to one third of the maintenance intravenous fluid requirement. Insensible loss is influenced by environmental conditions, the patient's activity level, the patient's body temperature (e.g., fever increases insensible fluid loss), and moisture content of the feces, which can be increased with diarrhea.

37. What is polyuria, and what is its clinical significance?

Polyuria is the excretion of excess urine and is suggested by urine production greater than 45 ml/kg/day in dogs and 40 ml/kg/day in cats.

The clinical significance of polyuria cannot be determined without knowledge of the patient's drug history, hydration status, physical examination, serum biochemical values, and urinalysis findings. Polyuria may be an appropriate response to excessive water intake or may be an inappropriate response seen with conditions that affect renal function.

38. What is the normal 24-hour water intake in dogs and cats?
Normal water intake should be less than 90 ml/kg/day in dogs and 45 ml/kg/day in cats.

39. What is polydipsia?
Water consumption in excess of normal values is evidence of *polydipsia.*

28. PHYSICAL AND CHEMICAL ASPECTS OF URINALYSIS

1. Why is urinalysis performed?
Urinalysis (UA) is performed in healthy patients to screen for occult disease. UA is an essential component in the diagnostic evaluation of a diseased patient. UA can also be used to monitor disease progression, response to therapy, and safety of potentially nephrotoxic drugs.

2. What are the components of a complete routine urinalysis, and why should all the components be done?
A complete UA includes assessment of several physical and chemical characteristics of urine by gross inspection of the urine, specific chemical testing, and microscopic examination of sediment.

Performance of a complete UA allows effective interpretation of data obtained from measurement of serum biochemical markers of renal function and of the individual components of the UA. For example, it is impossible to assess the importance of proteinuria without knowing the result of microscopic examination of the urine sediment. Also, in the presence of azotemia, knowledge of the urine specific gravity helps to localize the azotemia to prerenal, renal, or postrenal causes.

3. Describe ways that the urine collection method can influence results.
When interpreting the results of urine sediment examination, it is useful to consider the method of urine collection. Urine can be collected by cystocentesis, transurethral catheterization, and free catch of a voided sample.

Each method may be associated with contaminants. Urine obtained by *cystocentesis* should be free of bacteria and may contain low numbers (<5 per high-power field) of epithelial cells. A variable degree of iatrogenic microscopic hematuria is frequently induced by cystocentesis and cannot be readily distinguished from disease-induced hematuria. This contamination can be particularly pronounced when the bladder wall is inflamed. Samples collected by catheterization and free catch may be contaminated by variable amounts of epithelial cells, bacteria, and debris from the lower urinary tract. However, properly performed catheterization is ideally sterile. Voided urine collected from a tabletop or from the floor may contain additional contaminants (e.g., cleanser residue) that can affect results of chemical testing.

The collection method also influences the results of urine culture and sensitivity. Ideally, urine culture and sensitivity are performed on samples collected by cystocentesis. However, this is not always possible. When necessary, quantitative urine culture and sensitivity can be performed on samples collected by catheterization or free catch.

4. **Describe the optimal method of urine sample handling.**

For optimal results, urine should be analyzed within 30 minutes of collection. When this is not possible, urine may be refrigerated in a sterile, opaque, airtight container for up to 12 hours. Before analysis the urine should be allowed to warm to room temperature. The container in which the urine is placed can also affect UA results. Ideally, urine should be collected in a sterile container. The container should be airtight to prevent evaporation of volatile substances, such as the ketone acetone, and to prevent loss of carbon dioxide, which raises the pH. Containers that are contaminated with a detergent or food may affect the results of enzymatic and chemical tests, such as pH measurement. If UA will be delayed more than 30 minutes, use of an opaque container that prevents exposure of the urine sample to light may be useful; this will limit photodegradation of light-sensitive analytes such as bilirubin.

5. **What artifacts can refrigeration cause in urinalysis results?**

Before analysis of refrigerated urine samples, it is useful to allow them to warm to room temperature to avoid artifacts that refrigeration may induce. Refrigeration can decrease the solubility of crystallogenic substances that are in solution, which can cause in vitro crystal formation. The cold temperature of the sample may inhibit enzymatic reactions in the dipstick, such as the glucose test, leading to falsely decreased results. The specific gravity of cold urine is higher than that of room temperature urine, because cold urine is more dense.

6. **What artifacts may be observed when urine is stored for a prolonged period at room temperature before analysis?**

Prolonged storage at room temperature may cause an increase in pH due to the escape of carbon dioxide from the sample and in vitro bacterial overgrowth. The bacterial overgrowth not only will affect the sediment, but may affect other measurements as well. Bacterial overgrowth may falsely increase the turbidity of the sample. Bacteria may consume glucose that is present in the sample, leading to an in vitro reduction of this analyte. Depending on the type of bacteria, a variable in vitro change in pH may occur. If the overgrowth is caused by non-urease-producing bacteria, an acidic pH may result from their catabolism of glucose. If urease-producing bacteria are present, the urine may become alkaline. Alkalinization of urine may cause a false-positive dipstick protein reaction, lysis of cells, and degeneration of casts, and alter the type and amount of crystals present.

7. **What are the most common causes of discolored urine?**

Normal urine may be various shades of yellow due to the presence of urochromes. This color can be altered by the presence of substances not normally found in urine, such as the following:

a. Hemoglobin or myoglobin, which makes urine dark-reddish brown
b. Bilirubin, which imparts a dark-orange color to urine
c. Drugs and drug metabolites, which may cause the urine to turn various shades (e.g., blue or green)

Also, urine may become darker yellow with exposure to light, which causes urochrome degradation.

8. **What are the most common causes of cloudy urine?**

Urine is made cloudy by the presence of particulate matter that scatters light, such as cells, crystals, lipid, mucus, and bacteria.

9. **Why is horse urine normally cloudy?**

Horse urine is routinely cloudy due the presence of calcium carbonate crystals and mucus secreted by glands in the renal pelvis. The kidneys are the major route of calcium excretion in the horse. Consequently, a large number of calcium carbonate crystals are typically found in normal horse urine. Horses in renal failure will often develop hypercalcemia, unlike other domestic species, in which this is an uncommon finding associated with chronic renal failure.

10. What is urine specific gravity, and what portion of the nephron does it reflect?

Urine specific gravity is the ratio of the density of urine to the density of distilled water. Urine is denser than pure water because it contains excreted solutes. Therefore the urine specific gravity is always greater than 1.000. Specific gravity is affected by the number of solute particles in solution as well as their molecular weight. It is therefore a way to estimate a solution's osmolality, which is affected only by the number of solute particles in solution. The urine specific gravity primarily reflects the ability of the renal tubules to respond to the activity of antidiuretic hormone (ADH) to produce concentrated urine. To determine the clinical significance of a given urine specific gravity measurement, the value must be interpreted in light of the patient's hydration status, blood urea nitrogen (BUN), and serum creatinine.

11. Define isosthenuria, hyposthenuria, and hyperosthenuria.

Urine specific gravity is classified relative to the specific gravity of glomerular filtrate. The specific gravity of glomerular filtrate ranges from 1.008 to 1.012. Urine specific gravity within this range is classified as *isosthenuria.* Urine specific gravity less than this range is referred to as *hyposthenuria.* Urine specific gravity greater than that of the glomerular filtrate is classified as *hyperosthenuria.* However, hyperosthenuria does not necessarily indicate adequate concentrating function by the kidneys. The patient's signalment and hydration status and the degree of hyperosthenuria need to be considered when making this determination.

12. What urine specific gravity ranges in animals indicate the kidneys likely have adequate capacity to concentrate urine, and what degree of functional deficit must exist before abnormalities are detected by urine specific gravity?

A urine specific gravity of at least 1.025 to 1.030 in horses and bovines, 1.030 to 1.035 in dogs, and 1.035 to 1.045 in cats suggests that the kidneys likely have adequate capacity to concentrate the urine. However, urine specific gravity much lower than this may be seen in randomly collected samples, depending on the patient's hydration status.

The concentrating function of the kidneys must be compromised by at least two thirds before an abnormal result may be detected.

13. How can urine specific gravity be used to help localize the cause of azotemia (prerenal, renal, or postrenal)?

Azotemia can result from the following:

a. *Prerenal causes:* decreased delivery of nitrogenous waste to the kidneys due to renal hypoperfusion or increased generation of nitrogenous wastes
b. *Intrarenal causes:* decreased removal of nitrogenous wastes from circulation due to primary renal dysfunction
c. *Postrenal causes:* decreased elimination of nitrogenous wastes due to urethral obstruction or bladder rupture
d. Any *combination* of prerenal, intrarenal, or postrenal causes.

Urine specific gravity can be a useful tool in helping to localize the cause of azotemia. With *prerenal azotemia,* adequately functioning kidneys respond to decreased perfusion by producing a concentrated urine with urine specific gravity greater than 1.035 in dogs, 1.045 in cats, and 1.030 in cattle and horses.

With *renal azotemia,* urine specific gravity is usually between 1.008 and 1.029 in dogs and cattle and between 1.008 and 1.035 in cats. Renal azotemia is typically associated with a 75% reduction in renal function, whereas defective urine concentration typically occurs with a 68%

renal functional deficit. Therefore, renal azotemia is often found concurrently with inadequately concentrated urine. (However, some cats with renal azotemia maintain their concentrating ability and can have a specific gravity greater than 1.045.)

The urine specific gravity associated with *postrenal azotemia* is variable. Other clinical findings, such as oliguria or anuria with a firm, possibly distended bladder, can be used to distinguish this cause of azotemia.

14. Which molecule, creatinine or urea, more rapidly equilibrates in the total body water, and in which clinical situation is this knowledge important?

Urea is a smaller molecule than creatinine and therefore equilibrates more quickly within the total body water, for example, 1.5 hours for urea versus 4 hours for creatinine in nephrectomized dogs.

Application of this knowledge is useful when attempting to diagnose *uroabdomen* as a cause of postrenal azotemia. It is more useful to measure the concentration of creatinine within the abdominal fluid than to measure the urea concentration. With uroabdomen, abdominal fluid creatinine concentration will be significantly elevated compared with serum concentration.

15. Is hyposthenuria suggestive of renal failure?

Hyposthenuria does *not* suggest renal failure. Production of dilute urine is an active process performed by the renal tubules. Hyposthenuria suggests that there is adequate renal tubular function to dilute urine relative to the initial glomerular filtrate.

16. List diseases and drugs associated with hyposthenuria.

a. Diabetes insipidus (central or renal)
b. Psychogenic polydipsia
c. Hyperadrenocorticism
d. Hypercalcemia
e. Pyometra (endotoxin)
f. Hepatic disease
g. Glucocorticoids
h. Diuretics
i. Anticonvulsants
j. Excessive thyroid supplementation
k. Fluid therapy

17. What artifacts in urinalysis does hyposthenuria create?

Hyposthenuria refers to the production of dilute urine. Red blood cells (RBCs) in dilute urine are subject to an osmotic gradient that results in cellular uptake of water and in vitro erythrolysis. When hyposthenuria and hematuria are concurrent, only RBC ghosts may be visualized in the urine sediment. (Intact RBCs would be absent.) When a sample is hyposthenuric with a positive blood/heme reaction and no RBCs in the sediment, all three differential diagnoses for a positive blood/heme reaction—hematuria, hemoglobinuria, and myoglobinuria—should be considered.

18. What method of urine pH measurement is most often performed, and what is a more accurate method of urine pH measurement?

Urine pH is routinely measured by the urine dipstick test. However, when accurate measurements are critical to patient evaluation, a pH meter is necessary to measure urine pH. A pH measurement of 7.0 using a urine dipstick can be associated with a pH meter reading of 6.2 to 8.2. In cats, dipstick pH measurements are consistently lower than actual pH meter readings. There is no consistent alteration in dogs; dipstick readings are either below or above the reading from a pH meter.

19. What causes urine to be alkaline?

Urine pH is variable and reflects the animal's diet, the timing of urine collection relative to eating; and the patient's acid-base status, which can be affected by various disease states. Vegetable-based diets tend to result in alkaline urine. Additionally, because of gastric secretion of acid during digestion, a postprandial alkaline tide occurs, which may cause a transient increase in urine pH.

Diseases associated with alkaline urine include urinary tract infection by urease-producing bacteria (primarily *Staphylococcus* and *Proteus* spp.), metabolic or respiratory alkalosis, and vomiting. Administration of alkalinizing drugs, such as sodium bicarbonate, can also increase pH. In vitro conditions that may increase urine pH include overgrowth of urease-producing bacteria, loss of carbon dioxide from the sample due to prolonged storage before analysis, and exposure to detergent residues that may be present in the urine storage container.

20. What artifacts can alkaline urine create?

Alkaline urine may result in a false-positive protein dipstick reaction, lysis of red and white blood cells, deterioration of casts, and alteration of the number and type of crystals that may be present in the sample.

21. What causes urine to be acidic?

Meat-based diets tend to result in acidic urine. Many diseases that result in a metabolic or respiratory acidosis can cause the urine to be acidic, such as severe diarrhea, diabetic ketoacidosis, renal failure, severe vomiting, and protein catabolism. Administration of certain drugs, such as furosemide and methionine, can also acidify urine. In vitro conditions that may decrease urine pH include overgrowth of bacteria that metabolize glucose and create acidic metabolic byproducts. Also, during the dipstick test, urine from the protein test pad, which is adjacent to the pH test pad, may leach the acidic buffer from the protein test pad and contaminate the pH test pad, resulting in an artifactually decreased pH measurement.

22. What is the clinical significance of a metabolic alkalosis with a paradoxical aciduria?

In ruminants, paradoxical aciduria in metabolic alkalosis strongly suggests a displaced abomasum. This finding may be seen rarely in small animals that have severe vomiting. With ruminal displacement or severe vomiting, dehydration and hypokalemia may result from decreased intake and absorption of water and potassium. Additionally, the hydrochloric acid (HCl) secreted by the stomach is sequestered in the gastrointestinal tract or is lost with vomiting. This loss of HCl leads to a metabolic alkalosis. When a metabolic alkalosis is present, the urine is typically also alkaline. However, this is not the case with paradoxical aciduria. The presence of dehydration activates renal sodium and therefore water retention. Hydrogen ions are excreted in exchange for the sodium ions that are retained. The excretion of hydrogen ions results in an acidic urine, which is considered paradoxical because the patient has a concurrent metabolic alkalosis.

23. What is the renal threshold of glucose in dogs and cats?

The renal threshold for glucose is 180 mg/dl in dogs and 280 mg/dl in cats.

Typically, glucosuria is associated with a serum glucose concentration greater than or equal to its renal threshold; that is, the patient is also hyperglycemic. In some conditions, however, such as those that affect the proximal renal tubules, glucosuria can occur in the absence of hyperglycemia.

24. List differential diagnoses for hyperglycemic glucosuria.

a. Diabetes mellitus
b. Hyperadrenocorticism
c. Acute pancreatitis

d. Extreme stress
e. Pheochromocytoma
f. Glucagonoma
g. Drugs: dextrose, glucocorticoids, progesterone

25. List differential diagnoses for normoglycemic glucosuria.

a. Primary renal glucosuria
b. Fanconi's syndrome
c. Transient stress
d. Nephrotoxicity affecting the renal tubules (e.g., aminoglycoside administration)

26. What causes false results in glucose measurement by the dipstick method?

The presence of colored substances in the urine, such as pigmenturia and certain drugs, may interfere with interpretation of the dipstick test, because the endpoint of the reaction is a color change in the test pad. False-negative results may occur, especially when the glucose concentration is at the low end of what is detectable by the dipstick reaction, due to the presence of ascorbic acid or the ketone concentration being greater than 40 mg/dl. During the glucose dipstick test reaction, the presence of glucose results in the generation of hydrogen peroxide. This reaction causes oxidation of an indicator dye, which results in a visible color change. Therefore, false-positive results may occur when hydrogen peroxide, bleach, chlorine, or other oxidizing substances have contaminated the reaction. Proper storage and handling of urine samples and dipsticks decrease the risk of contamination.

27. Which ketones are produced in the body, and in what relative proportion and in response to what disordered states of energy metabolism are they excreted in the urine?

Listed in decreasing concentration, β-hydroxybutyrate (78%), acetoacetate (20%), and acetone (2%) are ketones excreted in the urine during states that result in decreased carbohydrate availability for energy metabolism, including the following:

a. Diminished use of carbohydrates (diabetes mellitus)
b. Increased use or loss of carbohydrates (lactation, pregnancy, renal glucosuria, fever)
c. Severely decreased dietary intake of carbohydrates (high-protein and high-fat diets)

28. What are the relative detection sensitivities for the different ketones by the dipstick reaction?

Beta-hydroxybutyrate, which is the predominant ketone present in urine, is not detected by the ketone dipstick reaction. The dipstick reaction is most sensitive to acetoacetate and is mildly sensitive to acetone. Approximately 96% of the color change associated with a positive reaction is caused by the presence of acetoacetate. Interpretation of the color change can be complicated by the presence of pigmenturia. Ketones in the sample can be decreased by the presence of a urinary tract infection, in vitro bacterial contamination, and in vitro evaporation of acetone.

29. During which disease state in small animals is it important to monitor urine ketone production?

Ketones can be monitored in diabetic dogs and cats to assist in monitoring the effectiveness of insulin therapy. Routine checking of the urine of unregulated, clinically ill diabetic animals for the presence of ketones can assist in the diagnosis of diabetic ketoacidosis.

30. List differential diagnoses for ketonuria without glucosuria.

a. Fever
b. Prolonged starvation
c. Glycogen storage disease

d. Lactation
e. Pregnancy
f. Carbohydrate restriction
g. Spurious causes

31. What differential diagnoses should be considered when the dipstick blood/heme reaction is positive, and how can they be distinguished from each other?

The blood/heme reaction on the urine dipstick detects heme groups found within myoglobin and hemoglobin, which is found either in RBCs or free in the urine. This test therefore may be positive due to hematuria, hemoglobinuria, or myoglobinuria. Additional laboratory data can be used to determine which of these possibilities is more likely. With *hematuria* the supernatant of the centrifuged urine sample should no longer be red-brown, and RBCs or RBC ghosts should be present in the sediment, unless the urine pH is extremely alkaline or the specific gravity is extremely low. With *hemoglobinuria* and *myoglobinuria* the supernatant will remain red-brown, and RBCs should be absent from the sediment. With hemoglobinuria the plasma may have a pink, hemolyzed appearance. For myoglobin to be present in the urine, significant muscle damage must also be present. Evidence of muscle damage can be found by measuring the serum creatine kinase concentration, which would be increased due to muscle damage.

32. Which test can be used to distinguish hemoglobinuria from myoglobinuria?

The presence of hemoglobin can be distinguished from myoglobin using an 80% saturated ammonium sulfate precipitation test. This is done by adding 2.8 g of ammonium sulfate to 5 ml of urine that has a neutral pH. After adding the ammonium sulfate, the sample is centrifuged. If present, hemoglobin will be precipitated by the ammonium sulfate, and the urine supernatant will return to yellow. Myoglobin is not precipitated by ammonium sulfate, and the supernatant will remain red-brown.

33. What degree of hemoglobinuria is associated with a positive dipstick protein reaction?

To cause a positive protein dipstick reaction resulting from the presence of hemoglobinuria, the blood/heme reaction must be at least 3+.

34. Is the clinical significance of bilirubinuria different in dogs and cats?

Bilirubinuria has different clinical significance in dogs and cats because the kidneys of each species handle bilirubin differently. Dogs readily eliminate bilirubin that is filtered by the glomerulus. Also, bilirubin is conjugated and excreted by the canine proximal renal tubules. In clinically normal dogs, especially male dogs with high urine specific gravity, a small amount of bilirubin is typically present in the urine. It is important to interpret the bilirubin in light of the urine specific gravity, which is a measure of how much solute is present in the urine sample. For example, a 2+ bilirubin reaction in a dog with a specific gravity of 1.020 is probably clinically significant, whereas the same value in a dog with a specific gravity of 1.040 is not likely to be clinically significant.

In cats the renal threshold for excretion of bilirubin is nine times that of dogs. Therefore any amount of bilirubinuria, regardless of the urine specific gravity, is considered abnormal. The presence of an abnormal amount of bilirubinuria in either species suggests prehepatic, hepatic, or posthepatic disease. Other clinicopathologic data can be used to help localize the problem of bilirubinuria.

35. How can urinalysis be used to help distinguish between intravascular and extravascular hemolysis?

The presence of intravascular hemolysis is suggested by the findings of a pink-red plasma color and a red-brown urine color with a positive blood/heme reaction, often in the absence of intact erythrocytes in the sediment. Hemoglobin casts may be present. Extravascular hemolysis can result in an orange urine color with a positive bilirubin reaction. In a given animal the two hemolytic processes may occur concurrently, and the UA findings may be useful in distinguishing which process is predominant.

36. Describe the difference in sensitivity between the dipstick protein reaction and sulfosalicylic acid protein precipitation.

The protein reaction on the dipstick is more sensitive to albumin than to globulins, hemoglobin, immunoglobulin light chains (Bence Jones proteins), and mucoproteins. The color change in the reaction depends on the binding of free amino groups of the proteins to the indicator dye. Of the proteins listed, albumin has the most abundant free amino groups available for this interaction with the indicator dye. For example, twice as much globulin is required to result in a similar color change induced by a given concentration of albumin. The sulfosalicylic acid test is able to precipitate most proteins, including Bence Jones proteins, resulting in cloudiness that is approximately proportional to the quantity of protein present.

False-positive reactions can be seen with the dipstick method when the urine is alkaline or if cleansers have contaminated the urine sample or dipstick (e.g., chlorhexidine, quaternary ammonium disinfectants). A false-negative protein dipstick reaction can be seen with a pure Bence Jones proteinuria. Highly alkaline urine can have the opposite affect on the sulfosalicylic acid test, causing a false-negative reaction. False-positive results can occur with this method if the test is performed using uncentrifuged urine or if exogenous substances are present, such as radiocontrast media and very high doses of some antibiotics.

37. What is the significance of a positive dipstick protein reaction?

Protein can enter the urine from any source along the genitourinary tract and may be present in the urine sample depending on the collection method. A small amount of protein (<20 mg/kg/day) is excreted in the urine normally along with other solutes. To determine the severity of proteinuria, the result should be interpreted in light of the urine specific gravity. For example, a 1+ protein reaction in a patient with a specific gravity of 1.020 may be clinically significant, whereas the same value in a patient with a specific gravity of 1.040 would not likely be clinically significant.

The results of urine sediment evaluation also are pivotal in the assessment of proteinuria. The findings can be useful when determining if the glomerulus or lower urinary tract is the likely source of protein within the urine. White and red blood cells and bacteria that may be present in the bladder or distal urinary tract can be a significant source of protein in the urine sample. When the sediment is inactive (i.e., free of cells and bacteria) and significant proteinuria is detected, glomerular dysfunction resulting in glomerular proteinuria should be considered. Tubular proteinuria due to defective resorption of low-molecular-weight proteins from the glomerular filtrate by the proximal tubules is another potential cause of proteinuria but is uncommon.

When the urine sediment is inactive and significant proteinuria is suspected, further testing (urine protein/creatinine ratio) can be done to qualify the degree of proteinuria.

38. What is a urine protein/creatinine ratio, and for what indications is this test performed?

A small amount of protein is excreted along with other solutes in the urine daily. Therefore, to qualify the degree of proteinuria and determine its significance, the urine protein concentration can be compared to that of creatinine, which passes freely through the glomerulus and is not modified by tubular excretion or reabsorption. A urine protein/creatinine ratio (UPC) is generally performed when the urine sediment is inactive (no cells or bacteria) during the initial evaluation of proteinuria. The UPC can be measured serially to stage the progression of disease and to evaluate the response to therapy. The UPC should be less than one. Values greater than one raise concern for glomerular disease (glomerulonephritis, glomerulosclerosis, canine amyloidosis), Bence Jones proteinuria, or less often tubular proteinuria.

39. What is Bence Jones proteinuria, and with what condition is it associated?

Bence Jones proteinuria is named for the English physician who first described it and denotes the presence of the light-chain portion of immunoglobulin molecules in urine. Bence Jones proteinuria can be seen with multiple myeloma and is one of the four potential criteria used in its diagnosis, along with presence of bone marrow infiltration by plasma cells, monoclonal gammopathy, and osteolytic lesions. Bence Jones proteins accumulate in the urine when the light-chain portion of an immunoglobulin molecule is synthesized by neoplastic plasma cells in excess of the heavy-chain portion of the molecule. This can be seen when the neoplastic cells only secrete the light-chain portion of the molecule and not the heavy-chain portion, in which case complete immunoglobulin molecules would not be assembled and a monoclonal gammopathy would not be detected. Alternatively, Bence Jones proteinuria can be seen when both light-chain and heavy-chain portions of the molecule are synthesized, but there is more light chain than can be assembled into complete immunoglobulin molecules. In this case, there would be concurrent monoclonal gammopathy and Bence Jones proteinuria.

40. What diseases can cause clinicopathologic abnormalities that mimic multiple myeloma?

Certain chronic infectious diseases, such as chronic ehrlichiosis and leishmaniasis, can cause bone marrow plasmacytosis and infrequently a monoclonal gammopathy. However, Bence Jones proteinuria is not found with these conditions.

41. How does feline amyloidosis differ from canine amyloidosis?

Canine amyloidosis results in amyloid deposition at the glomerulus, whereas feline amyloidosis affects the renal tubules. Therefore, glomerular proteinuria can be seen with canine amyloidosis but not with feline amyloidosis.

29. MICROSCOPIC ASPECTS OF URINALYSIS AND DISCUSSION OF SELECTED DISEASE PROCESSES

1. What is the clinical significance of crystalluria?

Crystalluria occurs when urine is saturated with crystallogenic substances. Various in vivo factors (e.g., urinary tract infection, diet) and several in vitro factors dictate whether crystal formation will occur. Factors that influence in vitro crystallogenesis include duration of sample storage, storage temperature, evaporation of water from the sample, urine pH, and the overgrowth of bacterial contaminants that may alter urine pH (e.g., urease-producing organisms).

To increase the likelihood that the crystals present in the urine sample represent those that may be present in the patient's bladder, fresh urine samples should be analyzed within 1 hour of collection. Increased duration of storage time, especially when samples are refrigerated, significantly increases in vitro crystal formation. However, refrigeration is the method of choice to preserve the chemical and other sediment components of the urine sample. When crystalluria is detected in a refrigerated urine sample, it is prudent to verify the finding by prompt analysis of a freshly obtained sample.

The finding of crystalluria does not necessarily indicate the presence of uroliths or even a predisposition to form uroliths. A small amount of struvite or amorphous phosphate crystalluria can occur in clinically normal dogs and cats. Calcium carbonate crystalluria is a common finding in equine, goat, rabbit, and guinea pig urine samples. Detection of crystalluria may be diagnostically useful when abnormal crystal types are identified (e.g., ammonium urate, calcium oxalate monohydrate), when large aggregates of struvite or calcium oxalate crystals are found, or when crystalluria is observed in a patient that has confirmed urolithiasis. Evaluation of the type of crystals present may be useful to estimate the mineral component of the urolith(s) while awaiting results of complete urolith mineral analysis. However, the type of crystalluria present is not a definitive indicator of a urolith's mineral content because uroliths are often heterogeneous. Additionally, sequential evaluation of crystalluria may aid in monitoring a patient's response to therapy for urolith dissolution.

2. **List crystals that form in acidic urine.**
   a. Ammonium urate (ammonium biurate)
   b. Amorphous urates
   c. Bilirubin
   d. Calcium oxalate monohydrate/dihydrate
   e. Cystine
   f. Sulfa metabolites
   g. Uric acid

3. **List crystals that form in neutral pH.**
   a. Ammonium urate (ammonium biurate)
   b. Calcium oxalate monohydrate/dihydrate
   c. Cystine
   d. Magnesium ammonium phosphate (struvite)

4. **List crystals that form in alkaline urine.**
   a. Amorphous phosphates
   b. Calcium carbonate
   c. Magnesium ammonium phosphate (struvite)

5. **What is the chemical composition of the crystal in Figure 29-1, and under what circumstances do these crystals occur?**
   Bilirubin may precipitate as orange to reddish brown granules or needlelike crystals. These crystals can be found in low numbers routinely in canine urine, especially in highly concentrated samples. When bilirubin crystals are found in other species or repeatedly in significant quantity in the urine of a canine patient, this suggests a disorder in bilirubin metabolism, which may be the result of a prehepatic (hemolysis), hepatic, or posthepatic disorder.

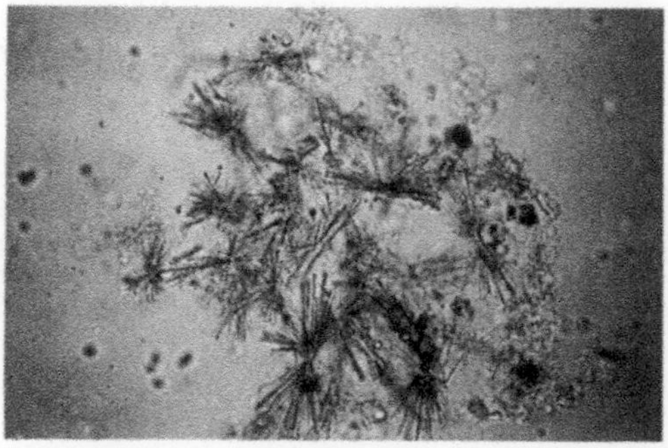

Figure 29-1 Bilirubin crystals in urine sediment from a dog with hepatic disease. These crystals appear as orange to reddish brown granules or needlelike crystals, often arranged in a "haystack" configuration. (Unstained; 125×.)

6. **What is the common name and chemical composition of the crystal in Figure 29-2, and under what circumstances do these crystals occur?**
   Magnesium ammonium phosphate crystals are referred to as *struvite* crystals or "triple phosphate" crystals (a misnomer). These are colorless and frequently form variably sized, coffin

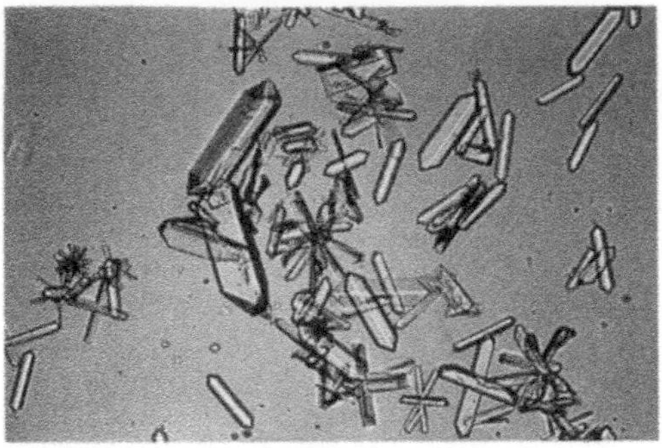

Figure 29-2 Magnesium ammonium phosphate crystals (struvite) in urine sediment from a cat. These crystals are usually three-dimensional, variably sized, and rectangular in shape with oblique ends. (Unstained; 125×.)

lid–shaped crystals. However, struvite crystals can have a variable appearance and may occur as three- to eight-sided prisms, needles, or flat crystals with oblique ends (see Figure 29-2). They form most often in alkaline urine. Struvite crystalluria may form in vitro in refrigerated, stored urine samples or in those that become alkaline with storage. When struvite crystals are detected in a stored urine sample, the finding should be verified by examination of a freshly obtained urine sample.

Magnesium ammonium phosphate crystals are seen frequently in dogs and occasionally in cats. When found in significant number, struvite crystals are most often associated with bacterial infection by urease-producing bacteria, such as *Staphylococcus* or *Proteus* spp. In cats, however, they can occur in the absence of infection, likely due to ammonia excreted by the renal tubules. Struvite crystals may be seen in clinically normal animals that have alkaline urine, animals that have sterile or infection-associated uroliths of potentially mixed mineral composition, or those with urinary tract disease in the absence of urolithiasis.

7. What is the chemical composition of the crystal in Figure 29-3, and under what circumstances do these crystals occur?

Calcium oxalate dihydrate crystals occur as colorless, variably sized octahedrons that resemble an envelope or a Maltese cross. They form most often in acidic urine. Prolonged storage, especially with refrigeration, significantly increases the potential of in vitro calcium oxalate formation. A sample that becomes acidic during storage also may lead to in vitro calcium oxalate formation. When the crystals are detected in a stored urine sample, the finding should be verified by examination of a freshly obtained urine sample. These crystals may be seen in clinically normal animals, in those with calcium oxalate urolithiasis, with hypercalciuria, (e.g., due to corticosteroids), or with hyperoxaluria, (e.g., ingestion of vegetables high in oxalates, or

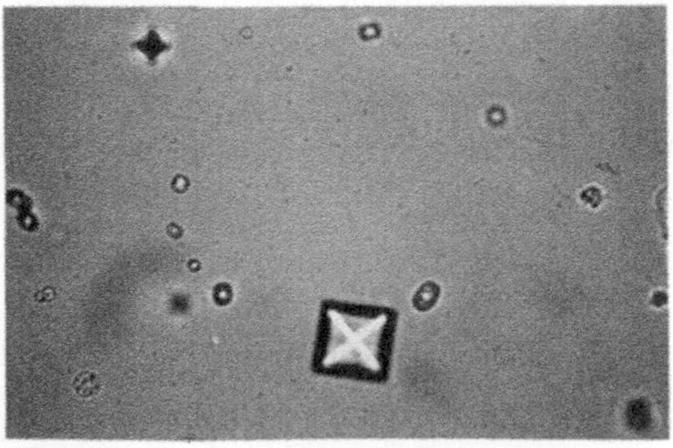

Figure 29-3 Calcium oxalate dihydrate crystals in urine sediment from a dog. Note the colorless, variably sized, octahedrons that, when viewed in a single plane, have the appearance of a square-shaped envelope. (Unstained; 125×.)

infrequently with ethylene glycol toxicosis). Calcium oxalate dihydrate crystals have been reported with increased frequency in cats as a complication of urine acidification to manage struvite formation.

8. What is the chemical composition of the crystal in Figure 29-4, and under what circumstances do these crystals occur?

Calcium oxalate monohydrate crystals are colorless and variably sized. These crystals typically are flat with pointed ends and appear similar to hemp seeds or picket fence boards (see Figure 29-4). Less often, they may occur as spindle- or dumbbell-shaped crystals. Although either calcium oxalate monohydrate or dihydrate crystals can be seen with acute ethylene glycol toxicity, the *monohydrate* form is more diagnostic of intoxication, since this form is usually only seen during acute ethylene glycol toxicity and is rarely found in clinically normal animals. Formation of crystals is time dependent and occurs only during the early phase of intoxication. Crystalluria may be observed within 3 hours of ingestion in cats and within 6 hours in dogs and may last up to 18 hours after ingestion.

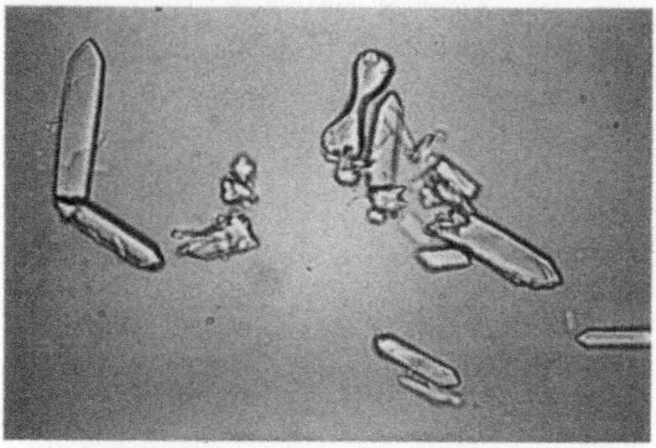

Figure 29-4 Calcium oxalate monohydrate crystals in urine sediment from a dog with acute ethylene glycol intoxication from ingestion of antifreeze. Note the long, rectangular, colorless, and variably sized crystals with pointed ends. These crystals are similar in appearance to magnesium ammonium phosphate crystals. However, unlike struvite, calcium oxalate monohydrate crystals are flat without the coffin lid–shaped, three-dimensional appearance. (Unstained; 125×.)

9. What serum biochemical information can also be used to support the diagnosis of ethylene glycol intoxication?

Ethylene glycol toxicosis is associated with signs of acute renal failure, including oliguria/anuria, marked azotemia, isosthenuria, hyperphosphatemia, hyperkalemia, hypocalcemia, and metabolic acidosis with greatly increased anion gap (40-50 mEq/L). Marked hyperglycemia (>350 mg/dl) may be observed in cats. The osmolal gap, which is calculated by subtracting the calculated serum osmolality from the actual measured serum osmolality, is normally 10 to 15 mOsm/kg. Values greater than 25 mOsm/kg suggest intoxication with osmotically active agents, such as ethylene glycol, mannitol, or ethanol. The formula for estimation of osmolality (expressed as mOsm/kg) follows:

$$1.86 \times [Na^+ \text{ (mEq/L)} + K^+ \text{ (mEq/L)}] + [\text{Glucose (mg/dl)} \div 18] + [\text{BUN (mg/dl)} \div 2.8] + 9$$

10. What is the chemical composition of the crystal Figure 29-5, and under what circumstances do these crystals occur?

Calcium carbonate crystals occur individually or in clusters and are variably sized, yellow-brown or colorless, radiant spheres or dumbbell shaped. They usually form in alkaline urine and are seen in clinically normal horses, goats, rabbits, and guinea pigs. Calcium carbonate crystals have rarely been observed in dogs.

11. What is the chemical composition of the crystal in Figure 29-6, and under what circumstances do these crystals occur?

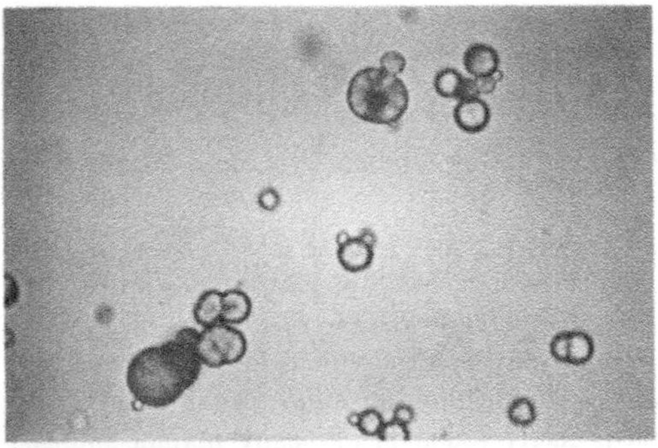

Figure 29-5 Calcium carbonate crystals in urine sediment from a normal horse. Note the variably sized, yellow-brown or colorless, radiant spheres and dumbbell shapes. (Unstained; 125×.)

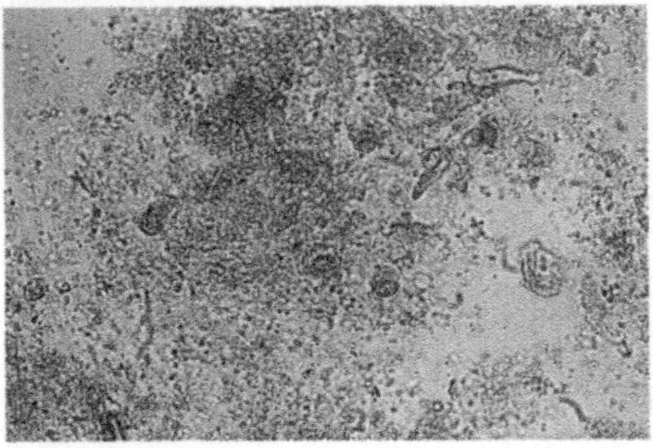

Figure 29-6 Amorphous urates in urine sediment from a Dalmatian dog. Amorphous phosphates and urates have a similar shape and may occur as amorphous debris or small spheroids. (Unstained; 125×.)

Amorphous phosphates and urates have a similar shape and may occur as amorphous debris or small spheroids. Amorphous phosphates are distinguished from amorphous urates in two ways: phosphates are colorless and precipitate in alkaline urine, whereas urates are yellow-brown to black and precipitate in acidic urine. Amorphous phosphates are a common finding in alkaline urine of clinically normal animals. They are of no known diagnostic significance. However, amorphous urates are uncommon in clinically normal dogs and cats. They may be seen in animals with portovascular malformation, severe hepatic disease, or ammonium urate urolithiasis. Amorphous urates are often seen in Dalmatians and English bulldogs and may represent a predisposition to urate urolithiasis in these breeds. Dalmatians have defective purine metabolism and do not convert uric acid to allantoin. (Most other breeds convert uric acid to allantoin, which is water soluble and excreted in urine.) Additionally, Dalmatians may also have decreased tubular resorption of uric acid.

12. What is the chemical composition of the crystal in Figure 29-7, and under what circumstances do these crystals occur?

Ammonium urate crystals may also be referred to as ammonium biurate crystals. They are golden to brown and spherical with irregular protrusions, giving the appearance of a thorn apple or sarcoptic mange mites (see Figure 29-7). In cats, they may occur as smooth aggregates of spheroids. Ammonium urate crystals are seen in animals with portovascular malformation and with severe hepatic disease and infrequently in clinically normal Dalmatians and English bulldogs.

13. What is the chemical composition of the crystal in Figure 29-8, and under what circumstances do these crystals occur?

Cystine crystals are colorless, flat hexagons that may have unequal sides. Cystine

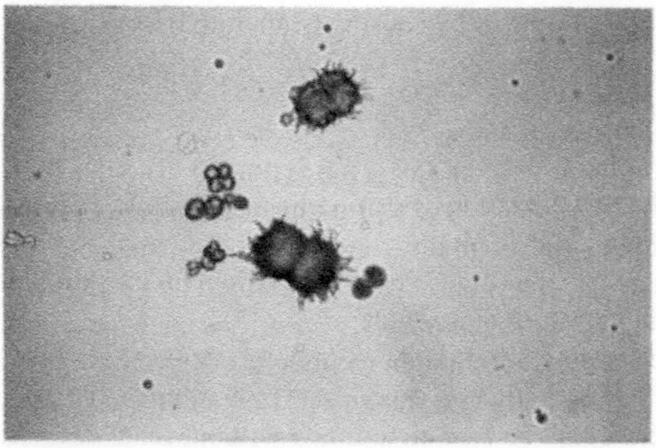

Figure 29-7 Ammonium urate crystals, also referred to as ammonium biurate crystals, in urine sediment from a dog with portocaval shunt. These crystals are golden to brown and spherical with irregular protrusions, suggesting a thorn apple or sarcoptic mange mites. (Unstained; 125×.)

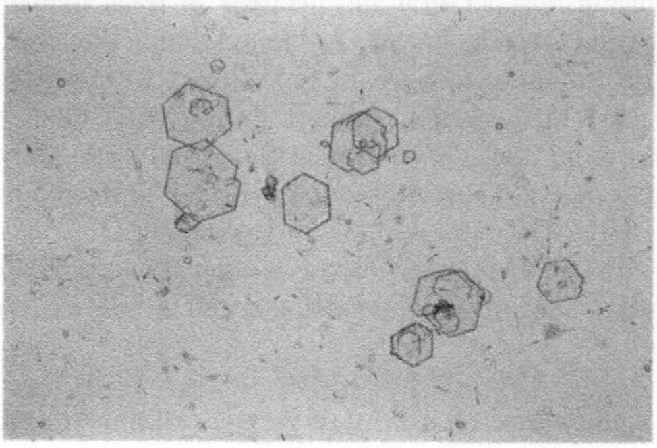

Figure 29-8 Cystine crystals in urine sedi ment from a dog. Note the colorless, flat hexagons that may have unequal sides. (Unstained; 125×.)

crystalluria is not considered a normal finding and is seen in animals that are cystinuric due to an inherited defect in renal tubular transport of the amino acid cystine. Crystals are prone to develop in cystinuric patients that have concentrated, acidic urine. Cystinuria is a predisposition for the development of cystine urolithiasis, although not all cystinuric individuals develop uroliths. Affected canine creeds include male dachshunds, English bulldogs, and Newfoundlands. Females and other breeds may also be affected. Among cats, cystinuria has been recognized in male and female Siamese and domestic shorthairs.

14. What are iatrogenic causes of crystalluria?

In vivo crystalluria can be seen with administration of radiocontrast media and drugs, such as antibiotics (e.g., sulfur containing compounds) or allopurinol (Figure 29-9). In vitro crystalluria may result from storage conditions that change the solubility of crystallogenic

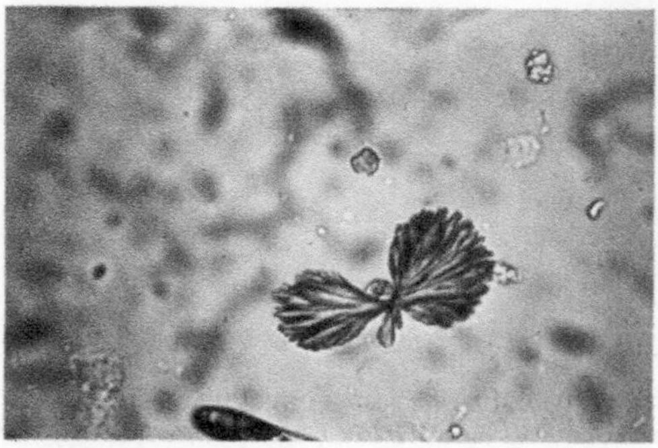

Figure 29-9 Sulfur crystals in urine sediment from a dog administered a sulfamethoxazole-trimethoprim product. Note the groups of wide, needlelike crystals bundled to the center of the stack. (Unstained; 125×.)

substance by altering the temperature or pH of the sample or by causing evaporative loss of water from the urine.

15. Define cylinduria and describe its clinical significance.

Cylinduria denotes the presence of renal tubular casts in the urine sediment. Tubular casts are imprints of renal tubules that form due to the accumulation of a proteinaceous matrix (Tamm-Horsfall mucoprotein) within the loop of Henle, distal tubules, and collecting ducts of the nephron, which results in hyaline casts. The proteinaceous matrix can be modified by the addition of renal tubular cells that exfoliate or by accumulation of leukocytes.

Once cells accumulate within a tubular cast, they are thought to undergo degeneration and progress from a cellular cast, to a granular cast, and finally to a waxy cast. Low numbers (<2 per high-power field, hpf) of hyaline or granular casts can be seen in animals without renal disease. However, when granular casts are present in increased numbers or when cellular casts are found, this suggests the presence of renal disease causing degeneration and necrosis of renal tubular epithelium. Renal tubular inflammation is suggested when leukocytes are found within the casts. The number of casts present does not reflect the duration, severity, or reversibility of the renal disease. Casts are formed on a regular basis and in increased numbers during renal tubular disease. When and whether they are dislodged depend on the renal tubular fluid flow rates. They may be dislodged immediately after formation or may remain within the tubule for an indefinite period, during which any cells that are present within the cast continue to degenerate.

Other specific types of casts may be seen with certain disease processes, such as hemoglobin casts with intravascular hemolysis, red blood cell casts with renal hemorrhage, and bilirubin casts with severe bilirubinuria.

16. Is there any difference in the clinical significance of granular versus cellular versus waxy cylinduria?

The type of cast present does not necessarily indicate the severity of the disease and should not typically be used as a prognostic indicator for the response to therapy or the potential for recovery. Rather, these types of casts represent various stages of development (Figures 29-10 and 29-11). When the cells in a cellular cast degenerate, they form an amorphous granular substance resulting in granular casts (Figure 29-12). With time, the membranes and other cellular material will form a homogeneous, cholesterol containing substance, which gives rise to a waxy cast (Figure 29-13). Therefore, these stages of cast development more accurately predict the length of time the cast has been lodged in the renal tubule, not necessarily the severity of the disease condition.

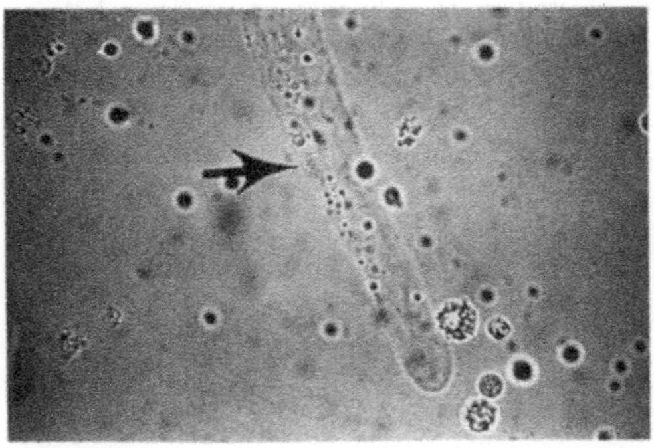

Figure 29-10 Hyaline cast *(arrow)* in urine sediment from a dog. These casts are colorless, clear, and composed of Tamm-Horsfall mucoprotein. (Unstained; 125×.)

17. Is urinalysis a definitive test for urinary tract infection?

The absence of urinalysis (UA) findings supportive of urinary tract infection (UTI) does not definitively exclude the possibility of infection. During some UTIs (e.g., pyelonephritis) the

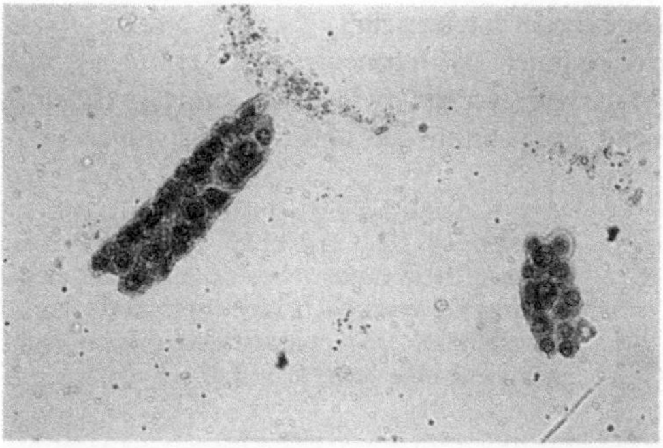

Figure 29-11 Tubular epithelial casts in urine sediment from a dog with renal disease. (New methylene blue stain; 125×.)

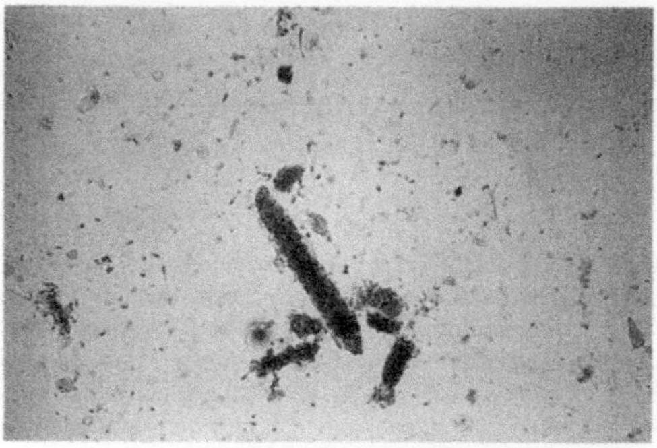

Figure 29-12 Granular casts (several small pieces) in urine sediment from a dog with renal disease. (Unstained; 125×.)

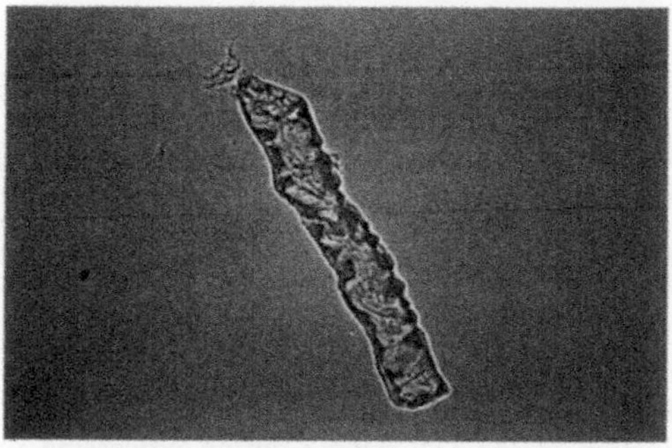

Figure 29-13 Waxy cast in urine sediment from a dog with renal disease. (Unstained; 125×.)

patient produces a high volume of dilute urine that may reduce the relative number of leukocytes present per volume of urine or cause those that may be present to lyse. A high volume of dilute urine can also reduce the number of bacteria present in the sediment below the concentration that is detectable by light microscopy (>10,000 bacilli/ml; >100,000 cocci/ml). Urine culture and sensitivity most directly address the possibility of a UTI. Even when bacteria are identified in a urine sediment, urine culture and sensitivity are useful to confirm the presence of a UTI, identify the organism, and select appropriate antimicrobial therapy.

18. List causes of bacteruria.

a. Urinary tract infection
b. Sample contamination during collection (free catch, catheterization) or processing
c. In vitro bacterial overgrowth

19. What is the significance of pyuria and concurrent bacteruria?

The finding of pyuria (leukocytes in the urine sediment) with concurrent bacteruria suggests active urinary tract inflammation with either a primary or a secondary bacterial infection (Figures 29-14 and 29-15). When these findings are present, urine culture and sensitivity are indicated.

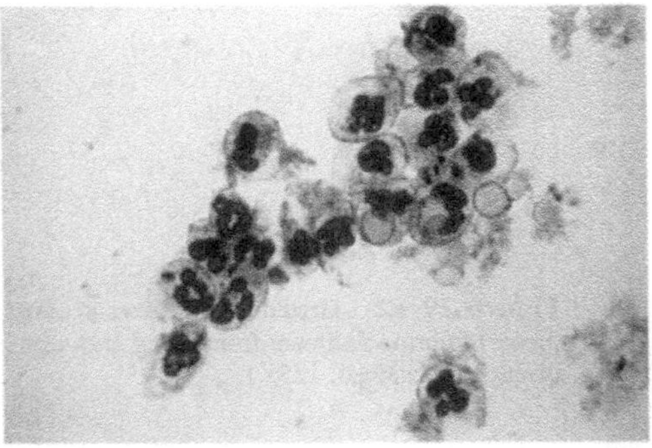

Figure 29-14 Bacterial cystitis in urine sediment from a dog. Note several neutrophils, with the neutrophil in the top right containing an intracellular, rod-shaped bacterium. (New methylene blue stain; 125×.)

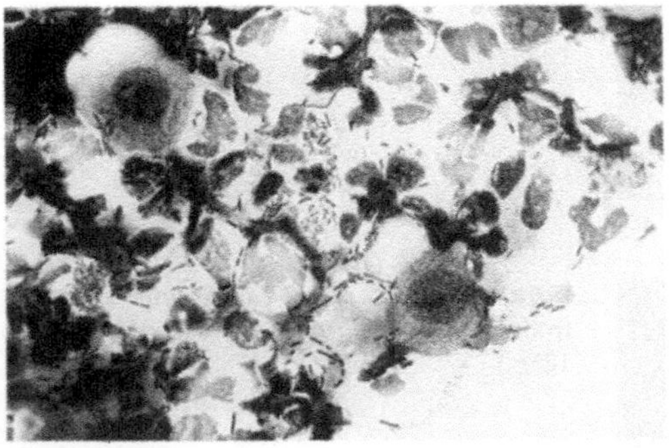

Figure 29-15 Bacterial cystitis in urine sediment from a dog. Note the numerous degenerate neutrophils and two large transitional epithelial cells. Several large, rod-shaped bacteria are seen in the background and within the cytoplasm of degenerate neutrophils. (Wright-Giemsa stain; 125×.)

20. List possible causes of a negative urine culture despite identification of bacteria in the urine sediment.

a. Observed bacteria may not be viable because of antimicrobial administration, prolonged urine storage, or fastidious nutritional and culture requirements.
b. Observed bacteria may not grow because of improper culture technique.
c. Observed bacteria represent contamination of the UA sample during processing or collection.
d. Observed bacteria may actually be nonbacterial structures in the sediment that were mistakenly identified as bacteria during examination.

21. Does a negative urine culture definitively rule out urinary tract infection?

A negative urine culture does not necessarily exclude the possibility of UTI. In addition to the causes of negative culture previously listed, UTIs infrequently result from viral, mycoplasmal, or ureaplasmal infection.

22. Does the absence of pyuria in a urine sediment rule out urinary tract infection?

The absence of pyuria does not definitively exclude the possibility of UTI. Silent UTIs (i.e., not eliciting an inflammatory response) can be seen with hyperadrenocorticism, diabetes mellitus, and immunosuppressed states (e.g., drug induced).

23. How can corticosteroids affect urinalysis?

Corticosteroids promote the development of UTI and may hinder its identification by routine UA. Corticosteroids (exogenously administered or endogenously produced in excess) predispose a patient to development of bacteruria associated with UTI, inhibit the migration of neutrophils into tissues, and induce hyposthenuria that can dilute urine sediment abnormalities. Therefore, urine culture and sensitivity are important in the evaluation of urine samples from animals exposed to excessive amounts of corticosteroids because they may have a silent UTI with a normal routine UA.

24. What is the difference between routine urine culture and sensitivity and quantitative culture and sensitivity; and when should the latter be performed?

With a *routine* urine culture and sensitivity, results simply identify the bacteria present with their respective antimicrobial sensitivities. With a *quantitative* urine culture and sensitivity, not only are the bacteria identified, but their quantity is also reported as colony-forming units per milliliter (CFUs/ml), which is determined by serial dilution and plating. The quantitative test is useful when determining if the bacteria cultured from a urine sample are likely contaminants or likely the result of a true infection. A sample collected by cystocentesis is preferred when the sample is to be cultured, although collection by this method is not always possible. Quantitative urine culture can be most important when the sample, out of necessity, has been collected by transurethral catheterization or by voiding. Additionally, isolation of more than one microorganism suggests bacterial contamination (Table 29-1).

Table 29-1 ***Interpretation of Quantitative Urine Culture Results***

COLLECTION METHOD	CONTAMINANT (CFUs/ml) DOG	CONTAMINANT (CFUs/ml) CAT	SUSPICIOUS (CFUs/ml) DOG	SUSPICIOUS (CFUs/ml) CAT	SIGNIFICANT (CFUs/ml) DOG	SIGNIFICANT (CFUs/ml) CAT
Cystocentesis	<100	<100	100-1000	100-1000	>1000	>1000
Catheterization	<1000	<100	1000-10,000	100-1000	>10,000	>1000
Voiding	<10,000	<1000	10,000-90,000	1000-10,000	>100,000	>10,000

CFUs/ml, Colony-forming units per milliliter.

25. Besides bacterial urinary tract infection, with what other conditions can pyuria be found?

Pyuria can be associated with any noninfectious or infectious cause of genitourinary tract inflammation, such as inflammation caused by the presence of uroliths, prostatitis, pyometra, neoplasms, and infection with viruses, mycoplasma, or ureaplasma.

26. Identify the cell type in Figure 29-16. In what portions of the urinary tract are these cells found; and what is their potential clinical significance?

Squamous epithelial cells are large, flat or rolled cells that have angular sides and small nuclei. They line the distal third of the urethra, the vagina, and the prepuce. These cells are usually found in variable numbers in the sediment of contaminated samples collected by catheterization or by voiding. However, squamous epithelial cells may rarely be observed in samples collected by cystocentesis, resulting from squamous cell carcinoma of the bladder or from squamous metaplasia of the bladder, which may be associated with transitional cell carcinoma or chronic bladder irritation.

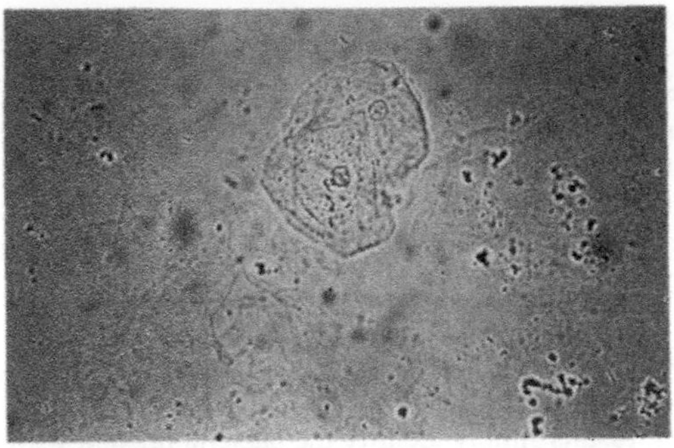

Figure 29-16 Two squamous epithelial cells *(top center)* in voided urine sample from a dog. (Unstained; 125×.)

27. Identify the cell type in Figure 29-17. In what portions of the urinary tract are these cells found; and what is their potential clinical significance?

Transitional epithelial cells are variably sized and smaller than squamous epithelial cells but larger than leukocytes. Transitional cells may be round, pear or spindle shaped, or polygonal and may have granular cytoplasm containing a single nucleus that is larger than that of squamous epithelial cells. Transitional cells line the bladder and proximal two thirds of the urethra. They can be found in low numbers (<5/hpf) in urine samples of clinically normal animals. These cells may be found in greater number in the urine sediment of samples collected by catheterization or in patients that have bladder irritation or inflammation. During these conditions the transitional epithelial cells undergo reactive hyperplasia, resulting in cytologic features that mimic malignancy. For this reason, in the presence of inflammation, neoplasia cannot be reliably diagnosed by urine sediment cytology. An increased number of atypical transitional epithelial cells may also be seen with transitional cell carcinoma.

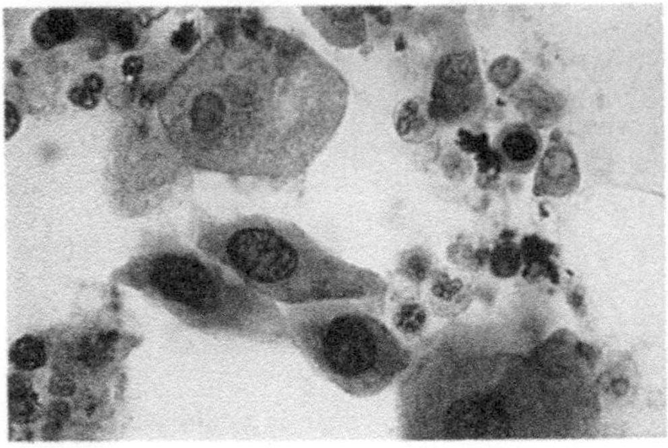

Figure 29-17 Three large transitional epithelial cells in urine sediment from a dog with cystitis. A large squamous epithelial cell *(top left)*, several neutrophils (lobulated nuclei), and renal epithelial cells (round nuclei) are also seen. (Sedi-Stain; 125×.)

28. What findings in the urine sediment suggest a transitional cell carcinoma?

In a veterinary patient that has a bladder or urethral mass, the urine sediment finding of atypical transitional epithelial cells in the absence of inflammation suggests transitional cell carcinoma. The cells may exfoliate in cohesive sheets or individually. They will display various malignant features, such as high nuclear/cytoplasmic ratio, variable cell and nuclear size, clumped chromatin with prominent nucleoli, and mitotic activity (Figures 29-18 and 29-19).

29. Identify substances that cause false-positive reactions with the v-bta test.

The *v-bta* (veterinary–bladder tumor antigen) *test* is designed as a screen for the early detection of transitional cell carcinoma by detecting an antigen present in the urine that is produced by the tumor. Urine samples that contain pyuria or hematuria can result in a false-

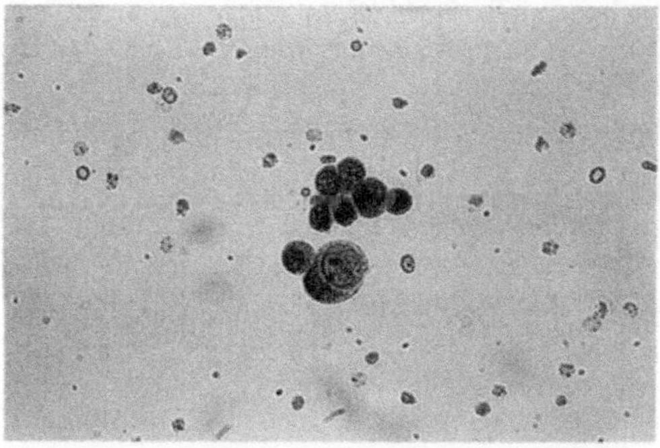

Figure 29-18 Transitional cell carcinoma in urine sediment from a dog. Note the small clumps of malignant transitional epithelial cells with high nuclear/cytoplasmic ratio, anisokaryosis, and prominent multiple nucleoli. (New methylene blue stain; 50×.)

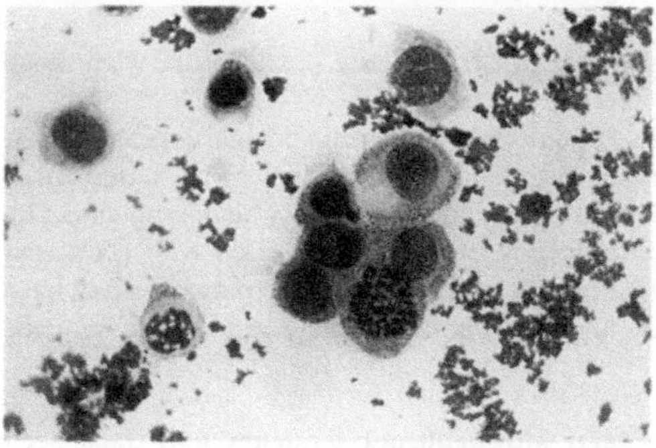

Figure 29-19 Transitional cell carcinoma in urine sediment from a dog. Note, among other malignant features, the mitotic figure *(bottom right)*. (Wright-Giemsa stain; 125×.)

positive result. Unfortunately, bladder tumors are often associated with secondary inflammation and hemorrhage. Therefore the v-bta test is not useful as a screening tool for the diagnosis of transitional cell carcinoma because pyuria and hematuria are also frequently present. Additionally, many investigators believe that the test has an unacceptable number of false-positive reactions, even in dogs with an otherwise-normal urine sediment, suspected to result from nonspecific reactivity of the diagnostic antigen used in this assay when applied to canine samples. Because of the low incidence of bladder tumors in dogs and the high incidence of false-positive reactions, an unacceptable number of animals may be subjected to invasive and costly diagnostic procedures only to prove a false reaction. A diagnosis of bladder cancer should not be made using this assay unless confirmatory diagnostic procedures are also performed.

30. Identify the structure in the urine sediment in Figure 29-20 and describe its clinical significance.

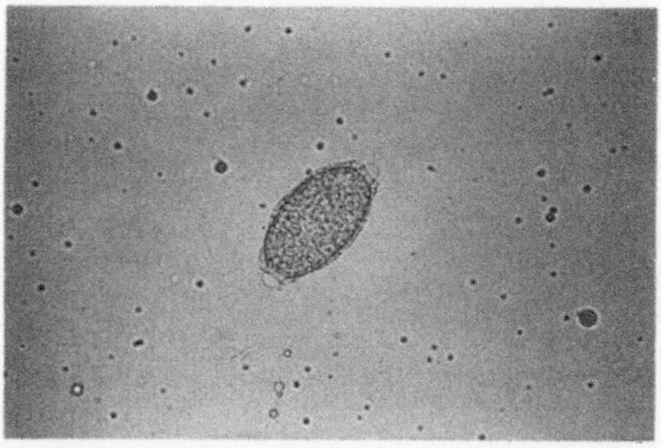

Figure 29-20 *Capillaria* eggs in urine sediment from a cat. Note the bipolar caps that are not parallel to each other and instead are slightly askew. (Unstained; 125×.)

Capillaria eggs are similar in appearance to those of *Trichuris vulpis,* which may be present in fecally contaminated urine samples. *Capillaria* can be distinguished from *Trichuris* eggs by the positioning of the bipolar caps, which in *Trichuris* are perfectly bipolar. The bipolar caps of *Capillaria* eggs are not perfectly bipolar and appear slightly askew (see Figure 29-20). *Capillaria* eggs are typically seen as an incidental finding in the urine of asymptomatic cats. However, *Capillaria* eggs are occasionally identified in cats that present with hematuria, which resolves with fenbendazole treatment.

31. List urinalysis findings seen with the potential toxicity associated with aminoglycoside administration.

a. Decreased urine specific gravity
b. Cylinduria
c. Normoglycemic glucosuria
d. Increased urine concentration of gamma-glutamyl transferase (GGT)

32. Contrast the clinicopathologic abnormalities seen during acute renal failure with those seen during chronic renal failure.

Acute and chronic renal failure may be associated with similar clinicopathologic findings, including azotemia, hyperphosphatemia, hyperkalemia, metabolic acidosis with increased anion gap, and abnormal urine specific gravity. Acute and chronic renal failure may be distinguished by the patient's packed cell volume. Chronic renal failure is frequently associated with decreased erythropoietin production by the kidneys. Consequently, chronic renal failure patients often have a normocytic, normochromic, nonregenerative anemia, whereas acute renal failure patients typically are not anemic.

33. List the clinicopathologic abnormalities seen with nephrotic tendency and those seen with nephrotic syndrome.

Nephrotic Tendency	Nephrotic Syndrome
Hypoalbuminemia	Hypoalbuminemia
Hypercholesterolemia	Hypercholesterolemia
Proteinuria	Proteinuria
	Edema

34. Why are veterinary patients that have nephrotic syndrome hypercholesterolemic?

Albumin is one of the major determinants of intravascular colloid osmotic pressure. The albumin molecule itself exerts osmotic pressure. Also, a major component of the osmotic effect exerted by albumin is caused by the positively charged cations (e.g., Na^+) that associate with the negatively charged albumin molecules due to the Gibbs-Donnan effect. Nephrotic patients are severely hypoalbuminemic and therefore have greatly decreased intravascular colloid osmotic pressure. Cholesterol is synthesized by the liver as a compensatory response to maintain colloid osmotic pressure.

35. Describe the pathogenesis of hypercoagulability seen with nephrotic syndrome.

Nephrotic syndrome is associated with glomerular disease that alters the "permselectivity" barrier function of the glomerulus and leads to protein loss into the urine. Albumin (molecular weight 69 kD) is lost, resulting in hypoalbuminemia and proteinuria. Smaller-molecular-weight proteins also accumulate in the urine, including antithrombin III (AT-III, molecular weight 65 kD), an anticoagulant that keeps coagulation in check by inhibiting the function of thrombin and coagulation factors IXa, Xa, XIa, and XIIa. Nephrotic patients typically are deficient in AT-III because of glomerular proteinuria, making them hypercoagulable and thus prone to thromboembolic disease.

36. During urethral obstruction, what clinicopathologic abnormality can be immediately life threatening, and what diagnostic methods can be used to detect it?

Moderate to severe hyperkalemia is a common abnormality associated with urethral obstruction that can be immediately life threatening due to its effect on the heart. Hyperkalemic animals may be lethargic, weak, and bradycardic with characteristic electrocardiogram abnormalities: tenting of T wave, decreased amplitude or absence of P wave, and prolonged QRS interval.

37. List clinicopathologic abnormalities seen with Fanconi's syndrome and predisposed breeds.

Clinicopathologic Abnormalities	Breeds
Normoglycemic glucosuria	Basenji
Aminoaciduria	Norwegian elkhound
Proteinuria	Shetland sheepdog
Renal tubular acidosis	Schnauzer
Azotemia	
Hyperphosphatemia	
Hypokalemia	

Renal Function and Urinalysis

BIBLIOGRAPHY

Albasan H, Lulich JP, Osborne CA, et al: Effects of storage time and temperature on pH, specific gravity, and crystal formation in urine samples from dogs and cats, *J Am Vet Med Assoc* 222:176-179, 2003.

Barsanti JA, Lees GE, Willard MD, et al: Urinary disorders. In Willard MD, Tvedten H, Turnwald GH, editors: *Small animal clinical diagnosis by laboratory methods,* ed 3, Philadelphia, 1999, Saunders, pp 108-135.

Finco DR: Kidney function. In Kaneko JJ, Harvey JW, Bruss ML, editors: *Clinical biochemistry of domestic animals,* ed 5, San Diego, 1997, Academic Press, pp 441-484.

Heuter KJ, Buffington CA, Chew DJ: Agreement between two methods for measuring urine pH in cats and dogs, *J Am Vet Med Assoc* 213:996-998, 1998.

Meyer DJ, Harvey JW: *Veterinary laboratory medicine: interpretation and diagnosis,* ed 2, Philadelphia, 1998, Saunders, pp 221-235.

Osborne CA, Stevens JB, editors: *Urinalysis: a clinical guide to compassionate patient care,* Shawnee Mission, Kan, 1999, Veterinary Learning Systems.

Section VI
Liver and Muscle

Douglas J. Weiss

30. TESTS FOR EVALUATION OF LIVER DISEASE

1. What are the major categories of enzymes used to evaluate liver disease?

There are two major categories of liver enzymes: leakage enzymes and cholestatic enzymes. *Leakage enzymes* are enzymes that leak into the plasma when hepatocyte injury or death occurs. Therefore, high activities in serum are an indication of hepatocellular injury. Commonly measured leakage enzymes include the following:

- Alanine aminotransferase (ALT; also alanine transaminase)
- Aspartate aminotransferase (AST; also aspartate transaminase)
- Sorbitol dehydrogenase (SDH)
- Lactate dehydrogenase (LDH)

Cholestatic enzymes are enzymes for which synthesis is increased as a result of bile retention or administration of drugs. Bile retention usually results from intrahepatic or extrahepatic bile duct obstruction. Commonly measured cholestatic enzymes include the following:

- Alkaline phosphatase (ALP)
- Gamma-glutamyltransferase (GGT; also gamma-glutamyltranspeptidase)

2. What are isoenzymes?

Isoenzymes are molecules with similar function but variable molecular structure. In general, these isoenzymes are produced in different tissues. For example, LDH (also LD) has five isoenzymes. LD_1 and LD_2 are primarily located in cardiac muscle, whereas LD_5 is primarily located in liver and skeletal muscle. By determining the specific isoenzyme increased in serum, the source of the cellular injury can be identified.

3. What determines the level of a liver enzyme in plasma?

Multiple factors are involved in determining the activity of an enzyme in plasma and include the following:

a. Amount of the enzyme in hepatocytes
b. Rate of synthesis of the enzyme
c. Number of hepatocytes injured
d. Molecular size
e. Intracellular location of the enzyme
f. Rate of clearance from the plasma
g. Rate of enzyme inactivation

4. Do liver enzyme tests evaluate liver function?

Enzyme tests provide information about hepatocellular injury or cholestasis but do *not* define how much functional liver is present. Therefore, specific liver function tests are needed to assess liver function.

5. What are the most clinically useful leakage enzymes?

Clinically useful leakage enzymes vary with the species tested. In dogs and cats, ALT is used as a liver-specific leakage enzyme. Horses, ruminants, and pigs have very little ALT in their liver, so serum ALT activity does not increase with liver disease; therefore SDH is used as a liver-specific leakage enzyme in these species. AST is used as a nonspecific indicator of tissue injury in all the species just listed.

6. How long do leakage enzymes remain elevated in blood of dogs and cats after transient hepatocellular injury?

ALT remains elevated for 1 to 3 weeks after a toxic insult in dogs and cats. AST remains elevated for 5 to 7 days (Figure 30-1).

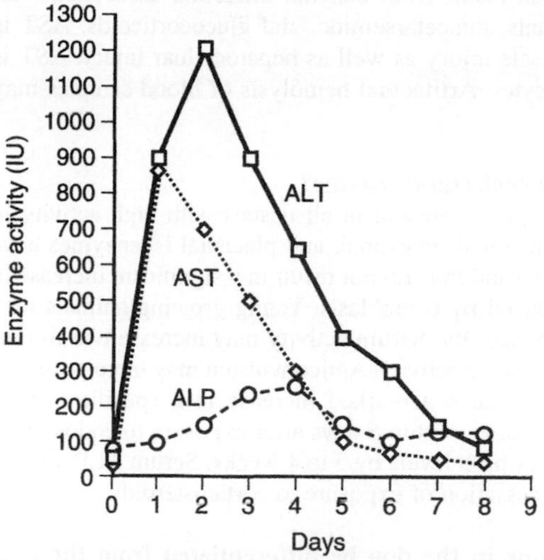

Figure 30-1 Serum enzyme activity after acute transient liver injury in dogs and cats. Alkaline phosphatase *(ALP)* increases slightly in dogs but may remain normal in cats. *AST,* Aspartate transaminase; *ALT,* alanine transaminase; *IU,* international units.

7. How long do leakage enzymes remain elevated in blood of horses and ruminants after transient hepatocellular injury?

SDH remains high for only 3 to 4 days. AST stays elevated for 1 to 2 weeks (Figure 30-2).

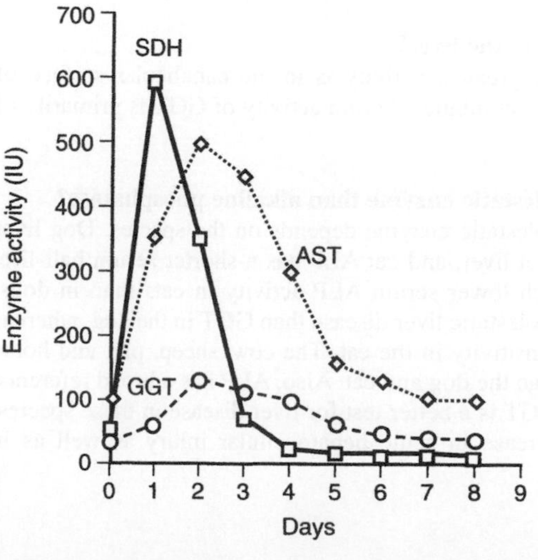

Figure 30-2 Serum enzyme activity after acute transient liver injury in horses and ruminants. *SDH,* Sorbitol dehydrogenase; *AST,* aspartate transaminase, *GGT,* γ-glutamyltransferase.

8. Does the magnitude of increase in leakage enzymes predict the number of hepatocytes injured?

In general, the higher the activity in the serum, the greater is the number of hepatocytes injured.

9. Do leakage enzymes predict whether liver injury is reversible?

Leakage enzymes do *not* predict reversible liver injury. Acute reversible toxic or traumatic hepatocellular injury can result in very high serum activities of leakage enzymes, whereas chronic fibrotic liver disease, which is irreversible, may result in only slight increases in leakage enzymes.

10. Are there other factors in addition to hepatocellular injury that increase serum enzyme activities?

A mild to moderate increase in ALT can result from enzyme induction associated with administration of drugs such as anticonvulsants, thiacetarsemide, and glucocorticoids. AST is present in most tissue and increases with muscle injury as well as hepatocelluar injury. AST is also present in kidney, pancreas, and erythrocytes. Artifactual hemolysis of blood samples may result in increased serum ALT activity.

11. Is alkaline phosphatase a liver-specific cholestatic enzyme?

ALP is not liver specific. ALP isoenzymes are present in all tissues with high activity in liver, bone, kidney, intestine, and placenta. The renal, intestinal, and placental isoenzymes have a very short half-life in the plasma (<6 minutes) and thus do not result in a significant increase in plasma activity. The bone isoenzyme is produced by osteoblasts. Young growing animals may have up to three times the normal adult serum activity. Serum activity may increase two to four times as a result of diseases that increase osteoblastic activity. Anticonvulsant may increase serum activity by two to six times. Corticosteroids induce a marked increase in a specific hepatic isoenzyme in dogs. The steroid isoenzyme increases within 6 days after exposure to endogenous or exogenous corticosteroids and can reach very high levels by 3 to 4 weeks. Serum ALP activity decreases slowly over weeks to months after cessation of exposure to corticosteroids.

12. How can the steroid-induced isoenzyme in the dog be differentiated from the liver isoenzyme?

The liver isoenzyme activity is greater than 90% inhibited by addition of levamisole, whereas the steroid-induced isoenzyme is relatively resistant to addition of levamisole. GGT is also present on some chemistry profiles. Because GGT is more liver specific than ALP, an increase in GGT in addition to ALP is consistent with cholestatic liver disease.

13. Is γ-glutamyltransferase only present in the liver?

GGT is present in most tissue, but the greatest activity is in the canalicular surface of hepatocytes, in bile duct epithelium, and in renal tubules. Serum activity of GGT is primarily of hepatic origin.

14. Is γ-glutamyltransferase a better cholestatic enzyme than alkaline phosphatase?

Whether GGT or ALP is the better cholestatic enzyme depends on the species. Dog liver contains about three times more ALP than cat liver, and cat ALP has a shorter serum half-life. Cholestatic liver disease thus results in much lower serum ALP activity in cats than in dogs. Therefore, ALP is a more sensitive test for cholestatic liver disease than GGT in the dog, whereas ALP and GGT have approximately equal sensitivity in the cat. The cow, sheep, pig, and horse have greater liver and serum GGT activity than the dog and cat. Also, ALP has a broad reference range in cattle, pigs, sheep, and horses, so GGT is a better test for liver disease in these species. In horses, cattle, and sheep, GGT may increase in acute hepatocellular injury as well as in cholestatic liver disease.

15. Do liver enzyme tests predict pathologic changes in the liver?

Enzyme tests predict liver changes only in very general terms. Serum leakage and cholestatic enzyme tests are sensitive indicators of hepatocellular injury and cholestatic disease, respectively. However, serum activities in a variety of diseases overlap and cannot be differentiated. In most cases, acute hepatocellular injury or necrosis can be differentiated from chronic fibrotic disease. In acute hepatocellular injury in dogs and cats, ALT and AST may increase 50 to 100 times the mean reference interval. A slight to moderate increase in ALP and little to no increase in GGT occurs. In acute diffuse hepatocellular injury in ruminant and horses, a marked increase in SDH and AST and a variable (mild to marked) increase in GGT occur. Alternatively, in extrahepatic bile duct obstruction or in chronic fibrotic liver disease, ALP and GGT are greatly increased, and leakage enzymes are only mildly increased. However, responses vary among the species. In cholestatic liver disease the magnitude of increase in ALP is marked for dogs, significantly less for cats and horses, and variable in ruminants. In my experience, attempting to predict other types of liver pathology solely on the serum enzyme activities is unreliable.

16. What defines a test of liver function?

A liver function test is a test that evaluates the capacity of the liver to perform a single function or multiple functions that are unique to the liver.

17. Can liver dysfunction be reversible?

Liver dysfunction can be reversed, particularly in acute hepatic disease. In acute toxic or traumatic liver disease, swelling or altered cellular metabolism may result in transient hepatocellular dysfunction. The liver also has the capacity to regenerate destroyed hepatocytes and thus regain functional mass. In chronic hepatitis, liver failure results from a combination of the opposing effects of hepatocellular destruction and liver regeneration. By the time liver dysfunction is detected, the destructive effects have overcome the regenerative effects. This condition is usually irreversible.

18. What are common liver function tests?

Because the liver has a very large number of unique metabolic functions, multiple liver function tests have been described. These tests can be subclassified as follows:

a. *Tests of peripheral blood uptake, conjugation, and secretion:* serum bilirubin and sulfobromophthalein (BSP) excretion test
b. *Tests of portal blood clearance:* ammonia tolerance and bile acids
c. *Tests of hepatic synthesis:* serum glucose, albumin, urea, and clotting factors

19. Do liver function tests vary in sensitivity?

Liver function tests vary greatly in their sensitivity in detecting liver dysfunction. The exact sensitivity of liver function tests has not been well defined and may vary among species. The most sensitive liver function test appears to be bile acids, which can detect 40% to 50% liver dysfunction. The BSP and ammonia tolerance tests are somewhat less sensitive. Liver function test included in serum chemistry profiles (e.g., total bilirubin, albumin) are very insensitive liver function tests, requiring 80% to 90% liver dysfunction before results are beyond reference limits.

20. What is the best liver function test for routine use?

Serum albumin and total bilirubin are the least expensive and easiest tests to perform but have significant limitations. Both are very insensitive tests and are not liver specific. Of the other tests, the serum bile acids test is the easiest to perform, the most sensitive, and liver specific. Therefore the bile acids test has largely replaced BSP and ammonia tolerance tests.

21. How is the serum bile acids test performed?

In dogs and cats, fasting (8-12 hours) and/or 2-hour postprandial blood samples are drawn.

During fasting, serum concentrations are lower because bile acids are removed from the blood and stored in the gallbladder. Feeding induces gallbladder contraction, which releases bile acids into the intestine. As bile acids are reabsorbed through the portal circulation, most are removed by the liver, but some enter the peripheral circulation. The 2-hour postprandial bile acids test increases the sensitivity of the test. It is particularly useful in detecting portosystemic venous shunts because fasting serum concentrations may be normal.

22. How does hepatocellular dysfunction result in increased bile acids in serum?

Reduced functional liver mass or shunting of portal blood away from the liver increases the number of bile acids that bypass the liver and enter the peripheral circulation. Also, intrahepatic bile duct obstruction, which is associated with liver disease, causes regurgitation of bile acids into the peripheral blood.

23. How do BSP and ammonia tolerance compare to bile acids as tests of liver function?

Both the BSP test and the ammonia tolerance test are more difficult to perform and have equal or lesser sensitivity for detection of liver dysfunction than the bile acids test. Therefore the bile acids test has largely replaced BSP and ammonia tolerance tests.

24. Is hyperbilirubinemia (icterus) a specific indicator of liver disease?

Hyperbilirubinemia can be caused by prehepatic, hepatic, or posthepatic causes; icterus is not a specific indicator for liver disease. Prehepatic causes are associated with hemolytic anemias. In animals with prehepatic icterus, hyperbilirubinemia is usually associated with a moderate to severe anemia, whereas the anemia associated with chronic liver disease is usually mild. Hepatic icterus is associated with diffuse hepatocellular swelling, severe acute hepatitis, and end-stage chronic hepatitis. Icterus is frequently accompanied by hepatic enzymopathy and low serum albumin. Posthepatic icterus results from extrahepatic bile duct obstruction.

25. In addition to determination of total bilirubin, is determination of direct (conjugated) and indirect (unconjugated) bilirubin useful in differentiating the cause of icterus?

In hemolytic anemias, unconjugated bilirubin is formed from the breakdown of heme. As a result, bilirubin in the blood is expected to be primarily *unconjugated.* In liver disease or extrahepatic bile duct obstruction, unconjugated bilirubin is conjugated by the remaining functional hepatocytes, but the conjugated bilirubin is regurgitated into the blood as a result of bile duct obstruction. Therefore the increase in serum bilirubin with liver disease and bile duct obstruction would be expected to be primarily *conjugated.* However, the relative concentrations of conjugated and unconjugated bilirubin in prehepatic and hepatic icterus frequently do not fit the expected patterns. Because of a high incidence of confusing results and the availability of other tests to differentiate hemolytic disease reliably from hepatic disease, conjugated and unconjugated bilirubin determinations are infrequently performed.

26. Are there species differences in bilirubin metabolism?

Dogs have a low renal threshold for bilirubin, and bilirubinuria frequently occurs without hyperbilirubinemia. Horses frequently become icteric, and bilirubin is primarily unconjugated despite the cause of hyperbilirubinemia. Unconjugated bilirubin is predominant in horses probably because uptake of bilirubin by the liver is the limiting step in bilirubin metabolism. With anorexia, uptake is reduced further, which can result in marked increases (5-10 mg/dl) in serum bilirubin concentration. Hyperbilirubinemia occurs infrequently in ruminants. When present, the magnitude of increase is slight and the cause more frequently related to hemolytic than hepatic disease.

27. What type of changes in serum proteins is expected in liver disease?

Hypoalbuminemia is an extremely late change in chronic liver failure. Hyperglobulinemia is a frequent finding in chronic liver disease and may result from increased numbers of enteric antigens bypassing the liver and entering the peripheral blood. A chronic immune response to these antigens results in a polyclonal gammopathy.

31. LABORATORY EVALUATION OF LIVER DISEASE IN DOMESTIC ANIMALS

1. What are the major types of inflammatory liver disease described in dogs?

Despite decades of study, the classification of canine inflammatory liver disease is poorly defined. Although many etiologic agents have been defined, a cause cannot be established for most cases of chronic hepatitis. The histopathologic classification of chronic liver disease is controversial. "Chronic hepatitis" is a general, all-inclusive categorization used by many clinicians. More specific terms include *chronic progressive hepatitis, chronic active hepatitis, chronic lobular dissecting hepatitis,* and *cirrhosis*.

2. List the known causes of acute hepatitis in the dog and cat.

a. *Infectious:* bacterial abscesses, cholangitis, cholangiohepatitis, canine adenovirus type 1, feline infectious peritonitis, histoplasmosis, toxoplasmosis
b. *Drugs:* thiacetarsemide, diethylcarbamazine, acetaminophen, mebendazole, halothane, methoxyflurane, aprinidine, ketoconazole, methotrexate, nalidixic acid, tetracycline, tolbutamide, trimethoprim-sulfadiazine, diazepam (cat)
c. *Chemicals:* carbon tetrachloride, dieldrin, chloroform, arsenic, chlorinated hydrocarbons, naphthalenes, chlorinated biphenyls, phosphorus, copper, mercury, iron, selenium, tannic acid

3. List the causes of chronic hepatitis in the dog.

a. *Infectious:* bacterial cholangitis or cholangiohepatitis, canine adenovirus type 1, leptospirosis, canine acidophil cell viral hepatitis, histoplasmosis, dirofilariosis
b. *Drugs:* primidone, phenytoin, phenobarbital, ketoconazole, methotrexate, milbolerone, methotrexate, trimethoprim-sulfadiazine, glucocorticoids
c. *Copper accumulation disorders:* Bedlington terriers, West Highland white terriers, Skye terriers, Doberman pinschers
d. *Autoimmune disorders*
e. *Alpha-1-antitrypsin disorder*

4. What are the major types of hepatitis described in cats?

Categorization of feline inflammatory liver diseases is controversial. Some authors prefer to use *cholangitis* or *cholangiohepatitis* to describe all inflammatory liver diseases. Other authors have used more specific categories, including *lymphocytic portal hepatitis, lymphocytic cholangitis/cholangiohepatitis, suppurative cholangiohepatitis, chronic cholangiohepatitis,* and *sclerosing cholangitis*. This categorization is complicated by evidence that lymphocytes accumulate in portal areas of aged cats.

5. What are the major clinical and laboratory abnormalities in acute hepatitis?

Clinical signs of acute hepatitis include anorexia, vomiting, icterus, and hepatic encephalopathy. A marked (>100-fold) increase in alanine transaminase (ALT) and aspartate transaminase

(AST) is a consistent finding. Alkaline phosphatase (ALP) is moderately increased in the dog but may not increase or may increase only slightly in the cat. Gamma-glutamyltransferase (GGT) may remain within reference limits or increase slightly. If lesions are diffuse, liver dysfunction may occur, as detected by increased serum bile acids or serum bilirubin and sulfobromophthalein (BSP) retention. Serum albumin and globulin concentrations are usually within reference limits but may be increased if hemoconcentration is present. Dogs with acute hepatitis are predisposed to development of disseminated intravascular coagulopathy.

6. What are the major clinical and laboratory abnormalities associated with canine chronic hepatitis?

Frequent clinical signs of canine chronic hepatitis include weight loss, anorexia, mild to moderate nonregenerative anemia, polyuria, polydipsia, and decreased liver size. In late-stage hepatic failure, icterus, ascites, or signs of hepatic encephalopathy may develop. Leakage enzymes are variably increased. The magnitude of increase roughly correlates with numbers of hepatocytes that are being destroyed. The term *chronic active hepatitis* has been used to describe chronic hepatitis in which large increases in leakage enzymes persist over time. Consistent large increases in cholestatic enzymes are present, and the magnitude of increase in cholestatic enzymes exceeds the magnitude of increase in leakage enzymes. Hepatocellular dysfunction can usually be identified at initial diagnosis. Polyclonal gammopathy and mild nonregenerative anemia are usually present. In late-stage liver failure, hypoalbuminemia, increased serum ammonia concentrations, and hyperbilirubinemia may be present.

7. What are the major clinical and laboratory abnormalities associated with canine steroid hepatopathy?

Clinical signs of steroid hepatopathy are usually not seen in the dog, although signs of hyperadrenocorticism or a history of glucocorticoid administration should be present. Lesions in the liver are characterized by multifocal areas of hepatocellular vacuolar change. Intracellular lipid content may also be increased. Leakage enzymes may be mildly to moderately increased due to altered cell membrane permeability and enzyme induction. A marked increase in ALP is present in dogs. Tests of liver function are usually within reference limits.

8. What are the major clinical and laboratory abnormalities associated with congenital portosystemic shunting of blood?

Clinical signs of congenital portosystemic shunting include microhepatia, hepatic encephalopathy, and hypoglycemic coma in young dogs. Leakage and cholestatic enzymes are usually within reference limits. Baseline plasma ammonia and postprandial bile acids are usually abnormal.

9. What are the major clinical and laboratory abnormalities associated with feline suppurative cholangiohepatitis?

Suppurative cholangiohepatitis tends to occur in young and middle-aged cats. Clinical signs include severe illness characterized by lethargy, fever, vomiting, and icterus. Liver size may be normal, increased, or decreased. Laboratory findings include neutrophilia, left shift, hyperbilirubinemia (mean 4.7 mg/dl), moderate to marked increase in ALT, and little or no increase in cholestatic enzymes. As cholangiohepatitis becomes more chronic, neutrophilia and left shift may not be present, ALT tends to be lower, and cholestatic enzymes may increase.

10. What are the major clinical and laboratory abnormalities associated with lymphocytic portal hepatitis?

Lymphocytic portal hepatitis tends to occur in old cats. Clinical signs include anorexia and vomiting. Liver size may be normal, increased, or decreased. Laboratory abnormalities include mild to moderate increases in ALT and normal to slight increases in ALP. Hyperbilirubinemia is mild (<3.0 mg/dl) when present.

11. What are the major clinical and laboratory abnormalities associated with feline hepatic lipidosis?

Clinical signs of hepatic lipidosis include anorexia (100% of cases), weight loss, lethargy, vomiting, and enlarged liver in the cat. Laboratory abnormalities include marked increases in ALT and ALP and marked hyperbilirubinemia (>5 mg/dl). Bile acids and BSP retention are usually abnormal, consistent with liver dysfunction. Serum albumin also is usually normal. Hyperglycemia may be present if hepatic lipidosis occurs secondary to diabetes mellitus.

12. What differences in complete blood counts and serum chemistry profiles may be useful in differentiating feline suppurative cholangiohepatitis from lymphocytic portal hepatitis and hepatic lipidosis?

Table 31-1 compares test results in differentiating feline suppurative cholangiohepatitis from lymphocytic portal hepatitis and hepatic lipidosis.

13. What additional tests are helpful in diagnosing canine and feline liver disease?

Hepatic biopsy or cytologic evaluation and imaging techniques are important tests for evaluation of liver diseases. A definitive diagnosis cannot be established without a hepatic biopsy or aspirate. Cytology has been used more frequently in recent years. Fine-needle aspiration is relatively safe compared with large-needle core biopsy. Both cytology and core biopsy techniques are frequently done under ultrasound guidance, which permits biopsy of focal lesions within the liver. The routine use of sonographic imaging has permitted evaluation of focal lesions in the liver and evaluation of the biliary system, leading to routine detection of bile duct obstruction.

14. List the major types of liver disease described in horses.

a. *Infectious:* Tyzzer's disease, equine herpesvirus type 1, septic cholangiohepatitis, abscesses
b. *Parasites:* nematodes, flukes
c. *Metabolic:* hyperlipemia and hepatic lipidosis, steroid hepatopathy
d. *Toxins:* pyrrolizidine alkaloid–containing plants, horsebrush, puncture vine, cycad palm, lupine, panic grass, blue-green algae, mushrooms, mycotoxins (moldy corn, moldy alfalfa), alsike clover
e. *Chemicals:* carbon tetrachloride, carbon disulfide, iron, copper, ferrous fumarate (foals)
f. *Drugs:* isoniazid, rifampin, halothane, dantrolene, phenothiazines
g. *Extrahepatic bile duct obstruction:* calculi, abscesses, neoplasia, colonic displacement, biliary atresia, parasitic disease
h. *Congenital:* portosystemic venous shunting of blood, biliary atresia
i. *Neoplasia:* hepatocellular carcinoma, biliary carcinoma, lymphosarcoma, hemangiosarcoma

Table 31-1 ***Test Results in Differentiating Feline Hepatic Disease***

TEST	SUPPURATIVE CHOLANGIOHEPATITIS	LYMPHOCYTIC PORTAL HEPATITIS	HEPATIC LIPIDOSIS
Neutrophilia	Present	Absent	Absent
Left shift	Present	Absent	Absent
ALT	Moderate to marked increase	Slight increase	Marked increase
ALP	Slight or no increase	Slight or no increase	Marked increase
Total bilirubin	Mild or moderate increase	Slight increase	Marked increase

ALT, Alanine transaminase (aminotransferase); *ALP,* alkaline phosphatase.

j. *Idiopathic:* Theiler's disease (serum hepatitis), chronic active hepatitis
k. *Secondary to other diseases:* portal vein thrombosis, pancreatitis, duodenal ulceration, large colon displacement

15. List the major types of liver disease described in ruminants.

a. *Infectious:* septic abscesses; *Chlamydia, Salmonella,* and *Listeria* spp.; tuberculosis; Johne's disease
b. *Parasites:* sarcosporidiosis, *Fasciola hepatica, Ascaris* spp.
c. *Metabolic:* hepatic lipidosis
d. *Toxins:* blue-green algae, pyrrolizidine alkaloid–containing plants, mycotoxins (moldy hay, moldy tall fescue), cottonseed meal, Klein grass
e. *Chemicals:* iron, copper, phosphorus, arsenic, carbon tetrachloride, hexachloroethane, gossypol, cresols, coal tar pitch, nitrite, chlorinated naphthylenes
f. *Drugs:* halothane
g. *Extrahepatic bile duct obstruction:* calculi, abscesses
h. *Congenital:* hepatic fibrosis, hemochromatosis of Salers cattle, portosystemic venous shunting of blood, congenital hyperbilirubinemia of Corrydale and Southdown sheep
i. *Idiopathic:* hepatic fatty cirrhosis (cattle, sheep)

16. What serum chemistry tests are appropriate for evaluation of equine liver disease?

Sorbitol dehydrogenase (SDH) is the most specific test for hepatocellular injury in horses. AST is a useful but nonspecific test for hepatocellular injury. ALP is a good test for cholestatic disease. GGT is also a good indicator of cholestasis but has also been reported to increase with hepatocellular injury.

17. What serum chemistry tests are appropriate for evaluation of ruminant liver disease?

In general, increases in leakage and cholestatic enzyme activity are less for ruminants than for other species. In ruminants as in horses, SDH is the most specific test for hepatocellular injury, and AST is a useful but nonspecific test. Again, ALP is not a good test for cholestatic disease, and GGT is the best indicator of cholestasis but may increase with hepatocellular injury. Total serum bilirubin is rarely increased with liver disease.

18. What liver function tests are appropriate for horses and ruminants?

BSP excretion tests have been used in horses and ruminants. The clearance time of BSP is determined by measuring the half-life of disappearance from the plasma. Bile acids have been used as tests of liver function in both horses and ruminants and appears to be useful in both.

19. What are the major clinical signs and laboratory abnormalities associated with pyrrolizidine alkaloid poisoning in the horse?

Clinical disease usually occurs acutely within 6 months after initial exposure to alkaloid-containing plants. Clinical signs associated with acute toxicity in the horse include depression, anorexia, icterus, ataxia, and skin lesions. If onset of signs occurs more slowly, weight loss may be seen. ALP, GGT, and AST are significantly increased. SDH may or may not be increased. Liver dysfunction is present, as determined by BSP retention and bile acids.

20. What are the major clinical signs and laboratory findings associated with Theiler's disease (serum hepatitis) in the horse?

Theiler's disease is associated with acute onset of signs 4 to 10 weeks after administration of whole blood or products containing equine serum. Lethargy, anorexia, icterus, and signs of hepatic encephalopathy are frequent findings in the horse. SDH, AST, ALP, and GGT activity and total bilirubin are usually increased at diagnosis. Bile acid concentrations are usually consistent with liver dysfunction.

21. What are the major clinical signs and laboratory findings associated with chronic hepatitis in the horse?

Clinical signs of chronic hepatitis include marked depression, weight loss, neurologic signs, and icterus in the horse. AST, ALP, GGT and sometimes SDH activities are increased. Total bilirubin concentration is increased, BSP retention is prolonged, and bile acids are increased, consistent with liver dysfunction.

22. What are the major clinical signs and laboratory abnormalities associated with cholangiohepatitis in horses?

Cholangiohepatitis is caused by an ascending infection within the biliary tree. *Salmonella* is the most frequent cause in the horse. In salmonellosis the most prominent clinical signs include acute diarrhea, fever, depression, and dehydration. SDH, AST, ALP, and GGT activity and total bilirubin concentration are usually increased.

23. What are the major clinical signs and laboratory findings associated with cholelithiasis in the horse?

Clinical signs of equine cholelithiasis include intermittent colic, fever, and icterus. Serum activities of ALP and GGT are usually increased. Ultrasonography is the most definitive diagnostic tool.

24. What are the major clinical signs and laboratory findings associated with hyperlipidemia and hepatic lipidosis in the horse?

The condition is usually associated with a negative energy balance secondary to pregnancy, lactation, exercise, or febrile illnesses. Clinical signs are nonspecific in equine hyperlipidemia and hepatic lipidosis. The serum is lipemic, and SDH, GGT, or ALP activities may be increased. Serum bilirubin concentration may also be increased depending on the severity of the hepatic lipidosis.

25. What are the major clinical signs and laboratory alterations associated with liver abscesses in feedlot cattle?

Hepatic abscesses are a frequent problem in feedlot cattle and result from absorption of enteric organisms into the enterohepatic circulation. The most frequently involved organisms are *Fusobacterium necrophorum* and *Actinomyces pyogenes*. The only consistent laboratory abnormality associated with hepatic abscesses is hyperglobulinemia.

26. What are the major clinical signs and laboratory findings associated with *Fasciola hepatica* infection in cattle and sheep?

Fluke-infected cattle rarely have evidence of clinical disease. Hepatic enzyme tests are usually within reference limits, and liver dysfunction is not present. Antemortem diagnosis is based on identification of ova in feces.

27. What are the major clinical signs and laboratory findings associated with hepatic lipidosis in cattle?

Fatty liver syndrome occurs in the periparturient period in heavily lactating dairy cows. The cause of hepatic lipidosis is thought to be a negative energy balance that results in mobilization of fatty acids more rapidly than they can be utilized. All periparturient dairy cows tend to accumulate fat in their liver, but some cows (particularly those that are overweight) have marked accumulation and develop hepatocellular disease. Concurrent diseases that lead to prolonged anorexia and perhaps congenital factors predispose to the condition. Decreased concentrations of protein kinase C, lecithin-cholesterol acyltransferase, and methionine have been reported in cows with fatty liver syndrome. Laboratory abnormalities are subtle. Slight increases in AST or ALP may occur. Slight decreases in albumin and albumin/globulin ratio have been reported. Bile acids are usually normal, and BSP retention may be normal or slightly increased.

28. What are the major clinical signs and laboratory findings associated with pyrrolizidine alkaloid–induced hepatic disease in cattle?

Clinical signs associated with pyrrolizidine alkaloid–induced hepatic disease include weight loss, weakness, anorexia, depression, and tenesmus. SDH, AST, ALP, and GGT activities are normal or slightly increased. In most cases, however, BSP retention and bile acids are abnormal, indicating liver dysfunction. In severe cases, hypoalbuminemia is present, but total serum protein is usually normal because of hyperglobulinemia.

29. What are the major clinical signs and laboratory findings associated with blue-green algae hepatotoxicosis in cattle?

Affected cows have clinical signs, including anorexia, unresponsiveness, and recumbency. These signs of blue-green hepatotoxicosis resemble those associated with milk fever. Slight increases in SDH, AST, ALP, or GGT may be present.

32. LABORATORY EVALUATION OF MUSCLE DISEASE IN DOMESTIC ANIMALS

1. What serum enzyme tests can be used to evaluate muscle degeneration or necrosis?

Creatine kinase (CK), aspartate transaminase (AST), and lactate dehydrogenase (LDH) have been used to evaluate muscle disorders in dogs, cats, ruminants, and horses. Alanine transaminase (ALT) has been used as a muscle specific enzyme in ruminant and horses because very little is present in liver. Serum activities increase with degenerative and necrotic lesions but do not increase with muscle atrophy or neoplasia.

2. Which of the muscle enzymes is the most specific for detection of muscle disease?

CK is highly specific for muscle injury. Although CK is present in low amounts in intestine, uterus, kidney, and urinary bladder, a substantial increase in serum CK activity is almost always an indication of skeletal or cardiac muscle degeneration or necrosis. CK activity increases within a few hours of onset of muscle necrosis. CK has a short half-life in plasma. As a result, CK activity returns to normal within 24 to 48 hours after cessation of muscle injury. Therefore a persistent increase in serum CK activity can be interpreted as continued muscle injury.

3. Which of the muscle enzymes is the most sensitive test of muscle injury?

CK is a very sensitive indicator of muscle injury. Even minor muscle injury, such as intramuscular injection, minor trauma associated with transportation of large animals, and strenuous exercise, will result in increased serum CK activity. AST activity increases more slowly in plasma. LDH activity increases rapidly, but the magnitude of increase is less than that of CK.

4. Does determination of creatine kinase (CK) and aspartate transaminase (AST) provide any additional information beyond determination of CK alone?

AST is present in most cells, but increased activity in serum is usually associated with liver or muscle disease. AST is also present in erythrocytes, so hemolysis may increase serum activity. The combination of CK and AST can be used to pinpoint the cause of the increase in AST activity. If both are increased, the disease process is probably related to muscle injury, whereas if AST activity is increased and CK activity is normal, the disease process is probably located in the liver. However, AST decreases more slowly after cessation of muscle injury. Therefore, previous muscle injury cannot be ruled out when increased AST activity and normal CK activity is observed.

5. Are creatine kinase (CK) isoenzymes useful in evaluating increased serum CK activity?

Two subunits of CK are present: *B* for brain and *M* for muscle. Each molecule of CK consists of two of these subunits. The *BB* isoenzyme (CK_1) is found in the brain, the *MB* isoenzyme (CK_2) primarily in cardiac muscle, and the *MM* isoenzyme (CK_3) in skeletal and cardiac muscle. CK_1 activity may increase in cerebrospinal fluid with brain injury but does not increase in plasma. Skeletal muscle injury primarily results in an increase in CK_3, whereas cardiac muscle injury results in an increase in CK_2 and CK_3.

6. Are lactate dehydrogenase (LDH) isoenzymes useful in evaluating muscle injury?

LDH (also LD) has five isoenzymes. Each isoenzyme consists of a tetrameric combination of two subunits: LD_1 (H_4), LD_2 (H_3M_1), LD_3 (H_2M_2), LD_4 (H_1M_3), and LD_5 (M_4). LD_5 is the major isoenzyme in skeletal muscle and erythrocytes. LD_1 is the major isoenzyme in cardiac muscle, and kidney. Therefore, skeletal muscle injury primarily results in an increase in LD_5, whereas myocardial injury primarily result in an increase in LDH_1.

7. How long do muscle enzymes remain elevated in serum after transient muscle injury?

CK increases rapidly after onset of muscle injury and returns to normal within 3 to 7 days. AST and LDH increase and decrease more slowly than CK (Figure 32-1).

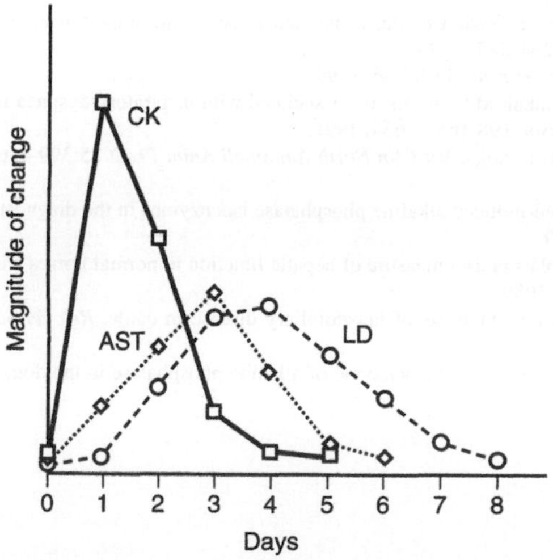

Figure 32-1 Serum enzyme activity after acute transient muscle injury in domestic animals. *CK*, Creatine kinase; *LD*, lactate dehydrogenase; *AST*, aspartate transaminase (aminotransferase).

8. What other chemistry tests may be altered with muscle injury?

Severe muscle injury may result in myoglobinuria and hyperkalemia. Myoglobin is released from degenerating and necrotic muscle and is rapidly excreted in the urine. Myoglobinuria can be differentiated from hemoglobinuria by addition of saturated ammonium sulfate. Ammonium sulfate clears the color associated with hemoglobin but not myoglobin. Muscle contains a high concentration of potassium, and severe muscle injury may result in hyperkalemia.

Liver and Muscle

BIBLIOGRAPHY

Aktas M, Auguste D, Concordet D, et al: Creatine kinase in dog plasma: preanalytical factors of variation, reference values, and diagnostic significance, *Res Vet Sci* 56:30-39, 1994.

Bergman JR: Nodular hyperplasia in the liver of the dog: an association with changes in the Ito cell population, *Vet Pathol* 22:427-438, 1985.

Bersso JG, Wrigley RH, Gliatto JM, et al: Ultrasonographic appearance and clinical findings in 14 dogs with gallbladder mucocele, *Vet Radiol Ultrasound* 41:261-271, 2000.

Boyd JW: Serum enzymes in the diagnosis of disease in man and animals, *J Comp Pathol* 98:381-393, 1988.

Bunch SE: Hepatotoxicity associated with pharmacologic agents in dogs and cats, *Vet Clin North Am Small Anim Pract* 23:659-670, 1993.

Cebra CK, Garry FB, Getzy DM, et al: Hepatic lipidosis in anorectic, lactating Holstein cattle: a retrospective study of serum biochemical abnormalities, *J Vet Intern Med* 11:231-237, 1997.

Center SA: Serum bile acids in companion animal medicine, *Vet Clin North Am Small Anim Pract* 23:625-648, 1993.

Center SA, Baldwin BH, Dillingham S, et al: Diagnostic value of serum gamma-glutamyl transferase and alkaline phosphatase activities in hepatobiliary disease in the cat, *J Am Vet Med Assoc* 188:507-512, 1986.

Center SA, Slater MR, ManWarren T, et al: Diagnostic efficacy of serum alkaline phosphatase and gamma glutamyltransferase in dogs with histologically confirmed hepatobiliary disease: 270 cases (1980-1990), *J Am Vet Med Assoc* 201:1258-1264, 1992.

Duncan JR, Prasse KW, Mahaffey EA: *Veterinary laboratory medicine,* ed 3, Ames, 1994, Iowa State University Press, pp 132-137, 184-187.

Fuentealba C, Guest S, Haywood S, et al: Chronic hepatitis: a retrospective study of 34 dogs, *Can Vet J* 38:365-373, 1997.

Jarrett WFH, O'Neil BW, Lindholm I: Persistent hepatitis and chronic fibrosis induced by canine acidophil cell hepatitis virus, *Vet Res* 120:234-235, 1987.

Messer NT, Johnson PJ: Idiopathic acute hepatic disease in horses: 12 cases (1982-1992), *J Am Vet Med Assoc* 204:1934-1937, 1994.

Nagaraja TG, Laudert SB, Parrott JC: Liver abscesses in feedlot cattle. 2. Incidence, economic importance, and prevention, *Compend Contin Educ Pract Vet* 18:S264-S277, 1996.

Pearson EG: Liver disease in the mature horse, *Equine Vet Educ* 11:87-96, 1999.

Pearson EG: Liver failure attributable to pyrrolizidine alkaloid toxicosis and associated with inspiratory dyspnea in ponies: three cases (1982-1988), *J Am Vet Med Assoc* 198:1651-1654, 1991.

Rolfe DS, Twedt DC: Copper-associated hepatopathies in dogs, *Vet Clin North Am Small Anim Pract* 25:399-416, 1995.

Teske E, Rothuizen J, deBruijne JJ, et al: Corticosteroid-induced alkaline phosphatase isoenzymes in the diagnosis of canine hypercorticism, *Vet Res* 125:12-21, 1989.

West HJ: Clearance of bromosulfophthalein from the plasma as a measure of hepatic function in normal horses and horses with liver disease, *Res Vet Sci* 46:264-269, 1989.

West HJ: Evaluation of total bile acid concentrations for diagnosis of hepatobiliary disease in cattle, *Res Vet Sci* 48:133-140, 1991.

Wilson SM, Feldman EC: Diagnostic value of the steroid-induced isoenzyme of alkaline phosphatase in the dog, *J Am Anim Hosp Assoc* 28:245-253, 1992.

Section VII
Lipids and Carbohydrates

Steven L. Stockham and Karen S. Dolce

33. TRIGLYCERIDES, CHOLESTEROL, AND OTHER LIPIDS

1. Define the following terms: lipid, lipoprotein, apolipoprotein, triglyceride, cholesterol, fatty acid, hyperlipemia, hyperlipidemia, hyperlipoproteinemia, and lipemia.

a. *Lipid:* class of compounds that are insoluble in water and soluble in organic solvents.

b. *Lipoprotein:* complex that is composed of a core of hydrophobic lipids (triglycerides) covered by a layer of phospholipids, apolipoproteins, and cholesteryl esters; the form in which lipids are transported in the blood. Four main classes are (1) chylomicrons, (2) very-low-density lipoproteins (VLDLs), (3) low-density lipoproteins (LDLs), and (4) high-density lipoproteins (HDLs). Some classifications include intermediate-density lipoproteins (IDLs) between VLDL and LDL molecules.

c. *Apolipoprotein:* protein component (apoprotein) of a lipoprotein. Five major families are designated apolipoprotein A, B, C, D, and E.

d. *Triglyceride:* storage form of lipids composed of three molecules of fatty acids bound with one molecule of glycerol. The molecule is more appropriately called triacylglycerol but is referred to as "triglyceride" in most medical literature.

e. *Cholesterol:* steroid alcohol synthesized in hepatocytes that is used to make steroidal molecules and is degraded to bile acids in hepatocytes.

f. *Fatty acid:* chain of carbon atoms with a carboxylic acid group at one end. Fatty acids combine with glycerol to form fat (e.g., mono-, di-, and triacylglycerol).

g. *Hyperlipemia* and *hyperlipidemia:* general terms that indicate increased concentration of lipids in the blood due to increased concentrations of free fatty acids, hypertriglyceridemia, hypercholesterolemia, or hyperlipoproteinemia.

h. *Hyperlipoproteinemia:* increased concentration of lipoproteins in the blood.

i. *Lipemia:* can be used as a synonym for hyperlipidemia and hyperlipoproteinemia; more often defined as the *lactescent* (milky) appearance of serum or plasma due to increased concentrations of large lipoprotein molecules.

2. Which two lipid compounds in the plasma of domestic mammals are most commonly measured by clinical laboratory assays?

The two major analytes are cholesterol and triglyceride (triacylglycerol). The triglyceride molecules and almost all the cholesterol molecules circulate in plasma lipoproteins.

Serum cholesterol concentration is the *total* cholesterol concentration. The reacting cholesterol molecules (cholesterol and cholesterol esters) were within lipoproteins, typically in cholesterol-rich LDL and HDL molecules. Likewise, serum triglyceride concentration is the *total* triglyceride concentration. The reacting triglyceride molecules were mostly within triglyceride-rich lipoproteins (chylomicrons, VLDLs, IDLs).

3. How are lipoproteins classified?

Lipoproteins are classified by either their electrophoretic mobility or by their density relative to water. Their electrophoretic migrations and their densities depend on their compositions. In the *electrophoretic* classification the large and poorly charged chylomicrons do not migrate from the application point (end of gamma region). However, the smaller lipoproteins with their external coating of charged protein and lipid molecules migrate into the alpha (α) and beta (β) regions, as designated by routine protein electrophoresis in which molecules are stained with a protein stain instead of a lipid stain. In the *density* classification, which uses the common lipoprotein names (e.g., VLDL, IDL), the lipoproteins are grouped by their relative density compared with water (Table 33-1).

Table 33-1 ***Classification, Content, and Properties of Human Lipoproteins***

	LIPOPROTEINS				
PROPERTY	CHYLOMICRON	VLDL	IDL	LDL	HDL
Density (g/ml)	<0.95	0.95-1.006	1.006-1.019	1.019-1.063	1.063-1.210
Major lipid	Dietary TG	Hepatic TG	Hepatic TG and CE	Phospholipid and CE	Phospholipid and CE
Electrophoretic migration	Origin	Pre-β	β to pre-β	β	α
Diameter (nm)	>70	25-70	22-24	19-23	4-10
Contribute to serum lactescence	Yes, floats with time	Yes	Maybe	No	No
Major site of formation	Small intestine enterocytes	Hepatocytes	Plasma	Plasma	Hepatocytes
Major sites of degradation or transformation	Plasma, hepatocytes	Plasma	Plasma	Nonhepatic cells, hepatocytes, macrophages	Hepatocytes

VLDL, IDL, LDL, HDL, Very-low-density, intermediate-density, low-density, and high-density lipoproteins; *TG,* triglyceride; *CE,* cholesterol ester; *β, α,* beta and alpha regions.

Data from Rifai N, Bachorik PS, Albers JJ: Lipids, lipoproteins, and apolipoproteins. In Burtis CA, Ashwood ER, editors: *Tietz textbook of clinical chemistry,* ed 3, Philadelphia, 1999, Saunders, pp 809-861.

4. How do the lipoproteins of human serum differ from the serum lipoproteins of domestic mammals?

The composition of the lipoproteins in human and domestic mammalian sera is similar; however, the relative amounts of the lipoproteins differ between species. For example, human sera typically have more VLDL and LDL molecules than HDL. However, dog sera typically have more HDL molecules than VLDL or LDL molecules.

5. Lactescence in lipemic blood samples is primarily caused by high concentrations of which lipoproteins?

The largest lipoproteins, chylomicrons and VLDLs, cause the *lactescence* (milky appearance) or turbidity seen in lipemic blood samples. These lipoproteins are large enough to interfere with light transmission through the serum or plasma and thus create lactescence.

6. How do clinical laboratory assays measure serum or plasma cholesterol and triglyceride concentrations?

Cholesterol assays typically are enzymatic assays that hydrolyze cholesterol esters and use cholesterol oxidase to oxidize cholesterol and generate hydrogen peroxide (H_2O_2), which reacts with an indicator dye. Other methods use oxygen-sensing electrodes to measure oxygen consumption. High serum concentrations of bilirubin and ascorbic acid may interfere with some assays.

Triglyceride assays involve reactions that generate products that are detectable by spectrophotometry. The glycerin that coats some red-top collection tubes interferes with some triglyceride assays.

7. What three major changes or alterations in physiologic processes produce hyperlipidemia?

Hyperlipidemia occurs when one or more of the following processes occur:

a. Increased production of lipoproteins by hepatocytes
b. Defective intravascular processing of lipoproteins, including defective lipolysis that is catalyzed by lipoprotein lipase
c. Defective cellular uptake of lipoproteins or lipoprotein remnants

8. What are the different lipases and what are their actions?

The breakdown of lipids in the body involves the following lipases:

a. *Gastric lipase* is produced by gastric mucosal cells and degrades ingested triglyceride.
b. *Pancreatic lipase* (triacylglycerol lipase) is produced by pancreatic acinar cells and catalyzes the hydrolysis of dietary triglyceride in the intestine. The action of pancreatic lipase requires the emulsification of dietary lipids by bile acids.
c. *Lipoprotein lipase* (LPL) is produced mainly by extrahepatic cells, including adipocytes and myocytes. Once produced, LPL migrates to the luminal surface of endothelial cells, where it catalyzes the hydrolysis of triglycerides in chylomicrons, VLDLs, and IDLs. The movement of LPL to the luminal surface is an insulin-dependent process.
d. *Hepatic lipase* is produced by hepatocytes, is present on endothelial cells of hepatic sinusoids, and hydrolyzes triglyceride in LDL molecules.
e. *Hormone-sensitive lipase* in adipocytes catalyzes the hydrolysis of stored triglyceride, which results in the liberation of fatty acids; it is stimulated by epinephrine and glucagon.
f. *Lysosomal acid lipase* is an intracellular lipase that catalyzes the hydrolysis of cholesterol esters.

9. What major physiologic processes result in the formation and degradation of lipoproteins?

Figure 33-1 illustrates and describes the major metabolic pathways for endogenous and exogenous lipids.

10. What are the two major physiologic or pathologic processes that produce hypercholesterolemia?

Hypercholesterolemia results from (a) increased cholesterol production by hepatocytes and/or (b) decreased intravascular lipolysis or processing of lipoproteins. In the healthy animal, these processes are influenced by hormones. Insulin promotes the storage of lipids; glucagon and catecholamines promote the mobilization of lipids; and thyroid hormones (thyroxine and triiodothyronine) promote cellular uptake and utilization of lipids.

11. What are the three major classifications of hyperlipidemic (or hyperlipoproteinemic) disorders or conditions, and what are the distinguishing features?

a. *Physiologic hyperlipidemia,* also called *postprandial lipemia,* is the increase in plasma lipoprotein concentrations that occurs after a fat-containing meal.

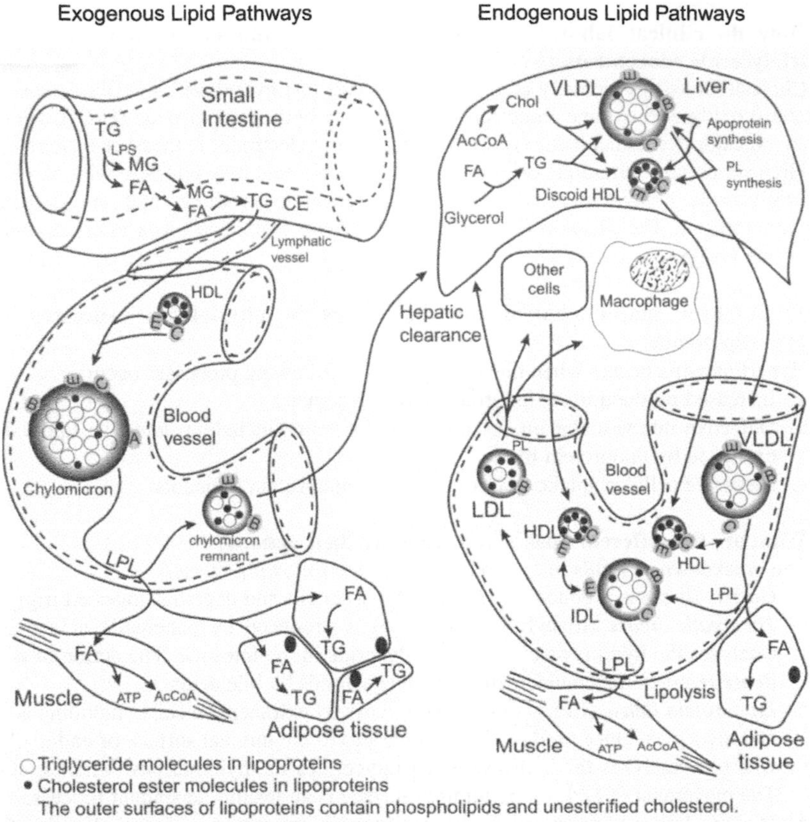

Figure 33-1 The three major processes that affect lipoprotein concentrations and thus triglyceride *(TG)* and cholesterol *(Chol)* concentrations are (1) synthesis of chylomicrons in enterocytes and very-low-density lipoprotein *(VLDL)* molecules in hepatocytes, (2) lipoprotein lipase *(LPL)*–catalyzed lipolysis on endothelial cell membranes, and (3) hepatocyte clearance of lipoprotein remnants. There are two major metabolic pathways for lipids, one for endogenous and one for exogenous lipids.
Exogenous or dietary lipids. Ingested TG in the presence of bile acids and pancreatic lipase undergoes lipolysis to form monoglyceride *(MG)* and fatty acid *(FA)*. After absorption by enterocytes, MG and FA are reassembled into TG. Enterocytes also produce cholesterol ester *(CE)*, phospholipids, and apolipoproteins A and B and then assemble the molecules into TG-rich lipoproteins called chylomicrons. The chylomicrons enter lymphatic vessels and then blood through the thoracic duct. In blood, chylomicrons obtain C and E apolipoproteins from circulating high-density lipoprotein *(HDL)*. In the presence of insulin, apolipoprotein C-II activates LPL (on endothelial cell membranes), which catalyzes the lipolysis of TG to generate FA. The FA enters adipocytes to be stored in TG or enters muscle fibers (or other cells) to undergo oxidation to generate energy. After removal of most TG molecules, the chylomicron remnants are cleared from plasma by hepatocytes in a process involving B apolipoproteins.
Endogenous lipids produced by hepatocytes. Hepatocytes produce TG, phospholipids, apolipoproteins, and CE, which may form from dietary cholesterol or de novo synthesis.
TG-rich VLDL molecules are assembled in hepatocytes and secreted into sinusoidal blood. In the presence of insulin, apolipoprotein C-II on VLDLs activates LPL on endothelial cells to initiate lipolysis and liberation of FA from TG. As VLDL molecules lose TG, they become denser to form intermediate-density lipoprotein *(IDL)*, which may also undergo additional lipolysis to form low-density lipoprotein *(LDL)*. LDL molecules deliver cholesterol to many cells for maintenance of cell membranes or steroid hormone synthesis. Hepatocyte clearance of LDL involves the action of hepatic lipase and the binding of a cholesterol-rich remnant to a B apolipoprotein receptor on hepatocytes. LDLs are also removed by macrophages in either receptor-mediated or non–receptor-mediated processes.

Figure 33-1, cont'd *Discoid HDL molecules* are produced by hepatocytes and then acquire their complete spherical form in blood. HDLs have two major functions: (1) serve as a source of C and E apolipoproteins for other lipoproteins and (2) accept cholesterol from plasma membranes or lipoproteins and transport it to hepatocytes for reutilization or degradation.
Shaded letters *A, B, C,* and *E,* apolipoproteins A, B, C, and E, respectively; *LPS,* pancreatic lipase; *PL,* phospholipid; *AcCoA,* acetyl coenzyme A; *ATP,* adenosine triphosphate.
(Modified from Stockham SL, Scott MA. *Fundamentals of veterinary clinical pathology,* Ames, 2002, Iowa State Press.)

---

b. *Primary hyperlipidemia* disorder is a pathologic state in which a congenital or hereditary defect in lipoprotein metabolism causes increased lipoprotein concentrations in plasma. Congenital (or hereditary) disorders in a Brittany spaniel, a mixed-breed pup, domestic cats, and possibly in miniature schnauzers have been reported.
c. *Secondary hyperlipidemia* disorder is a pathologic state in which an acquired disorder damages cells or alters hormone concentrations, causing defective lipoprotein metabolism and increased lipoprotein concentrations in plasma. Common secondary hyperlipidemia disorders include canine hypothyroidism, diabetes mellitus, pancreatitis, and protein-losing nephropathy.

12. What are the two major processes that produce hypertriglyceridemia?

Hypertriglyceridemia results from (a) increased triglyceride production by hepatocytes or enterocytes and/or (b) decreased intravascular lipolysis or processing of lipoproteins. These processes are influenced by hormones that affect metabolic pathways for body fuels.

13. Which diseases and conditions cause hypertriglyceridemia in domestic mammals?

Box 33-1 lists the diseases and conditions causing hypertriglyceridemia.

14. What are the three major processes resulting in hypercholesterolemia?

Hypercholesterolemia results from (a) increased cholesterol production by hepatocytes or enterocytes, (b) decreased intravascular lipolysis or processing of lipoproteins, and/or (c) defective hepatic uptake of LDLs. Again, these processes are influenced by hormones that affect metabolic pathways for body fuels.

15. What diseases and conditions cause hypercholesterolemia in domestic mammals?

Box 33-2 lists diseases and conditions causing hypercholesterolemia.

16. Why do many disorders or conditions cause both hypercholesterolemia and hypertriglyceridemia?

The disorders or conditions that cause hypercholesterolemia and hypertriglyceridemia are disorders that alter lipoprotein metabolism. Because lipoproteins contain cholesterol and triglyceride molecules, hyperlipoproteinemia may cause hypercholesterolemia, hypertriglyceridemia, or both, depending on the content of the lipoproteins that accumulate in plasma.

17. Describe the pathogenesis of postprandial hypercholesterolemia or hypertriglyceridemia.

After ingestion of a meal containing fat, triglycerides are digested to monoglyceride and fatty acid by the actions of pancreatic lipase. The monoglyceride and fatty acid are absorbed by intestinal mucosal epithelial cells and assimilated into triglyceride-rich chylomicrons. The chylomicrons that enter lymphatic vessels are dumped into blood through the thoracic duct. The plasma triglyceride concentration will be increased until the chylomicrons are cleared.

Box 33-1 ***Diseases and Conditions That Cause Hypertriglyceridemia***

Increased Triglyceride Production

By hepatocytes:
Equine hyperlipemia or hyperlipidemia
By enterocytes:
Postprandial hyperlipidemia

Decreased Lipolysis or Intravascular Processing of Lipoproteins

Hypothyroidism
Nephrotic syndrome
Lipoprotein lipase deficiency (rare in cats, very rare in dogs)

Other, Unknown, or Multiple Mechanisms

Acute pancreatitis
Diabetes mellitus (for types, see Chapter 34)
High-lipid diet
Hyperadrenocorticism or excess glucocorticoids
Hyperlipidemia in a Brittany spaniel
Idiopathic hyperlipidemia of miniature schnauzers

Data from Stockham SL, Scott MA: Lipids. In *Fundamentals of veterinary clinical pathology,* Ames, 2002, Iowa State Press, pp 521-537.

Box 33-2 ***Diseases and Conditions That Cause Hypercholesterolemia***

Increased Cholesterol Production

By hepatocytes:
Nephrotic syndrome or protein-losing nephropathy
By enterocytes:
Postprandial hyperlipidemia

Decreased Lipolysis or Intravascular Processing of Lipoproteins

Hypothyroidism
Nephrotic syndrome or protein-losing nephropathy
Lipoprotein lipase deficiency (very rare in dogs)

Other, Unknown, or Multiple Mechanisms

Acute pancreatitis
Cholestasis (obstructive)
Diabetes mellitus
Hyperadrenocorticism
Hypercholesterolemia in briards
Idiopathic hyperlipidemia of miniature schnauzers

Data from Stockham SL, Scott MA: Lipids. In *Fundamentals of veterinary clinical pathology,* Ames, 2002, Iowa State Press, pp 521-537.

Concurrently, increased production of VLDLs by hepatocytes probably occurs, but minimal amounts of lipid are contributed by the VLDLs compared with the fatty chylomicrons. Because chylomicrons and VLDLs contain relatively little cholesterol, plasma cholesterol concentration should not increase as much as triglyceride concentration.

18. When does postprandial hyperlipidemia indicate the presence of a pathologic condition?

In dogs and cats, physiologic processes should clear the postprandial hyperlipidemia within 8 hours and definitely within 16 hours. Delayed clearing indicates defective lipolysis or intravascular processing of the lipoproteins and thus the presence of either a primary or a secondary hyperlipidemia disorder.

19. Describe the pathogenesis of a hypercholesterolemia or hypertriglyceridemia associated with acute pancreatitis in dogs.

Hyperlipidemia is common in dogs with acute pancreatitis, but the mechanisms are not firmly established. Also, the hyperlipidemia from other disorders may predispose a dog to develop pancreatitis. Possible mechanisms involved in the hyperlipidemia included decreased insulin activity (and therefore decreased lipoprotein lipase activity), altered lipid metabolism created by inflammatory cytokines, and defective lipid metabolism associated with obstructive cholestasis. By whatever mechanism or process, decreased intravascular lipolysis or processing of plasma lipoproteins results in increased concentrations of VLDLs or chylomicrons. The higher concentrations of these molecules cause an increased triglyceride concentration and, to a lesser extent, increased cholesterol concentration.

20. Describe the pathogenesis of a hypercholesterolemia or hypertriglyceridemia associated with nephrotic syndrome or protein-losing nephropathy.

Hypercholesterolemia (sometimes accompanied by hypertriglyceridemia) is typically considered to result from increased hepatic production of VLDLs and defective lipolysis of lipoproteins in plasma. The defective lipolysis is thought to result from the renal loss of proteins that are needed for binding of lipoproteins to endothelial cells. With decreased binding of lipoproteins, there is defective intravascular lipolysis of lipoproteins. The lipoproteins that accumulate in animals with the nephrotic syndrome are large enough that they do not freely pass through the defective glomerular filtration barrier, whereas smaller proteins do pass and thus create the proteinuric state.

21. What is the pathogenesis of a hypercholesterolemia or hypertriglyceridemia associated with hypothyroidism?

The hypothyroid state results in the decreased production of thyroid hormones, primarily thyroxine. The lower concentration of thyroid hormones results in a decreased intravascular lipolysis or processing of lipoproteins (e.g., VLDLs, LDLs). These defects result in increased concentrations of cholesterol-rich LDLs and thus increased cholesterol concentration. The defective lipoprotein metabolism is probably caused by decreased LPL or decreased hepatic lipase activity. If the accumulating lipoproteins are rich in triglycerides, there would be a concurrent increase in triglyceride concentration.

22. What is the pathogenesis of a hypercholesterolemia or hypertriglyceridemia associated with lipoprotein lipase deficiency?

The decreased LPL activity may be congenital or acquired and results in decreased intravascular lipolysis or processing of lipoproteins, including chylomicrons and VLDLs, IDLs, and LDLs. The defective system may trigger hepatocytes to produce more VLDL molecules. Accumulation of these plasma lipoproteins results in increased concentrations of triglyceride and cholesterol.

23. What is the pathogenesis of a hypercholesterolemia or hypertriglyceridemia associated with cholestasis?

Hypercholesterolemia is a common finding in animals with cholestasis, which may have concurrent hypertriglyceridemia. The hypercholesterolemia appears to result from increased cholesterol synthesis by hepatocytes, defective excretion of cholesterol into bile, and defective uptake of LDLs by hepatocytes.

24. Describe the pathogenesis of a hypercholesterolemia or hypertriglyceridemia associated with diabetes mellitus.

As defined by the American Diabetes Association, "Diabetes mellitus is a group of metabolic diseases characterized by hyperglycemia resulting from defects in insulin secretion, insulin action, or both" (see Chapter 34, Glucose). The metabolic defects that produce the hyperglycemia frequently will also cause defective lipoprotein metabolism and thus development of hypercholesterolemia or hypertriglyceridemia. The cause of the defective lipoprotein metabolism varies with the cause of the diabetic state. The major mechanisms are as follows:

a. Lipoprotein lipase activity depends on the presence of insulin. Decreased plasma insulin concentration results in defective intravascular lipolysis or processing of plasma lipoproteins (e.g., chylomicrons, VLDLs, IDLs). When these lipoproteins accumulate in plasma, the plasma triglyceride and probably cholesterol concentrations increase.
b. With the defects in peripheral tissue utilization of glucose, metabolic pathways are signaled to mobilize lipids from adipose tissue by degrading triglycerides and releasing free fatty acids to plasma. The influx of free fatty acids into hepatocytes stimulates VLDL synthesis, which enhances the hyperlipidemia.

25. Describe the pathogenesis of a hypercholesterolemia or hypertriglyceridemia associated with hyperadrenocorticism.

The hyperlipidemia of hyperadrenocorticism can be directly and indirectly related to the excessive production of cortisol. Directly, cortisol stimulates the synthesis of VLDL molecules by hepatocytes. Cortisol also promotes the activity of hormone-sensitive lipase in adipocytes, which results in the release of free fatty acids and subsequently, increased production of VLDLs by hepatocytes. Indirectly, cortisol promotes the development of a diabetic state that involves defective lipoprotein metabolism.

26. Describe the pathogenesis of a hypercholesterolemia or hypertriglyceridemia associated with multiple conditions of equine hyperlipidemia.

The acquired defects in lipoprotein metabolism in disorders such as anorexia, pregnancy, lactation, renal failure, and endotoxemia vary but tend to have a common feature: creating a negative energy balance that results from altered hormonal control of lipoprotein metabolism. Catecholamines, glucagon, and cortisol stimulate hormone-sensitive lipase, which promotes the release of free fatty acids from adipose tissue. Progesterone promotes release of growth hormone, which decreases the uptake of glucose by peripheral tissues. Endotoxins (perhaps through cytokines) stimulate triglyceride and VLDL synthesis by hepatocytes and may also inhibit lipoprotein catabolism. The net result of these alterations is the increased synthesis of triglyceride-rich VLDL molecules by hepatocytes. Also, triglyceride molecules may accumulate in hepatocytes (fatty liver, hepatic lipidosis) if their production exceeds their packaging into VLDL molecules.

27. What is the major process that produces hypocholesterolemia?

Hypocholesterolemia results from decreased cholesterol synthesis by hepatocytes.

28. What diseases and conditions cause hypocholesterolemia in domestic mammals?

Box 33-3 lists diseases and conditions causing hypocholesterolemia.

29. What is the pathogenesis of hypocholesterolemia associated with a portosystemic shunt?

The hypocholesterolemia probably results from decreased cholesterol production by hepatocytes, which may be caused by two mechanisms. First, the shunting of portal blood results in

Box 33-3 ***Diseases and Conditions That Cause Hypocholesterolemia***

Decreased Cholesterol Production
Portosystemic shunts in dogs and cats
Protein-losing enteropathy

Other Mechanism
Hypoadrenocorticism

Data from Stockham SL, Scott MA: Lipids. In *Fundamentals of veterinary clinical pathology,* Ames, 2002, Iowa State Press, pp 521-537.

hepatic atrophy or hypoplasia, and thus fewer hepatocytes are available to make cholesterol. Second, the shunting allows bile acids to enter systemic blood, accumulate in hepatocytes, and then inhibit the synthesis of cholesterol in the remaining functional hepatocytes.

30. What relationships (if any) exist between presence/absence of plasma turbidity (lactescence) versus serum triglyceride concentration and plasma turbidity versus serum cholesterol concentration?

Lactescence of plasma is caused by the accumulation of the larger lipoproteins, chylomicrons and VLDLs. Because these are triglyceride-rich but relatively cholesterol-poor lipoproteins, lactescent plasma will have a hypertriglyceridemia, but there may not be a hypercholesterolemia. Also, there may be hypertriglyceridemia without lactescence if the number of large lipoproteins is insufficient to interfere with light transmission. High concentrations of the smaller but cholesterol-rich lipoproteins (HDLs and LDLs) may cause a hypercholesterolemia, but these are too small to cause lactescence.

31. Why are triglyceride concentrations in chylous effusions much higher than in serum triglyceride concentrations, and why is a cholesterol/triglyceride ratio much lower in chylous effusions than in nonchylous effusions?

By definition, a *chylous effusion* contains chylomicrons that formed in intestinal mucosa, entered intestinal lacteals, but then escaped from the lymph and entered a body cavity; chylothorax is more common than chyloabdomen. Because chylomicrons are triglyceride-rich molecules, their presence in the effusion will create a high triglyceride concentration. Assuming there is not a systemic defect in lipoprotein metabolism, the effusion will have a much higher triglyceride concentration than the plasma from a fasting animal.

The cholesterol/triglyceride ratio is much lower in chylous effusions than in nonchylous effusions because chylomicrons are cholesterol-poor but triglyceride-rich lipoproteins. Unless there is adipose tissue necrosis in the body cavity, the nonchylous effusion should have low triglyceride concentrations because the lipoprotein content of extravascular extracellular fluid is typically very low.

32. What is the difference between a lipid effusion and a chylous effusion?

Classifying an effusion as *lipid* indicates increased lipids in the fluid; the lipids may be triglycerides or cholesterol. A *chylous* effusion contains chylomicrons and is commonly assumed in lactescent effusions but is not documented. A chylous effusion is a lipid effusion, but a lipid effusion may not be a chylous effusion.

33. How can the presence of chylomicrons be confirmed in an effusion?

Chylomicrons have two properties that can be demonstrated. First, their low relative density (<0.95) makes them buoyant in aqueous fluids, and thus they tend to float after high-speed centrifugation. Second, chylomicrons remain at the application point during lipoprotein electrophoresis.

Before the frequent use of cholesterol/triglyceride ratios to document a chylous effusion, the simplest test was staining of the lactescent effusion with Sudan III or Sudan IV stain. The demonstration of sudanophilic droplets in the effusion documented the presence of triglyceride droplets in the sample, which were assumed to be from chylomicrons, just as the low cholesterol/triglyceride ratio is assumed to be from chylomicrons.

34. What is a lipiduria, and what does it indicate?

Lipiduria is the presence of lipid in urine and is typically seen as lipid droplets during the microscopic examination of urine sediment. The lipid droplets may be triglycerides in the urine or contaminants in the sample (e.g., lubricants, oils on equipment/glassware). The true lipiduria is most often seen in cats and, by itself, does not indicate pathologic state. Cats are unique among domestic animals because their renal tubular epithelial cells accumulate triglyceride, especially obese cats. Those triglyceride molecules are released to the tubular fluid during the physiologic turnover of epithelial cells.

All the triglyceride-rich lipoproteins of plasma are too large to pass through the glomerular filtration barrier. Molecules greater than 3.4 nm in diameter do not pass through the barrier; only the smallest cholesterol-rich HDL molecules approach this diameter (see Table 33-1). Therefore a lipiduria does not result directly from a hyperlipoproteinemia.

35. What does the presence of a creamy white layer on the top of serum indicate?

If a creamy white layer forms on top of serum, either at room temperature or in a refrigerator, chylomicrons are in the sample. In a standardized procedure, the serum is left undisturbed for 16 hours at 4° C to detect the creamy layer. However, the absence of the creamy layer does not mean that chylomicrons are not present. The lactescent sample may contain VLDLs (which do not float after 16 hours) or chylomicrons (which may float). Ultracentrifugation (e.g., 150,000 *g*) may be necessary to separate the chylomicrons from the aqueous serum.

36. Does the presence of a marked hyperlipidemia interfere with the accuracy of other laboratory assays?

Hyperlipidemia can interfere with clinical laboratory assays in two major ways: interference with light transmission and displacement of plasma water.

The lipids interfere with light transmission through a liquid and thus may interfere with assays that involve transmission (or absorbance) photometry or refractive properties. Because the diversity of the lipid molecules, it is difficult to predict how much the lipids may interfere. Use of patient blanks or kinetic photometric assays can reduce the interference.

The lipids displace plasma water and thus may result in falsely low concentrations of analytes in some assays. For example, lipemic serum will have a falsely low measured sodium concentration (pseudohyponatremia) if the sodium concentration is measured by flame photometry or indirect potentiometry. However, the lipids do not interfere with direct potentiometry.

34. GLUCOSE

1. Why does delayed processing or analysis of a blood sample result in a lower glucose concentration?

Prolonged exposure of serum or plasma to leukocytes, platelets, and erythrocytes allows the cells to consume glucose and lower the glucose concentration. The blood cells use the plasma glucose for their glycolytic pathways. The decline of plasma or serum glucose concentration is generally 5% to 10% per hour. This usually does not interfere with the interpretation of glucose concentrations because the processing of patient samples and the samples used for reference interval determination should be the same (i.e., removing serum or plasma from cells within 30 to 60 minutes after blood collection). The rate of glucose consumption can increase when there are more cells in the blood (marked leukocytosis, marked thrombocytosis, or possibly erythrocytosis). The rate of glucose consumption can be decreased by placing the blood sample in a cool environment, but clot formation and contraction are also reduced.

Serum separator tubes (tubes with gold or red/black stoppers) contain an activator and gel that enhance clot formation and allow easier separation of a blood clot and serum, respectively. After centrifugation, the serum glucose concentration remains stable in a refrigerator for at least 48 hours if the gel barrier is intact.

Erythrocytes from pigs are unique in that they lack a functional glucose transporter and therefore utilize glucose at a much lower rate than erythrocytes from other species. *Inosine* is the major energy substrate in pig erythrocytes, whereas *glucose* is the primary substrate in other domestic species.

2. If blood samples cannot be processed within an hour of collection, how can the glucose concentration in the sample be maintained?

Blood can be collected into evacuated tubes that contain sodium fluoride (NaF); these tubes have a gray stopper or cap. NaF tubes may contain potassium oxalate, sodium EDTA, or no anticoagulant. The fluoride ion enters the blood cells and reduces glycolysis by complexing with magnesium ion (Mg^{2+}), a cofactor for some enzymes (e.g., phosphopyruvate hydratase, or enolase). The oxalate or EDTA in some tubes binds free calcium ions (Ca^{2+}) to prevent the formation of fibrin through the coagulation pathways.

If NaF is not available, keeping the sample cool (not frozen) will reduce glycolysis. The blood sample should not be frozen because freezing will lyse blood cells and thus add their contents to the plasma.

3. What are the disadvantages of using sodium fluoride tubes?

Disadvantages of using NaF tubes include falsely lowering plasma glucose concentration, erythrocyte lysis, and limited use of the samples for other assays. Studies involving people, cats, and marine mammals have shown that plasma glucose concentrations decreased by 5% to 10% during the first hour after blood collection into NaF tubes. The decrease may result from the osmotic movement of water from erythrocytes to plasma when the blood is mixed with the hyperosmotic salts (NaF, potassium oxalate). Other data indicate that it takes about 1 hour for the fluoride to inhibit glycolysis completely. The antiglycolytic effect of fluoride depends on the fluoride concentration in the blood sample.

Erythrocytes are prone to lysis when exposed to the NaF and potassium oxalate, especially if an optimal amount of blood is not drawn into the evacuated blood tube. The release of erythrocyte contents (e.g., hemoglobin, phosphorus, potassium) may result in erroneous results in some clinical chemistry assays.

Besides inhibiting enolase in the glycolytic pathway, fluoride inhibits other enzymes, including the glucose oxidase of some glucose assays. Thus the NaF sample may not be an acceptable sample for determining glucose concentration.

4. **Why does a blood glucose concentration not equal a plasma/serum glucose concentration?**

The differences between blood glucose and plasma or serum glucose concentration typically will be slight, but differences can be caused by erythrocytosis, sample processing errors, or differences in assay methods. Erythrocytosis will increase the difference because the glucose concentration in erythrocytes is lower than in plasma/serum. The concentration of glucose in the plasma H_2O and erythrocyte H_2O is the same, but there is less H_2O in erythrocytes (most volume is occupied by hemoglobin) and thus less glucose in erythrocytes per unit volume. The greater the erythrocyte concentration in blood, the greater will be the difference between blood glucose concentration and plasma glucose concentration (blood glucose concentration will be lower). Plasma concentrations were calculated in Table 34-1 using the following conversion formula:

$$\text{Plasma [glucose]} = \frac{\text{Whole blood [glucose]}}{(1.0 - [0.0024 \times \text{Hematocrit \%}])}$$

Table 34-1 ***Calculated Plasma Glucose Concentrations in Blood Samples with Given Whole-Blood Glucose Concentrations (WBG) and Hematocrit (Hct) Values****

	WBG (mg/dl)				
HCT	50	100	400	800	INCREASE ABOVE WBG
10%	51	102	410	820	2%
45%	56	112	448	897	12%
60%	58	117	467	935	17%

Modified from Stockham SL, Scott MA: Glucose and related regulatory hormones. In *Fundamentals of veterinary clinical pathology,* Ames, 2002, Iowa State Press, pp 487-506.

*Agreement between calculated and measured plasma concentrations depends on the analytical properties (accuracy, precision, specificity, sensitivity) of the assays, sample handling, and amount of in vitro glycolysis.

5. **How do point-of-care glucose instruments measure glucose concentrations in whole blood?**

The analytical methods vary and include reactions catalyzed by glucose oxidase, glucose dehydrogenase, or hexokinase. Each type of assay method has it advantages and disadvantages.

Some blood glucose analyzers measure the blood glucose concentration but then convert it to a plasma glucose concentration assuming a normal hematocrit percentage or fraction. If the hematocrit value is either increased or decreased, the calculated concentration would not equal the true plasma concentration. In the blood glucose assays, erythrocytes are lysed so that a whole-blood glucose (plasma glucose + erythrocyte glucose) concentration is measured. In other assays, a barrier excludes erythrocytes from the reacting reagents, and thus the assays measure plasma glucose concentrations.

Other blood glucose analyzers determine glucose concentration by assessing plasma molality. Displacement of plasma water by proteins or lipids can result in incorrect values. For some glucose oxidase methods, high arterial oxygen tension (high PaO_2, as may occur during gas anesthesia) can produce a positive interference.

Because there are at least 12 point-of-care glucose instruments and each has its unique features, the user should closely follow the manufacturer's recommendations and know the limitations as described by the manufacturer or other resources.

6. How do most serum glucose assays measure glucose concentrations?

Most current serum glucose assays use hexokinase, glucokinase, glucose dehydrogenase, or glucose oxidase to catalyze the breakdown of glucose and the generation of products that can be measured by spectrophotometry, oxygen detection, or electron transfer. The glucose oxidase reaction is specific for glucose, but other factors can interfere with later stages of the assay (e.g., isopropyl alcohol can produce positive interference in reagent pad methods). Hexokinase can catalyze reactions with other hexoses, but rarely will there be another hexose in blood at sufficient concentration to increase the measured glucose concentration falsely.

7. How do most urine glucose assays estimate glucose concentrations?

In the *reagent pad method,* glucose reacts with glucose oxidase (which is glucose specific) to produce hydrogen peroxide (H_2O_2), which is detected when it reacts with a color indicator. The glucose concentration is proportional to color change in the reagent pad. Contamination of urine with H_2O_2 and sodium hypochlorite will produce false-positive reactions. False-negative reactions are caused by ascorbic acid, ketones, very concentrated urine samples, and possibly cold urine.

In the *copper-reduction method* (Clinitest), copper ion (Cu^{2+}) reacts with a reducing substance (e.g., a hexose) to produce cuprous (Cu^{+}) oxide and cuprous hydroxide and thus a color change. Cephalosporin and ascorbic acid may cause false-positive reactions.

8. In health, how similar are plasma/serum glucose concentrations and cerebrospinal fluid glucose concentrations?

Cerebrospinal fluid (CSF) glucose concentrations in health are approximately 60% to 80% of serum or plasma concentrations. CSF glucose concentrations may take 30 to 90 minutes to equilibrate with sudden changes in plasma/serum glucose concentration. In humans a decreased glucose concentration in the CSF (hypoglycorrachia) has been attributed to increased glucose metabolism by microorganisms or inflammatory cells (as in bacterial meningitis). However, this relationship is not a consistent finding in dogs.

9. How much does the plasma/serum glucose concentration contribute to plasma/serum osmolality?

The easiest way to understand the contribution of glucose to osmolality is to recognize that a glucose concentration of 1 mmol/L contributes 1 mOsm/L to osmolarity, which is approximately 1 mOsm/kg H_2O. Thus in healthy dogs and cats, a euglycemia of 5 mmol/L contributes about 5 mOsm/kg H_2O to the total plasma osmolality (almost 300 mOsm/kg H_2O). A marked hyperglycemia increases the plasma or serum osmolality; for example, increasing the glucose concentration from 5 to 25 mmol/L will increase the plasma osmolality about 20 mOsm/kg H_2O. Conversely, a marked hypoglycemia decreases the plasma or serum osmolality, but the minor changes (e.g., from 5 to 3 mmol/L) reduces the osmolality about 2 mmol/kg H_2O, a change of no clinical significance.

If glucose concentrations are reported in non-SI units (e.g., mg/dl), the glucose concentration is converted to mmol/L with the formula mg/dl $\times$ 0.05551 = mmol/L. The conversion is based on relative molecular weight of glucose (180 g = 1 mole) and the conversion of deciliters to liters.

10. What are the three major changes or alterations in physiologic processes that produce a hyperglycemia?

Hyperglycemia can be created by (a) increased glucose intake, (b) increased glucose production, and/or (c) decreased glucose uptake by peripheral tissues.

Increased glucose intake can result from ingestion of carbohydrate meal or the infusion of a glucose-containing fluid (e.g., 5% dextrose). Strictly speaking, *increased glucose production* is limited to increased gluconeogenesis within hepatocytes. However, hepatic glycogenolysis can also result in the release of glucose into blood. *Decreased glucose uptake by peripheral tissues* can result in a mild hyperglycemia by itself, but *increased glucose uptake* or *increased glucose production* can enhance the severity of the hyperglycemia. Figure 34-1 illustrates how these processes are influenced by activities of hormones and other factors.

11. What is diabetes mellitus?

According to a 2000 report of the American Diabetes Association, "Diabetes mellitus is a group of metabolic diseases characterized by hyperglycemia resulting from defects in insulin secretion, insulin action, or both." *Type 1* diabetes mellitus (DM) is caused by beta cell destruction, which usually leads to absolute insulin deficiency (formerly called insulin-dependent DM, type I DM, or juvenile-onset DM). *Type 2* DM is caused by insulin resistance with an inadequate compensatory insulin secretory response (formerly called non-insulin-dependent DM, type II DM, or adult-onset DM). The other forms of DM are referred to by the pathologic state or condition that created the carbohydrate metabolism defects (e.g., pancreatic, endocrine, drug-induced, infectious, and genetic DM).

12. What are the diagnostic criteria for diabetes mellitus?

A diagnosis of DM is appropriate when a hyperglycemia is associated with the clinical signs of polyuria (due to glucosuria), polydipsia, and weight loss. A hyperglycemia without the associated clinical signs is probably a transient hyperglycemia, and the animal probably does not have a disorder that is causing DM. However, the animal could be in a preclinical stage of DM. Diagnostic criteria in the preclinical stage include documentation of a carbohydrate (or glucose) intolerance.

13. What diseases and conditions cause hyperglycemia in domestic mammals?

Box 34-1 lists the diseases and conditions that may cause hyperglycemia.

14. What physiologic processes create a postprandial hyperglycemia?

After the ingestion of a meal containing carbohydrates, digestion results in the formation of glucose, which is absorbed by the intestinal mucosal epithelial cells and enters the portal blood. If hepatic extraction of glucose from portal blood is not complete, glucose enters the systemic blood to produce a hyperglycemia.

After the ingestion and digestion of proteins, amino acids are absorbed by the intestinal mucosal epithelial cells and enter the portal blood. The increased amino acid concentration stimulates the release of glucagon from alpha cells of pancreatic islets (also canine gastric mucosa). Glucagon promotes hyperglycemia by stimulating hepatic gluconeogenesis and antagonizing insulin activity in peripheral cells.

Animals with untreated DM will have a prolonged postprandial hyperglycemia because of defects in insulin secretion, insulin action, or both.

15. What physiologic processes create a hyperglycemia after excitement or fright?

Excitement or fright causes the release of catecholamines (epinephrine, norepinephrine) from the adrenal medulla. The catecholamines stimulate glycogenolysis within hepatocytes and the subsequent release of glucose to blood. Catecholamines also promote the release of growth hormone (GH), which reduces glucose uptake by myocytes and adipocytes and thus promotes or enhances hyperglycemia.

16. What physiologic processes create a hyperglycemia resulting from a physiologic increase in glucocorticoid hormone concentration?

Glucocorticoid hormones (e.g., cortisol and related steroids) can stimulate gluconeogenesis in hepatocytes. Excess hepatic glucose leaks out of the hepatocytes and enters peripheral blood to create a hyperglycemia.

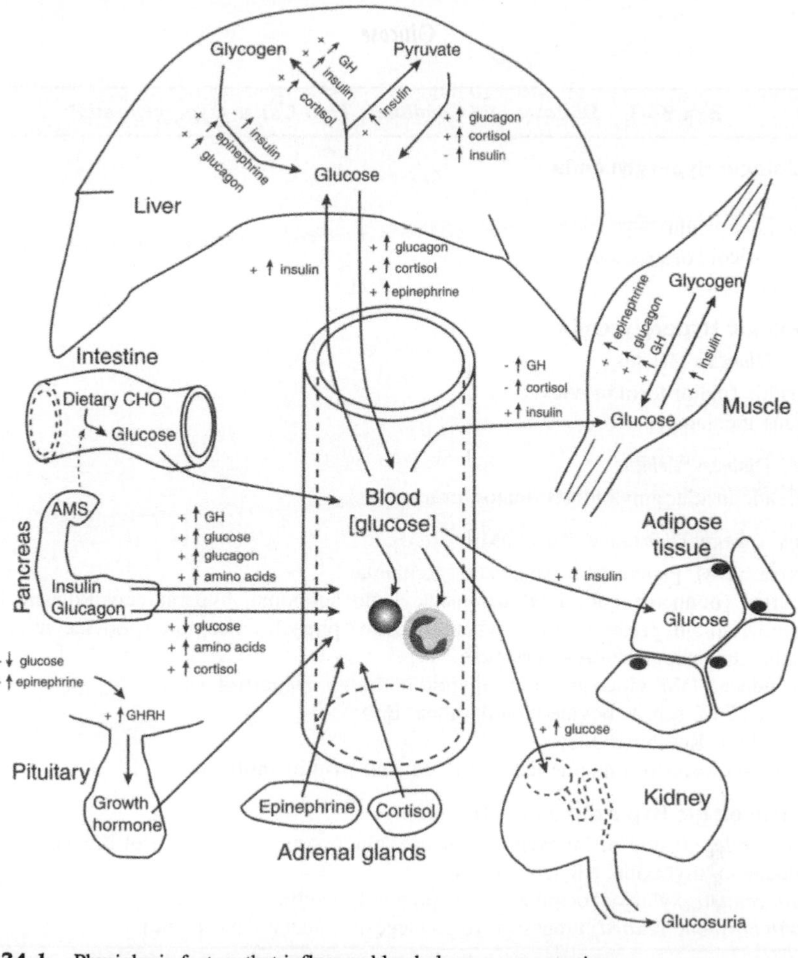

Figure 34-1 Physiologic factors that influence blood glucose concentration.
Intestine: In monogastric animals, dietary carbohydrates *(CHO)* are broken down to monosaccharides (including glucose) that are absorbed in the small intestine, from which they enter portal blood and then systemic blood if not removed by hepatocytes.
Pancreas: Insulin and glucagon are released from pancreatic islet cells (beta cells and alpha cells, respectively). Insulin secretion is stimulated by increased blood concentrations of glucose, growth hormone *(GH),* glucagon, and amino acids. Glucagon secretion is stimulated by increased blood concentrations of amino acids and cortisol or by decreased blood glucose concentrations.
Liver: Hepatocytes are the primary source of blood glucose during fasting. Glucose can be obtained from glycogenolysis (stimulated by epinephrine and glucagon but inhibited by insulin) or gluconeogenesis (stimulated by glucagon and cortisol but inhibited by insulin). Insulin also promotes glycolysis. Increased glucose release from hepatocytes is promoted by increased glucagon, cortisol, or epinephrine. Insulin promotes the uptake of glucose by promoting glucokinase activity.
Muscle: Glucose uptake by myocytes is promoted by insulin through specific insulin receptors and glucose transporters; GH and cortisol inhibit the uptake of glucose. Insulin promotes glycogen synthesis in myocytes, whereas GH, glucagon (in cardiac muscle), and epinephrine promote glycogenolysis.
Adipose tissue: Insulin promotes the uptake of glucose by adipocytes through specific insulin receptors and glucose transporters.
Kidney: If the renal threshold is exceeded, hyperglycemic glucosuria will develop.
Pituitary: GH release from the pituitary is stimulated by growth hormone–releasing hormone *(GHRH),* which is released from the hypothalamus during hypoglycemia or after epinephrine stimulation.
Blood cells: Glucose enters erythrocytes (except porcine), leukocytes, and platelets through insulin-independent processes and is used in glycolysis and the hexose monophosphate shunt. Pig erythrocytes lack a functional glucose transporter and use inosine as the major energy substrate.
(Modified from Stockham SL, Scott MA: *Fundamentals of veterinary clinical pathology,* Ames 2002, Iowa State Press.)

Box 34-1 ***Diseases and Conditions That Cause Hyperglycemia****

Physiologic Hyperglycemia
Postprandial
Excitement, fright
Glucocorticoid associated
Diestrus

Pathologic Hyperglycemia
Type 1 Diabetes Mellitus
Idiopathic (major form in dogs)
Immune mediated

Type 2 Diabetes Mellitus
Pancreatic insular amyloidosis (major form in cats)

Specific Types of Diabetes Mellitus (DM)
Pancreatic DM: pancreatitis, pancreatic carcinoma
Endocrine (nonpancreatic) DM: acromegaly, glucagonoma, hyperadrenocorticism, hyperpituitarism, hyperthyroidism, hypothyroidism, pheochromocytoma, bovine milk fever, canine hepatocutaneous syndrome
Drug-induced DM: glucocorticoids, thyroid hormone, megestrol acetate
Infectious DM: sepsis, bovine viral diarrhea (BVD)
Genetic DM: Keeshond dogs
Uncommon forms of immune-mediated DM: anti-insulin antibodies

Pharmacologic Hyperglycemia (Transient)
Glucose related: oral or intravenous glucose, glucocorticoids, megestrol acetate, ketamine, glucagon, thyroxine, ethylene glycol
Insulin related: xylazine, detomidine, propranolol, insulin
Growth hormone related: progestins (e.g., megestrol acetate, morphine)

Data from Stockham SL, Scott MA: Glucose and related regulatory hormones. In *Fundamentals of veterinary clinical pathology,* Ames, 2002, Iowa State Press, pp 487-506.
*Whole-blood glucose concentrations are lower than serum or plasma glucose concentrations, and thus appropriate reference intervals should be used to determine if hyperglycemic (see text). The classification system of an expert committee of the American Diabetes Association (2000) served as the basis of the DM categories.

Increased glucocorticoid hormone concentrations also can create a state of insulin resistance by decreasing the number or efficiency of glucose membrane transporters (e.g., GLUT-4) or by increasing glucagon and free fatty acid concentrations. The number of insulin receptors in target cell membranes may actually be increased because glucocorticoids stimulate their formation.

17. Describe the pathogenesis of a hyperglycemia that occurs after beta cell destruction in dogs.

Destruction of pancreatic beta cells results in decreased insulin production and release. With lower plasma insulin concentrations, there is decreased uptake of glucose by adipocytes, muscle fibers, and hepatocytes. The decreased tissue utilization of glucose results in a state of "tissue starvation," which triggers increased hepatic gluconeogenesis. The combination of increased gluconeogenesis and decreased cellular uptake produces the hyperglycemia. The severity of the hyperglycemia is reduced by renal excretion of glucose (glucosuria).

18. Describe the pathogenesis of a hyperglycemia that occurs in pancreatic amyloidosis in cats.

Amyloid accumulation in the islets results in damage to the pancreatic beta cells, which leads to decreased insulin production and release. As previously described, the diminished insulin activity alters glucose metabolism and produces a hyperglycemia. With a persistent hyperglycemia, there may be a reduction in glucose receptors on beta cells so that beta cells do not recognize hyperglycemia and thus do not produce or secrete insulin in the presence of hyperglycemia; this glucose resistance is sometimes called a *glucose toxicosis.*

19. Describe the pathogenesis of a hyperglycemia that occurs in hyperadrenocorticism in dogs.

Glucocorticoid hormones and drugs stimulate gluconeogenesis in hepatocytes and thus an increased release of glucose to blood. Also, glucocorticoid hormones create a state of insulin resistance by decreasing the number or efficiency of glucose membrane transporters (i.e., GLUT-4) or by increasing glucagon and free fatty acid concentrations.

20. Describe the pathogenesis of a hyperglycemia that occurs in equine hyperpituitarism.

A pituitary neoplasm produces excess adrenocorticotropic hormone (ACTH, corticotropin), which then stimulates the adrenocortical production of glucocorticoid hormones. As described previously, the excess glucocorticoid hormones results in both increased glucose production by hepatocytes and decreased utilization by target cells. The pituitary neoplasm may also produce excess GH, which reduces glucose uptake by myocytes and adipocytes.

21. Describe the pathogenesis of a hyperglycemia that occurs in cattle with bovine viral diarrhea.

The bovine viral diarrhea (BVD) virus infection damages islet beta cells and thus causes decreased insulin production and release. The lower insulin concentration reduces uptake of glucose by adipocytes, muscle fibers, and hepatocytes, which leads to hyperglycemia.

22. How do the following pharmacologic agents create a hyperglycemia?

a. **Intravenous glucose**

Hyperglycemia develops when the rate of glucose entry into the blood exceeds the rate of glucose removal from blood (by cells or renal excretion).

b. **Glucocorticoids**

The action of glucocorticoid drugs mimics the action of glucocorticoid hormones that create the hyperglycemia in hyperadrenocorticism or stress (see earlier).

c. **Ketamine**

Ketamine stimulates the release of epinephrine from the adrenal medulla. The epinephrine stimulates increased glycogenolysis, release of glucose from hepatocytes, and thus hyperglycemia.

d. **Xylazine or detomidine**

Xylazine and detomidine inhibit insulin release, which reduces glucose utilization by hepatocytes, myocytes, and adipocytes and thus creates a hyperglycemia.

e. **Excess injected insulin**

In response to excess injected insulin, an animal develops a hypoglycemia that stimulates the release of glucagon, epinephrine, and GH. These hormones promote development of a hyperglycemia. In a healthy animal, hyperglycemia is minimized by endogenous insulin release. In a diabetic animal, insulin release does not compensate adequately, and the animal develops a hyperglycemia that might be misinterpreted as evidence of insufficient insulin administration. The hyperglycemic response to excessive insulin injection is called the *Somogyi effect.*

f. **Progestins, e.g., megestrol acetate**
As a steroid, megestrol acetate promotes gluconeogenesis. As a progestin, it stimulates release of GH, which creates insulin resistance by causing insulin receptor and postreceptor defects. The combination of increased glucose release from hepatocytes and decreased glucose removal from blood causes a hyperglycemia.

23. What diseases and conditions cause hypoglycemia in domestic mammals?
Box 34-2 lists the diseases and conditions causing hypoglycemia.

Box 34-2 *Diseases and Conditions That Cause Hypoglycemia**

Pathologic Hypoglycemia

Increased insulin secretion: pancreatic beta cell neoplasia (insulinoma)

Decreased insulin antagonists
- Hypoadrenocorticism (decreased cortisol)
- Growth hormone (GH) deficiency
- Hypopituitarism (decreased cortisol and GH)

Decreased gluconeogenesis
- Hepatic insufficiency/failure: acquired, congenital
- Hypoadrenocorticism (decreased cortisol)
- Neonatal or juvenile hypoglycemia
- Starvation and severe malnutrition

Decreased glycogenolysis
- Glycogen storage diseases (rare)

Increased glucose utilization
- Lactational hypoglycemia (spontaneous bovine ketosis)
- Exertional hypoglycemia (hunting dogs, endurance horses)
- Leukocytosis, extreme
- Erythrocytosis, extreme

Other pathologic hypoglycemias with uncertain or unknown pathogenesis
- Hypoglycemia associated with non–beta cell neoplasms: epithelial and nonepithelial
- Sepsis, especially with endotoxemia
- Pregnancy hypoglycemia
- Chronic renal failure in a cat

Pharmacologic Hypoglycemia

Insulin

Sulfonylurea compounds (e.g., glipizide, glyburide)

Ethanol

Data from Stockham SL, Scott MA: Glucose and related regulatory hormones. In *Fundamentals of veterinary clinical pathology,* Ames, 2002, Iowa State Press, pp 487-506.

*Delayed analysis of blood samples or failure to remove serum or plasma from blood cells appropriately will result in falsely low glucose concentrations. Bromide ions will cause falsely low glucose concentrations using the i-STAT instrument. Whole-blood glucose concentrations are lower than serum or plasma glucose concentrations, and thus appropriate reference intervals should be used to determine if hypoglycemic.

24. List five major changes or alterations in physiologic processes that produce hypoglycemia.

a. Increased uptake of glucose by target cells stimulated by excess insulin
b. Decreased insulin antagonists, thus insulin activity more pronounced
c. Decreased gluconeogenesis
d. Decreased glycogenolysis
e. Increased glucose utilization by "hungry" cells (not insulin stimulated)

25. What is the pathogenesis of a hypoglycemia associated with pancreatic beta cell neoplasia (insulinoma)?

The uncontrolled and excessive release of insulin from neoplastic beta cells creates a state of hyperinsulinism, with increased glucose utilization by hepatocytes, myocytes, and adipocytes and decreased glucose production by hepatocytes; the combination produces a hypoglycemia.

26. What is the pathogenesis of a hypoglycemia associated with hypoadrenocorticism?

The bilateral adrenocortical hypoplasia results in decreased cortisol production. The hypocortisolemia results in decreased gluconeogenesis and increased insulin sensitivity in target cells; the combination produces a hypoglycemia.

27. What is the pathogenesis of a hypoglycemia associated with hepatic insufficiency?

Hypoglycemia develops when glucose production by the remaining functional hepatocytes cannot produce enough glucose to meet the demands of peripheral tissues. The liver has a large reserve capacity for producing glucose, and thus hypoglycemia solely due to liver disease occurs only when functional mass is greatly reduced.

28. Can anorexia cause a hypoglycemia?

It is unlikely that anorexia will cause a hypoglycemia as long as there is adequate liver function. During anorexia, hepatocytes attempt to maintain euglycemia by gluconeogenesis using fatty acids and amino acids. In a severely debilitated state, gluconeogenesis may not be able to produce enough glucose for physiologic needs.

29. What is the pathogenesis of a hypoglycemia associated with lactational hypoglycemia (bovine ketosis)?

Hypoglycemia develops when hepatic gluconeogenesis does not keep up with the need for glucose by mammary glands.

30. What is the pathogenesis of the hypoglycemia that occurs in swine eperythrozoonosis?

Available evidence indicates that *Eperythrozoon suis (Mycoplasma haemosuis)* consumes glucose at a rate that exceeds the gluconeogenesis pathways of the pig. It is not known if similar hypoglycemias occur with hemobartonellosis in cats and dogs.

31. Why should an animal's serum glucose concentration be known when interpreting an immunoreactive insulin concentration?

If increased, the immunoreactive insulin (IRI) concentration could represent an appropriate response to a hyperglycemia. However, the increased IRI concentration suggests an inappropriate release of insulin if the animal is normoglycemic or hypoglycemic.

If the IRI concentration is within an appropriate reference interval for normoglycemia but the animal is hyperglycemic, the IRI concentration indicates an inadequate response to the hyperglycemia. If the animal is hypoglycemic, the IRI concentration suggests an inappropriate release of insulin.

If the IRI concentration is decreased and the animal is hypoglycemic, the cause of the hypoglycemia is not insulin excess. If the animal is hyperglycemic, the results indicate defective production or release of insulin.

32. Why might published reference intervals for immunoreactive insulin (IRI) concentrations or IRI/glucose ratios *not* be appropriate intervals for the interpretation of these values in a veterinary patient?

Unfortunately, no uniform standardization of insulin assays exists, and thus two immunoassays for insulin may measure different insulin concentrations in the same sample. Minimal variations in glucose concentrations are measured by most serum glucose assays. However, blood glucose concentrations may be significantly different, varying with the assay method and hematocrit. When comparing a patient's results with reference intervals, the veterinary clinician should be sure to compare "apples to apples," that is, appropriate reference intervals and appropriate units.

33. Should the amended insulin/glucose ratio be used?

The amended insulin/glucose ratio should *not* be used. The subtraction of 30 from the glucose concentration was based on an invalid hypothesis, and the calculated value is no better than a simple insulin/glucose ratio if appropriate reference intervals are used.

34. What are fructosamine and glycated hemoglobin, and how are they measured?

A *fructosamine* is a ketoamine formed by the nonenzymatic addition of glucose to albumin or other serum proteins. The carbon backbone of this ketoamine is identical to fructose (thus "fructosamine"). *Glycated* (or glycosylated) *hemoglobin* is a ketoamine formed by the nonenzymatic addition of glucose to hemoglobin. The formation of ketoamines in blood depends on the magnitude and duration of hyperglycemia. Animals with DM thus have increased concentrations of fructosamine or glycated hemoglobin. Concentrations of these glycated proteins can be used to monitor the effectiveness of controlling the diabetic state. Because the fructosamine molecules have a shorter half-life (2-3 weeks) than glycated hemoglobin (2-3 months), fructosamine concentration is considered a better reflection of recent glucose concentration and thus a better analyte for assessing therapeutic or dietary control of DM.

Fructosamine concentrations can be measured by spectrophotometric assays. Hemolyzed and icteric serum or plasma can cause spectral interferences. Glycated hemoglobin percentages are determined by affinity chromatography, followed by spectrophotometric assays that measure the glycated and nonglycated hemoglobin fractions.

35. What are the two types or classifications of glucosuria?

a. *Hyperglycemic glucosuria* occurs when the renal tubular maximum (transport maximum, threshold) for glucose is exceeded because of a hyperglycemia. The hyperglycemia can be transient or persistent. The renal tubular maximum varies among domestic mammals: 180 to 220 mg/dl in dogs, about 290 mg/dl in cats, 150 mg/dl in horses and calves, and possibly lower in adult cattle.
b. *Renal glucosuria* results from an acquired or congenital defect in the resorption of glucose by the proximal tubular cells. Renal glucosuria is a diagnostic criterion for Fanconi's syndrome.

36. What is the difference between glycosuria and glucosuria?

The only "difference" is that "glycosuria" and "glucosuria" are spelled differently.

37. Where does ketone production fit into carbohydrate and lipid metabolism?

When there is decreased availability or utilization of carbohydrates (starvation, diabetes mellitus) by peripheral tissues, there is a mobilization of lipids from adipose tissue, which results in delivery of free fatty acids to hepatocytes. In hepatocytes, β-oxidation of the fatty acids results in the formation of acetyl coenzyme A (acetyl-CoA), which can be used for gluconeogenesis. If there is excessive formation of acetyl-CoA, there is increased ketogenesis (especially with glucagon stimulus), which results in the formation of ketoacids (acetoacetic acid, β-hydroxybutyric acid) and acetone. Acetone, acetoacetate, and β-hydroxybutyrate are commonly referred to as "ketone bodies," but chemically, β-hydroxybutyrate is not a ketone. Chemically, a ketone has a carbon atom that is double-bonded to an oxygen atom and also is bonded to two other carbon atoms; β-hydroxybutyrate does not meet these criteria.

38. How are ketone bodies measured in the urine and in the blood?

The presence of ketone bodies in the urine *(ketonuria)* is determined by a reagent strip or Acetest tablet test, both of which contain nitroprusside. Acetoacetate, and to a lesser extent acetone, react to form a colored complex with nitroprusside. The tablet test is considered to have a lower detection limit than the reagent strip method. False-positive reactions may occur if the urine is highly pigmented or if levodopa metabolites or sulfhydryl compounds are present in the urine. β-Hydroxybutyrate is not detected by these methods because it does not react with nitroprusside.

The presence of ketone bodies in the blood (*ketonemia)* can also be determined by using the reagent strip or Acetest tablet method on serum. The serum should be free of hemolysis because hemoglobin pigment may lead to a false-positive reaction or may discolor the reagent pad.

β-Hydroxybutyrate concentrations have been measured in whole blood, plasma, or serum using reactions that convert β-hydroxybutyrate to acetoacetate. High concentrations of acetoacetate inhibit the reaction. Some β-hydroxybutyrate assays have been developed for point-of-care instruments and others for automated chemistry instruments.

39. How does carbohydrate digestion and metabolism in ruminants and horses differ from that in dogs and cats?

In ruminants, ingested carbohydrates are fermented by rumen microflora to the volatile fatty acids acetate, propionate and butyrate, which are then transported to the liver to be metabolized. Glucose can be synthesized from propionate, and butyrate increases liver production of glucose. Acetate is not a glucogenic compound and is utilized for fat synthesis.

Up to 75% of the energy requirements of the horse are met by microbial fermentation of carbohydrates and production of the same volatile fatty acids in the cecum and colon.

Digestion of starches also occurs in the small intestines, where, as in the dog and cat, the carbohydrates are broken down into glucose and other monosaccharides by pancreatic amylase and by enzymes produced by the brush border of the jejunum, such as maltase and dextrinase.

40. What is the oral glucose tolerance test, and what does it measure?

The *oral glucose tolerance test* (oral GTT) is used to assess the ability of the animal to utilize a test dose of glucose. The test can be performed in monogastric animals suspected of having diabetes mellitus but do not have a persistent hyperglycemia. The oral GTT is not performed in ruminants because carbohydrates are fermented in the rumen.

A fasting blood sample is taken, followed by oral glucose administration. Serial blood glucose measurements are then performed over 3 hours. An animal that remains hyperglycemic 2 hours after the test dose of glucose suggests that the animal is diabetic. The blood glucose concentrations during the oral GTT depend on three major factors: (1) absorption of glucose by the intestine, (2) glucose utilization by tissues, and (3) renal excretion of glucose. All three factors should be considered when interpreting the results of an oral GTT.

41. What is the intravenous glucose tolerance test, and what does it measure?

The *intravenous glucose tolerance test* provides a more direct assessment of an animal's ability to utilize a test or challenge dose of glucose. Intravenous GTT also can be performed in animals with suspected DM but with no persistent hyperglycemia. This test can be performed in ruminants. The glucose disappearance rate, or the rate at which glucose is removed from the plasma (also known as the *k* value), is determined by the intravenous GTT. A diabetic animal will have a decreased glucose tolerance and therefore a slower glucose disappearance rate.

An insulin response curve may also be generated from the intravenous GTT. This curve assesses the beta cell response to the hyperglycemia.

42. What is the purpose of a glucose curve?

Glucose curves are generated during the initial regulation of diabetic animals to assess glycemic control and to determine if insulin therapy requires adjustment. Serial blood glucose measurements are performed every 1 to 2 hours throughout the day after feeding and insulin administration. The glucose curve can be used to determine insulin effectiveness, as well as *glucose nadir* (lowest glucose concentration) and duration of insulin effect. Ideally, insulin therapy should maintain glucose concentration between 100 and 300 mg/dl in diabetic cats and diabetic dogs with cataracts and between 100 and 200 mg/dl in diabetic dogs without cataracts. Alterations in insulin dosage, type, or frequency of administration are made based on results of the glucose curve.

Problems with glucose curves include variables such as stress (especially in cats) and inappetence. Also, the reproducibility of the glucose curve can vary from day to day or month to month in the same patient.

43. If pancreatic glucagon is an important regulatory hormone, why isn't its concentration routinely measured when investigating glucose and lipid disorders?

Although an important hormone in the regulation of plasma glucose concentration that also influences lipoprotein metabolism and ketogenesis, *pancreatic glucagon* is not routinely measured for the following reasons:

a. Alterations in plasma concentrations of pancreatic glucagon typically represent a compensatory or secondary process associated with a metabolic (or primary) disorder. Thus, plasma glucagon concentrations do not directly identify the primary disorder. Primary glucagon disorders (e.g., islet cell neoplasia producing glucagon) are rare in domestic mammals.
b. Pancreatic glucagon is a fragile polypeptide hormone, and special collection and handling conditions are needed to obtain accurate glucagon concentrations.
c. Very few valid assays are available for pancreatic glucagon. Some glucagon immunoassays detect pancreatic glucagon and glucagon-like peptides.

Lipids and Carbohydrates

BIBLIOGRAPHY

Bauer JE: Hyperlipidemias. In Ettinger SJ, Feldman EC, editors: *Textbook of veterinary internal medicine: diseases of the dog and cat,* ed 5, Philadelphia, 2000, Saunders, pp 283-292.

Bruss ML: Lipids and ketones. In Kaneko JJ, Harvey JW, Bruss ML, editors: *Clinical biochemistry of domestic animals,* ed 5, San Diego, 1997, Academic Press, pp 83-115.

Christopher MM, O'Neill S: Effect of specimen collection and storage on blood glucose and lactate concentrations in healthy, hyperthyroid and diabetic cats, *Vet Clin Pathol* 29:22-28, 2000.

Feldman EC, Nelson RW: Diabetes mellitus. In *Canine and feline endocrinology and reproduction,* ed 2, Philadelphia, 1996, Saunders, pp 339-391.

Gavin JR III: Report of the Expert Committee on the Diagnosis and Classification of Diabetes Mellitus, *Diabetes Care* 23:S4-S19, 2000.

Gross KL, Wedekind KJ, Cowell CS, et al: In Hand MS, Thatcher CD, Remillard RL, et al, editors: *Small animal clinical nutrition,* ed 4, Topeka, 2000, Mark Morris Institute, pp 21-107.

Hoenig M: Pathophysiology of canine diabetes, *Vet Clin North Am Small Anim Pract* 25:553-561, 1995.

Jeffcott LB, Field JR: Current concepts of hyperlipaemia in horses and ponies, *Vet Rec* 116:461-466, 1985.

Kaneko JJ: Carbohydrate metabolism and its diseases. In Kaneko JJ, Harvey JW, Bruss ML, editors: *Clinical biochemistry of domestic animals,* ed 5, San Diego, 1997, Academic Press, pp 45-81.

Lutz TA, Rand JS: Pathogenesis of feline diabetes mellitus, *Vet Clin North Am Small Anim Pract* 25:527-552, 1995.

Moller DE, Flier JS: Insulin resistance: mechanisms, syndromes, and implications, *N Engl J Med* 325:938-948, 1991.

Naylor JM: Hyperlipemia and hyperlipidemia in horses, ponies, and donkeys, *Compend Contin Educ Pract Vet* 4:S321-S326, 1982.

Rifai N, Bachorik PS, Albers JJ: Lipids, lipoproteins, and apolipoproteins. In Burtis CA, Ashwood ER, editors: *Tietz textbook of clinical chemistry,* ed 3, Philadelphia, 1999, Saunders, pp 809-861.

Sacks DB: Carbohydrates. In Burtis CA, Ashwood ER, editors: *Tietz textbook of clinical chemistry,* ed 3, Philadelphia, 1999, WB Saunders, pp 750-808.

Stockham SL, Scott MA: Glucose and related regulatory hormones. In *Fundamentals of veterinary clinical pathology,* Ames, 2002, Iowa State Press, pp 487-506.

Stockham SL, Scott MA: Lipids. In *Fundamentals of veterinary clinical pathology,* Ames, 2002, Iowa State Press, pp 521-537.

Watson TDG, Barrie J: Lipoprotein metabolism and hyperlipidaemia in the dog and cat: a review, *J Small Anim Pract* 34:479-487, 1993.

Whitney MS: Evaluation of hyperlipidemias in dogs and cats, *Semin Vet Med Surg Small Anim* 7:292-300, 1992.

Section VIII

Gastrointestinal Tract and Pancreas

Michel Desnoyers

35. GASTROINTESTINAL TRACT

1. What are the different components of the gastrointestinal tract?

Components of the gastrointestinal (GI) tract include the stomach, duodenum, jejunum, ileum, and colon. The duodenum, jejunum, and ileum form the small intestine, with the jejunum representing the longest segment.

2. Are antigens normally absorbed by the small intestine?

A small but significant percentage of dietary antigen (about 0.002%) is absorbed intact by the small intestine. These antigens probably play an important part of the normal local intestinal immune response.

3. Which clinical signs may be associated with small intestinal disease?

The most common clinical sign of small intestinal disease is diarrhea, which is an increase in the frequency, volume, and consistency of bowel movements. Less common signs include vomiting (although vomiting may be common in cats) especially in cases of inflammatory bowel disease (see Questions 58-63), weight loss (with chronic diarrhea), melena, hematemesis, polyphagia, coprophagia, pica, abdominal distention, abdominal pain, borborygmi, and flatus.

4. What are the major causes of diarrhea?

Diarrhea may be osmotic or secretory and may be caused by increased permeability, dysmotility, or malabsorption.

5. When should laboratory evaluation of diarrhea be undertaken?

Most cases of diarrhea are nonfatal and acute. However, laboratory evaluation should be performed in cases of acute severe and bloody diarrhea, with concurrent signs of systemic illness (e.g., fever), or in cases of chronic diarrhea.

6. Which basic tests should be performed in acute and chronic cases of diarrhea?

Tests should include fecal examination for parasites, hematology, and serum biochemistry.

7. Which gastrointestinal results can be expected on the complete blood count?

Red cell parameters

An increase in the packed cell volume (PCV) associated with increased total protein indicates hemoconcentration (dehydration). Conversely, a normocytic, normochromic, non-regenerative anemia may indicate chronic inflammation or, if the condition is acute, acute GI blood loss. This anemia of acute blood loss if frequently associated with a panhypoproteinemia. In cases of chronic GI blood loss (e.g., secondary to hookworms, ulcers, or tumors), an iron deficiency anemia may develop. Importantly, iron deficiency anemia secondary to blood loss may be regenerative, and therefore the mean corpuscular volume (MCV) may be within reference limits despite evidence of microcytosis on blood smears. Microscopic examination of a blood smear is always indicated in this case, since microcytosis will appear on a blood smear before the MCV begins to decrease.

Leukocyte parameters

A mild neutrophilia with or without a left shift may be seen in cases of inflammatory bowel disease, but this change is not always present. A leukopenia associated with a neutropenia and presence of a left shift is consistent with a severe acute GI infection, as in parvovirus in dogs or cats or *Salmonella* in small and large animal species. Eosinophilia may be seen in parasitism and less consistently in eosinophilic enteritis. Lymphopenia, especially if associated with hypocholesterolemia, may indicate lymphangiectasia.

Platelets

Platelets are usually within reference limits, except in cases of acute or, less frequently, chronic GI bleeding. This is secondary to increased platelet demand to prevent excessive blood loss.

8. Which gastrointestinal results can be expected on the biochemistry profile?

a. *Proteins* (albumin and globulins) are frequently decreased in cases of chronic diarrhea associated with protein-losing enteropathy (PLE) (see Question 56), but total protein values should always be interpreted in conjunction with the hydration status of the animal. The albumin/globulin ratio in cases of chronic diarrhea is frequently within reference limits.

b. Increased *blood urea nitrogen* (BUN) associated with creatinine within reference limits or a disproportionate increase in the BUN value compared with the creatinine value may suggest GI bleeding in the proximal portion of the small intestine. This change is secondary to hemoglobin degradation by intestinal enzymes.

c. *Hypocholesterolemia* associated with a lymphopenia and clinical signs of chronic diarrhea may suggest lymphangiectasia.

d. *Liver enzymes* (AST, ALT, ALP, GGT) may be increased in primary GI disease, presumably secondary to increased absorption of antigens and bacterial endotoxins due to GI damage. The liver plays an essential role in the detoxification process of intestinal toxins and antigens.

e. *Electrolyte* changes can vary. Hyperchloremic acidosis (decreased bicarbonates associated with a hyperchloremia and a strong ion difference (SID, <30) can be present in some cases, especially in acute diarrhea. If dehydration is severe enough, a high anion gap acidosis may be caused by decreased acids excretion by the kidneys (prerenal azotemia). In some cases of diarrhea (most notably hookworm infestation), electrolytic changes similar to those seen in hypoadrenocorticism may be seen (hyponatremia/hypochloremia and hyperkalemia). An adrenocorticotropic hormone (ACTH) stimulation test is always required to confirm hypoadrenocorticism, especially because diarrhea may be a clinical sign associated with this disease.

f. It is important to note that *routine hematology and biochemistry tests rarely allow for a final diagnosis of small intestinal or pancreatic disease,* and more sophisticated tests are required. However, hematologic and biochemistry tests are important to assess the hydration status and the general condition of the animal and to rule out extraintestinal or extrapancreatic causes.

9. If small intestinal bleeding is suspected and the animal does not show obvious signs of melena, how reliable are the tests for occult blood in feces?

All the tests available react with hemoglobin but also with any type of meat diet, which may result in false-positive results. It is strongly recommended to feed the patient a meat-free diet for at least 3 days before testing to increase the chances of having a reliable test result.

10. What is canine parvovirus?

Canine parvovirus type 2 (CPV-2) was discovered as a cause of acute hemorrhagic enteritis in dogs in the late 1970s. CPV-2 is highly contagious and is transmitted through the fecal-oral route. It is related to the feline parvovirus responsible for feline panleukopenia (see Question 23) and to mink enteritis virus. CPV-2 is very stable in the environment and can remain infectious for several months.

11. Describe the clinicopathologic changes associated with canine parvovirosis.

In addition to the clinical signs of acute hemorrhagic diarrhea, fever, and dehydration in young animals, dogs with parvovirosis are frequently leukopenic, neutropenic, and lymphopenic, with toxic neutrophils and a left shift (Figures 35-1 and 35-2). This hematologic change is present in up to 90% of infected animal. A leukopenia of less than 1500 to 2000 white blood cells per microliter (WBCs/μl) is common. The neutropenia is secondary to both increased losses of neutrophils in the gut and impaired bone marrow production of neutrophils, because the parvovirus is toxic to rapidly dividing bone marrow cells. Toxic neutrophils and left shift are secondary to the increased demand of neutrophils in the GI tract. Note that some breeds are more susceptible to parvovirus and include Rottweilers, Dobermans, pit bulls, and English Springer spaniels.

12. How is parvovirosis confirmed in a dog?

Demonstration of either the virus or viral antigens in the feces is required to confirm canine parvovirosis. Commercially available tests, such as enzyme-linked immunosorbent assay (ELISA; CITE Parvovirus test, IDEXX) or rapid immunomigration (RIM; WITNESS CPV, Synbiotics) can be used and are considered relatively specific and sensitive.

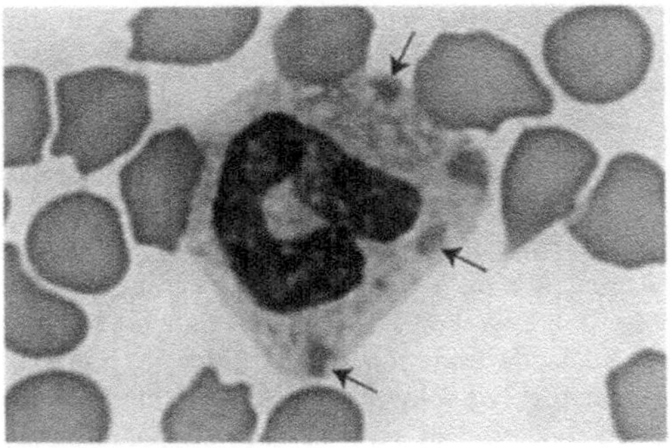

Figure 35-1 Toxic neutrophil in blood of a cat with panleukopenia. Note the presence of several Döhle bodies *(arrows)*. (Modified Wright's stain; 500×.)

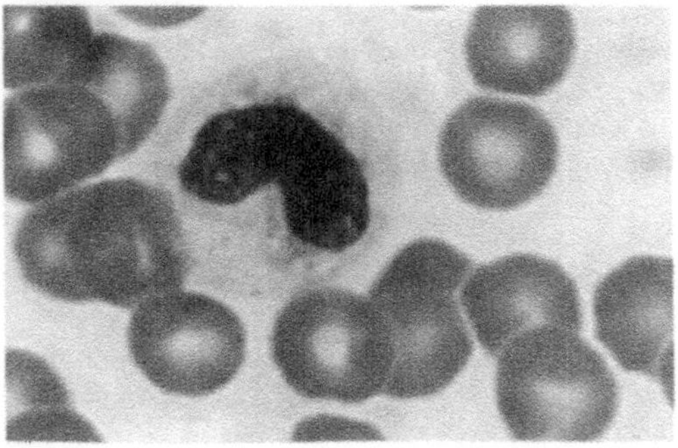

Figure 35-2 Metamyelocyte in blood of a dog with parvovirosis. (Modified Wright's stain; 500×.)

13. Can false-positive or false-negative results be obtained with the parvovirus detection test?

Virus shedding is relatively brief in the feces of infected animals, lasting less than 10 to 12 days after initial contact with the virus, which corresponds to 5 to 7 days of clinical signs; therefore, false-negative results can be obtained after that period. A false-positive result could be obtained 5 to 12 days after vaccination with a modified live virus.

14. Is *Salmonella* a common cause of acute diarrhea in dogs?

Salmonella infection (salmonellosis) occurs much less often in dogs than in other species, such as horses and humans. However, it can cause a life-threatening disease and is seen mainly in parasitized, kenneled, or immunosuppressed animals.

15. What are the clinical signs associated with acute salmonellosis in dogs?

Clinical signs of salmonellosis may be similar to those of parvovirosis: acute bloody diarrhea frequently associated with vomiting, fever, and dehydration.

16. What hematologic changes can be expected in canine salmonellosis?

Hematologic changes may be nonspecific, but frequently a severe leukopenia or, conversely, a neutrophilia can be present. In almost all cases, however, a left shift with toxic neutrophils is present, reflecting an increased demand in peripheral tissues (see Figures 35-1 and 35-2).

17. How is salmonellosis confirmed?

Bacterial culture of feces is essential for the final diagnosis of salmonellosis.

18. What is hemorrhagic gastroenteritis?

Hemorrhagic gastroenteritis is an acute syndrome characterized by diarrhea with severe hemoconcentration. Frequently, diarrhea has the aspect of raspberry jam and is often associated with vomiting and abdominal discomfort. In contrast with parvovirosis or salmonellosis, fever is uncommon in this syndrome.

19. What is the cause of hemorrhagic gastroenteritis?

The exact cause of hemorrhagic gastroenteritis is not known. The two current theories for the development of this type of diarrhea suggest either a type I hypersensitivity reaction or the production of enterotoxins by *Clostridium perfringens.*

20. Are there predisposed breeds for hemorrhagic gastroenteritis?

There is indeed a breed predisposition for this syndrome. Small breed dogs such as miniature and toy poodles, as well as miniature schnauzers, are predisposed.

21. Besides clinical signs, do clinicopathologic changes support a diagnosis of hemorrhagic gastroenteritis?

Probably the most common hematobiochemical change associated with hemorrhagic gastroenteritis is a marked hemoconcentration, with PCV frequently greater than 55% to 60%, despite GI blood loss. This increased PCV is not associated with a parallel increase in total protein. The absence of severe inflammation on the complete blood count (CBC) helps to differentiate hemorrhagic gastroenteritis from parvovirosis or salmonellosis.

22. How is hemorrhagic gastroenteritis confirmed?

Since the exact underlying cause for hemorrhagic gastroenteritis is not known, a confirmatory test does not exist. However, a positive fecal test for *Clostridium perfringens* spores or enterotoxin, in combination with consistent clinical signs, may support the diagnosis.

23. What is the cause of feline panleukopenia?

The cause of feline panleukemia is a parvovirus similar to the canine form. This means that clinical signs and transmission are also similar to its canine counterpart.

24. Describe the clinicopathologic changes in cases of feline panleukopenia?

As its name indicates, this virus causes a decrease in all WBC lines, primarily neutrophils and lymphocytes. A WBC count less than 2000/µl is common and frequently associated with a left shift and toxic neutrophils (see Figures 35-1 and 35-2).

25. Are parasitic infestations common in dogs and cats?

Canine and feline parasitic infections are common and include infestations by helminths (roundworms, hookworms, whipworms, cestodes, *Strongyloides*) and protozoa (coccidia, *Cryptosporidium, Giardia*).

26. Do all intestinal parasites cause hematologic or biochemical changes in their hosts?

Although parasites causing damage to the intestinal wall (e.g., hookworms) can result in a peripheral eosinophilia, parasites such as coccidia do *not* cause hematologic or biochemical changes. Therefore, eosinophilia is not a consistent finding in cases of parasitic infestation. Heavily parasitized animals may have a panhypoproteinemia, but this is also an inconsistent finding. Infestation with hookworms may result in blood loss anemia. If the infestation is severe and sufficiently prolonged, iron deficiency may occur. Fecal analysis remains the best way to confirm the presence of parasites.

27. Define malabsorption.

Malabsorption is a failure to either digest or absorb nutrients. Different pathologies can result in malabsorption.

28. Define the difference between maldigestion and malabsorption.

Even though maldigestion is defined as a failure of food digestion and malabsorption as a failure to absorb what was digested, the differentiation between the two is somewhat subjective. For example, malabsorption is inevitable if food is not digested. Therefore, for several authors, the global term *malabsorption* refers to a process where food is either not digested or absorbed properly.

29. What are the major causes of malabsorption?

Causes of malabsorption can be divided *arbitrarily* into luminal, mucosal, or postmucosal conditions, but there is major overlap between these different categories.

a. *Luminal* causes include exocrine pancreatic insufficiency (see Question 32), cholestatic liver disease, and small intestine bacterial overgrowth.
b. *Mucosal* causes include lactose deficiency, villous atrophy, and inflammatory bowel disease (see later).
c. *Postmucosal* causes include lymphangiectasia, neoplasia, and portal hypertension.

30. Which clinical signs can be expected in cases of malabsorption?

The most common clinical sign of malabsorption is probably chronic diarrhea associated with weight loss. Vomiting may also be present. However, it is important to note that diarrhea is *not* always present in cases of malabsorption.

31. Which clinicopathologic tests can be used to diagnose malabsorption?

Clinicopathologic tests for malabsorption depend on the suspected underlying cause. The two most common broad causes are intestinal and pancreatic problems (see following questions).

32. What are the causes of exocrine pancreatic insufficiency (EPI)?

The most common cause of EPI in adult dogs is chronic acinar atrophy. This atrophy seems idiopathic in several breeds and seems unique to dogs, even though some cases have been infrequently reported in other species. German Shepherd as well as rough-coated collies have a genetic predisposition for an immune-mediated condition called *atrophic lymphocytic pancreatitis*, resulting also in chronic acinar atrophy. Pancreatic hypoplasia is a possible but rare cause of EPI in dogs. Chronic pancreatitis seems to be a rare cause of EPI in dogs, whereas in *cats*, this condition seems to be the major cause of EPI.

33. Which clinical signs can be expected in cases of EPI?

Typical clinical signs of exocrine pancreatic insufficiency in dogs include large volumes of semiformed feces or diarrhea, often accompanied by weight loss and polyphagia, although the owner may report episodes of anorexia and hyporexia. Feces can have a greasy or discolored appearance, but these changes are not always present. Coprophagia and pica may also be reported. Animals are rarely depressed or lethargic. In cats, clinical signs are similar to the ones in dogs, even though vomiting and anorexia seem to be more common in feline than canine species.

34. Because clinical signs of EPI can resemble those seen in intestinal diseases, which tests can be used for diagnosis of EPI in dogs and cats?

Several tests are available to diagnose exocrine pancreatic insufficiency, and each has advantages and disadvantages. Tests include trypsin-like immunoreactivity (TLI), pancreatic elastase, oral triglyceride challenge (corn oil) test, BT-PABA (bentiromide) test, and tests for fecal fat (see later questions).

35. Is there a reason why hematology and routine serum biochemistry (amylase, lipase) are not listed in the series of tests for EPI in dogs and cats?

Hematology and routine serum biochemistry tests do not show specific changes in cases of exocrine pancreatic insufficiency and therefore are used more as a screening tool for the veterinary patient's overall health than for a specific diagnosis. Moreover, serum amylase and lipase are unreliable indicators of pancreatic function and should not be used to diagnose EPI (see later questions concerning pancreatitis).

36. Which is the most reliable test for the diagnosis of EPI?

Serum TLI is the most sensitive and specific test for exocrine pancreatic insufficiency in dogs and cats. Because TLI assays are species specific, it is important to perform the tests in veterinary and not human laboratories. Serum TLI measures the amount of trypsinogen that normally leaks from the pancreas into the bloodstream. Because trypsinogen is pancreas specific, the TLI test provides a good indication of the pancreatic tissue function. Sensitivity and specificity for TLI in cases of EPI are reportedly close to 100%.

37. What trypsin-like immunoreactivity (TLI) values should be expected if a dog or a cat has EPI, and what is the procedure to obtain TLI?

a. *Dogs:* less than 2.5 μg/L (reference value 5-35 μg/L)
b. *Cats:* less than 8 to 10 μg/L (reference value 17-49 μg/L)

Tests for serum TLI concentrations considered diagnostic for exocrine pancreatic insufficiency should be performed on an animal that has been fasted for at least 12 hours to prevent "gray zone" values. No special tubes are required, just a simple red-top tube.

38. Are any special procedures involved in submitting a serum sample for TLI?

TLI is quite thermoresistant, and therefore leaving the serum sample at room temperature for several hours before shipping to a laboratory should not influence the result, nor should refrigeration or freezing. Ideally, as for other biochemical analyses, serum should be separated 1 to 4 hours after clot formation. Mild to moderate hemolysis, lipemia, or icterus are not reported to influence results.

39. What are the TLI "gray zone" values in dogs and cats, and what should be done if such results are obtained?

TLI "gray zone" values vary between 2 and 5 μg/L in dogs and between 10 and 17 μg/L in cats. In cases of gray-zone results with clinical signs consistent with EPI, some authors recommend treating animals with pancreatic enzymes and retesting TLI in 1 or 2 months to see if TLI values decrease even further. Pancreatic enzyme supplementation does *not* affect the TLI value.

40. Is it possible to obtain a "normal" or even increased TLI value in an animal with exocrine pancreatic insufficiency?

In the one reported case of combined EPI and pancreatitis in dogs, the dog had clinical signs consistent both with pancreatitis (vomiting, anorexia) and with EPI (soft stools, weight loss). The TLI value was high (50 μg/L), but other tests (oral triglyceride test, fecal proteolytic digestion) were considered consistent with EPI. On necropsy the animal had evidence of chronic pancreatitis. It is therefore possible but rare to obtain a "normal" or high TLI in cases of EPI, but other clinical signs and abnormal tests besides TLI should also be present and should suggest another, concomitant pathology.

41. Because German Shepherd or rough-coated collies are predisposed to pancreatic acinar atrophy, what is done if a low TLI value is obtained in an animal that does not show typical signs of exocrine pancreatic insufficiency?

Some dogs may have repeatedly low TLI values (defined as <5 μg/L) despite sufficient pancreatic reserves that prevent or slow down the development of clinical disease (e.g., polyphagia, weight loss). Progression of EPI may vary greatly among individual animals, with some developing EPI and requiring enzyme supplementation while others do not. Immunosuppressive therapy is not recommended in these animals despite the immune-mediated nature of the problem. Enzyme supplementation in these animals should be instituted only if clinical signs of EPI appear.

42. Although pancreatic elastase 1 in stools is used as a gold standard for exocrine pancreatic insufficiency in human medicine, is it useful in dogs or cats?

Pancreatic elastase 1 in stool samples has become the noninvasive pancreatic function test with the highest sensitivity and specificity in human medicine. *Pancreatic elastase* is a zymogen produced exclusively by pancreatic acinar cells and eliminated in feces, and its value should decrease in cases of EPI. This zymogen is very stable and is resistant to proteolytic degradation in the gut.

Recently, a sandwiched-ELISA test has been developed for use in dogs and shows very good sensitivity and specificity. It is now available as a commercial test (ScheBo, Biotech AG). No studies have yet been done to develop a technique in cats.

43. Does elastase from other species, such as that present in pancreatic supplementation, interfere with the commercial test for canine pancreatic elastase?

Studies have shown that human, bovine, or porcine elastase is *not* detected with the sandwiched-ELISA test for canine EPI. This means that pancreatic supplementation can be provided without influencing the test results.

44. What pancreatic elastase results should be expected in a dog with exocrine pancreatic insufficiency?

Since few studies have been done on canine pancreatic elastase, only preliminary results can be given. Values less than 10 μg/g feces could suggest EPI, but further studies are required to confirm this value.

45. Is canine pancreatic elastase stable if the test cannot be done immediately?

It is better to keep feces frozen (preferably at –20° C) if the pancreatic elastase test cannot be performed immediately, to prevent degradation of the enzyme.

46. Is the gelatin (or x-ray film) fecal digestion test reliable?

Fecal proteolytic activity has been used for many years in veterinary medicine. However, this measurement is plagued by wide variation in results depending on the method used, and avoiding autodegradation of proteases during the interval between stool sample collection and analysis is important. The x-ray film, or gelatin, fecal digestion test is easy to perform but unfortunately is frequently unreliable because this procedure does not seem to be standardized among laboratories. Also, gelatin digestion is difficult to interpret, resulting in many false results. False-positive results may result from intestinal bacterial proteolytic activity. False-negative results may result from a delay between sampling and analysis or from severe diarrhea diluting pancreatic enzymes.

47. Are there other fecal proteolytic digestion tests that can be done besides the x-ray film test?

Other tests include determination of proteolytic activity on substrates such as azocasein or casein-containing agar gels. Theoretically, dogs and cats with EPI should have low protease activity, resulting in little or no protein digestion, but some normal dogs and cats can have intermittently low fecal protease activity. This means that the test must either be repeated on several stool samples, or if only a single sample can be obtained, dogs should be fed a crude soybean meal for 2 days before the test to increase chances of a true positive result.

48. Describe the oral triglyceride challenge (corn oil) test and the expected results in cases of exocrine pancreatic insufficiency.

The oral triglyceride challenge test is based on the assumption that dogs with EPI or primary small intestinal disease will have fat malabsorption. Dogs are given corn oil orally after a 12-hour fast, and if either a pancreatic or an intestinal problem is present, preprandial and postprandial serum triglyceride values should basically be the same. When the test is repeated with pancreatic enzyme supplementation (e.g., Viokase-V), postprandial triglycerides should increase at least twofold over baseline values if the animal has EPI. Unfortunately, false-positive and false-negative results are possible, and the corn oil test should not be used to confirm EPI. False-positive results can be found in dogs with EPI because up to 80% of triglycerides may still be absorbed, even when pancreatic enzymes are dramatically decreased or even absent. False-negative results may be found in some cases of EPI because intestinal free fatty acid absorption may be decreased, even when dogs receive supplementation with pancreatic enzymes.

The triglyceride challenge (corn oil) test does not seem to be used in cats.

49. Describe the BT-PABA test and the expected results in cases of exocrine pancreatic insufficiency.

The BT-PABA (*N*-benzoyl-L-tyrosyl-*p*-aminobenzoic acid) test, or bentiromide test, was a useful test for diagnosis of EPI before the introduction of TLI and pancreatic elastase testing. BT-PABA was administered orally to dogs suspected of EPI, and serum as well as urine values of PABA were measured. Low levels of serum or urine PABA were considered indicative of

EPI. However, interpretation was sometimes difficult, with possible overlap between results in dogs with EPI and dogs with small intestinal disease. Because the bentiromide test does not show advantages compared with TLI and fecal proteolytic assays, it is rarely used now, especially because it is expensive and technically challenging. The only potential advantage of BT-PABA versus TLI testing is in rare cases of EPI caused by pancreatic juice flow obstruction. In this situation, trypsinogen is released in blood but not in the gut, resulting in clinical signs of EPI, but with serum TLI values within reference limits; however, fecal proteolytic and pancreatic elastase tests should also be abnormal. The bentiromide test is not useful in cats because of the apparently wide variation in reference values in normal animals.

50. Are fecal fat tests useful in cases of exocrine pancreatic insufficiency, and how are the results interpreted?

Tests for fecal fat can be either qualitative or quantitative. In dogs and cats, the *qualitative* fecal fat test is unreliable because many false-positive results may be obtained. If used, fecal fat testing should be standardized by feeding the animal a diet containing moderate amount of fat (about 8%) for at least 48 to 72 hours before analysis and by analyzing at least two fecal samples. Qualitative fecal fat testing can be divided into direct and indirect tests. The direct test detects undigested fecal fats (triglycerides), and the indirect test detects split fats (e.g., fatty acids).

The *direct test* is performed by placing a small piece of fresh feces on a microscope slide mixed with a drop of Sudan III or IV, pacing a coverslip, and examining at 10× (low magnification). Positive results show more than three large, refractile orange droplets per field at low magnification.

The *indirect test* is performed by adding 1 or 2 drops of glacial acetic acid to the edge of the coverslip of the slide used for the direct test. The slide is then heated to near boiling, and heating is stopped when a few bubbles start to appear underneath the coverslip. The slide is examined under the microscope when still warm. Heat and acetic acid convert fecal soaps into insoluble free fatty acids that aggregate into large globules. Dogs with intestinal malabsorption should have more than three globules per field at low magnification.

Theoretically, animals with EPI should be positive for both the direct and indirect tests, whereas intestinal problems should result only in a positive indirect test. Practically, however, the fecal fat test does not seem to differentiate between pancreatic and intestinal causes of steatorrhea in either dogs or cats.

The quantitative fecal test is rarely used because it is time consuming, expensive, and unpleasant (feces collected for 72 hours). Moreover, this test could not accurately differentiate EPI from primary small intestinal problems in several studies.

Fecal fat tests cannot be used for a final diagnosis or even recommended as a screening test for EPI.

51. If EPI has been ruled out based on laboratory testing, and now small intestinal disease is suspected, which tests can be used to confirm it?

If parasites (fecal examination), systemic diseases (CBC, biochemistry profile, including thyroxine in older cats), and intestinal accidents (radiography, ultrasound) have been ruled out, more specific tests are required in dogs and cats. These tests may include D-xylose absorption, combined xylose/3-*O*-methyl-D-glucose, oral trigylceride challenge (discussed earlier with EPI), fecal fat excretion (also described with EPI), and serum folate and cobalamin (vitamin B_{12}) concentrations (see following questions).

52. Describe the D-xylose absorption test.

D-xylose is an exogenous pentose sugar that is absorbed by the small intestine through carrier-mediated transport. It is not metabolized after absorption, however, and is excreted intact in the urine. The test is performed by measuring either blood xylose after 3 hours or its urinary excretion after 5 hours (see Bibliography following Chapter 36 for sources detailing these procedures). If malabsorption is present secondary to a small intestinal problem, lower peaks in serum concentration and urine excretion are expected.

In humans, the D-xylose absorption test is considered a useful screening tool for primary intestinal disease. In dogs, however, the xylose test is not as accurate and shows relatively poor specificity and sensitivity. This may be the result of several factors, including a reduced dependence on active intestinal transport compared with humans, possibly associated with increased nonspecific absorption through tight junctions and aqueous pores. Also, up to 50% of D-xylose in dogs may be metabolized before being excreted. This means that plasma xylose concentrations are not always decreased in animals with small intestinal disease or may be decreased in animals not affected by small intestinal disease. Further, results may also be abnormal in dogs with EPI.

The D-xylose test also cannot be recommended for cats. There is tremendous individual variation, and the test seems quite insensitive to detect feline small intestinal disease.

53. Describe the combined xylose/3-*O*-methyl-D-glucose test.

The xylose/glucose test is not widely available and is technically demanding but shows promise for the diagnosis of small intestinal disease in dogs and cats. The rationale behind this test is that the absorption rates of these two sugars are different across the intestinal mucosa, and the uptake of 3-*O*-methyl-D-glucose is close to 100%, even in cases of severe small intestinal disease, giving a "constant" to which D-xylose can be compared.

54. Describe the measurement of serum folate and cobalamin concentrations.

The principle behind the measurement of folate and cobalamin for the diagnosis of small intestinal disease is that (a) folate is absorbed by specific carriers in the proximal jejunum and (b) cobalamin is absorbed by receptor-mediated endocytosis in the ileum. In cases of proximal intestinal disease, serum folate concentration should decrease. In cases of distal intestinal disease, serum cobalamin concentration should decrease. If extensive diffuse intestinal disease occurs, both folate and cobalamin concentrations should decrease. This test seems to be useful in dogs and cats, but it is only a *screening* tool and should not be used for final diagnosis of small intestinal disease.

55. Can false-positive or false-negative results be obtained when measuring folate and cobalamin?

Cobalamin values may falsely decrease when serum is exposed to bright light; proper handling is important. Serum folate values may increase if the sample is hemolyzed because erythrocytes are rich in folate. In small intestine bacterial overgrowth, which can result in small intestinal disease, increased numbers of bacteria can synthesize excess folate while binding cobalamin, possibly resulting in high-folate and low-cobalamin concentrations. Practically, however, bacterial overgrowth rarely seems to cause these changes. Increased serum folate and decreased serum cobalamin have been reported in dogs with EPI, possibly due to bacterial overgrowth secondary to decreased exocrine pancreatic activity. Also, however, pancreatic proteases are involved in the release of cobalamin from its protein binders, and the pancreas is a source of intrinsic factor, which is essential for cobalamin absorption. Thus it is important to rule out EPI before measuring folate and cobalamin serum values.

56. Describe the more specific small intestinal disease known as protein-losing enteropathy and the expected clinicopathologic changes.

Protein-losing enteropathy (PLE) is a general term indicating a small intestinal disease that results in the loss of plasma or other protein-containing tissues. Numerous conditions can cause PLE, including lymphoplasmocytic enteritis; eosinophilic enteritis; granulomatous enteritis; diffuse gastrointestinal neoplasia; foreign bodies; intussusception; small intestinal bacterial overgrowth; viral, bacterial or fungal enteritis; lymphangiectasia; and immune-mediated disease. Some of these conditions are described in greater detail later.

The most consistent change on the biochemical profile in cases of PLE is a *hypoproteinemia,* usually associated with both hypoalbuminemia and hypoglobulinemia. However, there are exceptions; for example, Basenji dogs have PLE characterized by hypoalbuminemia but also hyperglobulinemia, and dogs with diffuse intestinal histoplasmosis may have normal values or hyperglobulinemia despite increased intestinal protein loss. Also, ascites secondary to hypoalbuminemia rarely occurs until the albumin value drops below 1.0 to 1.2 g/dl.

Peripheral eosinophilia is not a consistent finding in cases of eosinophilic enteritis and should not be used to diagnose this condition. Peripheral eosinophilia is more often found in cases of parasitic disease.

Hypocholesterolemia, associated with *lymphopenia,* may be found in some cases of lymphangiectasia.

57. What is the best test to confirm a protein-losing enteropathy?

Intestinal biopsies remain the best diagnostic tool for confirmation of a PLE.

58. Are there alternatives in the diagnosis of PLE for a dog in poor physical condition that is not a good candidate for anesthesia, laparotomy, and intestinal biopsy?

Two noninvasive tests can be used to determine intestinal protein loss in the dog that is not a good candidate for biopsy: chromium-51 (^{51}Cr)–labeled albumin and fecal alpha-1 (α_1)-protease inhibitor.

The *^{51}Cr-labeled albumin test* is performed by either intravenous administration of ^{51}Cr chloride or exogenous ^{51}Cr-labeled human albumin. A known dose of either substance is injected intravenously, and feces are collected for 72 hours. The amount of radioactivity in the feces reflects the amount of albumin lost in the GI tract. A normal dog should excrete less than 5% of the labeled albumin or chloride. In dogs with PLE, losses greater than 50% have been reported. Because of the two major disadvantages of collecting feces for 72 hours and using radioactive material, this test now is rarely used.

Fecal α_1-protease inhibitor is an endogenous serum protein resistant to intestinal bacterial degradation. Fecal excretion of this inhibitor is increased in cases of PLE. Increases in fecal α_1-protease inhibitor may be sporadic in cases of PLE, and thus the testing of three stool samples is usually required.

59. What is inflammatory bowel disease?

Inflammatory bowel disease (IBD) is a heterogeneous group of disorders characterized by infiltration of the GI tract with inflammatory cells. Some types of IBD can result in protein-losing enteropathies. Inflammatory cells may be lymphocytes, plasma cells, eosinophils, neutrophils, or macrophages. This type of GI disease may represent the most common histologic diagnosis in dogs and cats presenting with signs of chronic vomiting and diarrhea.

60. Which form of inflammatory bowel disease is the most common?

Lymphoplasmocytic enteritis (LPE) represents the most common form of IBD in small animals. The exact etiology for LPE is still unknown, but local immune stimulation caused by enteric bacteria has been shown. Certain breeds of dogs (Basenjis, boxers, German Shepherds, Shar-Pei) and perhaps purebred cats seem to be predisposed to LPE.

61. Are there hematologic or biochemical changes that suggest lymphoplasmocytic enteritis?

A mild neutrophilia and a mild left shift have infrequently been reported in cases of LPE but may also be found in other types of inflammatory intestinal disease, so these changes are not pathognomonic. Hypoalbuminemia and hypoglobulinemia may be seen in cases of LPE but may also be found in other causes of PLE. About 25% of cats with LPE may show elevated liver enzymes, including alanine transaminase (ALT), aspartate transaminase (AST), and alkaline phosphatase (ALP). These enzymes may be elevated due to a hepatic response to the intestinal inflammation. Lymphocytosis or hyperglobulinemia are not reported in cases of LPE. Final diagnosis is made by intestinal biopsy.

62. What is the most common form of inflammatory bowel disease besides lymphoplasmocytic enteritis?

Eosinophilic enteritis seems to represent the second most common form of IBD. It is present in both dogs and cats (less common in feline species), and the etiology is still unclear. Eosinophilic enteritis frequently involves the stomach and colon in addition to the small intestine and, as with LPE, can result in a PLE. In cats, eosinophilic enteritis may be part of the more severe hypereosinophilic syndrome, in which multiple organs are infiltrated with eosinophils.

63. Because there is eosinophilic infiltration of the GI tract in eosinophilic enteritis, can an eosinophilia be expected on the complete blood count?

Unfortunately, peripheral eosinophilia is not always present in eosinophilic enteritis. Moreover, if an eosinophilia is present, it is important to discern this eosinophilia from one caused by parasites, intestinal neoplasia (e.g., mast cell tumor, lymphoma), or even hypoadrenocorticism. As with LPE, final diagnosis of eosinophilic enteritis is made by intestinal biopsy.

36. PANCREAS

1. How is pancreatitis classified?

Pancreatitis is inflammation of the pancreas that may be classified as acute or chronic. *Acute pancreatitis* is marked by inflammatory episodes that often have a sudden onset. *Chronic pancreatitis* is defined as an ongoing inflammatory process that may lead to exocrine pancreatic insufficiency (EPI) and diabetes mellitus (DM) if not controlled.

2. What mechanisms lead to the development of pancreatitis?

The pancreas is rich in digestive enzymes that are essential for food digestion and absorption. To prevent pancreatic autodigestion, several of these enzymes are stored in an inactive form *(zymogens)* in the pancreas and are activated only when released in the intestine under physiologic conditions. Moreover, when synthesized, these zymogens are contained into granules that are physically segregated from lysosomal enzymes, preventing their accidental activation within the pancreas itself. In cases of pancreatitis, however, it is believed that abnormal fusion of zymogen granules and lysosomal enzymes results in the intrapancreatic activation of zymogens, most notably trypsinogen, which is converted to *trypsin.* Once trypsin has been activated, a domino effect ensues, resulting in more activation of pancreatic enzymes inside the gland. This results in autodigestion of the gland with secondary activation of inflammatory mediators, including tumor necrosis factor alpha (TNF-α), interleukin-1 (IL-1), IL-2, IL-6, IL-8, IL-10, interferon-α (IFN-α), INF-γ, nitrous oxide (NO), and platelet-activating factor (PAF). These mediators play an important role in the progression of the inflammation.

3. Is it true that only dogs can develop acute pancreatitis?

Until the early 1990s, acute feline pancreatitis was thought to be rare. With the development of more sophisticated tests (see Questions 9 to 13), however, feline pancreatitis is now more common than previously thought, although its prevalence is much lower than for canine pancreatitis.

4. What are the clinical signs that suggest acute pancreatitis in dogs and cats?

Most **dogs** with pancreatitis are overweight, middle-aged to older animals. Clinical signs may be related to recent ingestion of a large amount of fatty meals and may vary depending on whether the pancreatitis is acute or chronic. In cases of *acute* pancreatitis, clinical signs may include anorexia, depression, vomiting, and possibly marked abdominal pain. Diarrhea may occur but is not as common as vomiting. Some animals may even be in shock on presentation. Clinical signs of *chronic* pancreatitis, if present, are variable and frequently nonspecific, rendering the diagnosis more difficult.

In **cats**, clinical signs may be subtler. In some cases, cats show no clinical signs, and pancreatitis is diagnosed only at necropsy; others display signs that are not recognized by the owner. In cases of severe pancreatitis, lethargy is the most common clinical sign reported by owners, followed by anorexia. Vomiting, which is a common sign in dogs with pancreatitis, seems to be present in only about one third of feline cases. Abdominal pain is present in about one fourth of feline cases.

5. What hematologic changes are found in cases of acute canine pancreatitis?

Neutrophilic leukocytosis is a common finding in cases of acute canine pancreatitis. If pancreatitis is severe (usually reflected by more severe clinical signs), the neutrophilia may be associated with a left shift and toxic neutrophils. Erythrocytosis (increased hematocrit, hemoglobin, and red blood cell [RBC] count) is common and is secondary to clinical dehydration. If a hemorrhagic pancreatitis is present, a slight anemia (nonregenerative or regenerative depending on duration of condition) may be present, but the anemia may be masked by clinical dehydration, resulting in RBC parameters within reference limits. If pancreatitis is extremely severe, disseminated intravascular coagulation (DIC) may result, possibly causing a thrombocytopenia as well as RBC pathologies on the blood smear, including schizocytes (Figure 36-1), keratocytes (Figure 36-2), and acanthocytes (Figure 36-3).

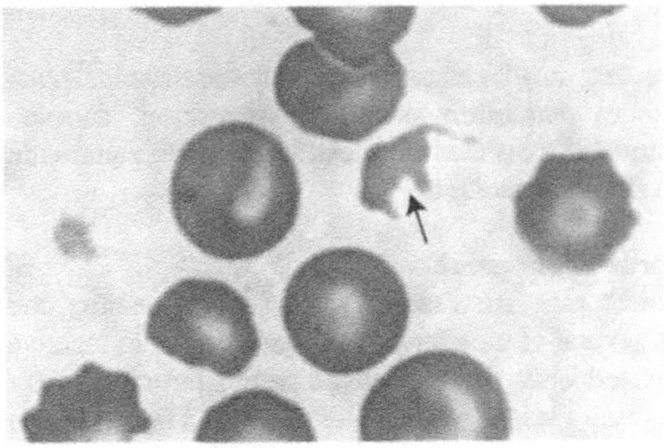

Figure 36-1 Schizocyte *(arrow)*, a red blood cell fragment, in a dog with acute pancreatitis. (Modified Wright's stain; 500×.)

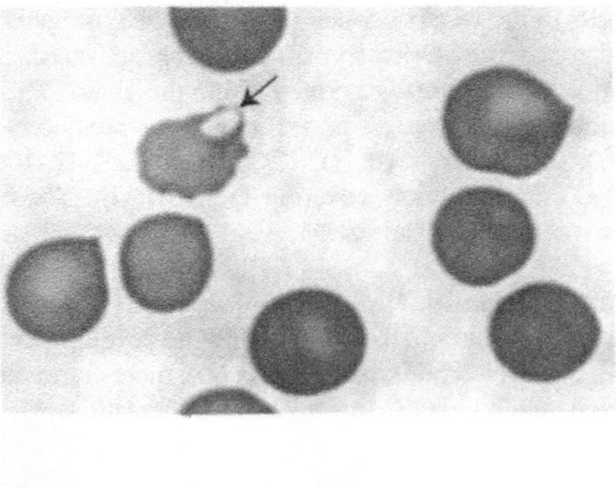

Figure 36-2 Keratocyte *(arrow)* in a dog with acute pancreatitis. Note the projections resembling blunt horns. (Modified Wright's stain; 500×.)

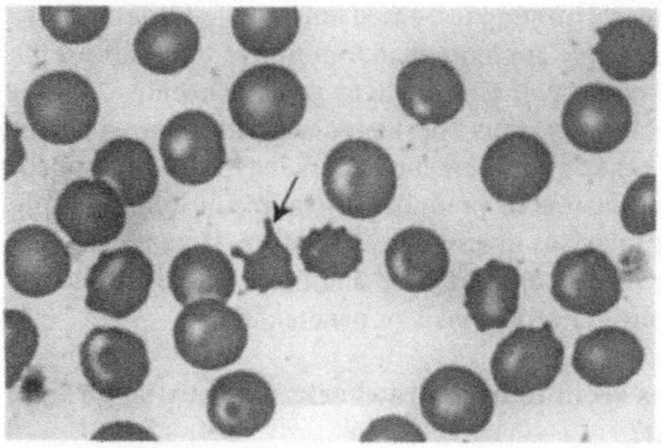

Figure 36-3 Acanthocyte *(arrow)* in a dog with acute pancreatitis. This red blood cell pathology has projections varying in length and width, allowing its differentiation from an echinocyte. (Modified Wright's stain; 500×.)

6. What changes can be expected on a routine biochemistry panel in cases of acute canine pancreatitis?

a. *Hyperglycemia* is common in dogs with acute pancreatitis and is associated with a combination of stress and increased glucagon production in relation to insulin production. Glucose monitoring is important in cases of pancreatitis because DM may be a transient or permanent consequence.

b. *Increased liver enzymes,* including alanine transaminase (ALT), aspartate transaminase (AST), alkaline phosphatase (ALP), and gamma-glutamyl transferase (GGT), are frequently seen. Increases in liver enzyme concentrations result from a combination of hepatic damage, secondary to exposure to toxic products released by the pancreas and delivered through portal blood, and hepatic ischemia. If hepatic damage is severe enough, intrahepatic and extrahepatic cholestasis may occur, resulting in increased total bilirubin and possibly clinical icterus.

c. *Hypercholesterolemia* and *hypertriglyceridemia* are common, and a milky appearance of the serum is possible if hypertriglyceridemia is severe.

d. *Hypocalcemia* may occur, especially in cases of necrotizing pancreatitis, but usually is not severe enough to cause clinical signs. The cause of the hypocalcemia is still obscure but may be related to calcium deposition as soaps, resulting from fat breakdown by pancreatic enzymes released in the abdominal cavity. Another explanation is a calcium shift into soft tissues (e.g., muscles) through altered membrane integrity.

e. *Increased blood urea nitrogen* (BUN) and *creatinine* are frequently seen due to prerenal azotemia secondary to dehydration. It is important to monitor BUN and creatinine in dogs with acute pancreatitis, since acute renal failure is an uncommon but possible consequence of pancreatitis and may be related to severe vasoconstriction or prolonged hypovolemia.

f. *Electrolytic changes* are relatively common in acute canine pancreatitis. Hypokalemia may be present and is secondary to vomiting. If transient DM is present in a dog with pancreatitis, serum potassium values may be within reference limits, despite vomiting, because increased glucagon/insulin ratio can impede intracellular potassium shift from serum to cells. Chloride may be elevated (if the animal is dehydrated), within reference limits, or low if the animal is vomiting (HCl loss). Sodium may also be increased (dehydration), within reference limits, or low if there is diarrhea or if there is ascites secondary to the pancreatitis (third space loss).

7. Are amylase and lipase useful in the diagnosis of canine pancreatitis?

Both amylase and lipase can originate from pancreatic factors but also from extrapancreatic sources, such as the small intestinal and gastric mucosa. Both amylase and lipase are eliminated by the kidneys, and thus renal failure may result in a twofold to threefold increase in these parameters. Whether prerenal azotemia can result in increased amylase and lipase values is controversial. Clinicians should be careful about interpreting increased amylase and lipase values in a severely dehydrated animal except if the increases are more than four to five times above the upper reference limit, where pancreatitis is more likely, if clinical signs are consistent.

Because of its more limited tissue distribution, lipase is considered superior to amylase for the diagnosis of pancreatitis in dogs. However, other nonpancreatic factors may result in a lipase increase. Corticosteroid administration (dexamethasone or prednisone) can result in a threefold to fivefold increase in lipase without a parallel increase in amylase. Therefore, if pancreatitis is suspected in a dog receiving dexamethasone or prednisone, amylase and lipase values should be determined, and both should be increased to consider a diagnosis of pancreatitis.

8. Since amylase and lipase determinations seem to have drawbacks for the diagnosis of canine pancreatitis, is there a better test?

Yes, two tests could theoretically be used to confirm pancreatitis in dogs: trypsinlike immunoreactivity (TLI) and pancreatic lipase immunoreactivity (PLI). Surprisingly, TLI is less sensitive than total lipase for the diagnosis of pancreatitis, having a sensitivity of only 35%. In cases in which TLI is increased, the enzyme value is usually high (>35 μg/L). However, there seems to be a poor correlation between TLI serum level and clinical severity of the disease. A recent study has shown that only 3 out of 20 dogs with pancreatitis had TLI values greater than the highest concentration in control dogs, confirming that several dogs with pancreatitis may have TLI values within reference limits. As for amylase and lipase, the kidneys excrete TLI, and renal function evaluation (BUN, creatinine, and urine specific gravity) is essential for good interpretation of the TLI value since renal failure can cause a two- to threefold increase in its value. TLI assays are species specific; it is therefore very important to have its value determined in a veterinary laboratory.

The best test available thus far for the diagnosis of canine pancreatitis is PLI. The reference range for canine PLI is 2.2 to 102.1 μg/L. If a cutoff value of 200 μg/L is used for the diagnosis of pancreatitis in dogs, PLI has a sensitivity of 82%, which is better than total lipase (55%), TLI (35%), and abdominal ultrasound (68%). Moreover, dehydration, renal failure, and prednisone administration do not result in an increased PLI value.

9. What hematologic changes may be present in cases of feline pancreatitis?

On presentation, some cats show a neutrophilia that may be associated with a left shift. Some animals may be anemic, but after rehydration the proportion of anemic cats tends to be higher, indicating that anemia can be masked by dehydration on initial presentation. The anemia can be either regenerative or nonregenerative and may be secondary to gastrointestinal or intra-abdominal blood loss or intensive fluid administration for the treatment of dehydration and shock. Platelet count is frequently within reference limits.

10. What biochemical changes may be present in cases of feline pancreatitis?

Most biochemical changes seen in dogs can also be seen in cats with pancreatitis (see Question 6). Hyperbilirubinemia and clinical icterus reportedly are more common in cats than in dogs with pancreatitis. In contrast with cats that develop hyperglycemia in cases of necrotizing pancreatitis, cats with suppurative pancreatitis tend to develop hypoglycemia. Hypocalcemia in cats, in contrast to dogs, seems to be associated primarily with hypoalbuminemia.

11. Can amylase and lipase be used for the diagnosis of pancreatitis in the cat?

Several studies have shown that amylase and lipase are not useful for the diagnosis of feline pancreatitis.

12. Which tests are best for the diagnosis of feline pancreatitis, and what are the expected results?

Abdominal ultrasound, abdominal computed tomography, and serum TLI have been studied in the diagnosis of pancreatitis in the cat. TLI was considered the most sensitive, even though the sensitivity was much less than 100%. If a TLI value of greater than 49 μg/L was used, the sensitivity to diagnose feline pancreatitis was 86%. If a value of 100 μg/L was used (suggested as a "real-life" clinical cutoff value), a sensitivity of 33% was determined. Despite this low percentage, TLI was considered the most sensitive of all the diagnostic tests evaluated.

13. Given study results, does this mean that cats with pancreatitis may have TLI values within reference limits?

Cats may have TLI values with reference limits because of the nature of feline pancreatitis. Large amounts of enzymes may be released during the initial phase of the disease, followed by smaller amounts, which may result in TLI values within reference limits.

14. Because TLI is not always increased in cases of feline pancreatitis, will pancreatic lipase immunoreactivity be increased in those cases?

Preliminary studies have shown that PLI is superior to TLI for the diagnosis of feline pancreatitis. PLI will increase during the first 4 days of feline pancreatitis (compared with 2 days for TLI), but additional studies are required to confirm the usefulness of PLI for the diagnosis of this disease.

15. What are the reference and cutoff values for PLI in cats?

Preliminary results indicate a reference range of 2.0 to 6.7 μg/L for PLI in cats. A cutoff value of 12 μg/L is considered suggestive of pancreatitis but, as stated in question 14, additional studies are required to confirm these findings.

Gastrointestinal Tract and Pancreas

BIBLIOGRAPHY

Archer FJ, Kerr ME, Houston DM: Evaluation of three specific protein assays, TLI (tryspin-like immunoreactivity), PASP (pancreas specific protein) and CA 19-9 (glycoprotein) for use in the diagnosis of canine pancreatitis, *J Vet Med* 44:109-113, 1997.

Batt RM: Exocrine pancreatic insufficiency, *Vet Clin North Am Small Anim Pract* 23:595-608, 1993.

Gerhardt A, Steiner JM, Williams DA, et al: Comparison of the sensitivity of different diagnostic tests for pancreatitis in cats, *J Vet Intern Med* 15:329-333, 2001.

Hall EJ, Simpson KW: Diseases of the small intestine. In Ettinger SJ, Feldman EC, editors: *Textbook of veterinary internal medicine: diseases of the dog and the cat,* ed 5, Philadelphia, 2000, Saunders, pp 1182-1239.

Hall EJ: Clinical laboratory evaluation of small intestinal function, *Vet Clin North Am Small Anim Pract* 29:441-469, 1999.

Jergens AE: Inflammatory bowel disease: current perspectives, *Vet Clin North Am Small Anim Pract* 29:501-522, 1999.

Melgarejo T, Williams DA, Asem EK: Enzyme-linked immunosorbent assay for canine alpha 1-protease inhibitor, *Am J Vet Res* 59:127-130, 1998.

Ruaux CG, Atwell RB: Levels of total α-macroglobulin and trypsin-like immunoreactivity are poor indicators of clinical severity in spontaneous canine acute pancreatitis, *Res Vet Sci* 67:83-87, 1999.

Spillmann T, Wittker S, Teigelkamp C, et al: An immunoassay for pancreatic elastase 1 as an indicator for exocrine pancreatic insufficiency in dogs, *J Vet Diagn Invest* 13:468-474, 2001.

Steiner JM, Williams DA: Serum feline trypsin-like immunoreactivity in cats with exocrine pancreatic insufficiency, *J Vet Intern Med* 14:627-629, 2000.

Wiberg ME, Westermarck E: Subclinical exocrine pancreatic insufficiency in dogs, *J Am Vet Med Assoc* 8:1183-1187, 2002.

Williams DA: Exocrine pancreatic disease. In Ettinger SJ, Feldman EC, editors: *Textbook of veterinary internal medicine: diseases of the dog and the cat,* ed 5, Philadelphia, 2000, Saunders, pp 1345-1367.

Section IX
Endocrine System
Susan J. Tornquist

37. LABORATORY TESTING FOR THYROID DISEASE

1. What is the best diagnostic test for feline hyperthyroidism?

The majority of hyperthyroid cats have serum total thyroxine (T_4) concentration above reference ranges. For about 90% of hyperthyroid cats, measuring serum total T_4 will be diagnostic.

2. How useful is measuring serum total triiodothyronine in diagnosis of feline hyperthyroidism?

Although usually elevated in feline hyperthyroidism, serum total triiodothyronine (T_3) may be within reference ranges in up to 33.5% of hyperthyroid cats and thus is less diagnostically useful than measurement of total T_4. In virtually all cats with elevated total T_3, total T_4 is also elevated.

3. Why do some hyperthyroid cats have total T_4 concentration within the reference range?

Total T_4 concentration may be within the reference range in some hyperthyroid cats for the following reasons:

a. A very early stage of hyperthyroidism is present, with overproduction of thyroxine just beginning.
b. Normal fluctuation in T_4 levels over time bring total T_4 within reference range at the time of sample collection.
c. Concurrent nonthyroid illness in hyperthyroid cats may decrease total T_4 to within reference range.

4. How can one diagnose the 10% of hyperthyroid cats with total T_4 concentration within reference range?

Three methods can be used to diagnose hyperthyroid cats with total T_4 within the reference range:

a. Retest total T_4 concentration a few weeks later.
b. Measure free T_4 concentration.
c. Use one of the dynamic thyroid function tests, either T_3 suppression or thyrotropin-releasing hormone (TRH) stimulation.

5. Why would repeating the total T_4 assay a few weeks later help with the diagnosis of hyperthyroidism?

Concentrations of total T_4 in hyperthyroid cats may vary significantly over a 2-week period and may be within reference range at one or more times during that period. The peak of T_4 does not occur at any particular time of day. In a cat with clinical signs consistent with hyperthyroidism and total T_4 in the reference range, repeating the total T_4 on a different day may be diagnostic.

6. How accurate is measurement of free T_4 in diagnosis of hyperthyroidism?

Free T_4 concentration appears to be a more sensitive diagnostic test for feline hyperthyroidism than total T_4 concentration. Unfortunately, free T_4 is also less specific. In other words, some euthyroid cats with nonthyroid illness will have high free T_4 concentrations but total T_4 values below the reference range. It is recommended that free T_4 assay results in cats be interpreted in the context of total T_4 results as well as clinical signs and physical examination findings. A high free T_4 along with a total T_4 that is within or above the reference range is most consistent with hyperthyroidism.

7. Does the method used to measure free T_4 affect test sensitivity?

The method used does affect test sensitivity; free T_4 concentration should be measured by equilibrium dialysis.

8. When should dynamic tests of thyroid function be performed?

If repeated total T_4 testing and measurement of free T_4 are not diagnostic in a cat with clinical signs of hyperthyroidism, the T_3 suppression or the TRH stimulation test might be used.

9. How does the T_3 suppression test work?

In a normal cat, exogenous T_3 should suppress thyroid-stimulating hormone (TSH) secretion from the pituitary and thus decrease T_4 production by the thyroid. T_4 is typically suppressed by more than 50% in euthyroid cats after administration of T_3. In hyperthyroid cats, T_4 concentration does not decrease to this degree, primarily because TSH is already suppressed due to negative feedback by the excess circulating T_4.

To administer the T_3 suppression test, a baseline blood sample is taken for measurement of serum T_3 and T_4, then 15 to 25 μg of liothyronine sodium is given orally to the cat every 8 hours for the next 2 days. On the morning of the third day, a seventh dose is given, and a blood sample taken 2 to 4 hours later for T_3 and T_4 assay. An increase in the T_3 level above baseline indicates that the synthetic T_3 was successfully administered and absorbed. This test is not associated with adverse clinical effects.

10. How is the thyrotropin-releasing hormone (TRH) stimulation test performed and interpreted?

Blood for baseline serum T_4 is obtained, then 0.1 mg of TRH/kg body weight is given intravenously. A second blood sample for serum T_4 is obtained 4 hours after TRH administration. Adverse reactions seen in cats include salivation, urination, defecation, vomiting, tachycardia, and tachypnea. Results after stimulation are generally interpreted as follows:

- Increase of less than 50% over baseline serum T_4 is consistent with hyperthyroidism.
- Increase of greater than 60% over baseline is normal.
- Increase of 50% to 60% over baseline T_4 is nondiagnostic.

11. Can one measure endogenous thyroid-stimulating hormone (TSH) to assist in the diagnosis of feline hyperthyroidism?

There is currently no validated assay for feline TSH, although there seems to be some cross-reactivity between feline TSH and the reagents used for assay of canine TSH.

12. If a laboratory reports T_3 and T_4 in different units from those used in another laboratory, how is nmol/L converted to µg/dl?

Table 37-1 lists conversion factors for units used in T_3 and T_4 assays.

Table 37-1 *Unit Conversions in Thyroxine (T_4) and Triiodothyronine (T_3) Assays*

ANALYTE (UNITS)	CONVERSION FACTOR (DIVIDE BY)	UNITS OBTAINED
Total T_4 (nmol/L)	12.87	µg/dl
Total T_3 (nmol/L)	1.536	ng/ml
Free T_4 (pmol/L)	1.287	pg/ml
Free T_4 (pmol/L)	12.87	ng/dl
Free T_3 (pmol/L)	1.536	pg/ml
Free T_3 (pmol/L)	15.36	ng/dl

Units: *nmol,* nanomoles; *pmol,* picomoles; *µg,* micrograms; *ng,* nanograms; *pg,* picograms
Per *(/)* liter *(L),* deciliter *(dl),* or milliliter *(ml).*

13. What are the reference ranges for thyroid hormones?

Results should always be interpreted using the reference ranges generated by the laboratory running the assay because differences in assay methods and reagents may affect the reference ranges.

14. Are there typical changes in the hemogram or serum biochemical profile in feline hyperthyroidism?

Although hemogram abnormalities occur in some hyperthyroid cats, none occurs consistently enough to be useful diagnostically. Alkaline phosphatase (ALP), alanine transaminase (ALT) and aspartate transaminase (AST) are often increased in hyperthyroid cats; activities of these enzymes usually return to reference ranges with successful management of hyperthyroidism. Other serum biochemical changes, such as azotemia and hyperphosphatemia, are common but not as consistent as the changes in liver enzymes.

Complete blood count (CBC), serum biochemical profiles, and urinalysis can be very useful in detection of nonthyroid illness that may affect serum total T_4 and free T_4 concentrations.

15. How will concurrent nonthyroid illness affect total T_4 and free T_4?

In a study that included large numbers of hyperthyroid cats, normal cats, and cats with nonthyroid disease, none of the cats with nonthyroid disease had total T_4 values above reference ranges, but almost 40% had total T_4 concentration below reference ranges. In the group of cats with nonthyroid disease, free T_4 concentrations were mostly within reference ranges (about 75%), but some were high, and about three times as many were low.

16. What's the best way to monitor hyperthyroid cats after therapy?

For hyperthyroid cats treated with radioiodine, measurement of serum free T_4 may be more sensitive than total T_4 for detection of persistent hyperthyroidism, but results of long-term studies have not been published. Cats that are medically managed with methimazole or carbimazole generally become euthyroid, based on serum total T_4 concentrations, within a week. With continued therapy, total T_4 concentration in many cats drops below the reference range, but clinical signs of hypothyroidism are not apparent, and serum free T_4 may remain within reference range.

17. How useful is an in-house ELISA test for total T_4 in the diagnosis of hyperthyroidism in cats?

In a comparison of serum total T_4 concentrations measured with an in-house enzyme-linked immunosorbent assay (ELISA) test kit and those obtained by radioimmunoassay (RIA), considered to be the gold standard for thyroid testing, correlation coefficients were low (0.59) for cats. The ELISA test kit consistently gave higher results than the RIA, with potential incorrect diagnosis and treatment suggested in half the cases.

18. What is the best approach for testing for canine hypothyroidism?

Testing for canine hypothyroidism can be fairly straightforward in dogs that have typical clinical signs and laboratory findings on hemogram and serum biochemical profile, no concurrent illness, and no recent history of drugs such as glucocorticoids, anticonvulsants, or sulfonamides being given. In these dogs, low serum total T_4 concentration is considered consistent with hypothyroidism, especially if total T_4 is very low. Unfortunately, it is not always possible to rule out concurrent nonthyroid illness or drug administration, and clinical signs and laboratory results may mimic those of other conditions. Also, some percentage of dogs produce autoantibodies to T_4, T_3, or thyroglobulin, and total T_4 levels are not always low enough to be definitively diagnostic. In these cases, additional tests, a combination of tests, or alternative testing protocols are indicated for diagnosis of canine hypothyroidism.

19. How do you interpret serum total T_4 in dogs?

Total T_4 concentration includes T_4 that circulates bound to proteins as well as the free, or metabolically active, form of T_4. A total T_4 concentration that is within reference range indicates that it is unlikely that the dog is hypothyroid. Thus the total T_4 can be a useful way to rule out hypothyroidism. If the total T_4 is below reference range, the dog could be hypothyroid, or it could be affected by nonthyroid illness, drugs, or normal fluctuations in serum T_4 levels.

20. How would a dog with low total T_4 be tested further?

Measurement of free T_4 using the equilibrium dialysis method is a much more specific method of diagnosing hypothyroidism in dogs. In other words, free T_4 is less affected by factors such as drugs and nonthyroid illness than is total T_4. Thus a low free T_4 is more diagnostic for hypothyroidism than a low total T_4, although free T_4 may also be falsely lowered by glucocorticoids, phenobarbital, and nonthyroid illness. Because free T_4 measured by equilibrium dialysis is more labor and time intensive, the assay is more expensive than the total T_4 assay. However, free T_4 may be the preferred screening test in many situations.

21. What information can measurement of TSH add to the diagnosis of canine hypothyroidism?

TSH should be increased in hypothyroid dogs that lack the negative feedback on the pituitary that normal or increased circulating T_4 levels would provide. Although elevated in most hypothyroid dogs, TSH has not been shown to be extremely sensitive or specific for hypothyroidism. This test appears to be most useful for diagnosis of hypothyroidism when combined with the free T_4 by equilibrium dialysis assay.

An estimated 5% of hypothyroid dogs have secondary hypothyroidism caused by a deficiency of TSH. Of course, TSH concentrations would be decreased to undetectable levels in these dogs.

22. Given all the problems with sensitivity and specificity of tests, can the diagnosis of canine hypothyroidism be accurately made?

Currently, the best combination of findings for diagnosis of canine hypothyroidism appears to be high serum TSH and low free T_4 by equilibrium dialysis in a dog that shows typical clinical signs of hypothyroidism without evidence of concurrent nonthyroid illness or drug administration.

23. How useful is measurement of total T_3 in the diagnosis of canine hypothyroidism?

Measurement of serum total T_3 does not appear to have much benefit because there is great overlap in values obtained from hypothyroid dogs, dogs with nonthyroid illness, and clinically healthy dogs.

24. How do autoantibodies to thyroid hormones affect thyroid testing in dogs?

Primary hypothyroidism in dogs apparently is often associated with immune-mediated destruction of thyroid gland. Thus some dogs have circulating antibodies to thyroglobulin, T_3, and/or T_4. Of these, autoantibodies to thyroglobulin are the most common, although the significance of these autoantibodies is unclear because they are present in up to half of hypothyroid dogs but also in some apparently euthyroid dogs.

Autoantibodies to T_3 are more common than those to T_4, but the frequency of both is reported to be quite low (<1%). Because they can compete for hormone binding in assays, autoantibodies may affect assay results for T_3 and T_4, with falsely elevated values being the most common effect. This could result, for example, in normal or high total T_4 concentration in a hypothyroid dog. False decreases in T_3 have also been reported.

The free T_4 assay, when performed using equilibrium dialysis, is not affected by autoantibodies to T_4.

25. Is the TSH stimulation test valuable in the diagnosis of canine hypothyroidism?

Most authors consider the TSH stimulation test to be the gold standard in testing for canine hypothyroidism, although it is not always able to distinguish truly hypothyroid dogs from those with nonthyroid illness or receiving drug therapy. The TSH test measures the ability of the thyroid gland to produce T_4 in response to exogenous TSH stimulation. Hypothyroid dogs typically fail to respond to TSH with a relative or absolute increase in T_4 that is considered adequate by the laboratory performing the testing. Since TSH is no longer readily available for a reasonable cost, the TSH stimulation test is usually not performed for clinical purposes, although it is still used in many research settings.

26. Is the TRH response test used in the diagnosis of canine hypothyroidism?

The TRH response test is not used in diagnosis of hypothyroidism in dogs because it does not reliably distinguish between hypothyroid and euthyroid dogs.

27. What is the best way to monitor the effects of T_4 therapy in dogs?

The effects of thyroxine therapy in dogs can be monitored by assaying total T_4 in serum taken 4 to 6 hours after T_4 administration. If dosage level is appropriate and the medication is being administered and absorbed, total T_4 concentration should be high normal to increased. In addition, finding a TSH concentration within the reference range indicates adequate control for the several days before testing.

28. Can one make an accurate diagnosis of hypothyroidism in dogs that are already receiving T_4?

Exogenous thyroxine has a suppressive effect on a dog's normal thyroid production. For accurate results that do not reflect the effects of administered T_4, therapy should be discontinued for 6 to 8 weeks before testing.

29. What are the effects of phenobarbital, corticosteroids, and sulfonamides on thyroid test results in dogs?

Phenobarbital has been shown to decrease serum total T_4 concentration and increase TSH concentration, with no association with clinical signs of hypothyroidism found. In the same study, free T_4 was also decreased in dogs receiving phenobarbital, suggesting that the low T_4 levels were not caused by changes in protein binding resulting from the presence of the drug.

Corticosteroids inconsistently decrease total T_4, free T_4 and total T_3 levels in dogs, with the effects dependent on the dose and specific corticosteroid given.

Some forms of sulfonamides actually cause reversible hypothyroidism by decreasing iodination of thyroglobulin, so decreased T_4 and T_3 concentrations and increased TSH may be found in dogs that received sulfonamides in the previous 3 weeks.

Many other drugs are known to affect thyroid tests in humans and may have similar effects on dogs.

30. Are other laboratory abnormalities associated with canine hypothyroidism?

The most common hemogram abnormality in hypothyroid dogs is a mild to moderate nonregenerative anemia. Hypercholesteremia and fasting lipemia are the serum biochemical abnormalities most often present.

31. What is the prevalence of canine hyperthyroidism?

Hyperthyroidism is uncommon in dogs because only about 25% of thyroid neoplasms produce T_4 at levels high enough to cause clinical signs or increased serum T_4 levels.

32. What are the sample and handling requirements for thyroid testing?

Most thyroid testing is done on serum, but some laboratories may use EDTA plasma. Total T_4 is stable in frozen serum or plasma in plastic tubes, but free T_4 may increase in frozen plasma, depending on the assay used. Both serum total T_4 and free T_4 are stable in plastic tubes at room temperature for up to 5 days, which allows time for shipping to a diagnostic laboratory.

33. How are horses tested for hypothyroidism?

True hypothyroidism is not well documented in adult horses, although neonatal hypothyroidism occurs in foals born to mares that ingest excess iodine or plant goitrogens. There is also an idiopathic neonatal form that is most common in western Canada. Diagnosis of hypothyroidism in horses is associated with the same problems as in dogs; that is, nonthyroid factors such as concurrent illness, food deprivation, and drug administration may decrease serum thyroid hormone concentrations. In horses made hypothyroid experimentally, serum TSH concentrations increased, and total T_4 and free T_4 concentrations decreased. Similar findings might be expected in natural equine hypothyroidism. An equine-specific TSH assay is not available commercially at this time.

38. LABORATORY TESTING FOR ADRENAL DISEASE

1. What causes canine hyperadrenocorticism?

Hyperadrenocorticism (HAC) in dogs is a condition in which serum cortisol levels are persistently elevated due to either an adrenal tumor that secretes cortisol or a pituitary tumor that secretes adrenocorticotropic hormone (ACTH, adrenocorticotropin), thus continuously stimulating release of cortisol from the adrenal gland. *Pituitary-dependent* hyperadrenocorticism (PDH) accounts for about 85% of canine HAC cases and *adrenal-dependent* hyperadrenocorticism (ADH) for about 15%. It is important to determine which type is present in dogs with HAC because therapy options differ.

2. What is the best test to screen for canine hyperadrenocorticism?

No consensus exists regarding the best test to screen for canine HAC. The tests used most often are the *low-dose dexamethasone suppression test* (LDDST) and the *ACTH stimulation test.* Other tests used less often are the urine cortisol/creatinine ratio and the combination LDDST/ACTH stimulation test. None of these tests has both extremely high sensitivity (ability to detect disease when present) and specificity (ability to rule out disease when absent). When dogs with typical clinical signs and other laboratory findings consistent with HAC are tested with one of the screening tests, the results are often conclusive, but in some cases, more than one assay is required or other diagnostic modalities are needed.

3. How is the low-dose dexamethasone suppression test performed and interpreted in dogs?

The LDDST is best started between 8 and 9 AM. A baseline blood sample for cortisol assay is taken, then 0.01 mg/kg body weight of dexamethasone or dexamethasone sodium phosphate is given intravenously (IV). Blood samples for cortisol assay are taken 3 to 4 hours and 8 hours after dexamethasone injection. Cortisol levels in normal dogs are decreased to less than 1.0 μg/dl at both 4 and 8 hours. Dogs with HAC generally have cortisol concentrations greater than 1.4 μg/dl at 8 hours, with cortisol levels of 1.0 to 1.4 μg/dl considered nondiagnostic.

The cortisol concentration 4 hours after dexamethasone injection may help distinguish between PDH and ADH in some dogs. If the cortisol level is *suppressed* (defined as <1.4 μg/dl or <50% of baseline concentration) at 4 hours, the dog most likely has PDH because dogs with ADH will not be suppressed at 4 hours. About 40% of PDH dogs also will not be suppressed at 4 hours, so lack of suppression at 4 hours is not diagnostic.

4. What are the advantages and disadvantages of the LDDST?

The low-dose dexamethasone suppression test probably has a higher sensitivity (ability to detect presence of HAC) and lower specificity (ability to rule out HAC) than the ACTH stimulation test. LDDST is relatively easy to perform and interpret and may distinguish between PDH and ADH, thus eliminating the need for further testing. LDDST cannot be used to diagnose iatrogenic HAC. The test is affected by stress, non-HAC illnesses, and drugs such as phenobarbital. The LDDST takes 8 hours to complete.

5. How is the ACTH stimulation test performed and interpreted?

A baseline blood sample is collected for cortisol assay, then 2.2 units/kg of aqueous ACTH gel is given intramuscularly (IM), or 250 μg of synthetic ACTH (cosyntropin) is given IM or IV. Lower doses of synthetic ACTH have also been used successfully for this test, but a single vial contains 250 μg, so this amount is most often used regardless of the dog's size. A second blood sample for cortisol assay is collected 2 hours after ACTH injection, if the gel is used, or 1 hour after injection if synthetic ACTH is used. Interpretation of results may vary between laboratories. In general, normal dogs will stimulate to a cortisol level of 6 to 18 μg/dl. Stimulation to18 μg/dl or greater may be interpreted as being consistent with HAC, depending on the reference ranges and interpretation provided by the laboratory performing the assay.

6. What are the advantages and disadvantages of the ACTH stimulation test?

The ACTH stimulation test appears to have a somewhat lower sensitivity but higher specificity for diagnosis of canine HAC than does the LDDST; that is, a relatively high percentage of dogs with HAC, especially those with ADH, do not stimulate to higher than reference ranges. However, the ACTH test reportedly is better at ruling out HAC when it is not present, especially when nonadrenal illness causes a false-positive LDDST response. The ACTH stimulation test is the only test used to detect iatrogenic HAC and to monitor medical therapy for HAC. It does not distinguish between ADH and PDH. The amount of time necessary to do the ACTH stimulation test is less than that needed for the LDDST, and the ACTH stimulation test may be performed at any time of the day.

7. Is the combined LDDST/ACTH stimulation test a good way to test for and differentiate between types of canine hyperadrenocorticism?

Although it seems a convenient way to combine screening for HAC and testing for ADH versus PDH, the combined LDDST/ACTH stimulation test does not appear to be as accurate for either purpose than other available tests and is generally not recommended.

8. How useful is the urine cortisol/creatinine ratio in screening for canine hyperadrenocorticism?

Urinary cortisol excretion is increased in HAC, but cortisol concentration in urine varies with the amount of urine produced at any given time. Urine creatinine is excreted at a constant rate throughout the day, so measurement of creatinine concentration in the same sample provides a method of canceling out the effects of urine volume. The sensitivity of this test appears to be very high, that is, the ratio will be elevated in almost all dogs with HAC. Because many non-HAC conditions also result in an elevated urine cortisol/creatinine ratio, the test has very low specificity and has value only in ruling out HAC.

9. Can an assay for the corticosteroid-induced isoenzyme of alkaline phosphatase be useful in diagnosis of canine hyperadrenocorticism?

The isoenzyme of alkaline phosphatase induced by corticosteroids may be assayed. This isoenzyme may be induced by nonadrenal disease as well as by drugs such as phenobarbital, so this assay is not specific for HAC. In addition, it has not been shown to be particularly sensitive for diagnosis of HAC. Therefore, this assay is not recommended.

10. Which tests can be used to differentiate adrenal-dependent and pituitary-dependent hyperadrenocorticism in dogs?

In addition to the 4-hour LDDST cortisol concentration, which may be diagnostic in some dogs, two laboratory tests are used.

The *high-dose dexamethasone suppression test* (HDDST) is performed like the LDDST except that dexamethasone is given at 0.1 mg/kg IV. Normal animals will have cortisol levels suppressed at both 4 hours and 8 hours. Dogs with ADH do not have suppression at 4 or 8 hours. Approximately 25% of dogs with PDH also do not have suppressed cortisol levels at these times. Thus, suppression with the HDDST is virtually diagnostic for PDH rather than ADH, but failure to suppress is not diagnostic. This test is often done with sampling only at baseline and 8 hours as there is little evidence that the 4 hour sample provides additional information in most cases. Suppression is defined as it is in the LDDST (<1.4 μg/dl or <50% of baseline concentration).

Endogenous ACTH measurement is another test used to distinguish PDH from ADH. Dogs with HAC that is adrenal dependent most often have plasma ACTH concentrations less than 10 pg/ml (some use <20 pg/ml as the cutoff). Hyperadrenocorticoid dogs with greater than 45 pg/ml ACTH (depending on the laboratory, 15-40 pg/ml may be used as the cutoff) most often have HAC that is pituitary dependent. The range of concentrations between the two groups is nondiagnostic. If a value is in this nondiagnostic range, measuring ACTH in a second sample is often diagnostic. ACTH is quite labile and should be collected into a chilled syringe, plastic tube, or siliconized glass tube containing heparin or EDTA. The sample should be centrifuged immediately, preferably at 4° C, and plasma separated and frozen in plastic tubes, then shipped frozen on dry ice to a reference laboratory. A protease inhibitor, aprotinin, may be added to EDTA-anticoagulated blood to preserve ACTH immunoreactivity in glass and at room temperature for centrifugation and 4° C for shipping. This use of aprotinin may not apply to all ACTH assays.

11. What type of sample is needed for cortisol testing?

Blood for cortisol testing should be collected into EDTA or heparin. The plasma should be collected and frozen or shipped on cold packs. Cortisol may also be assayed in serum, although it is less stable in serum than in plasma and must be kept cold. The animal does not need to be fasted before blood collection.

12. What conversion factors are used for the different units in adrenal testing?

- To convert cortisol in μg/dl to nmol/L, multiply by 27.6.
- To convert μg/dl to ng/ml, multiply by 10.
- To convert ACTH in pg/ml to pmol/L, multiply by 0.22.

See also Table 37-1.

13. Are there typical complete blood count and serum biochemical profile findings in canine hyperadrenocorticism?

The most common abnormalities on the complete blood count (CBC) are those of the typical stress leukogram: mature neutrophilia, lymphopenia, monocytosis, and eosinopenia. The most typical biochemical profile abnormality is increased alkaline phosphatase (ALP). Increased alanine transaminase (ALT), gamma-glutamyl transferase (GGT), cholesterol, and glucose are also seen.

14. What is the best test for feline hyperadrenocorticism?

HAC is less common in cats than in dogs, but feline and canine HAC are similar in that the majority of cats with HAC have the PDH rather than the ADH form. As with the dog, no ideal screening test exists for the cat with HAC, but both ACTH stimulation and dexamethasone suppression tests have been used. There are some differences in the protocols and interpretation when used in cats.

When performing the ACTH stimulation test in cats, the use of synthetic ACTH is preferred because it appears to stimulate the adrenal cortex more consistently than the gel. A baseline sample is taken for cortisol assay, then 125 μg of synthetic ACTH is given either IM or IV, followed by sampling at 30 and 60 minutes. A cortisol concentration greater than 13 μg/ml at either 30 or 60 minutes suggests HAC. Reports vary, but only 50% to 60% of HAC cats may stimulate to that degree with this test, so sensitivity is relatively low. In addition, increased cortisol levels after stimulation may occur in cats with many different chronic illnesses.

Although the LDDST can be used in cats, it is considered even less sensitive and specific than it is in dogs. Recommendations often suggest using the HDDST to screen cats for HAC. In cats, it is performed as in dogs, with 0.1 mg/kg of dexamethasone given IV and baseline and 4-hour and 8-hour samples taken. It may be helpful to obtain 2-hour and 6-hour samples as well. Cortisol concentrations less than 1.4 μg/ml again are usually interpreted as suppressed, with failure of suppression at any of the sampling times suggestive of HAC.

15. How is feline PDH distinguished from feline ADH?

Distinguishing pituitary-dependent from adrenal-dependent HAC in cats may not be easy. Some advocate the use of ultrahigh-dose dexamethasone testing using 1.0 mg/kg dexamethasone IV. ADH cats will not show suppressed cortisol levels at this dose, whereas some PDH cats will suppress with this higher dose. Measurement of endogenous ACTH may also be useful, with sampling and interpretation of results similar to those in the dog, although ACTH ranges in normal cats apparently overlap significantly with ranges in cats with adrenal tumors.

16. What causes canine hypoadrenocorticism?

Canine hypoadrenocorticism most often results from destruction of the adrenal cortex, with an immune-mediated etiology often proposed. This type is called *primary hypoadrenocorticism,* or Addison's disease, and is associated with both mineralocorticoid and glucocorticoid deficiencies. Secondary hypoadrenocorticism occurs when the pituitary gland secretes insufficient ACTH, so glucocorticoid production is decreased, but mineralocorticoid production is usually normal.

17. What are the typical complete blood count and serum biochemical abnormalities seen in canine hypoadrenocorticism?

CBC findings are often unremarkable, except for the lack of an expected stress leukogram in a sick dog and sometimes a mild, nonregenerative anemia. The most typical biochemical abnormalities are hyperkalemia, hyponatremia, and sodium/potassium ratio less than 27:1. These changes are not always present in hypoadrenocorticism and may occur in diseases of other systems. Other abnormal laboratory findings may include prerenal azotemia, hypochloremia, hyperphosphatemia, hypercalcemia, mild hypoglycemia, and metabolic acidosis.

18. How is canine hypoadrenocorticism confirmed with laboratory tests?

The ACTH stimulation test is used to confirm hypoadrenocorticism. The protocol is the same as that used in screening for HAC. Dogs with hypoadrenocorticism have low to normal resting cortisol levels and show no or negligible response to ACTH stimulation.

19. Does administration of glucocorticoids affect the ACTH stimulation test?

Serum cortisol assays are not affected by dexamethasone but are affected by prednisone, prednisolone, cortisone, and hydrocortisone, which cross-react in the assay. Because dogs showing signs of hypoadrenocorticism often are presented with acute clinical signs, treatment with fluids and dexamethasone may precede ACTH stimulation testing. If other forms of glucocorticoid have been used, ACTH stimulation testing should be delayed by at least 24 hours.

20. How are primary and secondary hypoadrenocorticism differentiated in dogs?

No electrolyte abnormalities are usually seen in secondary hypoadrenocorticism, but this cannot always be used to differentiate the two conditions, and hyponatremia may occur in secondary hypoadrenocorticism. Measurement of plasma ACTH levels should show elevation in dogs with primary hypoadrenocorticism and very low to undetectable levels in dogs with secondary hypoadrenocorticism.

21. Which tests and laboratory findings are used to diagnose feline hypoadrenocorticism?

Primary hypoadrenocorticism is extremely uncommon but does occasionally occur in cats. Secondary hypoadrenocorticism may occur when pituitary ACTH production is suppressed by administration of glucocorticoids or progestagens. Serum biochemical findings tend to be like those seen in dogs, with CBC abnormalities being inconsistent. ACTH stimulation is the best diagnostic test to confirm feline hypoadrenocorticism, and it is performed as described for feline HAC testing. Cats with hypoadrenocorticism have low or low-normal resting cortisol levels and minimal if any response to stimulation. Endogenous ACTH can be measured and interpreted as in dogs for distinguishing primary and secondary hypoadrenocorticism, with levels very high in primary hypoadrenocorticism.

22. Is there a laboratory test to diagnose pheochromocytomas?

Pheochromocytomas (tumors of the adrenal medulla) are rarely functional (catecholamine secreting) in dogs and cats. In humans these tumors are diagnosed by finding increased levels of plasma and urine catecholamines or vanillylmandelic acid, which is the metabolite of catecholamine. These assays are not readily available, and interpretation is difficult because reference ranges and values associated with disease have not been clearly established. In addition, catecholamine release is episodic, so a single sample may not be diagnostic.

39. LABORATORY TESTING FOR EQUINE PITUITARY DISEASE

1. What causes equine Cushing's syndrome?

Equine Cushing's syndrome is due to the presence of chronic excessive circulating glucocorticoids. The syndrome is almost always associated with a tumor or hyperplasia of cells in the pars intermedia of the anterior lobe of the pituitary gland. The tumor causes production of excess adrenocorticotropic hormone (ACTH, adrenocorticotropin) and related peptides. These stimulate the adrenal gland to overproduce glucocorticoids and results in loss of the normal circadian regulation of cortisol in affected horses.

2. Are there typical complete blood count and serum biochemical abnormalities in equine Cushing's syndrome?

Complete blood count (CBC) often, but not always, shows a mature neutrophilia and lymphopenia. Mild to moderate hyperglycemia is the most common serum biochemical abnormality in this equine pituitary dysfunction, often accompanied by glucosuria.

3. What is the best test to diagnose pituitary pars intermedia dysfunction in horses?

As with other endocrine diseases, several different tests and protocols may be used to diagnose equine pituitary pars intermedia dysfunction, and none of them is always accurate in making the diagnosis. The tests are most diagnostic when used in conjunction with observation of appropriate clinical signs and history.

The test recommended most often is the *dexamethasone suppression test* (DST). In horses, DST is best performed as an overnight test, with a baseline plasma sample taken before intramuscular injection of 40 μg/kg body weight of dexamethasone. Because of the normal diurnal pattern of cortisol production, DST should be started in the late afternoon at around 5 PM. A single follow-up plasma sample is taken at 19 hours after stimulation. Normal horses will have plasma cortisol levels suppressed to less than 1.0 μg/dl at this time. Cortisol concentrations greater than 1.0 μg/dl at 19 hours are considered diagnostic for equine pituitary pars intermedia dysfunction. Some horses show partial suppression and may be in earlier stages of disease or have less severe disease, although this has not been well documented.

Although concerns about exacerbation of laminitis have been reported with this DST protocol, it does not appear to be a common finding.

4. Is the ACTH stimulation test useful for diagnosing equine Cushing's syndrome?

Although this test has been used in horses, ACTH stimulation does not reliably distinguish between normal and affected horses and is not recommended.

5. Can measurement of endogenous plasma ACTH diagnose equine pituitary pars intermedia dysfunction?

Mean plasma concentrations of ACTH have been shown to be significantly higher in affected horses than in normal horses. An ACTH concentration greater than 50 pg/ml may be used as an indicator of disease, although this varies among laboratories. This test appears to have fairly good sensitivity and specificity. Although equine ACTH may be somewhat more stable than canine ACTH when not immediately frozen, samples still need to be handled with care, including collection into plastic tubes, prompt separation, and timely shipping of frozen samples to the laboratory. There is variability in the assay, and the reagents used and interpretation of results should be based on validation and reference range studies performed at each laboratory.

The plasma ACTH test may be a good substitute for the DST in horses considered at high risk for the development of laminitis.

6. What other tests have been used for the diagnosis of equine Cushing's syndrome?

Other laboratory tests that have been investigated in equine pituitary pars intermedia dysfunction include the urine cortisol/creatinine ratio, serum insulin measurement, thyrotropin-releasing hormone (TRH) stimulation test, and combined DST/TRH stimulation test. None of these is widely used because of problems with sensitivity, specificity, convenience, and cost.

7. What tests should be used to monitor horses being treated for pituitary pars intermedia dysfunction?

Several different drugs may be used to treat horses with Cushing's syndrome, along with changes in management and diet. Clinical improvement may be seen in treated horses without accompanying improvement in laboratory test results, so periodic laboratory testing is important in evaluating response to treatment. Blood glucose and DST or ACTH assay should be performed about 1 month after changes in treatment regimens or twice a year in horses that appear to be stable.

Endocrine System

BIBLIOGRAPHY

Behrend EN, Kemppainen RJ: Diagnosis of canine hyperadrenocorticism, *Vet Clin North Am Small Anim Prac* 31:985-1003, 2001.

Behrend EN, Kemppainen RJ, Young DW: Effect of storage conditions on cortisol, total thyroxine, and free thyroxine concentrations in serum and plasma of dogs, *J Am Vet Med Assoc* 212:1564-1568, 1998.

Breuhaus BA: Thyroid-stimulating hormone in adult euthyroid and hypothyroid horses, *J Vet Intern Med* 16:109-115, 2002.

Couetil L, Paradis MR, Knoll J: Plasma adrenocorticotropin concentration in healthy horses and in horses with clinical signs of hyperadrenocorticism, *J Vet Intern Med* 10:1-6, 1996.

Duesberg C, Peterson ME: Adrenal disorders in cats, *Vet Clin North Am Small Anim Pract* 27:321-347, 1997.

Dybdal NO, Hargreaves KM, Madigan JE, et al: Diagnostic testing for pituitary pars intermedia dysfunction in horses, *J Am Vet Med Assoc* 204:627-632, 1994.

Feldman EC, Nelson RW, Feldman JS: Use of low- and high-dose dexamethasone tests for distinguishing pituitary-dependent from adrenal tumor hyperadrenocorticism in dogs, *J Am Vet Med Assoc* 209:772-775, 1996.

Gaskill CL, Burton SA, Gelens HC, et al: Effects of phenobarbital treatment on serum thyroxine and thyroid-stimulating hormone concentrations in epileptic dogs, *J Am Vet Med Assoc* 215:489-496, 1999.

Guptill L, Scott-Moncrieff JC, Widmer WR: Diagnosis of canine hyperadrenocorticism, *Vet Clin North Am Small Anim Pract* 27:215-235, 1997.

Kemppainen RJ, Behrend EN: Diagnosis of canine hypothyroidism: perspectives from a testing laboratory, *Vet Clin North Am Small Anim Pract* 31:951-962, 2001.

Kintzer PP, Peterson JE: Primary and secondary canine hypoadrenocorticism, *Vet Clin North Am Small Anim Pract* 27:349-357, 1997.

Lurye JC, Behrend EN, Kemppainen RJ: Evaluation of an in-house enzyme-linked immunosorbent assay for quantitative measurement of serum total thyroxine concentration in dogs and cats, *J Am Vet Med Assoc* 221:243-249, 2002.

Mooney CT: Feline hyperthyroidism: diagnostics and therapeutics, *Vet Clin North Am Small Anim Pract* 31:963-983, 2001.

Peterson ME, Graves TK, Cavanaugh I: Serum thyroid hormone concentrations fluctuate in cats with hyperthyroidism, *J Vet Intern Med* 1:142-146, 1987.

Peterson ME, Melian C, Nichols R: Measurement of serum total thyroxine, triiodothyronine, free thyroxine, and thyrotropin concentrations for diagnosis of hyperthyroidism in dogs, *J Am Vet Med Assoc* 211:1396-1402, 1997.

Peterson ME, Melian C, Nichols R: Measurement of serum concentrations of free thyroxine, total thyroxine, and total triiodothyronine in cats with hyperthyroidism and cats with nonthyroidal disease, *J Am Vet Med Assoc* 218:529-536, 2001.

Schott HC: Pituitary pars intermedia dysfunction: equine Cushing's disease, *Vet Clin North Am Equine Pract* 18:237-270, 2002.

Scott-Moncrieff JCR, Nelson RW, Bruner JM, et al: Comparison of serum concentrations of thyroid-stimulating hormone in healthy dogs, hypothyroid dogs, and euthyroid dogs with concurrent disease, *J Am Vet Med Assoc* 212:387-391, 1998.

Section X
Cytology

40. SAMPLE COLLECTION AND PREPARATION

Rick L. Cowell, Ronald D. Tyler, and James H. Meinkoth

1. Why is cytology performed?

Cytology allows for the rapid determination of a diagnosis or identification of a process so that appropriate therapy can be provided quickly and cost effectively. Cytology is safe, with only minimal risks in most cases. Cytology is not a replacement for histopathology, but rather a complementary procedure.

2. Should the smears for cytology be stained or fixed before submitting them to the laboratory?

Generally, smears need not be stained and require no other special preparation before submitting them to the laboratory. Because most cytopathologists use a Romanowsky-type stain, the smears are simply allowed to air-dry and then packaged well to prevent breakage. There is no need to "fix" the smears in alcohol or other preservatives before mailing. Most laboratories want some if not all smears *unstained* in case special stains are needed, and many cytopathologists prefer using the stain they are most familiar with and staining the smears at the laboratory. If specific instructions are needed, however, the laboratory or the cytopathologist who will analyze the sample should be contacted with any questions.

3. What important considerations should one remember when mailing cytology smears?

A major problem is breakage in transit, so one should be sure to package the smears well. When submitting fluid samples, one should be sure to send the fluid in an EDTA tube and to send some premade smears from the fluid. Using premade air-dried smears of the fluid preserves the cells so that they can be evaluated better. Smears made from the fluid after arrival at the laboratory can have many artifacts in the cells that occurred in transit. The names of the owner and patient and the location where the sample was collected must be labeled in pencil on the frosted end of the slide to help prevent samples from being mixed up. Also, unstained cytology smears should never be mailed with histopathology samples. Formalin fumes fix the cells on cytology smears and inhibit their staining with Romanowsky stains and may make them uninterpretable.

4. Is special preparation of the collection site needed?

For cutaneous masses the site is prepared as is done for an injection. If a microbiologic culture is to be performed on the sample or if a body cavity is to be entered (e.g., abdominal, thoracic, or pericardial cavities; joints; transtracheal washes through cricothyroid ligament), the area of needle insertion should have a surgical scrub preformed.

5. List the common techniques used to collect cytology samples.

a. Fine-needle aspiration technique
b. Fine-needle nonaspiration biopsy technique

c. Impression smears
d. Scrapings
e. Swabs

6. Which size of needle and syringe should be used with the fine-needle technique (aspiration and nonaspiration)?

A small-gauge needle, between 25 and 22 gauge, should be used for fine-needle technique. Using a larger needle often results in more blood contamination and occasionally the collection of a core of tissue rather than individual cells.

Size of syringe is not a factor with the nonaspiration technique but varies with the aspiration technique. If one is aspirating a tissue that exfoliates cells easily, such as a lymph node, a smaller syringe (5 ml) can be used. For most tissues, however, a 12- or 20-ml syringe is needed to have sufficient negative pressure to collect tissue cells.

7. How is fine-needle aspiration performed?

For fine-needle aspiration of cutaneous masses, the mass is stabilized between the thumb and index finger of one hand while the needle (with syringe attached) is introduced into the mass. Negative pressure is applied by rapidly withdrawing the syringe plunger two-thirds to three-fourths the syringe volume. Multiple areas of the mass should be aspirated. If the mass is large enough and the animal calm enough, the needle may be redirected in the mass while negative pressure is maintained. If the mass is small or the animal difficult to restrain, the negative pressure should be released, the needle redirected, and negative pressure reapplied (Figure 40-1).

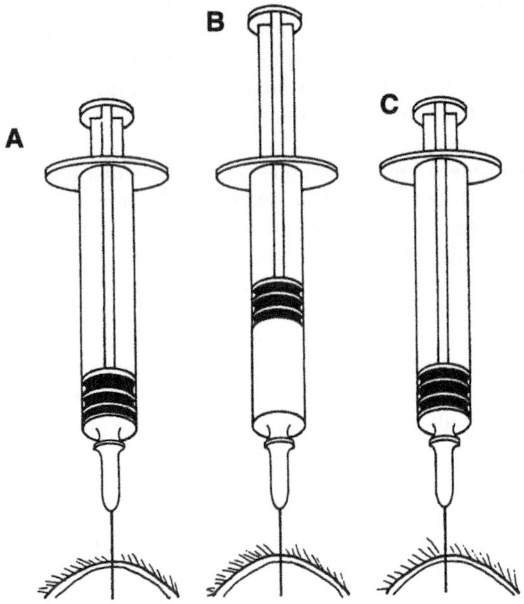

Figure 40-1 Fine-needle aspiration from a solid mass. After the needle is within the mass **(A),** negative pressure is placed on the syringe by rapidly withdrawing the plunger **(B),** usually half to three-fourths the volume of the syringe barrel. The needle is redirected several times while negative pressure is maintained, if done without the point leaving the mass. Before removing the needle from the mass, the plunger is released, relieving negative pressure on the syringe **(C).** (From Cowell RL, Tyler RD, Meinkoth JH: *Diagnostic cytology and hematology of the dog and cat,* ed 2, St Louis, 1999, Mosby.)

It is important to release negative pressure before exiting the mass because aspirating surrounding tissues may contaminate the sample. Also, if the sample collected is small, it may be aspirated into the barrel of the syringe and may not be retrievable. Whenever blood becomes visible in the needle hub or syringe, aspiration at that site should cease. If aspiration continues, the sample will be diluted by excessive blood contamination. After several areas of the mass have been sampled, the negative pressure is released, the needle is removed from the mass and then from the syringe, air is drawn into the syringe, the needle is replaced on the syringe, and the collected material is forced onto a clean glass slide by rapidly depressing the plunger. The material is smeared (by one of several techniques) and allowed to air-dry. The cytology samples may be stained and evaluated or may be sent stained or unstained to a cytopathologist.

8. How is fine-needle nonaspiration biopsy performed?

In fine-needle nonaspiration biopsy, no negative pressure is applied during collection of the sample. A small-gauge needle is attached to a 3-ml or larger syringe (size of syringe is unimportant because no negative pressure is applied) and 2 or 3 ml of air are drawn into the syringe, allowing the collected material to be expelled quickly onto a glass slide. The syringe with attached needle is grasped at or near the needle hub with the thumb and forefinger (as in grasping a pencil or throwing dart). The mass is stabilized as described in the aspiration technique, and the needle is inserted into the mass. The needle is moved back and forth in a stabbing motion 8 to 10 times while trying to stay in the same tract with each stab. This allows cells to be collected into the bore of the needle by cutting and capillary action. Care should be taken to keep the tip of the needle in the mass during the stabbing to avoid contamination by surrounding tissues.

The needle is then withdrawn from the mass, and the material in the bore of the needle is expelled onto a glass slide by rapidly depressing the plunger. The material is spread and allowed to air-dry. The technique typically collects enough material for only one smear and collects material from only one area of the mass. Therefore the procedure should be repeated in multiple areas of the mass.

9. How is an impression smear collected?

Impression smears may be collected from cutaneous ulcers or exudative lesions, from masses that have been surgically removed, and from tissues at necropsy. Ulcers should be imprinted, cleaned, and reimprinted. To collect impression smears from tissues collected at surgery or necropsy, the tissue to be imprinted should first be cut in half to have a fresh surface. The fresh surface is then blotted (e.g., paper towel, surgical gaze) to remove as much of the blood and tissue fluid as possible. The fresh surface is then touched to a clean glass slide. No further smearing is needed. One must not slide the tissue around on the glass slide, but simply press down and lift directly up. The material is allowed to air-dry.

10. How is a scraping collected?

Scrapings can be collected from cutaneous lesions or from tissues removed surgically or at necropsy. Scrapings are prepared by gently rubbing a scalpel blade across the cutaneous lesions or the fresh-cut surface of tissues surgically removed or collected at necropsy. The material collected on the blade is then transferred to a glass slide, smeared, and allowed to air-dry.

11. When is a swabbing for cytology collected?

Swabs are generally used only when other collection methods are not practical (e.g., ear canal, vaginal cytology, fistulous tracts). If the area to be swabbed is dry, it is best to wet the swab with sterile saline. Also, if culture is to be done, a sterile cotton swab should be used. After swabbing the area, the cotton swab is simply rolled on a glass slide and the smear allowed to air-dry.

12. What common smearing techniques are used on cytology samples?

a. Cytology samples collected from solid tissues
   (1) "Squash" preparation (slide-over-slide technique)
   (2) Blood smear technique
   (3) "Starfish" preparation (needle spread technique)

b. Cytology samples collected from fluid-filled masses or body cavity fluid
   (1) Blood smear technique
   (2) Line smear technique

13. Describe the "squash" preparation (slide-over-slide technique).

For the squash preparation, material collected by one of many techniques (e.g., aspiration or nonaspiration fine-needle biopsy, scrapings) is placed in the middle of a clean glass slide *(smear slide)*. A second glass slide *(spreader slide)* is placed over the sample perpendicular to the smear slide. The sample will begin to spread out due to the weight of the spreader slide. Once the sample has begun to spread, the spreader slide is gently drawn across the sample slide, smearing the sample (Figure 40-2). One must be careful not to put any downward pressure on the spreader slide. Excessive pressure will cause cells to rupture.

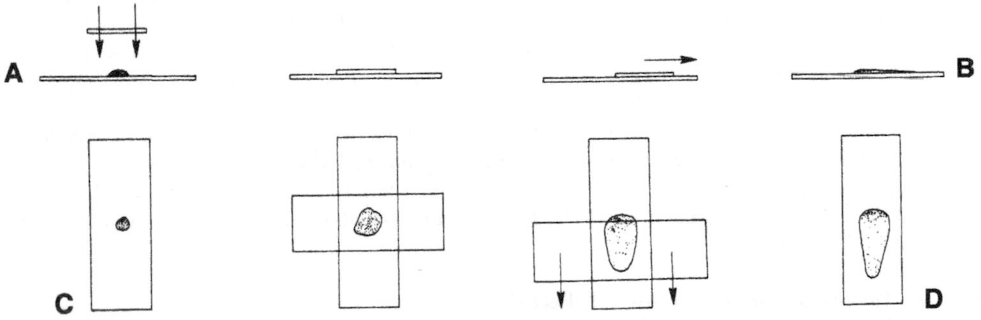

Figure 40-2 "Squash" preparation (slide-over-slide technique). **A**, A portion of aspirate is expelled onto a glass microscope slide, and another slide is placed over the sample. **B**, This spreads the sample. If the sample does not spread well, gentle digital pressure can be applied to the top slide. Care must be taken not to place excessive pressure on the slide, causing the cells to rupture. **C**, Slides are smoothly slid apart. **D**, This usually produces well-spread smears but may result in excessive cell rupture. (From Cowell RL, Tyler RD, Meinkoth JH: *Diagnostic cytology and hematology of the dog and cat,* ed 2, St Louis, 1999, Mosby.)

The slide-over-slide technique works well for spreading samples from nonfragile tissues (e.g., carcinomas). However, squash preparation tends to rupture excessive numbers of cells from more fragile tissues (e.g., lymph nodes). Once spread, the material is allowed to air-dry. No fixative is needed.

14. Describe the blood smear technique.

The blood smear technique is performed in the same manner as making a blood smear. The collected material is placed near one end of a glass slide (smear slide). A second slide (spreader slide) is placed on the smear slide at a 45-degree angle and backed up until it encounters one half or more of the material on the smear slide. The spreader slide is then quickly moved forward, as if making a blood smear (Figure 40-3).

The blood smear technique has much less shearing force than squash preparation and causes less cell rupturing. However, blood smearing does not spread cells as well as using slide over slide.

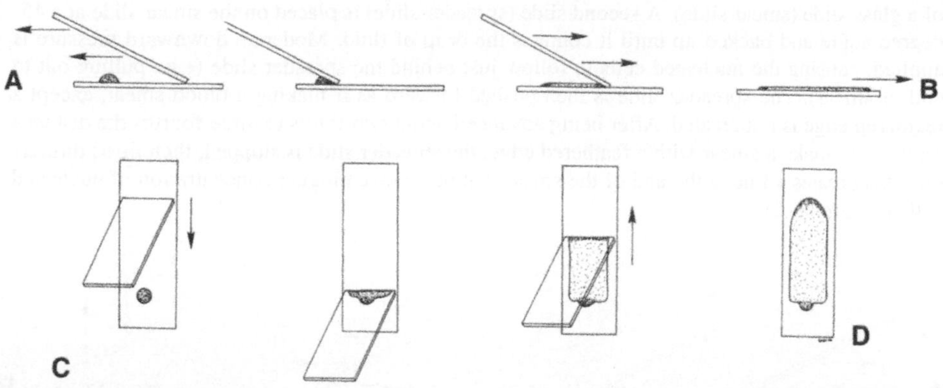

Figure 40-3 Blood smear technique. **A,** A drop of fluid sample is placed on a glass microscope slide close to one end, then another slide is slid backward to contact the front of the drop. **B,** When contacted, the drop rapidly spreads along the juncture between the two slides. **C** and **D,** The spreader slide is then smoothly and rapidly slid forward the length of the slide, producing a smear with a feathered edge. (From Cowell RL, Tyler RD, Meinkoth JH: *Diagnostic cytology and hematology of the dog and cat,* ed 2, 1999, Mosby.)

15. Describe the "starfish" preparation (needle spread technique).

After material is placed on a glass slide, the point of the needle is used to drag the aspirated material in several different directions, producing a starfish shape. Starfish preparation is gentle and tends not to rupture cells; rather, it leaves a thick layer of tissue fluid around the cells that may inhibit their spreading to normal size and shape. Some acceptable areas are usually present on the smear (Figure 40-4).

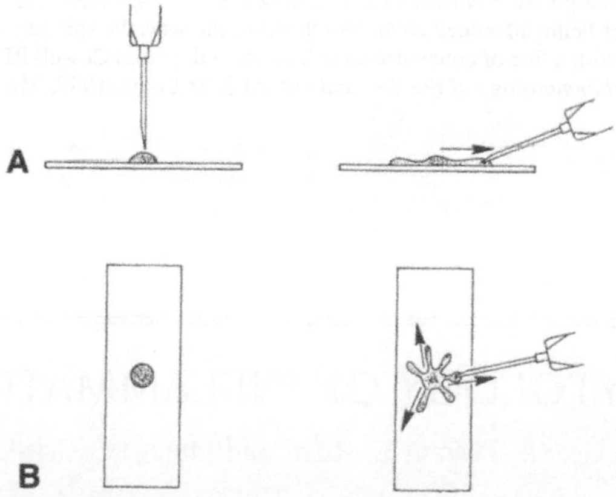

Figure 40-4 "Starfish" preparation (needle spread technique). **A,** A portion of aspirate is expelled onto a glass microscope slide. **B,** A needle tip is placed in the aspirate and moved peripherally, pulling a trail of the sample with it. The procedure is repeated in several directions, resulting in a preparation with multiple projections. (From Cowell RL, Tyler RD, Meinkoth JH: *Diagnostic cytology and hematology of the dog and cat,* ed 2, St Louis, 1999, Mosby.)

16. Discuss the line smear technique.

The line smear technique is useful for concentrating cells in a fluid sample when the sample cannot be centrifuged to make smears from the sediment. A drop of fluid is placed near one end of a glass slide (smear slide). A second slide (spreader slide) is placed on the smear slide at a 45-degree angle and backed up until it contacts the drop of fluid. Moderate downward pressure is applied, causing the nucleated cells to follow just behind the spreader slide (e.g., pulling out to end of smear). The spreader slide is then pushed forward as if making a blood smear, except a feathered edge is not created. After being advanced about two-thirds to three-fourths the distance required to make a smear with a feathered edge, the spreader slide is stopped, then lifted directly up. This creates a line at the end of the smear that has a much higher concentration of nucleated cells (Figure 40-5).

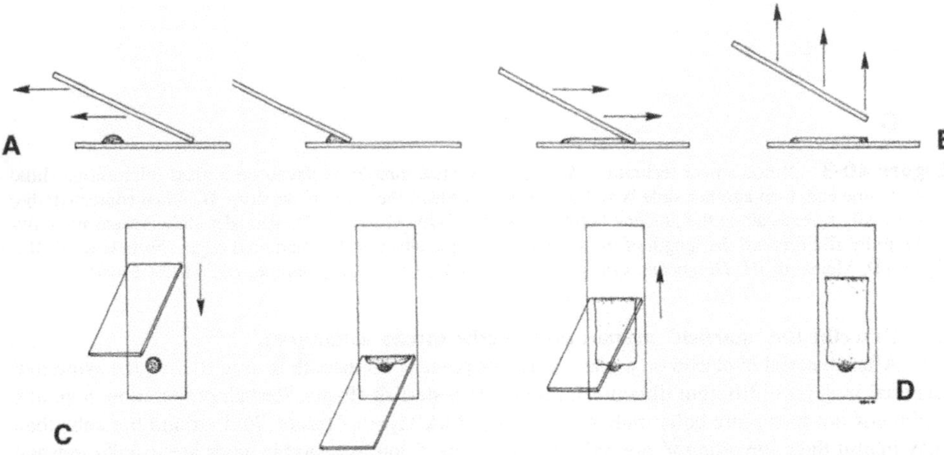

Figure 40-5 Line smear technique. **A,** A drop of fluid sample is placed onto a glass microscope slide close to one end, and another slide is slid backward to contact the front of the drop. **B,** When contacted, the drop rapidly spreads along the juncture between the two slides. **C,** The spreader slide is then smoothly and rapidly slid forward. **D,** After being advanced about two thirds of the way, the spreader slide is raised directly upward, producing a smear with a line of concentrated cells at its end. (From Cowell RL, Tyler RD, Meinkoth JH: *Diagnostic cytology and hematology of the dog and cat,* ed 2, St Louis, 1999, Mosby.)

41. CYTOLOGY OF INFLAMMATION

Rick L. Cowell, Theresa E. Rizzi, and James H. Meinkoth

1. What is neutrophilic inflammation?

Preparations in which greater than 70% to 75% of the cells are neutrophils are referred to as having *neutrophilic inflammation* (Figure 41-1). *Suppurative inflammation* and *purulent inflammation* are other terms for a marked predominance of neutrophils (>85%). The terms "active" or "acute" inflammation are occasionally used for this type of cellular reaction, but in this case the terms relate only to the cell type and not to a time frame.

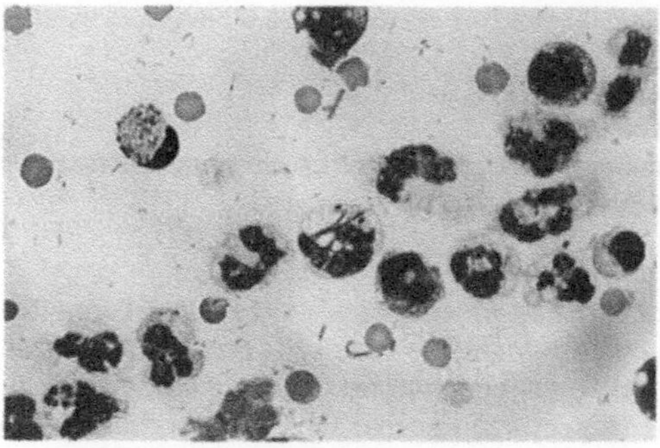

Figure 41-1 Septic neutrophilic inflammation. Aspirate of mass from a dog showing high numbers of degenerate neutrophils and mixed bacteria. Bacteria are present both intracellularly and extracellularly. (Wright's stain; 250×.)

2. What causes neutrophilic inflammation?

The most common cause of neutrophilic inflammation is a bacterial infection. Other organisms (e.g., *Sporothrix*) and many noninfectious disorders (e.g., necrotic areas in tumors, immune mediated disorders) can also cause neutrophilic inflammation.

3. What is pyogranulomatous inflammation?

Preparations with an inflammatory population that contains both neutrophils and a prominent fraction of macrophages (15% to 50% macrophages) are referred to as showing *pyogranulomatous inflammation* (Figure 41-2). The term "chronic active inflammation" is sometimes used for this type of inflammatory reaction, although it is falling out of usage because it relates only to the cell reaction and should not be interpreted in relation to a time frame. Multinucleated giant cells, reactive fibroblasts, and lymphocytes may also be present in pyogranulomatous inflammation.

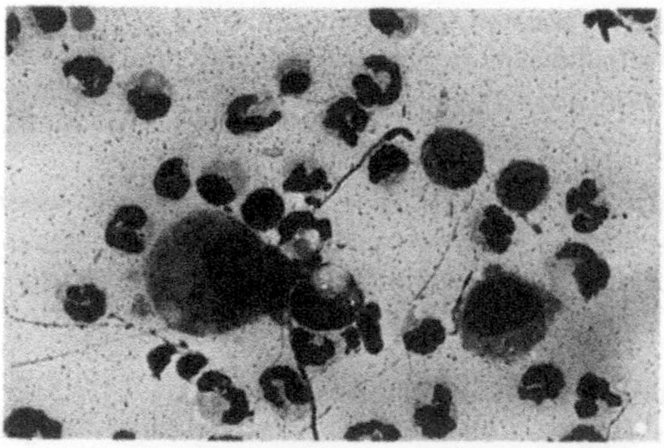

Figure 41-2 Pyogranulomatous inflammation. Aspirate from cutaneous lesion on a dog showing many neutrophils and moderate numbers of macrophages in stippled mucoprotein background. (Wright's stain; 250×.)

4. What are the diagnostic implications of pyogranulomatous inflammation?

Pyogranulomatous inflammation suggests a cause other than "routine" bacterial infection. Fungal infections (e.g., blastomycosis), higher bacteria (e.g., *Actinomyces*), mycobacteria, protozoa, and noninfectious disorders (e.g., foreign bodies, necrosis) are common causes of pyogranulomatous inflammation.

5. What is granulomatous (chronic) inflammation?

Preparations in which greater than 50% of the cells are macrophages are often referred to as having *granulomatous inflammation*. The term "chronic inflammation" is occasionally used, but this term relates only to the cell types present and does not indicate a time frame; thus it is falling out of usage. Multinucleated inflammatory giant cells, reactive fibroblasts, and lymphocytes may also be seen in granulomatous inflammation.

6. What causes granulomatous inflammation?

Causes of granulomatous inflammation are similar to those that cause pyogranulomatous inflammation (e.g., fungal, mycobacteria, protozoa, foreign bodies, necrosis).

7. What is eosinophilic inflammation?

Preparations in which large proportions of the cells are eosinophils (>10%-20%) are often referred to as showing *eosinophilic* (or mixed) *inflammation.* The other cells present are often an admixture of neutrophils, macrophages, mast cells, and lymphocytes. Occasionally, eosinophil granules may stain tan or muddy brown in tissue preparations, making them more difficult to recognize. However, their distinct granules allow for eosinophil identification. Also, neutrophils occasionally have a fine eosinophilic stippling in thick exudates and should not be confused with eosinophils.

8. What causes eosinophilic inflammation?

Common causes of eosinophilic inflammation include immune/allergic reactions, parasitic disorders (e.g., lungworms, some arthropod bites), certain fungal infections (e.g., phycomycosis), and some neoplasias (e.g., mast cell tumors).

9. What is lymphocytic or lymphocytic/plasmacytic inflammation?

Preparations from nonlymphoid tissue that contain a large proportion of mature lymphocytes (small lymphocytes and plasma cells) are referred to as having *lymphocytic* or *lymphocytic/plasmacytic inflammation.* This is differentiated from cutaneous lymphoma (lymphosarcoma) in that cutaneous lymphoma usually consists almost totally of large lymphoblasts. When small cell lymphoma is present, biopsy and histopathology for the evaluation of architecture generally are needed to obtain a definitive diagnosis.

10. What causes of lymphocytic or lymphocytic/plasmacytic inflammation?

Lymphocytic or lymphocytic/plasmacytic inflammation occurs with some injection site reactions, some insect bites, feline stomatitis/gingivitis, and lymphocytic/plasmacytic gastroenteritis.

11. What are degenerative neutrophils?

Degenerative neutrophils are neutrophils that have lost their ability to control water homeostasis and are undergoing hydropic degeneration. As water diffuses into the cell, it causes the cell to swell. Water also diffuses into the nucleus through nuclear pores and causes the nucleus to swell, fill more of the cytoplasm, and stain homogeneously eosinophilic.

12. What is the diagnostic significance of degenerative neutrophils?

The presence of degenerative neutrophils suggests a bacterial cause because these changes are caused primarily by toxins produced by bacteria (e.g., endotoxin). However, the absence of degenerative neutrophils does not rule out a bacterial cause because bacteria may be present in low numbers and some bacteria produce low levels of toxin. Therefore, when degenerative neutrophils are present, suspicion of a bacterial infection is increased. Although all cell types are subjected to the same toxin, degenerative change is evaluated only in neutrophils. Also, degenerative changes can be induced by autolysis (rot). Therefore, samples made from dead animals or samples collected and held for a long time before smears are made may show degenerative as well as pyknotic changes.

13. What are nondegenerative neutrophils?

Neutrophils with tightly clumped, basophilic nuclear chromatin are termed *nondegenerative neutrophils.* A few or many neutrophils may be hypersegmented or pyknotic (nuclear chromatin broken into tight, round spheres), representing aging changes that may occur in vivo or in vitro.

14. How do bacteria appear cytologically, and what is their interpretive significance?

With the routine blood stains (e.g., Wright's, Diff-Quik, Dip-Stat), all bacteria (gram positive and negative) stain blue to purple (basophilic); the few exceptions include mycobacteria that do not stain. *Intracellular* bacteria indicate bacterial infection (primary or secondary), whereas *extracellular* bacteria may represent bacterial infection or contamination. Bacterial infections often have bacteria intracellularly and extracellularly, whereas contamination has only extracellular bacteria. Also, the bacteria should be evaluated to determine if only one population exists (e.g., monomorphic population of cocci or rods) or if a mixture of rods and cocci or variably sized rods exists (e.g., pleomorphic population). Pleomorphic bacteria are common with, for example, infections of gastrointestinal origin and bite wounds.

15. How are mycobacteria recognized?

Infection with any of the *Mycobacterium* species tends to cause a granulomatous inflammatory reaction. These organisms have a lipid cell wall and therefore do not stain with routine cytologic stains but appear as nonstaining small rods within the cytoplasm of macrophages and giant cells. Nonstaining organisms may also be present in the background of the smear. Mycobacterial organisms stain positively with acid-fast stains. Culture is needed to determine the species of *Mycobacterium* present.

16. Are Gram stains typically used on cytology preparations?

Gram stains can be used, but it is difficult to obtain reproducible, accurate staining of bacteria when they are in exudative effusions. Cells and exudative proteins stain red with Gram stain. Bacteria, whether gram positive or negative, tend to stain red in exudative effusions. Thus Gram stain is a poor choice when trying to confirm the presence of bacteria because it is difficult to see red bacteria in a red-staining background.

17. What common genera of coccoid bacteria are seen cytologically?

Pathogenic bacterial cocci in veterinary medicine are typically gram positive (*Staphylococcus* and *Streptococcus* spp.). *Dermatophilus congolensis* replicates by transverse and longitudinal division, producing long chains of coccoid bacterial doublets that resemble small, blue, railroad tracts.

18. What are the distinctive characteristics of some pathogenic bacterial rods?

Small bacterial rods are typically gram negative, and all pathogenic small, bipolar rods are gram negative. Common small bacterial rods include *Escherichia coli* and *Pasteurella.* Large spore-forming bacterial rods usually indicate *Clostridium.* Filamentous rods are usually *Actinomyces* or *Nocardia* (Figure 41-3). These rods are characterized by long, slender (filamentous) strands that stain pale blue and have intermittent, small, pink or blue areas.

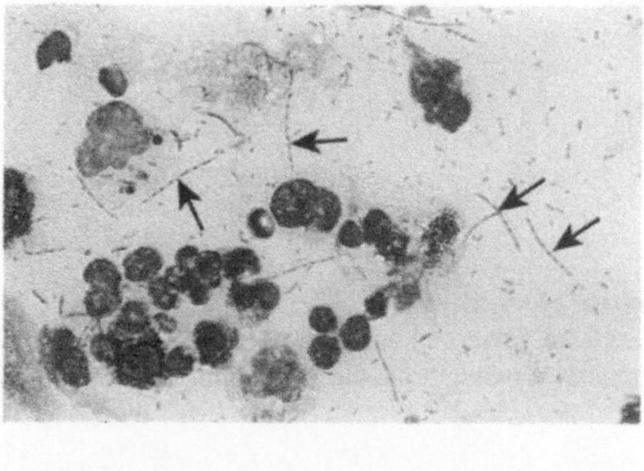

Figure 41-3 Actinomycosis. Aspirate of thoracic fluid from a dog showing many degenerate neutrophils and high numbers of mixed bacteria. Filamentous rods *(arrows)* suggest either *Actinomyces* or *Nocardia* organisms. (Wright's stain; 250×.)

19. What common fungi produce only yeast at body temperature in the common domestic animals?

The fungi that are specific enough to identify cytologically and produce only yeast at body temperature in domestic animals are subdivided into those that produce small yeasts, medium yeasts, or large yeasts. Some common fungal diseases that produce only small yeasts are sporothricosis and histoplasmosis. Some common fungal diseases that produce medium-sized yeasts are blastomycosis and cryptococcosis. A common fungal disease that produces large yeasts is coccidioidomycosis.

20. How are *Sporothrix schenckii* organisms recognized?

Sporothrix schenckii organisms are round to oval to fusiform (cigar shaped) and are about 3 to 9 micrometers (μm; or microns, μ) long and 1 to 3 μm wide. They stain pale to medium blue with a slightly eccentric pink or purple nucleus. *S. schenckii* organisms are usually surrounded by a thin, clear halo (Figure 41-4).

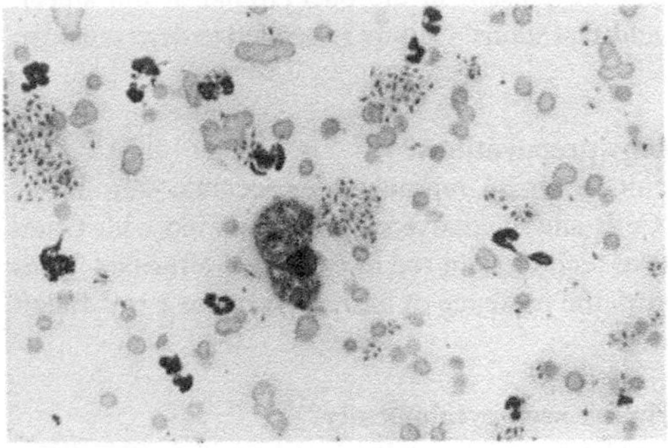

Figure 41-4 Sporothricosis. Swab of draining tract from a cat showing moderate numbers of *Sporothrix* organisms both within macrophages and free in smear. (Wright's stain; 250×.)

21. How are *Histoplasma capsulatum* organisms recognized?

Histoplasma capsulatum organisms are round to slightly oval but are **not fusiform**, a major feature in differentiating *H. capsulatum* from *Sporothrix* organisms. *H. capsulatum* organisms are about 2 to 4 μm in diameter, stain pale to medium blue, and contain an eccentric, pink- to purple-staining nucleus that is often crescent shaped. A thin, clear halo resulting from artifactual shrinkage is usually present around the yeast (Figure 41-5).

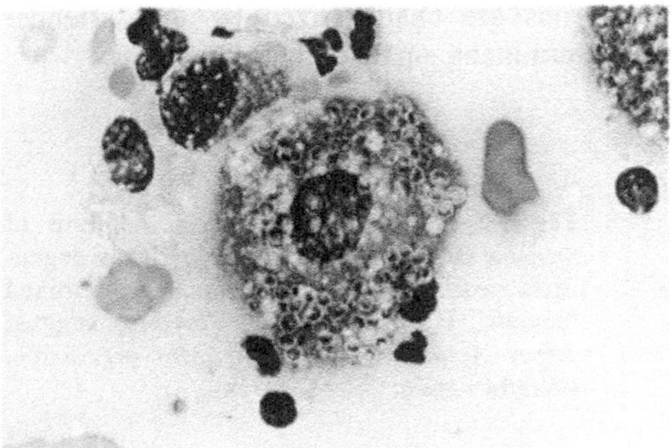

Figure 41-5 Histoplasmosis. Aspirate from a dog showing macrophage containing moderate numbers of *Histoplasma* organisms. (Wright's stain; 250×.)

22. How are *Blastomyces dermatitidis* organisms recognized?

Blastomyces dermatitidis organisms are dark blue, spherical, and 7 to 20 μm in diameter and have a thick, refractile outer wall. Occasional organisms showing broad-based budding may be found.

23. How are *Cryptococcus neoformans* organisms recognized?

Cryptococcus neoformans organisms are extremely variable in size but are generally 4 to 15 μm in diameter without their capsule and 8 to 40 μm in diameter with their capsule (thick mucoid). The organism stains pink to blue purple and may be slightly granular. The capsule is usually clear and homogeneous (Figure 41-6). Also, nonencapsulated forms of *Cryptococcus* may be found. These appear similar to encapsulated forms but have a thin, clear capsule. Occasional organisms showing narrow-based budding may be found. Often, only minimal cellular response is observed.

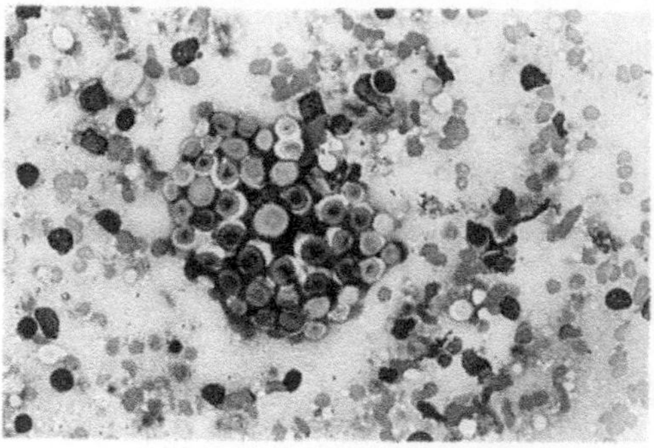

Figure 41-6 Cryptococcosis. Aspirate of mass on a cat showing a group of light- to dark-staining *Cryptococcus* organisms with medium-sized clear capsules. Red blood cells are also present. (Wright's stain; 125×.)

24. How are *Coccidioides immitis* organisms recognized?

Coccidioides immitis organisms range from 10 to 100 μm or greater in diameter. They appear as blue or clear, double-contoured spheres with finely granular protoplasm and often appear folded or crumpled. Round endospores 2 to 5 μm in diameter may be seen in some of the larger organisms. Occasionally, endospores may be released from ruptured spherules and observed free in the background of the smear (Figure 41-7).

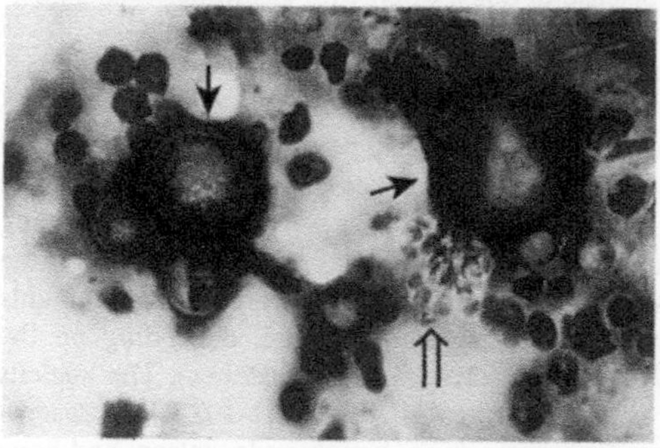

Figure 41-7 Coccidioidomycosis. Lung aspirate from a dog showing several large *Coccidioides* spores *(arrows)* and some endospores *(double arrow)* from a ruptured spore that are free in the background. (Wright's stain; 250×.)

25. How is the protozoal organism *Leishmania donovani* recognized?

Leishmania donovani organisms (amastigote) are oval and 2 to 4 μm in diameter. They have a blue to light-purple nucleus and a small, dark-blue to purple, rod-shaped kinetoplast. Although variable, the kinetoplast tends to be located between the nucleus and greatest volume of cytoplasm (Figure 41-8). Leishmaniasis tends to be associated with a granulomatous or pyogranulomatous reaction.

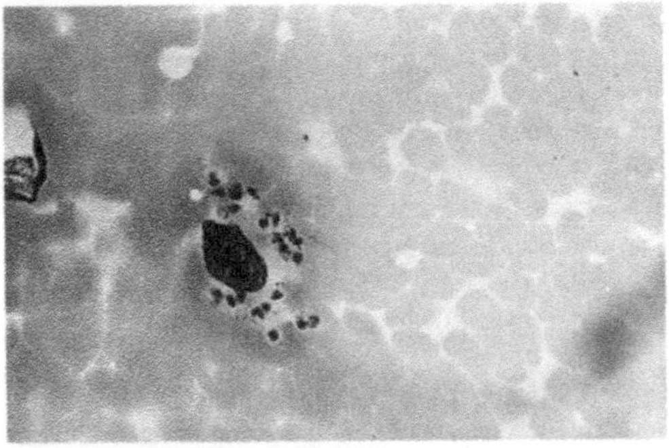

Figure 41-8 Leishmaniasis. Aspirate from cutaneous mass on a dog showing numerous red blood cells and macrophage containing *Leishmania* organisms. (Wright's stain; 250×.)

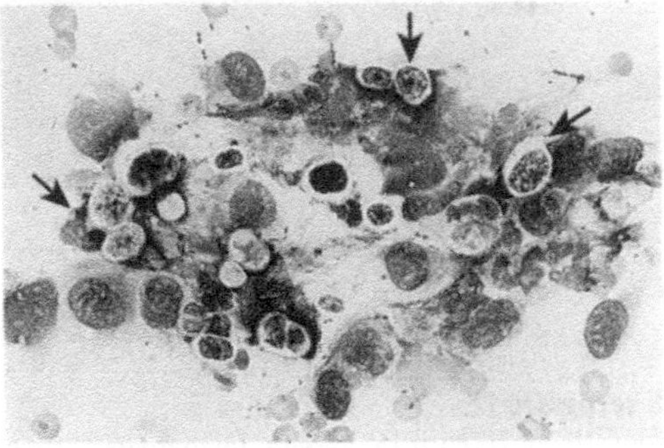

Figure 41-9 Protothecosis. Rectal scraping from a dog showing extracellular bacteria, red blood cells, epithelial cells, neutrophils, and *Prototheca* organisms *(arrows)*. (Wright's stain; 250×.)

26. How are protothecal infections recognized?

Protothecal infections tend to be associated with a granulomatous or pyogranulomatous reaction. *Prototheca* spp. are round to oval organisms 1 to 14 μm wide and 1 to 16 μm long, with a granular basophilic cytoplasm and thin, clear cell wall (Figure 41-9). They are associated with cutaneous infections in cats and disseminated disease in dogs, often with gastrointestinal signs.

27. How is cytauxzoonosis recognized in tissue aspirates?

Cytauxzoonosis is caused by the protozoal parasite *Cytauxzoon felis.* Diagnosis may be made by finding characteristic signet ring, intraerythrocytic red cell parasites (may be absent or in very low numbers early in disease) or by tissue aspirates. In cytauxzoonosis, schizogony occurs in macrophages throughout the body, and finding macrophages containing developing merozoites on tissue aspirates or impression smears provides a definitive diagnosis. These macrophages appear as extremely enlarged mononuclear cells with moderate to large amounts of intracytoplasmic basophilic material or eosinophilic stippled material, depending on the degree of development of the organisms (shizonts full of developing merozoites). The nucleus of the macrophage usually contains a greatly enlarged nucleolus (Figure 41-10). These macrophages can usually be found in cytology smears from liver, lung, lymph node, spleen, and bone marrow.

28. How is toxoplasmosis recognized on cytology?

Toxoplasmosis is caused by the protozoan *Toxoplasma gondii.* Cytologic diagnosis is made by finding the small (5 × 2 μm), crescent-shaped tachyzoites. The tachyzoites stain pale blue to blue purple and have an eccentrically placed, dark-staining nucleus (Figure 41-11). Unfortunately, *Toxoplasma* cannot be reliably differentiated from *Neospora* cytologically.

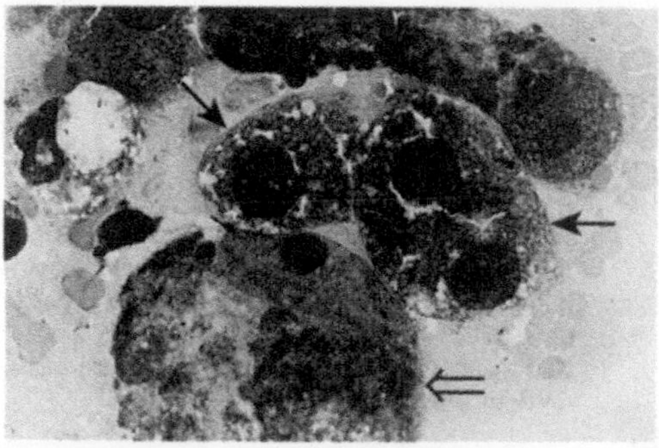

Figure 41-10 Cytauxzoonosis. Liver aspirate from a cat showing hepatocytes *(arrows)* and large macrophages full of developing merozoites of cytauxzoon *(double arrow).* (Wright's stain; 250×.)

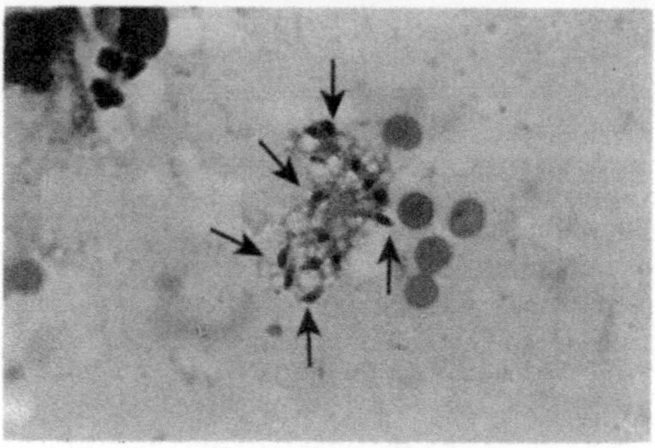

Figure 41-11 Toxoplasmosis. Transtracheal wash from a cat showing a few red blood cells and many *Toxoplasma* organisms *(arrows).* (Wright's stain; 250×.)

29. How is *Neospora caninum* recognized?

Cytologically, the tissue stage of *Neospora caninum* appears similar to the tissue stage of *Toxoplasma,* and therefore these organisms cannot be differentiated based on morphology alone. *N. caninum* is recognized using immunofluorescent assay (IFA) with specific antibodies and by polymerase chain reaction (PCR).

30. Are all inflammatory reactions associated with infections?

Many inflammatory reactions are *not* associated with an infectious organism. Examples of noninfectious inflammatory reactions include cysts, neoplasia, injection site reactions, eosinophilic granuloma, steatitis, and immune-mediated disease.

31. What is the cytologic appearance of cystic lesions?

Fluid from a variety of cystic lesions (e.g., salivary mucocele, seroma, hygroma) is typically evaluated cytologically. Most cystic fluids contain numerous macrophages, although some cysts are of low cellularity. The macrophages may be relatively small, unstimulated macrophages resembling blood monocytes or large, actively phagocytic macrophages with abundant vacuolated cytoplasm. Neutrophils may be present in variable numbers resulting from inflammation induced by the pressure of the cyst (neutrophils mean *inflammation,* not infection). Intracystic hemorrhage occasionally occurs and is recognized by the presence of red blood cell breakdown products (hemosiderin, hematoidin). Fluid from a salivary mucocele can often be recognized by the presence of amorphous, blue, mucous "tufts" scattered among the cells.

32. How does neoplasia cause inflammation?

Tumors often outgrow their blood supply and create necrotic areas that contain many inflammatory cells (neutrophils with or without macrophages).

33. What is the cytologic appearance of injection site reactions?

Injection site reactions may be neutrophilic, pyogranulomatous, granulomatous, or lymphocytic. Occasionally, amorphous, homogeneous, brightly eosinophilic material may be seen extracellularly or within macrophages with vaccine reactions (Figure 41-12).

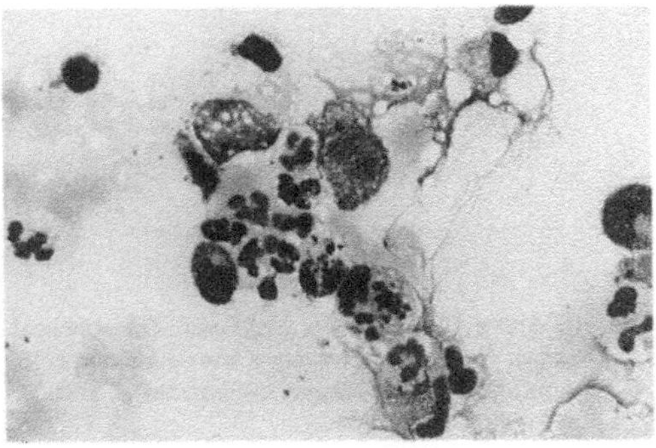

Figure 41-12 Injection site reaction. Mixed inflammatory response with neutrophils, macrophages, and lymphocytes. Large macrophage near center contains red intracytoplasmic material typically seen with vaccination reactions. (Wright's stain; 250×.)

34. What is the cytologic appearance of eosinophilic granulomas?

Scrapings or aspirates from eosinophilic granulomas usually contain high numbers of eosinophils. Often, especially in scrapings, numerous free eosinophil granules are present in the background of the smear. Fibroblasts and macrophages are present in variable numbers.

35. What is the cytologic appearance of steatitis?

Aspirates from areas of inflamed fat typically consist of inflammatory cells admixed with high numbers of variably sized lipid vacuoles (Figure 41-13). Granulomatous (macrophagic) inflammation is most common, although pyogranulomatous and purulent inflammation may be seen. The macrophages often contain numerous small, clear, lipid vacuoles within their cytoplasm. Large, multinucleated macrophages are often seen and must not be confused with neoplastic cells.

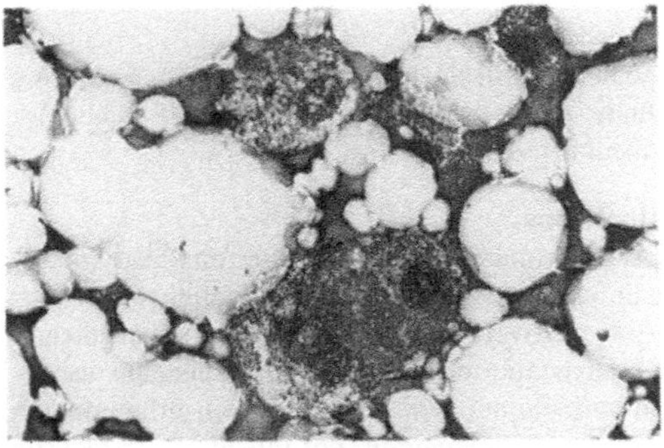

Figure 41-13 Steatitis. Aspirate from cutaneous mass on a dog showing red blood cells, many fat spaces, and moderate numbers of macrophages. (Wright's stain; 250×.)

36. What is the cytologic appearance of aspirates from the pustules of immune-mediated skin lesions?

Aspirates from immune-mediated skin lesions associated with pemphigus foliaceus consist of many nondegenerative neutrophils and some necrotic debris. Occasionally, acantholytic cells (rounded squamous epithelial cells) are observed.

42. CYTOLOGY OF NEOPLASIA

Rick L. Cowell, Debbie J. Cunningham, and James H. Meinkoth

1. What is a good general approach to evaluation and classification of tissue cells in cytologic preparations?

a. Tissue cells found on cytologic smears may be from normal, hyperplastic, dysplastic, or neoplastic tissues. Although architecture is lost with cytology, evaluation of the cell pattern, cell population, and any extracellular material present allows for a diagnosis in many cases.

b. Tissue cells should be evaluated for their general characteristics of size, shape, and distribution pattern (individual discrete cells or cells in groups and clusters). Cells are classified as round, spindle, or epithelial based on the following (Table 42-1):

(1) Morphology (size and shape)
(2) Tendency to cluster (cohesiveness)
(3) Production of extracellular matrix

c. Tissue cells are then evaluated for criteria of malignancy. Application of criteria of malignancy is primarily for epithelial and spindle cell tumors.

Table 42-1 ***General Appearance of Cells in Basic Tumor Categories***

TUMOR TYPE	GENERAL CELL SIZE	GENERAL CELL SHAPE	SCHEMATIC REPRESENTATION	CELLULARITY OF ASPIRATES	CLUMPS OR CLUSTERS COMMON
Epithelial	Large	Round to caudate	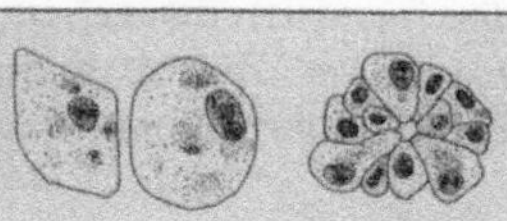	Usually high	Yes
Mesenchymal (spindle cell)	Small to medium	Spindle to stellate	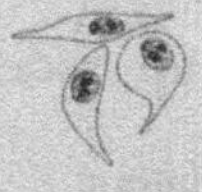	Usually low	No
Discrete round cell	Small to medium	Round	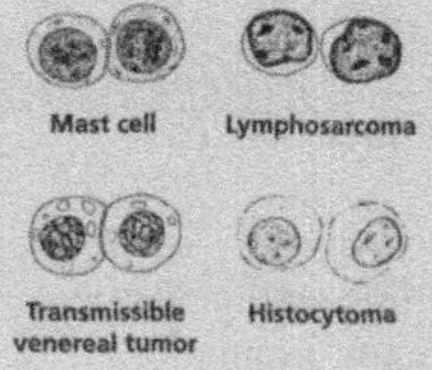	Usually high	No

From Cowell RL, Tyler RD, Meinkoth JH: *Diagnostic cytology and hematology of the dog and cat,* ed 2, St Louis, 1999, Mosby.

(1) Epithelial cells with adequate criteria of malignancy are classified as carcinomas or adenocarcinomas.
(2) Spindle cells with adequate criteria of malignancy are classified as sarcomas.
(3) Round cell tumors are generally readily recognized by cell morphology and classified accordingly.

2. Discuss the cytologic criteria of malignancy.

In general, a uniform population of cells suggests the mass is benign, whereas variation in cells suggests malignancy. An important exception is lymphoma (lymphosarcoma), which consists of a fairly uniform population of lymphoblasts, whereas lymphoid hyperplasia typically has marked variation due to the mixed population of small lymphocytes, prolymphocytes, lymphoblasts, and plasma cells. Nuclear criteria of malignancy are considered diagnostic, whereas cytoplasmic criteria of malignancy are only supportive of malignant neoplasia. It is important to find more than three of the following nuclear criteria of malignancy in a few cells to many cells to call a mass "malignant neoplasia" (Table 42-2).

Nuclear Criteria of Malignancy

a. *Anisokaryosis:* variation in nuclear size
b. *Macrokaryosis:* increased nuclear size (>10 μm)
c. *Increased nuclear/cytoplasmic ratio:* large nucleus and less cytoplasm (normal in some cell types, e.g., small lymphocyte)
d. *Marconucleoli:* nucleoli that are greater than 5 μm in diameter
e. *Abnormally prominent nucleoli* with variable shapes. Nucleoli are angular instead of round or oval.
f. *Abnormal mitosis:* improper alignment of chromosomes
g. *Coarse chromatin pattern:* ropy or cordlike chromatin
h. *Nuclear molding:* nucleus deformed (molded) around other nuclei within the same cell or other cells; indicates loss of contact inhibition

Cytoplasmic Criteria of Malignancy

a. *Cytoplasmic basophilia:* increased ribonucleic acid (RNA) synthesis/content
b. *Abnormal vacuolization* and/or *secretory granules*
c. *Relatively little cytoplasm* for the cell type: scant cytoplasm in large epithelial cells

General Criteria of Malignancy

a. *Anisocytosis:* variation in cell size
b. *Macrocytosis:* cells larger than expected for cell type

3. List the round (discrete) cell tumors.

a. Mast cell tumor
b. Histiocytoma
c. Transmissible venereal tumor (TVT)
d. Lymphosarcoma
e. Plasmacytoma

Occasionally, basal cell tumors and melanomas may appear to exfoliate round cells but are not included in the round cell tumor group.

4. What are the general characteristics of round cell tumors?

Round cell tumors tend to exfoliate high numbers of individual cells (e.g., cells not in sheets or clumps) that are generally round in shape and have distinct cell borders. Cell nuclei are roundish and may be indented (e.g., lymphocytes). Round cells are typically smaller than epithelial cells.

Table 42-2 *Criteria of Malignancy in Tissue Cells*

CRITERIA	DESCRIPTION	SCHEMATIC REPRESENTATION
General Criteria		
Anisocytosis and macrocytosis	Variation in cell size, with some cells ≥1.5 times larger than normal	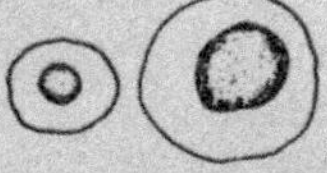
Hypercellularity	Increased cell exfoliation due to decreased cell adherence	Not depicted
Pleomorphism (except in lymphoid tissue}	Variable size and shape in cells of the same type	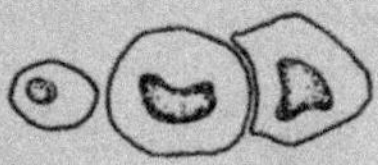
Nuclear Criteria		
Macrokaryosis	Increased nuclear size	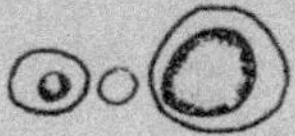
Increased nuclear/ cytoplasm (N/C) ratio	Normal nonlymphoid cells usually have N/C of 1:3-1:8 depending on the tissue; increased ratios (e.g., 1:2, 1:1) suggest malignancy.	See Macrokaryosis.
Anisokaryosis	Variation in nuclear size; especially important if nuclei of multinucleated cells vary in size	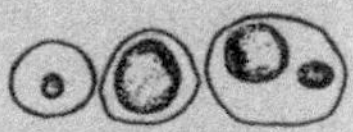
Multinucleation	Multiple nuclei in a cell; especially important if nuclei vary in size	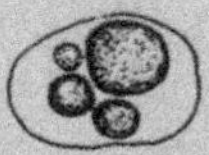
Increased mitotic figures	Mitosis is rare in normal tissue.	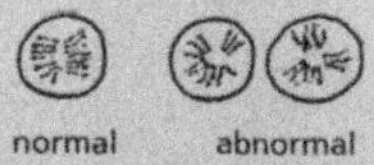
Abnormal mitosis	Improper alignment of chromosomes	See Increased mitotic figures.
Coarse chromatin pattern	Chromatic pattern is coarser than normal and may appear ropy or cordlike.	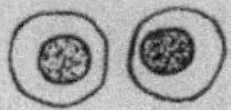
Nuclear molding	Deformation of nuclei by other nuclei within same cell or adjacent cells	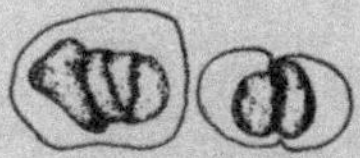
Macronucleoli	Nucleoli increased in size; nucleoli ≥5 μm strongly suggest malignancy. For reference, RBCs are 5-6 μm in cat and 7-8 μm in dog.	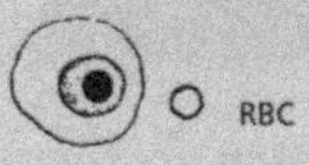
Angular nucleoli	Nucleoli are fusiform or have other angular shapes instead of normal round to oval shape.	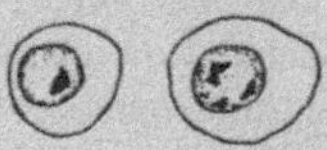
Anisonucleoliosis	Variation in nucleolar shape or size; especially important if variation is within same nucleus.	See Angular nucleoli.

Modified from Cowell RL, Tyler RD, Meinkoth JH: *Diagnostic cytology and hematology of the dog and cat,* ed 2, St Louis, 1999, Mosby.

5. How are mast cell tumors recognized cytologically?

Mast cell tumors exfoliate high numbers of cells that have a moderate amount of cytoplasm, which contains a few or many small, red-purple (metachromatic) granules (Figure 42-1). These granules are the most distinctive feature of mast cell tumors. The cells have a round to oval nucleus that may be obscured by the granules. Variable numbers of eosinophils are present. It is important to remember that some stains (e.g., Diff-Quik) occasionally will not stain the mast cell granules.

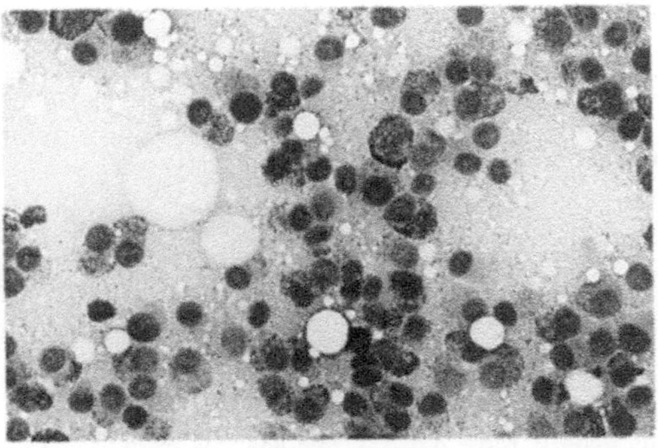

Figure 42-1 Mast cell tumor. Cutaneous mass on a dog showing high numbers of discrete round cells in a tissue fluid background. Many round cells contain reddish purple intracytoplasmic granules. (Wright's stain; 125×.)

6. How are histiocytomas recognized cytologically?

Histiocytomas exfoliate small, benign-appearing, round, discretely oriented cells. These cells have a round to oval nucleus, finely stippled chromatin, and indistinct nucleoli. Histiocytomas have a moderate amount of homogeneous clear to gray to blue-gray cytoplasm that often stains lighter than the surrounding tissue fluid background (Figure 42-2). Lymphoid cells (none to many) may also be present. Moderate to high numbers of small lymphocytes suggest an immune response and that the histiocytoma is about to regress spontaneously.

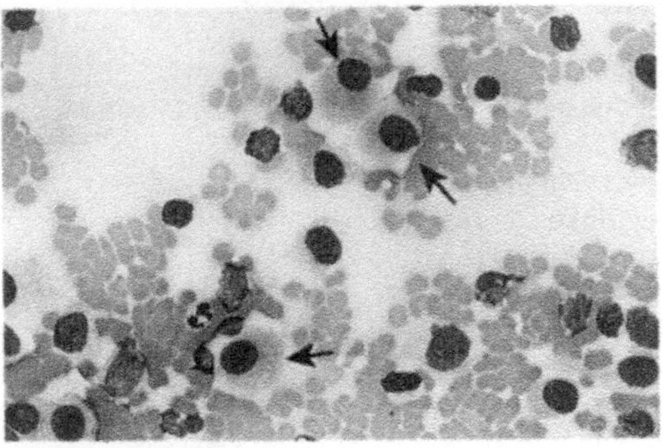

Figure 42-2 Histiocytoma. Cutaneous mass on a dog showing high numbers of red blood cells (RBCs) and scattered discrete round cells. These cells have a round to oval nucleus, finely stippled chromatin, and indistinct nucleoli compatible with histiocytoma cells *(arrows)*. Some small lymphocytes are also present. (Wright's stain; 125×.)

7. How are transmissible venereal tumors recognized cytologically?

Transmissible venereal tumors (TVTs) exfoliate high numbers of round cells that have a moderate amount of basophilic cytoplasm, which often contains a few or many clear intracytoplasmic vacuoles (Figure 42-3). Clear vacuoles may also be present in the background of the smear. Cells from TVTs have round nuclei with coarse (ropy) nuclear chromatin and one or more prominent nucleoli. Moderate to marked variation in cell and nuclear size (anisocytosis, anisokaryosis) is common. Mitotic figures may be observed.

8. How are cutaneous lymphomas recognized cytologically?

Cutaneous lymphomas (lymphosarcomas) usually consist of a uniform population of

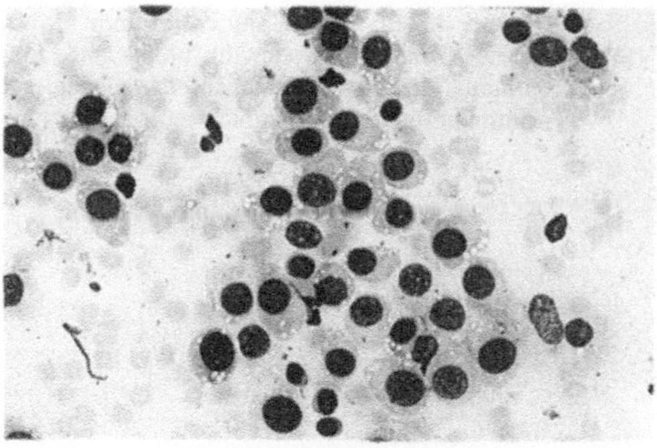

Figure 42-3 Transmissible venereal tumor (TVT). Cutaneous mass on a dog showing high numbers of RBCs and moderate numbers of round cells that have a moderate amount of basophilic cytoplasm, which contains moderate number of clear intraocytoplasmic vacuoles. (Wright's stain; 125×.)

lymphoblasts that have an oval to variably shaped nucleus with finely granular chromatin and one to multiple nucleoli. These cells generally have a slight to moderate amount of lightly basophilic cytoplasm that is not visible all the way around the nucleus because it runs confluent with the nucleus for part of its course. Cytoplasmic fragments are present in the background of the smear. Occasionally the lymphoblasts appear histiocytic.

9. How are cutaneous plasmacytomas recognized cytologically?

Cutaneous plasmacytomas exfoliate many plasmacytoid cells that have round, eccentric nuclei and a moderate amount of deeply basophilic cytoplasm. A perinuclear clear area (Golgi area) is often seen, generally located between the nucleus and greatest volume of cytoplasm. Binucleated and multinucleated cells are common. Anisocytosis and anisokaryosis are typical features (Figure 42-4).

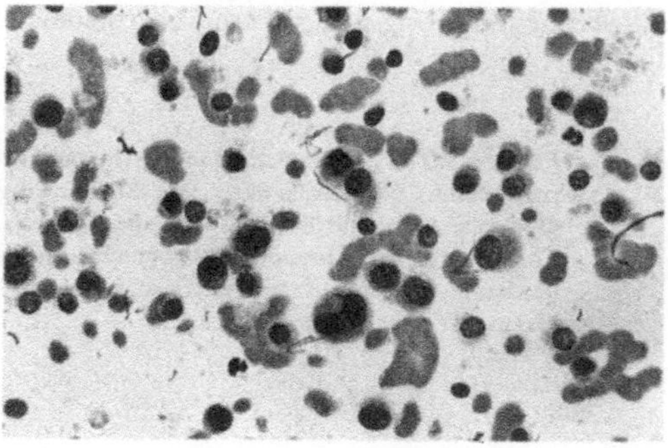

Figure 42-4 Plasmacytoma. Cutaneous mass on a dog showing high numbers of RBCs and moderate numbers of round cells that appear plasmacytoid and have round, eccentric nuclei and moderate amount of deeply basophilic cytoplasm. (Wright's stain; 125×.)

10. What are epithelial cells?

Epithelial cells arise from lining surfaces (e.g., skin), parenchymal tissues (e.g., liver), or glandular tissues (e.g., mammary gland) and are typically large cells that have a roundish to polygonal shape with distinct cytoplasmic borders (Figure 42-5). Epithelial cells tend to have cell-to-cell adherence and therefore frequently exfoliate in sheets (monolayer of cells) or clusters (ball arrangement), although some individual cells may be present as well.

11. What are some of the epithelial cell tumors?

Epithelial cell tumors can be benign or malignant and can be cystic or noncystic. Benign epithelial cell tumors are "oma"s (e.g., hepatoma, adenoma) whereas malignant epithelial cell tumors are *carcinomas* or *adenocarcinomas*. Examples include mammary gland adenoma and mammary gland adenocarcinoma, thyroid adenoma and thyroid adenocarcinoma, perianal adenoma and perianal adenocarcinoma, and transitional cell carcinoma.

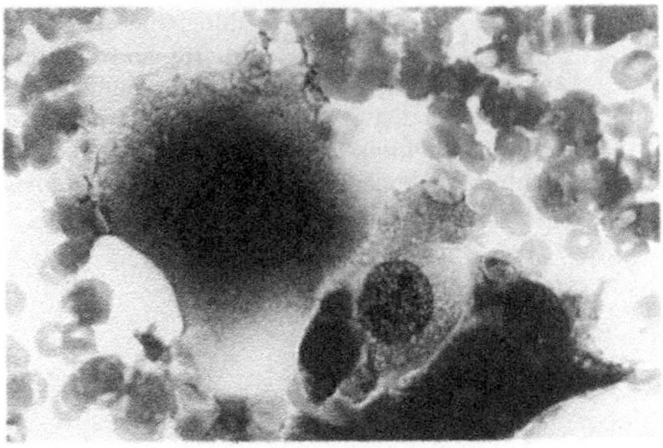

Figure 42-5 Epithelial cell tumor. Mass aspirate from a dog showing blood and large epithelial cells with abundant cytoplasm and prominent nucleoli. (Wright's stain; 250×.)

12. How are benign epithelial cell tumors differentiated from malignant tumors?

In general, malignant epithelial cell tumors have three or more malignant criteria in many of the cells present. Benign tumors have few or no malignant criteria present. As with all rules, this is not 100% accurate. Some malignant tumors (e.g., adenocarcinoma of perianal sac, some bile duct adenocarcinomas) do not show much in the way of malignant criteria. Familiarity with which malignant tumors occasionally show minimal malignant criteria helps increase diagnostic accuracy.

13. What are mesenchymal (spindle) cell tumors?

Spindle cell tumors are often referred to as *mesenchymal cell tumors* because they often have a fusiform, stellate, or spindled shape resembling the embryonic connective tissue, mesenchyme (Figure 42-6). Nuclei are typically round to oval, and the cytoplasmic border is often indistinct. Spindle cell tumors typically exfoliate individual cells, but cell clumps are occasionally present. An eosinophilic extracellular matrix may be present between the cells. Some spindle cell tumors exfoliate poorly. Spindle cells are typically of connective tissue origin (e.g., fibroblast, osteoblast, myocyte, endothelial cell, adipocyte).

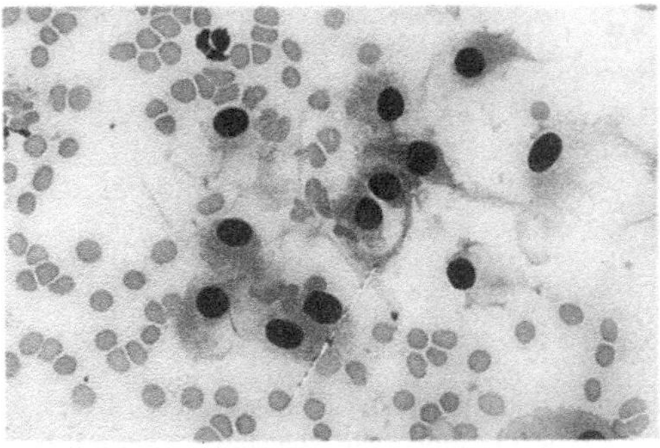

Figure 42-6 Spindle cell tumor (hemangiopericytoma). Cutaneous mass on a dog showing moderate numbers of RBCs and spindle cells. These cells have round to oval nuclei and a moderate amount of tapered basophilic cytoplasm. (Wright's stain; 125×.)

14. What are some of the mesenchymal (spindle) cell tumors?

In general, benign tumors are "oma"s, whereas malignant tumors are *sarcomas*. Examples include osteosarcoma, hemangiopericytoma, fibroma and fibrosarcoma, lipoma and liposarcoma, and hemangioma and hemangiosarcoma.

15. Adipocytes aspirated from lipomas look like large epithelial cells, so why are they classified as mesenchymal cell tumors?

Lipomas, consisting of fat-filled adipocytes, are a mesenchymal cell tumor. Normal adipocytes (before being filled with fat) are spindle cells. However, once they fill with fat, they become very large and lose their spindled shape. *Liposarcomas* often exfoliate some spindle-shaped cells because the cells generally contain less fat. It is important to remember that the routine cytologic stains (e.g., Romanowsky type) contain alcohol and dissolve fat. Therefore, free lipid from ruptured cells does not stain. However, stains such as oil red O stain fat well.

16. Do melanomas and malignant melanomas always contain spindle-shaped cells?

Melanomas and malignant melanomas are among the few tumors that do *not* consistently have a single cell shape. Cells from melanomas and malignant melanomas may have the cytologic features of spindle, round, or epithelial cells (Figure 42-7).

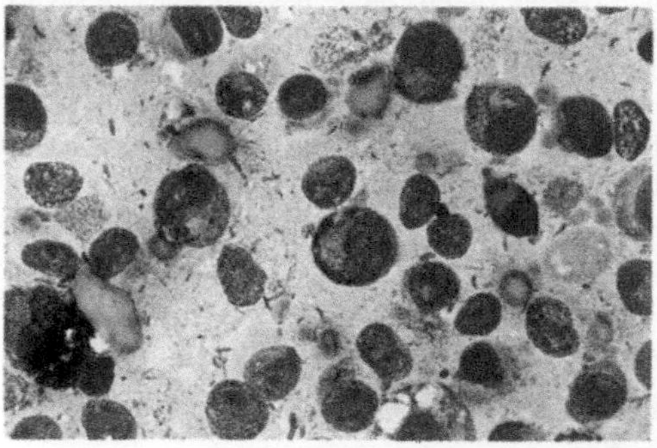

Figure 42-7 Malignant melanoma. Aspirate from mass in mouth of a dog showing many malignant-appearing cells (large nucleoli, anisocytosis) that contain melanin granules and have a round shape. Melanomas and malignant melanomas may appear as round, spindle, or epithelial cell tumors. (Wright's stain; 250×.)

17. Do melanomas and malignant melanomas always contain recognizable pigment?

Well-differentiated tumors tend to be heavily granulated, and the numerous greenish black granules may obscure the nucleus, making cytologic evaluation of malignant criteria impossible. Poorly differentiated tumors may contain few to no granules. Some tumors contain only a fine dusting of grayish pigment.

18. Are all cystic lesions associated with tumors?

Although some are so associated, many cystic lesions are *not* associated with tumors. Cystic lesions occur for many reasons, including secondary to blocked ducts (e.g., salivary cysts) and secondary to trauma (e.g., seroma).

43. CYTOLOGY OF LYMPH NODES AND THYMUS

Rick L. Cowell, Debbie J. Cunningham, and James H. Meinkoth

1. When should a lymph node be aspirated for cytology?

Lymph node aspiration is useful whenever one or multiple lymph nodes are enlarged. Aspiration of a nonenlarged node is difficult and usually results in aspiration of perinodal fat with little or no lymphoid tissue present. However, aspiration of a nonenlarged node is sometimes attempted to check for metastatic neoplasia.

2. List some diagnoses made from lymph node aspirates.

a. Reactive or hyperplastic lymphadenopathy
b. Lymphadenitis (neutrophilic, histiocytic or macrophagic, eosinophilic)
c. Lymphoma
d. Metastatic neoplasia
e. Aspiration of extranodal tissues (fat, salivary gland)
f. Infectious agents (e.g., bacterial, mycotic, algal, protozoal, rickettsial)

3. What is the cytologic appearance of an aspirate from a normal lymph node?

Aspirates from normal lymph nodes consist of 75% to 95% (usually about 90%) small mature lymphocytes (Figure 43-1). Small lymphocytes are slightly larger than the size of a canine red blood cell (RBC) and about 1.5 to 2 times the size of a feline RBC. They have a dark staining, roundish nucleus with densely aggregated chromatin and no visible nucleoli. Small lymphocytes have a scanty amount of clear to light-blue cytoplasm that is generally visible only on one side of the nucleus (not visible all the way around nucleus). Other cell types are present in low numbers and may include lymphoblasts, prolymphocytes, plasma cells, macrophages, neutrophils, and mast cells. Lymphoglandular bodies, bare nuclei, and strands of nuclear chromatin are often present as well.

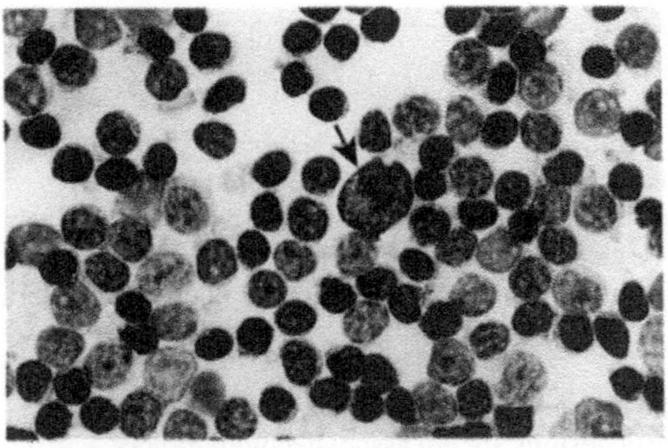

Figure 43-1 Normal lymph node. Lymph node aspirate from a dog showing high numbers of small lymphocytes and one lymphoblast *(arrow)*. (Wright's stain; 250×.)

4. What are lymphoglandular bodies?

Lymphoglandular bodies are cytoplasmic fragments from lymphoid cells. This is a normal finding in all lymphoid tissues. The main concern is not to confuse lymphoglandular bodies with an organism or cell.

5. What is the cytologic appearance of a hyperplastic lymph node, and how does it differ from a normal lymph node?

Cytologically, no clear line of separation exists between a normal and a hyperplastic lymph node. Both may look identical to the other, and the cytologic evaluation of the lymph node aspirate is reported as "hyperplastic" because the node is enlarged.

6. What is a reactive lymph node, and how does it differ from a hyperplastic lymph node?

Often the term "reactive" is used instead of "hyperplastic" when there are mildly increased numbers of inflammatory cells (macrophages, neutrophils, eosinophils), lymphoblasts, or prolymphocytes. Plasma cell numbers may be mildly to greatly increased.

7. What is a Mott cell?

A *Mott cell* is a plasma cell that has its cytoplasm filled with roundish vacuoles that stain clear to light blue (Figure 43-2). These vacuoles, termed *Russell bodies,* are packets of immunoglobulin.

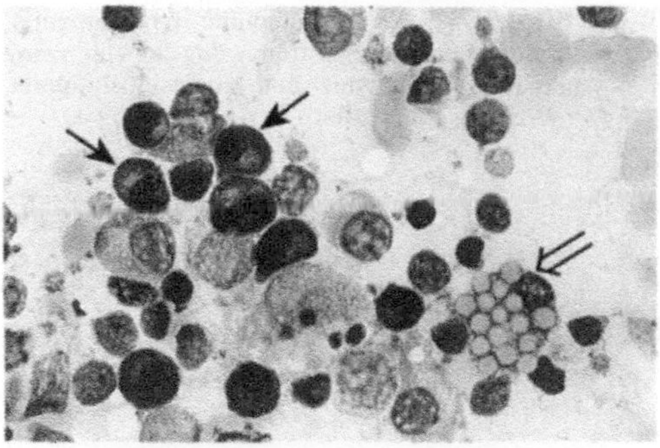

Figure 43-2 Mott cell. Lymph node aspirate showing many small lymphocytes and plasma cells *(arrows)*, a macrophage, and a Mott cell *(double arrow)*. Many lymphoglandular bodies are present in the background of the smear. (Wright's stain; 250×.)

8. List the different types of lymphadenitis.

a. Neutrophilic lymphadenitis
b. Eosinophilic lymphadenitis
c. Histiocytic (macrophagic) or granulomatous lymphadenitis
d. Any combination (e.g., pyogranulomatous lymphadenitis, neutrophilic and eosinophilic lymphadenitis)

9. How is neutrophilic lymphadenitis recognized cytologically?

When neutrophils make up more than 5% of the nucleated cells present on a lymph node aspirate or impression smear, neutrophilic lymphadenitis is present. This is a common finding in lymph nodes draining areas of neutrophilic inflammation. When neutrophils account for more than 20% of the nucleated cells present, some use the term *purulent* or *suppurative* lymphadenitis, whereas others use these terms synonymously with neutrophilic lymphadenitis. Most bacterial infections of lymph nodes cause marked numbers of neutrophils (Figure 43-3), and often the lymph node aspirate looks more like an abscess than a lymph node. One major exception is mycobacterial infections of lymph nodes, which cause a granulomatous reaction. Other causes of neutrophilic lymphadenitis include neoplasia and immune-mediated conditions. Blood contamination can mimic neutrophilic lymphadenitis, especially if a peripheral blood neutrophilia is present.

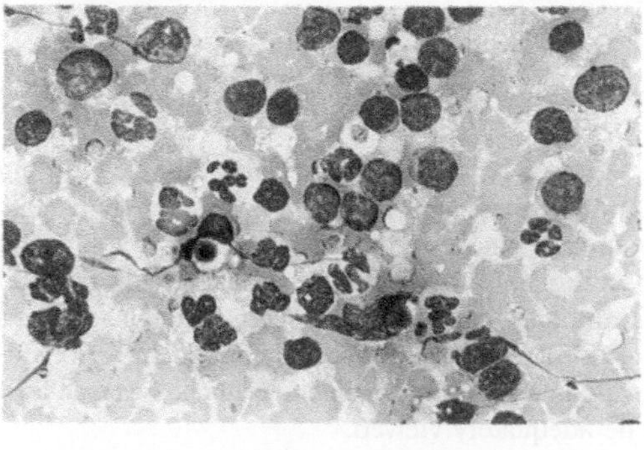

Figure 43-3 Neutrophilic lymphadenitis secondary to cryptococcosis. Lymph node aspirate from a dog showing many red blood cells (RBCs), small lymphocytes, and neutrophils. A single *Cryptococcus* organism is also present. (Wright's stain; 250×.)

10. How is eosinophilic lymphadenitis recognized cytologically?

When eosinophils constitute more than 3% of the nucleated cells present on a lymph node aspirate or impression smear, eosinophilic lymphadenitis is present (Figure 43-4). Some causes of eosinophilic lymphadenitis are allergic or parasitic conditions, feline eosinophilic skin disease, hypereosinophilic syndrome, and neoplasia (e.g., mast cell tumors, carcinoma, some lymphomas).

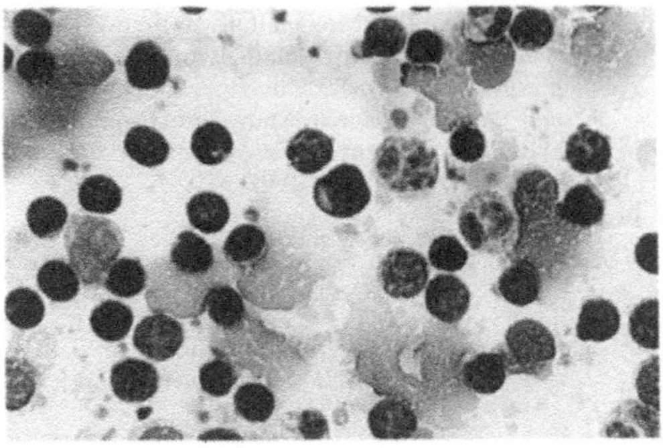

Figure 43-4 Eosinophilic lymphadenitis. Lymph node aspirate from a dog showing many small lymphocytes and some eosinophils. (Wright's stain; 250×.)

11. How is histiocytic (macrophagic) lymphadenitis recognized cytologically?

Increased numbers of macrophages in a lymph node aspirate or impression smear indicates histiocytic lymphadenitis. What constitutes increased numbers of macrophages is difficult to define. Whenever one can find more than five macrophages per oil power field, histiocytic lymphadenitis is present. Histiocytic lymphadenitis occurs at lower numbers of macrophages, but the number listed here helps keep this disorder from being overdiagnosed. Also, neutrophil numbers are often increased along with macrophages, resulting in a pyogranulomatous inflammatory reaction. Causes of histiocytic lymphadenitis include fungal infections, protozoal infections, mycobacterial infections, and rickettsial infections (Salmon disease).

12. How is lymphoma (malignant lymphoma, lymphosarcoma) recognized cytologically?

A neoplastic lymphoid cell cannot be differentiated from a nonneoplastic lymphoid cell cytologically. Criteria of malignancy apply to epithelial cells (carcinomas) and spindle cells (sarcomas) but not to lymphoid cells. Lymphoma is recognized cytologically by the ratio of blastic/nonblastic lymphoid cells. The cytologic hallmark of lymphoma is the presence of excessive numbers of blastic lymphocytes. When blastic lymphoid cells represent more than 50% of all nucleated cells throughout the smear, a diagnosis of lymphoma *(high grade)* can be made. Small cell lymphoma *(low grade)* is difficult to recognize on lymph node aspirates because normal nodes consist almost totally of small lymphocytes. Small cell lymphoma generally requires surgical removal of a node and histopathology for the evaluation of nodal architecture for a definitive diagnosis.

13. What is the major obstacle in diagnosing a blastic (immature lymphocyte, high-grade) lymphoma cytologically?

Lymphoblasts and prolymphocytes are extremely fragile and readily rupture during collection and/or smearing. The main difficulty in diagnosing blast cell (e.g., lymphoblastic, centroblastic, immunoblastic) lymphoma is obtaining smears with sufficient numbers of intact cells. It is important to try different smearing techniques (blood smear, squash, starfish) to find the technique that works best for the person making the smear. Most lymphomas in dogs and cats are blast cell (high-grade) lymphomas (Figure 43-5). Another problem is insufficiently spread-out samples that are too thick. Smears that are thick are often impossible to evaluate because they often stain poorly, and individual cells cannot be adequately viewed.

14. How are large granular lymphomas recognized cytologically?

Large granular lymphoma (LGL) is a subtype of lymphoma characterized by a predominance of large lymphoid cells with azurophilic (eosinophilic) intracytoplasmic granules. Large granular lymphocytes may be either cytotoxic T cells or natural killer (NK) cells (Figure 43-6).

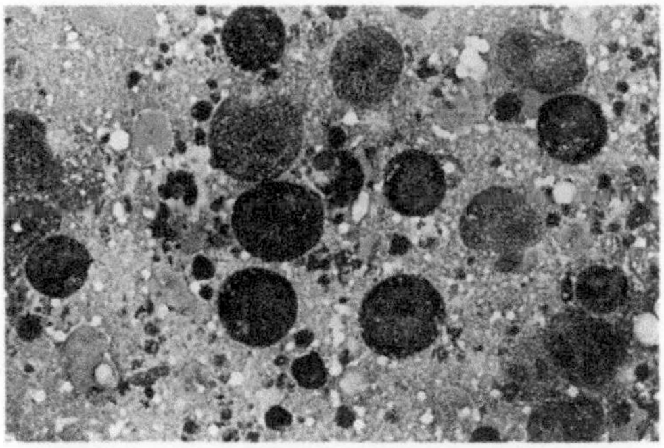

Figure 43-5 Lymphoma. Lymph node aspirate from a dog showing several large lymphoblasts. Numerous lymphoglandular bodies are present in background of smear. (Wright's stain; 250×.)

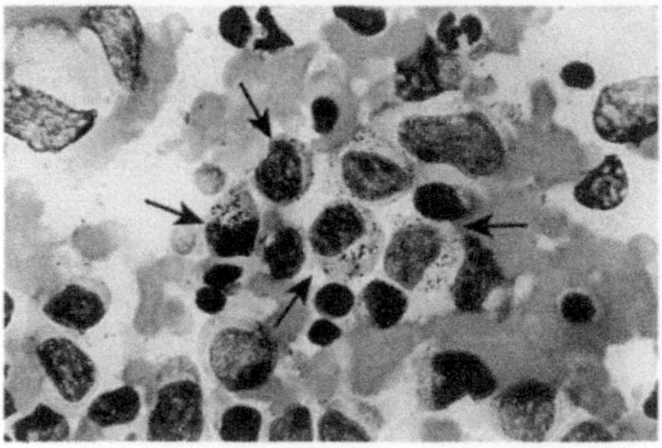

Figure 43-6 Large granular lymphoma. Image shows many RBCs, moderate numbers of large granular lymphocytes *(arrows)*, and a few small lymphocytes. (Wright's stain; 250×.)

15. How are T cell and B cell lymphomas differentiated?

Immunostaining and cytochemical staining of cytologic aspirates can be used to differentiate T cell and B cell lymphomas. B cell lymphomas are often positive for CD21, CD79a, and surface immunoglobulin. T cell lymphomas are often positive for CD3, CD4, CD8, and nonspecific esterases (CD4 and CD8 are subset markers).

16. How is neoplasia metastatic to a lymph node recognized cytologically?

Metastatic neoplasia is recognized by finding greatly increased numbers of cells that should be present only in *low* numbers (e.g., mast cells) or by finding cells that should *not* be present in lymph node aspirates that have three or more malignant criteria (e.g., epithelial cells, spindle cells) (Figure 43-7).

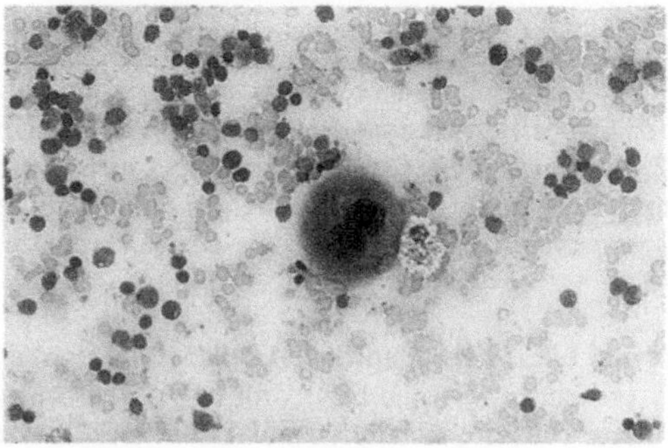

Figure 43-7 Metastatic carcinoma. Lymph node aspirate from a dog showing RBCs, scattered lymphocytes, single large epithelial cell with large prominent nucleoli, and a macrophage. (Wright's stain; 250×.)

17. What are the common nonlymphoid tissues that are accidentally aspirated when attempting a lymph node aspirate?

Perinodal fat is the most common nonlymphoid tissue accidentally aspirated (Figure 43-8). In some cases the smear consists only of fat, and in others there is a mixture of fat and lymphoid tissue. The salivary gland frequently is aspirated accidentally when attempting to aspirate a submandibular lymph node.

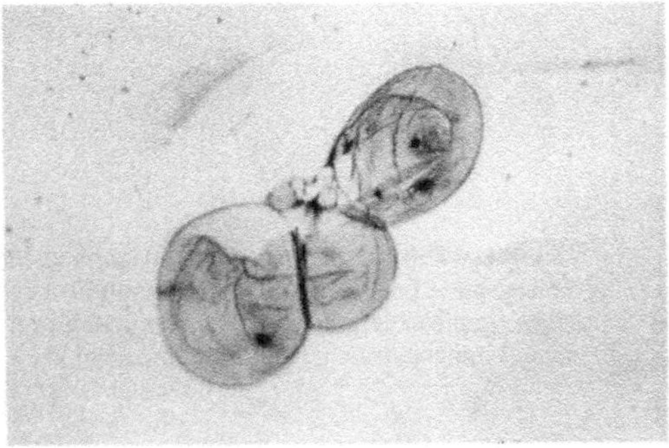

Figure 43-8 Perinodal fat. Attempted aspirate of popliteal lymph node in a dog showing cluster of large adipocytes. (Wright's stain; 50×.)

44. LIVER CYTOLOGY

Rick L. Cowell, Sylvie Beaudin, and James H. Meinkoth

1. What cell types are seen in aspirates from normal liver?

a. Hepatocytes
b. Biliary tract epithelial cells
   (1) Cuboidal cells from small ductules
   (2) Columnar cells from large ductules
c. Blood (with associated blood leukocytes)
d. Macrophages (rare)
e. Mast cells (rare)

Sheets of mesothelial cells (lining cells) may be present in aspirates from normal liver as an incidental finding. It is important not to mistake these cells for neoplastic cells.

2. What is the cytologic appearance of normal hepatocytes?

Normal hepatocytes will be present in small to large clusters or groups as well as individually in the smear. *Hepatocytes* are large epithelial cells with abundant, light-blue cytoplasm that is generally oval to polyhedral in shape. The cytoplasm often appears grainy because of the contrast between high numbers of blue-staining ribosomes and clear to lightly pink–staining organelles. Hepatocytes generally have round, uniform nuclei with moderately coarse chromatin and one or multiple small nucleoli (Figure 44-1).

3. What is the cytologic appearance of normal biliary tract epithelial cells?

Biliary tract epithelial cells are generally present in low numbers, with only a few small groups or sheets of 15 to 20 cells observed. These cells are usually cuboidal to low columnar

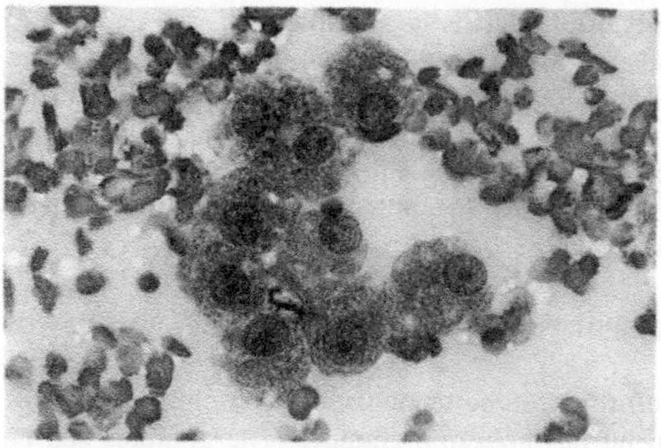

Figure 44-1 Normal hepatocytes. Liver aspirate from a dog showing a group of normal-appearing hepatocytes and red blood cells (RBCs). (Wright's stain; 250×.)

cells. They tend to have a round nucleus that is often centrally placed in a small amount of light-blue cytoplasm. Nucleoli are not visible.

4. List the main pigments seen in liver aspirates.

a. Bile pigments
b. Hemosiderin
c. Lipofuscin
d. Copper
e. Ultrasound gel contamination

5. How is bile pigment recognized cytologically?

Bile pigment appears as bright- to dark-green granules within the cytoplasm of hepatocytes or as dark-green to black bile casts between hepatocytes (in bile canaliculi) (Figure 44-2). Increased amounts of bile pigment indicates cholestasis, however, the cholestatic process may not be severe enough to cause hyperbilirubinemia or jaundice. Some bile pigment may be present in the cytoplasm of normal hepatocytes. The presence of bile casts indicates cholestasis. Pigment can be confirmed as bile pigment by staining some smears with Hall's stain, which causes bile pigments to stain green. Staining to confirm bile pigment is seldom done.

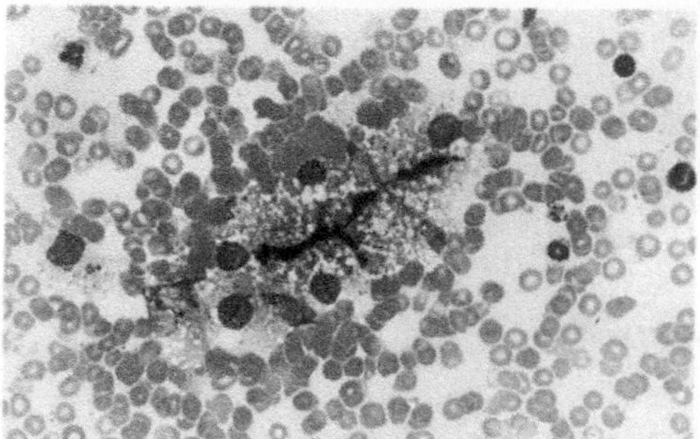

Figure 44-2 Cholestasis. Liver aspirate from a dog showing blood and a cluster of vacuolated hepatocytes with bile casts. (Wright's stain; 125×.)

6. How is hemosiderin recognized cytologically, and what are some causes of hemosiderosis?

Hemosiderin appears as golden to golden-brown granules within the cytoplasm of hepatocytes or macrophages. Smears stained with Prussian blue can confirm the presence of hemosiderin, which stains blue.

Hemosiderosis occurs with chronic hemolysis and excessive iron supplementation (especially iron injections).

7. How is lipofuscin recognized cytologically, and what is its significance?

Lipofuscin appears as blue-green granules within the cytoplasm of hepatocytes. The presence of lipofuscin can be confirmed by the Luxol fast blue procedure, which stains lipofuscin blue (this procedure is seldom performed).

Lipofuscin is a common finding in hepatocytes of older animals. The accumulation of lipofuscin does not represent a pathologic process but rather an aging process, since lipofuscin is derived from degenerate lipids as the cell ages.

8. How is hepatic copper accumulation recognized cytologically, and in what dog breeds is it most often found?

Copper accumulation must be marked before it can be recognized on cytology smears. It appears as refractile, pale-green to blue-green intracytoplasmic granules. The granules can be confirmed as copper with a rubeanic acid stain.

Excessive hepatic copper accumulation is most often seen in Bedlington terriers, West Highland white terriers, and Doberman pinschers.

9. How is ultrasound gel contamination recognized cytologically?

Ultrasound gel contamination appears as a magenta pigment (Figure 44-3). It may be mild, moderate, or marked contamination. Marked contamination of ultrasound gel can cause a cytology smear to be nondiagnostic. The ultrasound gel stains so deeply that it masks cells and other structures. It is important when collecting cytology samples by ultrasound-guided methods to be sure to clean off the gel in the area of needle insertion. Alcohol may be used instead of ultrasound gel when cytology is to be collected.

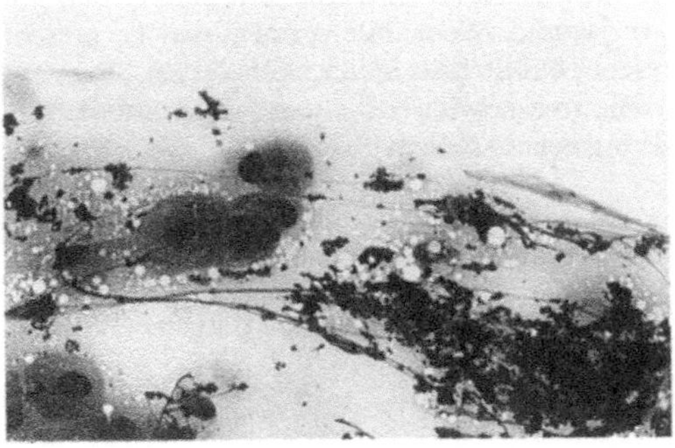

Figure 44-3 Ultrasound gel contamination. Liver aspirate from a dog showing a few normal-appearing hepatocytes and a large amount of dark-magenta–colored material (ultrasound gel). (Wright's stain; 125×.)

10. List nonneoplastic disorders seen in liver aspirates.

a. Cellular degeneration or injury
   (1) Lipidosis
   (2) Glucocorticoid induced (glycogen accumulation)
   (3) Amyloid
b. Inflammation
   (1) Neutrophilic
   (2) Histiocytic or macrophagic
   (3) Lymphocytic-plasmacytic
   (4) Eosinophilic
c. Extramedullary hematopoiesis
d. Hyperplastic nodules

11. How is feline hepatic lipidosis recognized cytologically?

Fatty change in hepatocytes appears as discrete, clear, round intracytoplasmic vacuoles. Mild and moderate fat deposition does not equal a cytologic diagnosis of hepatic lipidosis. The fatty deposition must be marked to make a cytologic diagnosis. Often the hepatocytes will be so filled with fat that it is difficult to recognize them as hepatocytes (Figure 44-4). Also, the background of the smear typically contains much fat. The presence of fat can be confirmed by applying Sudan III stain (which stains fat red) to fresh (unstained) smears of liver aspirates.

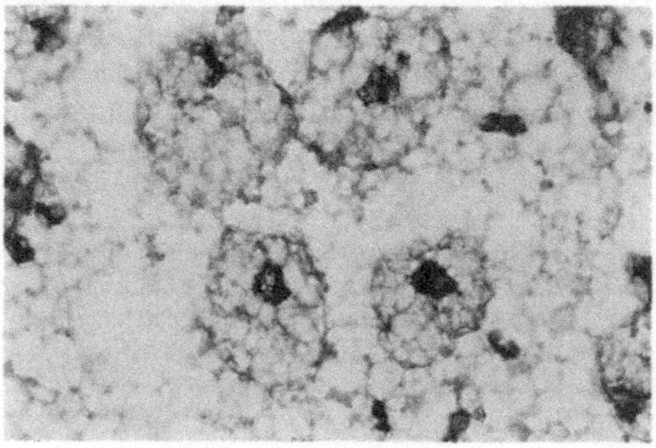

Figure 44-4 Hepatic lipidosis. Liver aspirate from a cat showing hepatocytes with marked fatty deposition and many fat spaces in the background of the smear. (Wright's stain; 250×.)

12. How is glycogen accumulation recognized cytologically?

Excessive *glycogen accumulation* in hepatocytes appears as indistinct (wispy) vacuoles (Figure 44-5). The hepatocytes may be much larger than normal because of the glycogen and water accumulation. The presence of glycogen can be confirmed with periodic acid–Schiff (PAS) stain. In dogs, a high level of plasma glucocorticoids is a common cause of excessive glycogen accumulation (steroid hepatopathy).

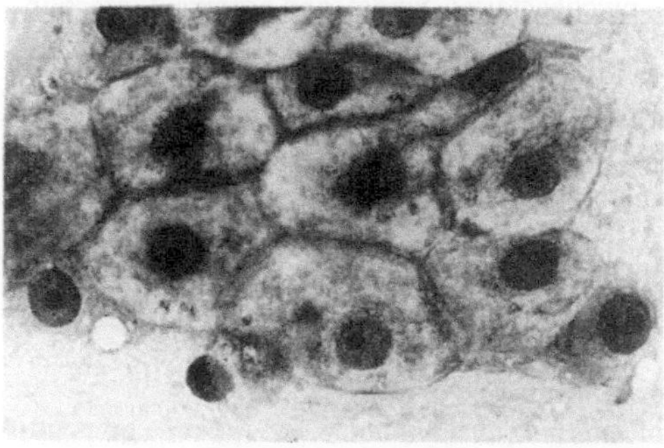

Figure 44-5 Glycogen deposition. Liver aspirate from a dog showing a group of hepatocytes with marked glycogen deposition. (Wright's stain; 250×.)

13. How is amyloid recognized cytologically?

Amyloid appears as swirls of extracellular, eosinophilic, amorphous material in close association with hepatocytes. Amyloid stains a birefringent apple green under polarized light with Congo red stain. Amyloid is an uncommon finding.

14. List types of inflammation seen in liver aspirates.

a. Neutrophilic inflammation
b. Histiocytic or macrophagic inflammation
c. Lymphocytic or lymphoplasmacytic inflammation
d. Eosinophilic inflammation

15. How is neutrophilic inflammation recognized cytologically?

The presence of high numbers of mature neutrophils relative to the number of red blood cells (RBCs) suggests *neutrophilic inflammation.* However, blood contamination from an animal with a peripheral leukocytosis will appear similar. The presence of neutrophils in hepatocellular clumps supports neutrophilic inflammation.

16. What are some causes of neutrophilic inflammation?

Common causes of neutrophilic inflammation include necrosis, bacterial infection (Figure 44-6), sterile inflammatory processes (e.g., pancreatitis-induced hepatitis), feline infectious peritonitis (FIP), and feline suppurative cholangiohepatitis. Blood contamination, especially from animals with peripheral blood neutrophilia, can artifactually appear to represent increased numbers of neutrophils in the cytology smear and may be mistaken for neutrophilic inflammation.

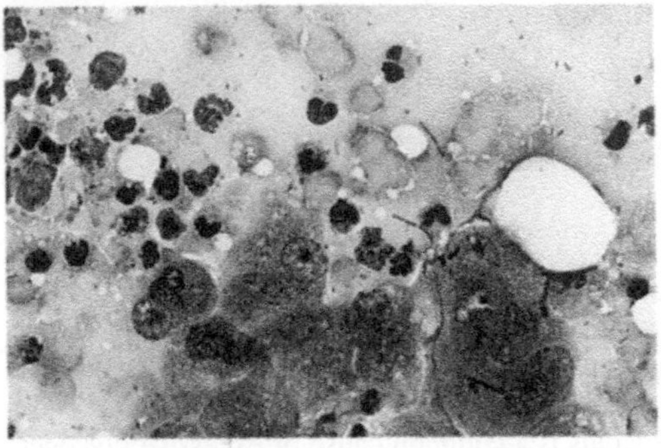

Figure 44-6 Septic neutrophilic inflammation. Liver aspirate from a dog showing many neutrophils, a group of hepatocytes, and bacterial rods. A moderate number of RBCs is also present. (Wright's stain; 250×.)

17. What are some causes of histiocytic or macrophagic inflammation?

Causes of histiocytic inflammation include mycobacterial, fungal, and protozoal infections; FIP; and immune-mediated disorders.

18. What are some causes of lymphocytic or lymphoplasmacytic inflammation?

Small lymphocytes, with or without plasma cells, are typically seen in older cats with lymphocytic cholangitis or cholangiohepatitis and may be seen in dogs with chronic progressive hepatitis. A lymphocytic or lymphoplasmacytic inflammation may be difficult to differentiate from small cell lymphoma. Often, biopsy and histopathology are needed to rule out small cell lymphoma.

19. What is mixed-cell inflammation, and what are some causes?

Mixed-cell inflammation is the presence of multiple inflammatory cell types (e.g., neutrophils, small lymphocytes, macrophages) in variable numbers. Causes of mixed-cell inflammation include infectious disorders (e.g., mycotic, protozoal, viral [FIP]), chronic neutrophilic cholangiohepatitis, and nodular regenerative hyperplasia in older dogs.

20. What are some causes of eosinophilic inflammation?

Causes of eosinophilic inflammation include hypereosinophilic syndrome in cats, liver flukes, and occasionally, eosinophilic enteritis and disseminated mast cell tumors.

21. How is extramedullary hematopoiesis recognized cytologically?

Although an occasional hematopoietic precursor cell may be found in aspirates from normal liver, *extramedullary hematopoiesis* is recognized by the presence of hematopoietic cells at all stages of maturation, with a predominance of the more mature stages. Cells of the erythroid series usually predominate when associated with anemia. Granulocytic and megakaryocytic cell types may be present, and granulocytes may be the predominant cell type, especially with nodular regenerative hyperplasia in dogs. If immature hematopoietic precursor cells predominate, neoplastic disease (not extramedullary hematopoiesis) is indicated. Myelolipoma is a rare, benign neoplasm that contains lipid and hematopoietic cells and may be confused cytologically with extramedullary hematopoiesis.

22. What are the cytologic characteristics of hyperplastic nodules and hepatic adenomas, and how are they distinguished?

Both hyperplastic nodules and hepatic adenomas may occur as single or multiple masses. Cytologically, they may appear similar to or indistinguishable from normal hepatocytes. Mild anisocytosis and anisokaryosis, increased cytoplasmic basophilia, binucleate hepatocytes, and increased numbers of intranuclear inclusions may be seen. In some cases, cytology, clinical findings, diagnostic imaging, and history can be correlated to help differentiate hyperplastic nodules from hepatocellular tumors. However, it is not possible to differentiate hyperplastic nodules from hepatic adenomas cytologically, and biopsy and histopathology are needed for a definitive diagnosis.

23. Can hepatocellular carcinomas be recognized cytologically?

Hepatocellular carcinomas are uncommon. They may be composed of hepatocytes that appear relatively normal and cannot be definitively recognized cytologically as malignant, or they may be composed of atypical hepatocytes that are easily recognized as malignant. Therefore, hepatocellular carcinomas that have extremely anaplastic hepatocytes can be diagnosed cytologically, but many cannot and require histopathology.

24. Can bile duct tumors be diagnosed cytologically?

Because of the diffuse nature of many bile duct tumors, the potential for cytologic diagnosis is good. Both bile duct adenomas and carcinomas tend to exfoliate relatively normal-appearing bile duct epithelial cells. These cells tend to be in tightly adhered clusters or sheets. Occasionally, acinar formation is observed. Some adenocarcinomas will have malignant criteria that allow for a diagnosis, whereas others will require histopathology for a definitive diagnosis.

25. Can infectious canine hepatitis be diagnosed cytologically?

Canine adenovirus type 1, the etiologic agent for infectious canine hepatitis (ICH), produces large eosinophilic intranuclear inclusions in hepatocytes that are readily seen cytologically.

26. What is the significance of the rhomboid crystals seen within the nucleus of some hepatocytes?

These rhomboid crystals have no known significance. They tend to occur more often in older dogs.

45. TRANSTRACHEAL WASH AND BRONCHOALVEOLAR LAVAGE

Rick L. Cowell, James H. Meinkoth, and Sylvie Beaudin

1. What are some indications for transtracheal wash and bronchoalveolar lavage (TTW/BAL)?

TTW/BAL is indicated to obtain material for culture and cytologic evaluation in animals with a chronic cough or unresponsive or undiagnosed bronchopulmonary disease.

2. What are the common findings on TTW/BAL from normal animals?

Washes from normal animals typically consist primarily of alveolar macrophages. In TTW, ciliated columnar epithelial cells are often present in moderate to high numbers (Figure 45-1). Cuboidal epithelial cells may also be observed. Small lymphocytes are present in variable numbers (low to moderate) with BAL. A small amount of mucus may be present. Some red blood cells (RBCs) may be present as well as occasional neutrophils, eosinophils, lymphocytes, and mast cells. Also, rare goblet cells may be observed.

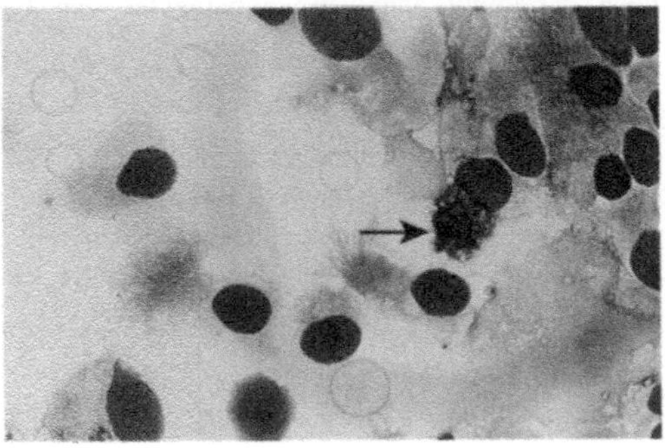

Figure 45-1 Transtracheal wash from a dog showing scattered ciliated columnar epithelial cells and a goblet cell *(arrow)*. (Wright's stain; 250×.)

3. List the common cytologic interpretations from TTW/BAL.

a. Oropharyngeal contamination
b. Eosinophilic infiltrate
c. Neutrophilic infiltrate
d. Histiocytic or macrophagic infiltrate
e. Presence of atypical cells
f. Identification of various organisms

An insufficient sample means no cells or an inadequate number of cells for evaluation.

4. What are goblet cells, and how are they recognized?

Goblet cells are mucus-producing cells. They are epithelial cells that are generally columnar in shape with a basally placed nucleus and medium-sized, roundish, intracytoplasmic granules of mucus (see Figure 45-1). Occasionally the granules will distend the cytoplasm so greatly that the cell may appear round. The granules may stain red, blue, or clear with various stains. Goblet cell numbers may increase secondary to any chronic airway irritant.

5. What are Curschmann spirals?

Curschmann spirals are mucous casts of small bronchioles. They appear as spiral, twisted masses of mucus that may have perpendicular radiations, giving the spirals a "test tube brush-like" appearance (Figure 45-2). Curschmann spirals may be found with any disease or disorder that results in chronic, excessive production of mucus.

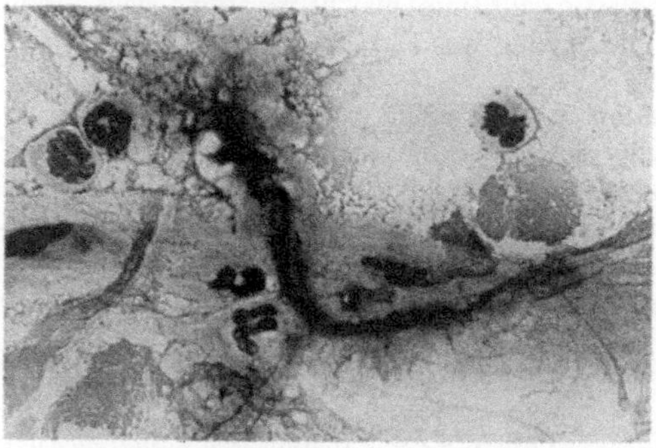

Figure 45-2 Transtracheal wash from a dog showing a Curschmann spiral, mucus, and some neutrophils. (Wright's stain; 250×.)

6. How is oropharyngeal contamination recognized cytologically?

The hallmark of oropharyngeal contamination is the presence of superficial squamous epithelial cells and/or *Simonsiella* organisms. Often the superficial squamous epithelial cells are coated with a population of mixed bacteria that represent the normal flora of the oropharyngeal area and esophagus. If oropharyngeal contamination is present, culture results are of questionable significance. Neutrophils may be present secondary to oropharyngeal contamination if inflammation affects the oropharyngeal area (e.g., dental disease, ulcers). When oropharyngeal contamination and inflammation are present, the source of inflammation (lungs, oropharyngeal area) may be difficult or impossible to determine.

7. What are *Simonsiella* organisms, and how are they recognized?

Simonsiella organisms are rod-shaped bacteria that divide lengthwise and line up in parallel rows, giving the appearance of a single large bacterium (Figure 45-3). These are nonpathogenic organisms and indicate oropharyngeal contamination. They may adhere to the surface of superficial squamous epithelial cells or may be free in the background of the smear.

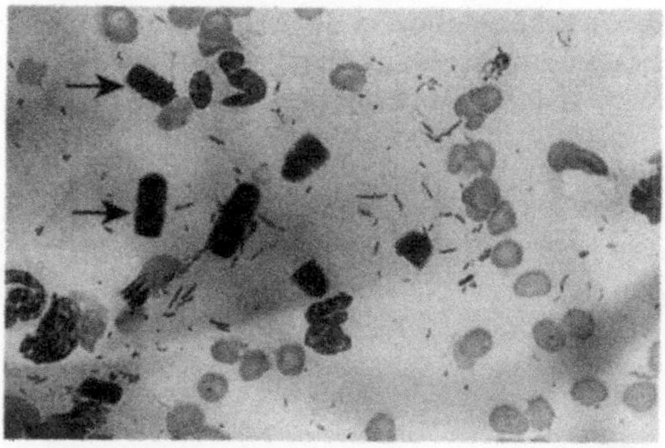

Figure 45-3 Transtracheal wash from a dog showing red blood cells, bacterial rods, and scattered *Simonsiella* organisms *(arrows)*. (Wright's stain; 250×.)

8. How long should one wait before repeating a TTW/BAL wash?

Generally, when TTW/BAL needs to be repeated for any reason, the wash should be repeated either immediately or after waiting 48 hours. A TTW/BAL wash, even though sterile saline solution is used, will induce a neutrophilic response that will peak at about 24 hours but will have abated by 48 hours. Therefore, if the wash is repeated the next day, it will be difficult to differentiate mild to moderate neutrophilic inflammation secondary to the previous wash from inflammatory lung disease. The wash can be repeated immediately, and although some contaminants from the previous wash may be collected, they should be minimal if the second wash is done without further contamination. Waiting 48 hours allows time for the lungs to clear the oropharyngeal contaminants, but the time delay may be problematic by delaying a diagnosis. TTW/BAL washes performed to search for fungal organisms (e.g., *Histoplasma, Blastomyces*), protozoal organisms (e.g., *Toxoplasma*), or neoplastic cells (rare) may be rewarding even during the period when the washes are influenced by the previous wash.

9. What constitutes eosinophilic inflammation in TTW/BAL?

Eosinophilic inflammation (hypersensitivity reaction) is characterized by the presence of increased numbers of eosinophils in the wash (Figure 45-4). Eosinophil numbers as high as 20% to 25% have been reported in bronchial washes from some normal cats, but greater than 5% eosinophils in dogs or 10% eosinophils in cats is considered an increased number and supportive of eosinophilic inflammation. Eosinophilic inflammation in the lungs may be present with or without a peripheral blood eosinophilia.

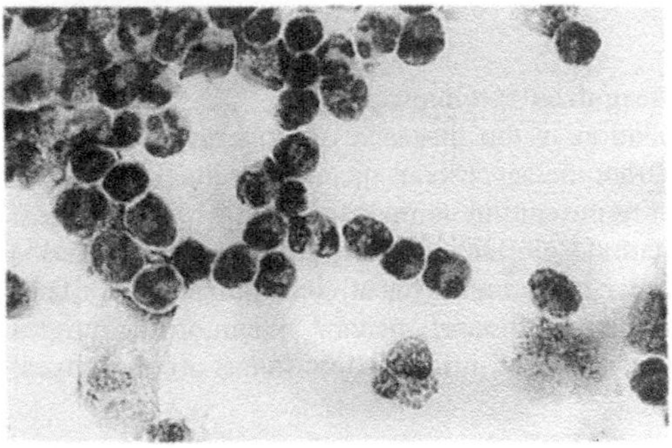

Figure 45-4 Transtracheal wash from a dog showing high numbers of eosinophils and a rare neutrophil. (Wright's stain; 250×.)

10. What are some causes of eosinophilic inflammation in TTW/BAL?

Common causes of eosinophilic inflammation (hypersensitivity reaction) in dogs and cats include allergic bronchitis/pneumonitis, feline asthma, lung worms, heartworms, some mycotic infections, and pulmonary eosinophilic granulomatosis.

11. What constitutes neutrophilic (suppurative) inflammation in TTW/BAL?

Greater than 5% neutrophils in the wash indicates neutrophilic inflammation (Figure 45-5). Neutrophilic inflammation may result from infectious or noninfectious causes.

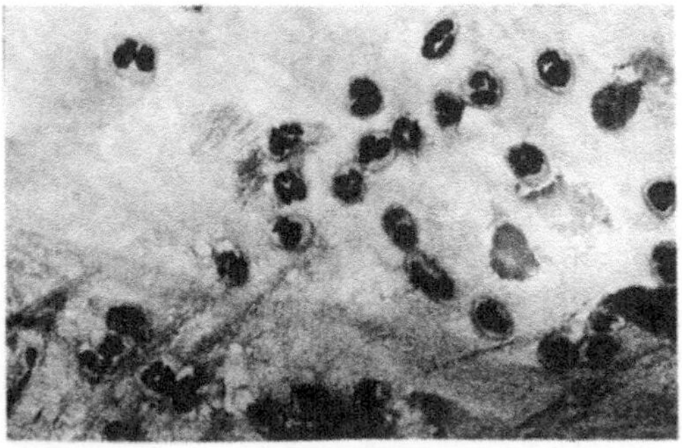

Figure 45-5 Transtracheal wash from a dog showing much mucus and moderate numbers of neutrophils. (Wright's stain; 250×.)

12. What constitutes histiocytic or macrophagic inflammation in TTW/BAL?

Histiocytic or macrophagic inflammation is often difficult to recognize because alveolar macrophages are usually present in normal washes. Recognizing the presence of increased numbers of macrophages is difficult and often impossible. With chronic inflammation, macrophages become activated, and binucleated macrophages are often observed. The presence of multinucleated inflammatory giant cells is an indication of histiocytic or macrophagic inflammation. Some classify the reaction as "granulomatous" if multinucleated inflammatory giant cells are present.

13. What are some causes of histiocytic or macrophagic inflammation?

Histiocytic or macrophagic inflammation may be associated with many different disorders, such as mycotic infections, viral infections (e.g., feline infectious peritonitis [FIP]), protozoal infections, bacterial infections (e.g., *Mycobacterium*), congenital abnormalities of the airway, abnormal function of cilia, and inhalation of noxious substances (e.g., smoke).

14. What constitutes mixed inflammation in TTW/BAL?

A mixed inflammatory response consisting of neutrophils and macrophages may be present in many disorders, including inhalation pneumonia, lung lobe torsion, some mycotic infections, FIP, and protozoal infections.

15. How is intrapulmonary hemorrhage recognized cytologically?

Intrapulmonary hemorrhage is differentiated from blood contamination in TTW/BAL the same way it is differentiated in other cytologic samples. The presence of phagocytized RBCs and RBC breakdown products (hematoidin, hemosiderin) indicate true intrapulmonary hemorrhage. If washes are left undisturbed for a time or shipped overnight, some erythrophagocytosis may occur in the tube. Making smears from the sediment and sending premade smears eliminate this artifact.

16. How can neoplasia be present in the lungs and neoplastic cells not be present on TTW/BAL?

To find neoplastic cells in wash fluid, the neoplasia must be accessible by washing (e.g., in bronchial tree), and the bronchi/bronchioles must not be blocked by mucus. Many pulmonary tumors are interstitial and not accessible by TTW/BAL. In these cases, transthoracic fine-needle biopsy (aspiration or nonaspiration technique) is often used to collect a cytology sample.

17. What tumors are most likely to exfoliate cells into TTW/BAL?

The two pulmonary tumors that are most likely to exfoliate cells into the wash fluid and to be found cytologically are primary bronchiolar adenocarcinoma (Figure 45-6) and lymphosarcoma. The absence of tumor cells does not rule out these or other tumors.

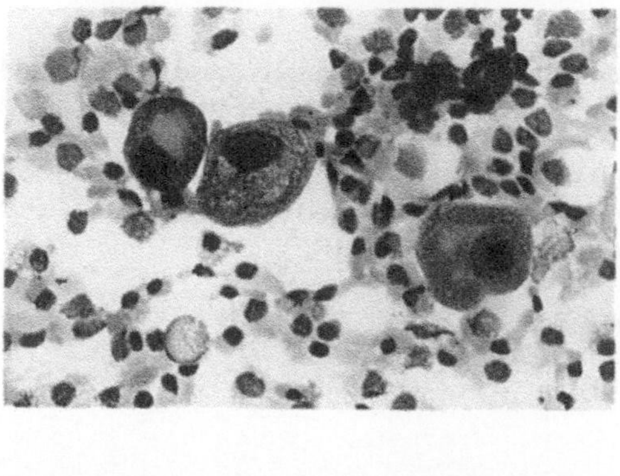

Figure 45-6 Transtracheal wash from a dog showing high numbers of alveolar macrophages and columnar cells, scattered red blood cells, and three large epithelial cells with marked criteria for malignancy (e.g., extremely large, prominent nucleoli; coarse nuclear chromatin). (Wright's stain; 125×.)

46. BODY CAVITY EFFUSIONS (ABDOMINAL, THORACIC, PERICARDIAL)

Rick L. Cowell, Theresa E. Rizzi, and James H. Meinkoth

1. List the three major classifications of effusions.

a. Transudates
b. Modified transudates
c. Exudates

2. What is a transudate?

Transudates are clear, colorless effusions of low protein concentration (<2.5 g/dl) and low total nucleated cell counts (<1500 cells/µl; some use 1000 cells/µl as the cutoff point). These effusions are often referred to as *pure transudates.*

3. How are transudates or pure transudates formed?

Generally, transudates are formed by leakage of protein-poor fluids from small vessels as a result of increased hydrostatic vascular pressure or low plasma oncotic pressure. In the early stages of uroabdomen, the fluid may be in the transudate range since urine is typically low in protein concentration and has a low cell count.

4. What are some causes of pure transudates?

Since plasma albumin concentration is the dominant factor in control of plasma oncotic pressure, severe hypoalbuminemia is a common cause of pure transudates. Other causes include hypertension, early myocardial insufficiency, hepatic insufficiency, and portosystemic shunts.

5. What is a modified transudate?

Modified transudates are transudates that are modified by higher total protein concentrations and cell counts. Reference numbers for modified transudates vary slightly among authors. In general, modified transudates have total protein concentrations greater than 2.5 g/dl and nucleated cell counts between 1000 and 7000/µl in dogs and cats (some use range of 1000-5000 cells/µl). Cell counts in horses are often allowed to be higher and are generally from 1000 to 10,000 nucleated cells/µl. Some overlap between pure transudates and modified transudates exists. In general, if the protein is greater than 2.5 g/dl, the fluid is classified as a modified transudate even if the cell count is in the transudate range.

6. How are modified transudates formed?

Modified transudates are formed by leakage of fluid from small vessels caused by increased vascular permeability and increased hydrostatic pressure within local vascular beds.

7. List common causes of modified transudates.

a. Congestive heart failure (increased hepatic and splanchnic blood pressure)
b. Nonseptic inflammation (e.g., pancreatitis, hepatitis, splenitis)
c. Sterile irritants (e.g., uroabdomen)
d. Vascular insults (e.g., pulmonary thrombosis)
e. Feline infectious peritonitis (FIP)
f. Neoplasia (exfoliative or nonexfoliative)

8. What is an exudate?

Exudates are effusions of high total protein concentration and high nucleated cell count. Again, actual numbers vary among authors. Generally, total protein concentration is greater than 3 g/dl and nucleated cell count greater than 7000 cells/μl in dogs and cats (some use >5000/μl). In horses, nucleated cell count is typically greater than 10,000 cells/μl.

9. How are exudates formed?

Exudates are formed by leakage (exudation) of protein-rich fluid through highly permeable vessels and migration of leukocytes into the cavities in response to chemotactic factors.

10. What are some causes of exudates?

Exudates have both *septic* causes (e.g., bacterial, fungal, protozoal, viral) and *nonseptic* causes (e.g., bile peritonitis, pancreatitis, steatitis, abscesses, inflammation associated with neoplasia).

11. What is a chylous effusion?

Chylous effusions are effusions that contain high amounts of chylomicron-rich lymph fluid. They occur most often in the thoracic cavity. The classic chylous effusion is milky white and consists primarily of small mature lymphocytes (Figure 46-1). Generally, scattered foamy macrophages, neutrophils, and some eosinophils are also present. However, not all chylous effusions are milky white, and small lymphocytes do not always predominate.

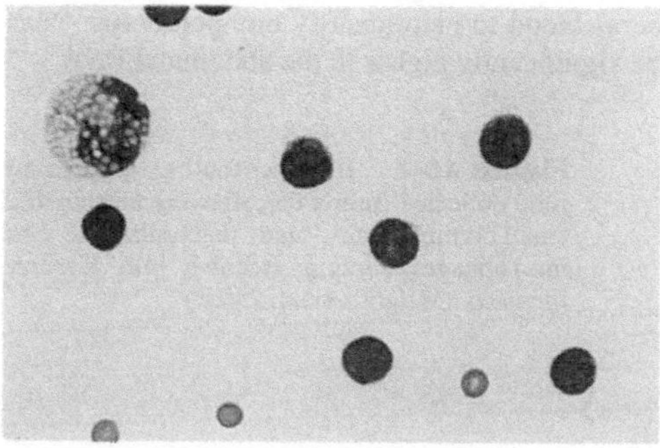

Figure 46-1 Chylous effusion. Milky-white thoracic fluid collected from a cat showing small lymphocytes, two red blood cells, and a single foamy macrophage. (Wright's stain; 250×.)

12. How are chylous effusions formed?

Chylous effusions are formed by leakage of chyle from lymphatics as a result of increased pressure in the lymphatic bed or because of rupture of a major lymphatic vessel.

13. What tests can be performed to confirm fluid as being chylous?

A cholesterol/triglyceride ratio less than 1.0 in the effusion is generally considered diagnostic of a chylous effusion. Other tests include an effusion triglyceride concentration greater than 100 mg/dl in chylous effusions and triglyceride concentrations higher in chylous effusions than in serum at a ratio greater than 3:1.

14. What are some causes of chylous effusions?

Causes of thoracic chylous effusions include cardiovascular disease, neoplasia (generally nonexfoliating neoplasia), dirofilariasis, mediastinal granuloma, diaphragmatic hernia, lung torsion, chronic coughing, vomiting, and thoracic duct rupture.

A chylous effusion in the abdominal cavity is much less common but does occur. Causes include neoplasia, biliary cirrhosis, lymphatic rupture, congenital lymphatic defects, and intra-abdominal steatitis.

15. What is uroperitoneum?

Uroperitoneum refers to the presence of urine within the peritoneal cavity.

16. What are some common causes of uroperitoneum?

Causes of uroperitoneum include ureteral, urinary bladder, and urethral rupture.

17. How is uroperitoneum recognized cytologically?

Acute cases of uroperitoneum often produce effusions in the pure transudate range because urine is of low protein concentration and has a low nucleated cell count. In cases of chronic or longstanding uroperitoneum, a chemical peritonitis may develop, and the effusion may be in the modified transudate or exudate category. Also, if cystitis or protein-losing renal disease preexisted, this will often cause the uroperitoneum to be in the modified transudate or exudative category. Uroperitoneum is typically diagnosed by measuring creatinine levels in the abdominal fluid and peripheral blood. With uroperitoneum, creatinine level is significantly higher in the abdominal fluid than in the blood (generally in 2:1 ratio). Rarely, urine crystals will be identified cytologically to help aid in the diagnosis of uroperitoneum.

18. How is bile peritonitis recognized cytologically?

The first feature often noticed with *bile peritonitis* is the color of the effusion, typically greenish or yellow-orange (bile colored). The effusion is typically in the modified transudate or exudative range. Macrophages containing phagocytized bile pigments (blue-green to yellow-green) can be seen cytologically and indicate bile peritonitis (Figure 46-2). Bilirubin levels can be measured in the abdominal fluid and peripheral blood to help identify bile peritonitis. With bile peritonitis, bilirubin concentration should be significantly higher in the abdominal fluid.

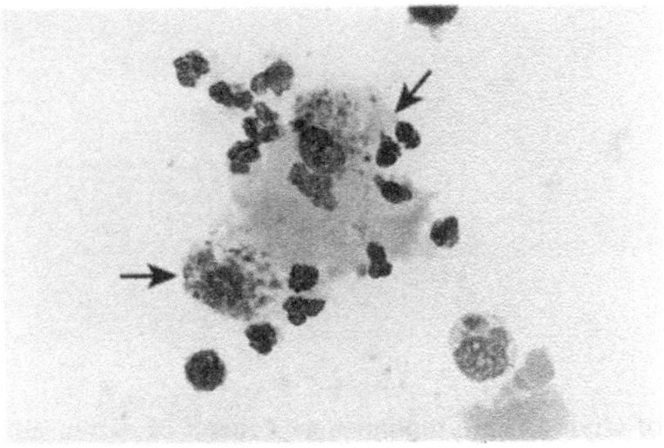

Figure 46-2 Bile peritonitis. Abdominal fluid collected from a dog showing neutrophils, small lymphocytes, and macrophages. The macrophages contain greenish bile pigment *(arrows)*. (Wright's stain; 250×.)

19. What is the typical cytologic appearance of an effusion secondary to cardiovascular disease?

Effusions secondary to cardiovascular disease are usually in the modified transudate category. However, occasional effusions will be in the pure transudate range. Ascites secondary to right-sided heart failure is a common problem in veterinary medicine. The ascites develops secondary to the increased intrahepatic pressure and subsequent leakage of high-protein lymph from hepatic lymphatics. No cytologic findings in the effusion are diagnostic of heart failure. Simply an effusion in the modified transudate range in an animal with heart failure suggests the effusion is secondary to the cardiovascular disease.

20. What is the cytologic appearance of an effusion secondary to feline infectious peritonitis?

The effusion of FIP is typically an odorless, straw-colored to golden, tenacious fluid that foams when shaken. Fibrin strands and flecks may be present in the effusion, and the effusion may clot. The effusion typically has a high protein concentration (>3.5 g/dl) and a moderate cell count (2000-6000 nucleated cells/µl) and is in the modified transudate category. However, the effusion may be in the exudate category, with nucleated cell counts greater than 25,000/µl reported. Cytologically, smears typically consist primarily of nondegenerative neutrophils in a thick, precipitous eosinophilic background with protein crescents. The cytologic appearance of the effusion is not pathognomonic for FIP but is presumptive of FIP.

21. How is a hemorrhagic effusion differentiated from blood contamination?

Hemorrhage into a body cavity quickly results in red blood cells (RBCs) being phagocytized and RBC breakdown products forming over time. Also, platelets in a body cavity quickly aggregate, degranulate, and are removed. Therefore, blood contamination tends to have platelets and no RBC phagocytosis or RBC breakdown products. While intracavity hemorrhage tends to have RBC phagocytosis (with or without RBC breakdown products depending on duration) and no platelets (Figure 46-3).

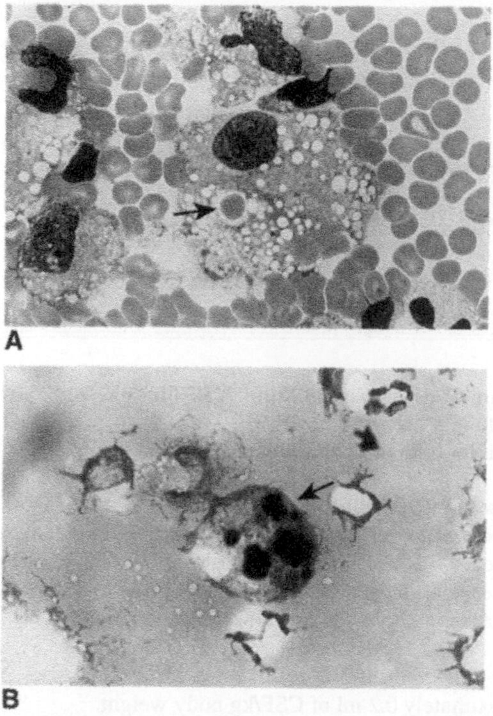

Figure 46-3 Intraabdominal hemorrhage. **A,** Cytospin smear of abdominal fluid showing many red blood cells (RBCs), a few small lymphocytes, and macrophages. Erythrophagocytosis is present *(arrow).* **B,** Same case as in *A* showing a macrophage with RBC breakdown products (hemosiderin) *(arrow).* (Wright's stain; 250×.)

However, chronic active hemorrhage or blood contamination of a hemorrhagic effusion can result in the presence of platelets along with phagocytized RBCs. Also, if blood contamination is present and the fluid is allowed to sit in the tube for a prolonged period before smears of the fluid are made, RBC phagocytosis may occur in the tube.

22. How is a neoplastic effusion recognized cytologically?

Tumor cells in effusions are generally recognized by finding high numbers of immature (blastic) cells (e.g., lymphoblasts) in the effusion or by finding epithelial cells (or rarely spindle cells) with sufficient criteria of malignancy to make a diagnosis of neoplasia (Figure 46-4). It is important not to confuse reactive mesothelial cells with carcinoma cells, especially in pericardial effusions. Many neoplastic effusions do not exfoliate neoplastic cells into the fluid, and in these effusions, neoplasia cannot be diagnosed cytologically.

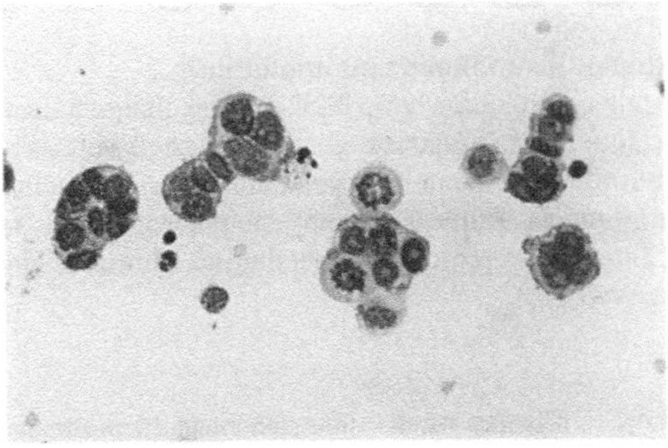

Figure 46-4 Adenocarcinoma. Thoracic fluid collected from a cat showing clusters (acini) of large epithelial cells with many criteria of malignancy. Metastatic mammary adenocarcinoma was final diagnosis at necropsy. (Wright's stain; 250×.)

47. CEREBROSPINAL FLUID ANALYSIS

Rick L. Cowell, James H. Meinkoth, and Theresa E. Rizzi

1. **List the two common sites for collection of cerebrospinal fluid (CSF) in dogs and cats.**
   a. Atlantooccipital space (cerebellomedullary cistern)
   b. Lumbar subarachnoid space: between the fifth and sixth lumbar vertebrae (L5-6)

2. **What determines which location to use for CSF collection?**
   Selection is based on the neurologic localization of the lesion. The atlantooccipital space (cerebellomedullary cistern) is used to collect CSF when the lesions are above the foramen magnum or for lesions of the extreme craniocervical spinal cord. The lumbar subarachnoid space, L5-6, is used as the site of CSF collection for lesions below the craniocervical spinal cord.

3. **How much cerebrospinal fluid can be collected safely?**
   CSF can be collected safely up to approximately 0.2 ml of CSF/kg body weight.

4. **Are there times when CSF collection is contraindicated?**
   CSF collection is contraindicated when anesthesia is contraindicated and in animals with increased intracranial pressure (ICP) because of the risk of brain herniation.

5. **Describe normal cerebrospinal fluid.**
   CSF is a clear, colorless, transparent fluid with very low cellularity (almost acellular). Reference ranges are 0 to 5 cells/µl for dogs and 0 to 8 cells/µl for cats. Most normal dogs and cats have between 0 and 2 cells/µl. CSF also has very low protein concentration (10-20 mg/dl for CSF from atlantooccipital space; <40 mg/dl for CSF from L5-6).

6. List the components of a routine CSF analysis.

a. Examination of physical characteristics of CSF (e.g., color, turbidity)
b. Total nucleated cell count (TNCC)
c. Erythrocyte count
d. Protein concentration
e. Cytologic evaluation of sediment smears

7. What other tests are sometimes performed on a CSF analysis?

Other tests done on the CSF analysis include the Pandy test, various biochemical measurements (e.g., glucose, creatine kinase, lactate dehydrogenase), electrophoresis, and culture.

8. What is the Pandy test?

The *Pandy test* is a procedure to determine the presence of immunoglobulins in CSF. In normal animals, the Pandy test should be negative.

9. How is the Pandy test performed, and what is its sensitivity?

The Pandy test is performed by adding a few drops of CSF to 1 ml of 10% carboxylic acid (Pandy reagent). If turbidity develops, the test is positive (presence of immunoglobulins). The test has a sensitivity of about 50 mg immunoglobulin/dl CSF.

10. How quickly should cerebrospinal fluid be processed?

Cell counts and cytology smears should be done within 30 to 60 minutes of CSF collection.

11. Why does the CSF sample need to be processed so quickly?

The low protein concentration of CSF causes the cells to lyse quickly.

12. What if the CSF sample cannot be processed quickly?

If the CSF sample cannot be processed within 30 minutes, 40% ethanol can be added in a 1:1 ratio with the CSF to help preserve the cells. Other choices are adding plasma, 20% albumin, 4% to 10% neutral buffered formalin, or 50% to 90% alcohol in a 1:1 ratio with CSF. Also, adding 1 drop of 10% formalin to 1 to 2 ml of CSF has been suggested. Formalin will interfere with staining of the sample (Romanowsky stains), and many laboratories do not recommend its use. All these preservation measures will interfere with other tests (e.g., biochemical analysis) and will falsely decrease the cell count (dilution effect). The cell count is multiplied by two to correct for the dilution effect.

In addition, CSF samples are often split, and 40% ethanol (or one of the other choices) is added to one of the two sample halves to help preserve cells for cell counts and cytology. Ethanol (or other) is not added to the other sample half so that it can be used for other testing, such as protein concentration and biochemical analysis, which are relatively stable. Refrigeration of the sample also helps to slow down cell lysis.

13. How is a total nucleated cell count performed on CSF?

Cell counts can be performed by drawing a small amount of new methylene blue (NMB) into a microhematocrit tube, removing the tube from the NMB, and tilting the tube to create a small air pocket. CSF is then drawn into the tube (CSF and NMB are separated by the small air pocket), and the tube is gently rocked back and forth several times so that the two columns of liquid move back and forth. A small amount of dye will line the inside surface of the tube as it is rocked and will stain the cells as CSF passes by. The tube is allowed to sit for a short time undisturbed (no longer than 10 minutes). Then the CSF is loaded directly into a hemocytometer, and the cells are counted. With practice, one can perform a count without using the NMB. This method is used because the TNCC of normal CSF is too low to be performed on an automated hematology analyzer or by a standard Unopette system.

14. Can CSF protein concentration be accurately determined by a refractometer reading or by the techniques used to determine total protein concentration of serum or plasma?

The protein concentration of CSF is too low to be accurately determined by a refractometer or by the methods used for serum proteins.

15. How is the CSF protein concentration determined in the laboratory?

One of the microprotein assays, such as Coomassie brilliant blue, is used to measure the protein concentration of cerebrospinal fluid in the laboratory. One of the microprotein assays must be used because CSF protein concentrations are typically extremely low.

16. Can CSF protein concentration be performed in the clinic?

Although most clinics do not have the machines to perform quantitative microprotein levels, a semiquantitative CSF protein measurement can be determined using a urine dipstick. The protein pads on urine dipsticks are made to measure very low concentrations of albumin. The pads are very insensitive to globulins, however, so the protein concentration will be underestimated, especially if globulins account for much of the protein in the CSF (some inflammatory conditions). Urine dipsticks allow for an estimate of CSF protein levels when a quantitative microprotein assay cannot be performed.

17. How is a cytology smear made from cerebrospinal fluid?

Because normal CSF is of very low cellularity, some type of concentrated smear must be made. Most laboratories will make concentrated smears using a cytocentrifuge. If CSF cytology is being evaluated in the clinic, most practitioners make concentrated smears by sedimentation techniques. Several techniques are available, but most practitioners use one of the syringe barrel sedimentation techniques.

18. What is cytoalbuminemic dissociation?

An increased CSF protein concentration often is associated with an elevated TNCC. The term *cytoalbuminemic dissociation* is used when the CSF protein concentration is increased but the TNCC is within the reference range.

19. List some causes of cytoalbuminemic dissociation.

a. Blood contamination
b. Intervertebral disk disease
c. Trauma
d. Fibrocartilaginous embolism
e. Cervical spondylomyelopathy
f. Degenerative spinal cord disease (e.g., degenerative myelopathy of German shepherds)
g. Neoplasia, especially primary central nervous system tumors deep within parenchyma of brain

20. Will cytoalbuminemic dissociation be evident from either site used for CSF collection?

Whether cytoalbuminemic dissociation will be evident depends on the location of the lesion. CSF protein levels are more likely to be elevated or more significantly elevated when CSF is collected at a site caudal to the lesion. Therefore, CSF collected from L5-6 is more likely to have an elevated protein concentration than CSF from the atlantooccipital space.

21. What causes cerebrospinal fluid to be turbid?

Turbidity is caused by particles suspended in the fluid. It takes approximately 200 nucleated cells or 400 red blood cells (RBCs) per microliter of CSF before turbidity is visible grossly.

22. Are erythrocytes (RBCs) present in normal CSF?

Erythrocytes are not found in normal CSF. The presence of RBCs in CSF indicates either blood contamination during sample collection *(traumatic tap)* or true intracavity hemorrhage (*hemorrhage by rhexis:* vessel wall not intact; *hemorrhage by diapedesis:* vessel wall intact).

23. How is hemorrhage from a traumatic tap differentiated from true intracavity hemorrhage?

Hemorrhage from a traumatic tap will generally be a pink to red color that clears with centrifugation of the CSF (clear supernatant and red pellet of erythrocytes at bottom of tube). CSF generally starts out clear and then develops a red discoloration, or starts out red and then becomes clear.

True intracavity hemorrhage tends to have RBC breakdown products, producing a yellow to orange *(xanthochromic)* color to the fluid that does not clear with centrifugation. Macrophages may be observed containing phagocytized RBCs or RBC breakdown products (hemosiderin, hematoidin). CSF it typically discolored throughout its collection.

24. What is pleocytosis?

An elevated total nucleated cell count in CSF is termed a *pleocytosis*. Pleocytosis can be subclassified as either neutrophilic, mononuclear, mixed, or eosinophilic.

25. Will a CSF sample collected 8 hours after a negative myelogram be abnormal?

The CSF sample will be abnormal because myelography induces an inflammatory response within 90 minutes that lasts for at least 24 hours. The inflammatory response is usually mixed but may be neutrophilic.

26. List some causes of a neutrophilic pleocytosis.

a. Steroid-responsive meningitis
b. Necrotizing vasculitis
c. Infection
   (1) Feline infectious peritonitis (FIP)
   (2) Bacterial
   (3) Rickettsial (e.g., *Ehrlichia ewingii*)
   (4) Mycotic (e.g., cryptococcosis)
d. Intervertebral disk disease
e. Spinal trauma
f. Necrosis
g. Neoplasia (primarily meningioma)
h. Cervical spondylomyelopathy

27. List some causes of a mononuclear pleocytosis.

a. Canine distemper virus
b. Granulomatous meningoencephalitis (GME)
c. Necrotizing meningoencephalitis (pug encephalitis)
d. *Ehrlichia canis*
e. Toxoplasmosis
f. Neosporosis
g. Bacterial meningitis after treatment with antibiotics

28. What are some causes of a mixed pleocytosis?

Causes of a mixed pleocytosis include granulomatous meningoencephalitis (GME) and many of the same diseases that cause a neutrophilic pleocytosis.

29. List some causes of an eosinophilic pleocytosis.

a. Idiopathic, eosinophilic meningoencephalitis
b. Protozoal encephalitis (toxoplasmosis, neosporosis)
c. Larval migration
d. Protothecosis
e. Some mycotic infections (e.g., cryptococcosis)

48. VAGINAL CYTOLOGY

Rick L. Cowell, James H. Meinkoth, and Debbie J. Cunningham

1. List the four types of normal vaginal epithelial cells identified on cytology smears.

a. Basal cells
b. Parabasal cells
c. Intermediate cells
d. Superficial cells

2. What are basal cells?

Basal cells are located on the basement membrane and are the precursor cell for the other vaginal epithelial cells (parabasal, intermediate, superficial). Basal cells are seldom observed on vaginal cytology smears and appear as small cells with a small amount of basophilic cytoplasm.

3. What are parabasal cells?

Parabasal cells are the smallest and most immature of the epithelial cells typically observed on cytology smears. They appear as small round cells with a small amount of basophilic cytoplasm and a roundish nucleus. Parabasal cells with cytoplasmic vacuoles are called *foam cells.*

4. What are intermediate cells?

Intermediate cells are larger than parabasal cells, often being twice as large or larger. Depending on their size, intermediate cells are subclassified into small and large intermediate cells. The size of intermediate cells depends on the amount of their cytoplasm because the nucleus of both large and small intermediate cells is about the same size and typically roundish. The cytoplasm of small intermediate cells is usually smooth and round to slightly oval. The cytoplasm of large intermediate cells tends to be angular and occasionally may also be irregular and folded. The cytoplasm is typically blue to blue-green in both small and large intermediate epithelial cells. The terms *superficial* and *transitional* are occasionally used for *large* intermediate cells.

5. What are superficial cells?

Superficial cells are the most mature cells of vaginal epithelial stages. They are large cells with abundant, angular or folded, blue to blue-green cytoplasm. The cytoplasm may contain a few to many vacuoles, and some cells may contain dark-staining bodies of unknown significance. The nucleus is smaller than that of intermediate cells and may be faded or even absent (anucleate). The maturation process and development of superficial cells are often referred to as *cornification,* and superficial epithelial cells are sometimes referred to as *cornified cells.*

6. List the cytologic stages of the estrous cycle.

a. Proestrus
b. Estrus
c. Diestrus
d. Anestrus

7. What are the cytologic features of proestrus in dogs?

a. Admixture of parabasal cells, small and large intermediate cells, and superficial epithelial cells
   (1) In *early proestrus,* parabasal cells and small intermediate cells greatly predominate.
   (2) As proestrus advances closer to estrus, the absolute number and percentage of large intermediate cells and superficial cells increase, and these cells become the predominant cell types present on the cytology smears.
   (3) About 4 days before the *luteinizing hormone* (LH) *peak,* parabasal and small intermediate cells are no longer observed on cytology smears.
b. Usually a few up to many red blood cells (RBCs) and neutrophils are present, although they may be absent. Their numbers decrease in late proestrus.
c. *Bacteria,* generally small bacterial rods, often are present in high numbers both adhered to the epithelial cells and free throughout the smear. Although generally present in high numbers, bacterial numbers may range from none to many on cytology smears.
d. *Mucus* may increase sufficiently to give the background of the smear a "dirty" appearance.

8. Are the red blood cells observed on proestrus vaginal cytology smears from vaginal vessels?

RBCs observed during proestrus are not from vaginal vessels; they are erythrocytes exiting *uterine* capillaries by diapedesis.

9. What is the duration of proestrus in dogs?

In normal dogs, proestrus ranges from 2 to 17 days (depending on the reference source) with a mean duration of 9 days.

10. How do the cytologic features of proestrus in cats differ from those in dogs?

In cats, RBCs and neutrophils are absent, so only the epithelial cells are present. The epithelial cell changes are similar to those in dogs. Also, bacteria may be present.

11. What are the cytologic features of estrus in dogs?

a. Greater than 90% of the epithelial cells are *superficial* cells (Figure 48-1). These may all be superficial epithelial cells with small pyknotic nuclei, all anucleate cells, or any mixture of the types. Occasionally the cells more closely resemble large intermediate cells (larger nucleus).
b. Neutrophils should be absent. The presence of neutrophils is an abnormal finding and suggests inflammation.
c. RBCs may be present or absent. When present, RBCs come from uterine capillaries.
d. Bacteria are often present in high numbers, although the numbers are variable and bacteria may be absent.

12. How do the cytologic features of estrus in cats differ from those in dogs?

The cytologic features are similar except that superficial epithelial cells may comprise less than 90% (40%-88%) in feline estrus and RBCs are absent. Anucleate superficial epithelial cells generally make up 10% to 40% of the epithelial cells. Also, a prominent clearing of the background is observed in most cases of feline estrus, which some suggest is a sensitive indicator of estrus in the cat.

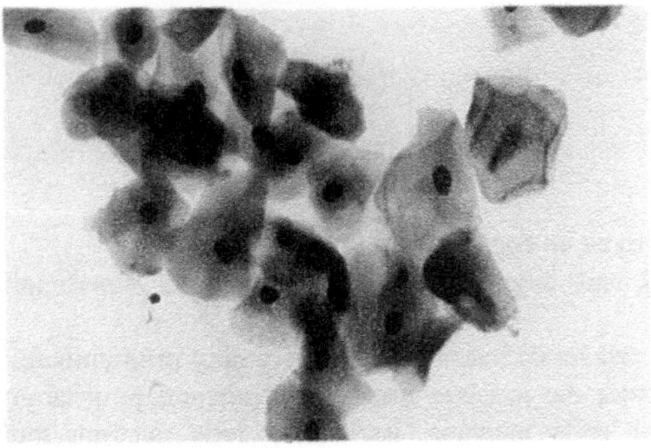

Figure 48-1 Estrus. Vaginal smear from a dog consisting of approximately 100% large superficial epithelial cells. (Wright's stain; 125×.)

13. Is cytology a good predictor of the luteinizing hormone peak and time of ovulation in dogs?

Cytology is *not* a good predictor of LH peak and canine ovulation because too much variation exists. The occurrence of cytologic estrus may range from 6 days before to 3 days after the LH peak. Ovulation usually occurs 1 to 3 days after the LH peak.

14. What is the duration of estrus in dogs?

Duration of estrus in mature dogs has a broad range of 3 to 21 days, with an average duration of 9 days.

15. What is the duration of estrus in cats?

Duration of estrus in cats ranges from 3 to 16 days, with an average duration of 8 days.

16. Is the estrus cycle the same in dogs and cats?

The estrus cycle is not the same in cats and dogs. Cats are seasonally *polyestrus,* with the interval between estrus periods ranging from 4 to 22 days (average of 9 days) unless ovulation occurs. All stages other than estrus may occur during this interval period.

17. Since cats are induced ovulators, can collecting a vaginal swab induce ovulation?

Vaginal swabbing can induce ovulation, but only rarely.

18. When ovulation occurs in a cat, does it delay onset of the next estrus?

Ovulation and pseudopregnancy, which generally follows ovulation, will delay the next estrus for about 45 days.

19. What are the cytologic features of diestrus in the dog?

In canine diestrus there is an abrupt decrease in superficial epithelial cells and an increase in parabasal cells and intermediate cells. Although the number is variable (absent to high numbers), neutrophils are often present in the cytology smear in moderate numbers. Neutrophils also may be observed within the cytoplasm of epithelial cells (see next question). RBCs may be present or absent during diestrus in the dog.

20. What are metestrous cells?

Metestrous cells are epithelial cells that have neutrophils within their cytoplasm. They may occur in any stage of the estrous cycle except estrus in normal dogs and therefore are not specific for diestrus (metestrus). Metestrous cells are more likely to be observed in diestrus because neutrophil migration across epithelial cells typically occurs during diestrus in dogs.

21. When does diestrus occur in the dog?

Canine diestrus occurs about 6 to 10 days after the LH peak, with a mean of 8 days.

22. How do the cytologic features of diestrus in cats differ from those in dogs?

Vaginal cytology smears from cats in diestrus do not contain RBCs. Neutrophils are usually absent, but a few neutrophils may be observed. The epithelial changes are similar to those in dogs.

23. Is the lack of neutrophils and red blood cells a problem in evaluating vaginal cytology smears from cats?

If serial smears are not evaluated, lack of neutrophils and RBCs may be a problem. Feline vaginal cytology smears made during the transition period from estrus to diestrus appear similar to those in proestrus. It is often necessary to evaluate smears daily for several days to identify the stage of estrus accurately.

24. What are the cytologic features of anestrus in the dog?

Vaginal cytology smears during canine anestrus consist primarily of parabasal and intermediate epithelial cells. Neutrophils and bacteria are absent or present only in low numbers.

25. Do the cytologic features of anestrus in the cat differ from those in the dog?

The cytologic features of anestrus in the cat are the same as those in the dog, except neutrophils are absent.

26. What is the cytologic appearance of vaginal smears from prepubertal dogs?

Vaginal cytology smears from prepubertal dogs are similar to those from anestrus dogs, except the smears may have very high numbers of parabasal cells, which occasionally exfoliate in sheets. When parabasal cells exfoliate in sheets, it is important not to confuse them with neoplastic cells.

27. Can spermatozoa be found on vaginal cytology to confirm mating?

The closer the sample collection time is to mating time, the higher the percentage of positive samples to confirm mating. Intact spermatozoa or sperm heads are reportedly present in approximately 65% of the vaginal cytology smears collected 24 hours after mating and 50% of samples collected 48 hours after mating (Figure 48-2). Negative findings cannot be used to rule out mating.

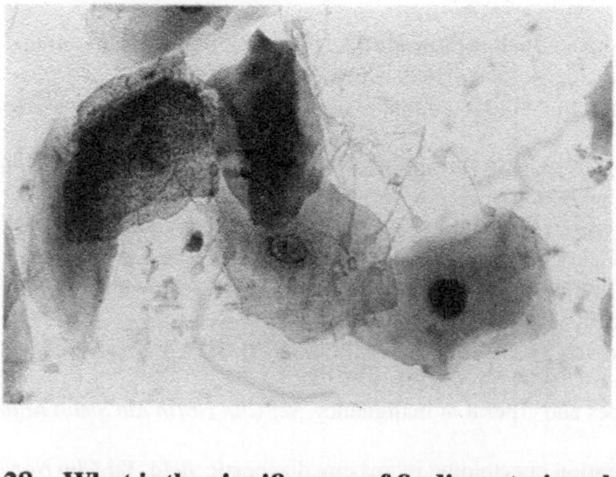

Figure 48-2 Spermatozoa (after mating). Vaginal swab from a cat showing large superficial epithelial cells and many spermatozoa. (Wright's stain; 250×.)

28. What is the significance of finding uterine glandular epithelial cells on a vaginal cytology?

Uterine glandular epithelial cells are occasionally found in vaginal smears, especially soon after whelping and in dogs with subinvolution of placental sites.

29. What is the cytologic appearance of a vaginal smear from a dog with an open pyometra?

The vaginal smear would be of high cellularity and consist primarily of degenerative neutrophils in a dog with an open pyometra. Bacteria may be observed within the cytoplasm of some or many of the neutrophils.

30. How would diestrus be differentiated from pyometra cytologically?

Cytologically, one would expect to see degenerative neutrophils and phagocytized bacteria in an open pyometra and nondegenerative neutrophils with or without phagocytized bacteria in diestrus. (Phagocytized bacteria may be observed in vaginal smears from some dogs during diestrus.)

Cytology

BIBLIOGRAPHY

Baker R, Lumsden JH: Cerebrospinal fluid. In Baker R, Lumsden JH, editors: *Color atlas of cytology of the dog and cat,* St Louis, 2000, Mosby, pp 95-115.

Baker R, Lumsden JH: The gastrointestinal tract: intestines, liver, and pancreas. In Baker R, Lumsden JH, editors: *Color atlas of cytology of the dog and cat,* St Louis, 2000, Mosby, pp 179-181.

Baker R, Lumsden JH: Infectious agents. In Baker R, Lumsden JH, editors: *Color atlas of cytology of the dog and cat,* St Louis, 2000, Mosby, pp 23-29.

Baker R, Lumsden JH: Pleural and peritoneal fluids. In Baker R, Lumsden JH, editors: *Color atlas of cytology of the dog and cat,* St Louis, 2000, Mosby, pp 159-164.

Baker R, Lumsden JH: The reproductive tract: vagina, uterus, prostate, and testicle. In Baker R, Lumsden JH, editors: *Color atlas of cytology of the dog and cat,* St Louis, 2000, Mosby, pp 235-238.

Baker R, Lumsden JH: The respiratory tract: nasal, bronchial, and tracheal wash and lung. In Baker R, Lumsden JH, editors: *Color atlas of cytology of the dog and cat,* St Louis, 2000, Mosby, pp 133-140.

Blue JT, French TW, Meyer DJ: The liver. In Cowell RL, Tyler RD, Meinkoth JH, editors: *Diagnostic cytology and hematology of the dog and cat,* St Louis, 1999, Mosby, pp 183-194.

Burkhard MJ, Valenciano A, Barger A: Respiratory tract. In Raskin RE, Meyer DJ, editors: *Atlas of canine and feline cytology,* Philadelphia, 2002, Saunders, pp 157-182.

Cowell RL: Cytology of neoplasia. In Proceedings of the North American Veterinary Conference, Small Animal and Exotic, Orlando, Fla, 2002, Eastern States Veterinary Association, pp 154-155.

Cowell RL, Dorsey KE, Meinkoth JH: Lymph node cytology, *Vet Clin North Am Small Anim Pract* 33:47-67, 2003.

Cowell RL, Thrall MA, Rebar AH: Cytology of skin masses. In Proceedings of the North American Veterinary Conference, Small Animal and Exotic, Orlando, Fla, 2003, Eastern States Veterinary Association, pp 171-172.

Cowell RL, Tyler RD, Baldwin CJ, Meinkoth JH: Transtracheal/bronchoalveolar washes. In Cowell RL, Tyler RD, Meinkoth JH, editors: *Diagnostic cytology and hematology of the dog and cat,* St Louis, 1999, Mosby, pp 159-173.

Cowell RL, Tyler RD, Meinkoth JH: Abdominal and thoracic fluid. In Cowell RL, Tyler RD, Meinkoth JH, editors: *Diagnostic cytology and hematology of the dog and cat,* St Louis, 1999, Mosby, pp 142-158.

Duncan JR: The lymph nodes. In Cowell RL, Tyler RD, Meinkoth JH, editors: *Diagnostic cytology and hematology of the dog and cat,* St Louis, 1999, Mosby, pp 97-103.

Freeman KP, Raskin RE: Cytology of the central nervous system. In Raskin RE, Meyer DJ, editors: *Atlas of canine and feline cytology,* Philadelphia, 2001, Saunders, pp 325-365.

Henson KL: Reproductive system. In Raskin RE, Meyer DJ, editors: *Atlas of canine and feline cytology,* Philadelphia, 2001, Saunders, pp 289-297.

Lumsden JH, Baker R: Cytopathology techniques and interpretation. In Baker R, Lumsden JH, editors: *Color atlas of cytology of the dog and cat,* St Louis, 2000, Mosby, pp 7-20.

Meinkoth JH, Crystal MA: Cerebrospinal fluid analysis. In Cowell RL, Tyler RD, Meinkoth JH, editors: *Diagnostic cytology and hematology of the dog and cat,* St Louis, 1999, Mosby, pp 125-141.

Meinkoth JH, Cowell RL: Recognition of basic cell types and criteria of malignancy, *Vet Clin North Am Small Anim Pract* 32:1209-1235, 2002.

Meinkoth JH, Cowell RL: Sample collection and preparation in cytology: increasing diagnostic yield, *Vet Clin North Am Small Anim Pract* 32:1187-1207, 2002.

Menard M, Papageorges M: Fine-needle biopsies: how to increase diagnostic yield, *Comp Contin Educ Pract Vet* 19:738-740, 1997.

Meyer DJ: The acquisition and management of cytology specimens. In Raskin RE, Meyer DJ, editors: *Atlas of canine and feline cytology,* Philadelphia, 2001, Saunders, pp 1-17.

Meyer DJ: The liver. In Raskin RE, Meyer DJ, editors: *Atlas of canine and feline cytology,* Philadelphia, 2001, Saunders, pp 231-252.

Raskin RE: General categories of cytologic interpretations. In Raskin RE, Meyer DJ, editors: *Atlas of canine and feline cytology,* Philadelphia, 2001, Saunders, pp 27-33.

Raskin RE: Lymphoid system. In Raskin RE, Meyer DJ, editors: *Atlas of canine and feline cytology,* Philadelphia, 2001, Saunders, pp 93-134.

Raskin RE: Skin and subcutaneous tissues. In Raskin RE, Meyer DJ, editors: *Atlas of canine and feline cytology,* Philadelphia, 2001, Saunders, pp 35-56.

Shelly SM: Body cavity fluids. In Raskin RE, Meyer DJ, editors: *Atlas of canine and feline cytology,* Philadelphia, 2001, Saunders, pp 187-205.

Taylor JA, Baker R: The lymphoid system: lymph nodes, spleen, and thymus. In Baker R, Lumsden JH, editors: *Color atlas of cytology of the dog and cat,* St Louis, 2000, Mosby, pp 71-94.

Thrall MA, Olson PN: The vagina. In Cowell RL, Tyler RD, Meinkoth JH, editors: *Diagnostic cytology and hematology of the dog and cat,* St Louis, 1999, Mosby, pp 240-248.

Tyler RD, Cowell, RL, Baldwin CJ, Morton, RJ: Introduction. In Cowell RL, Tyler RD, Meinkoth JH, editors: *Diagnostic cytology and hematology of the dog and cat,* St Louis, 1999, Mosby, pp 1-19.

Tyler RD, Cowell RL, Meinkoth JH: Cutaneous and subcutaneous lesions: masses, cysts, ulcers, and fistulous tracts. In Cowell RL, Tyler RD, Meinkoth JH, editors: *Diagnostic cytology and hematology of the dog and cat,* St Louis, 1999, Mosby, pp 23-51.

Weiss DJ, Moritz A: Liver cytology, *Vet Clin North Am Small Anim Pract* 32:1267-1291, 2002.

Section XI

Avian and Reptilian Clinical Pathology

Armando R. Irizarry-Rovira

The chapters in this section are not intended as a definitive or extensive discourse on normal avian hematology and diagnosis of avian hematologic disorders (Chapter 49), avian biochemical analysis (Chapter 50), normal reptilian hematology and diagnosis of reptilian hematologic disorders (Chapter 51), reptilian biochemical analysis (Chapter 52), or avian and reptilian cytology (Chapter 53). These chapters are solely intended as quick reference guides to these fascinating areas of avian and reptilian medicine. The discussions focus on the use of hematologic and biochemical principles to help diagnose diseases in pet birds (Chapters 49 and 50) and pet reptiles (Chapters 51 and 52) and the use of cytologic principles to diagnose diseases in live and dead birds and reptiles (Chapter 53). Diseases of wild birds and poultry are mentioned where appropriate to complement the discussion in Chapters 49 and 50.

For detailed discussions on the subjects addressed in these chapters, refer to the Bibliography following Chapter 53.

49. AVIAN HEMATOLOGY

1. How are avian blood cells different from the blood cells of mammals?

Avian blood cells are similar to mammalian blood cells in some aspects but differ significantly in others, particularly morphology. As in mammals, avian blood cells include erythrocytes, leukocytes, and thrombocytes (platelets), all of which are easily evaluated by examination of air-dried, Romanowsky-stained blood smears.

2. What are some important principles to understand about the identification of avian leukocytes by blood smear evaluation?

a. Proper identification of leukocytes depends on familiarity with the morphology of leukocytes and the species of bird, prompt processing of the blood sample, quality of the blood smear, and staining techniques used to visualize the leukocytes.
b. Fresh blood (no anticoagulant) and ethylenediaminetetraacetic acid (EDTA) or heparin anticoagulated blood samples are both satisfactory for use in the identification of leukocytes, but fresh blood smears are preferred. When cell enumeration is required, it is best to keep samples at a cool temperature when shipping. Long transit times may result in inaccurate leukocyte counts, abnormal morphology, or hemolysis (e.g., ostrich erythrocytes in EDTA).
c. Gaining familiarity with leukocyte morphology requires frequent examination of blood samples from normal and sick patients of various species. Staining affinity of cytoplasmic granules may vary between species of birds.
d. Use of consistent staining techniques and methods is important to avoid excessive variation in cell staining and to ensure consistent and accurate leukocyte identification.

e. Formalin fumes, even if the source is a few feet away, will alter cellular proteins in such a way that the staining intensity and affinity of leukocytes will be altered. Therefore, blood smears should be kept away from formalin sources and stained promptly.
f. If a blood smear must be stored for longer periods, either for later examination or for archiving, immersion oil should be removed with appropriate solvents and the slide permanently coverslipped.

3. Describe the various avian leukocytes.

Avian leukocytes include the heterophil, basophil, monocyte, lymphocyte, and eosinophil. Descriptions are based on Romanowsky-stained (e.g., Wright-Giemsa, Diff-Quik) blood smears.

a. The *heterophil* is the predominant leukocyte in health in many avian species and predominates in many disease conditions (Figure 49-1). It has a lobulated, condensed nucleus, although the degree of lobulation is less than that of mammals. The heterophil of most bird species has a cytoplasm that is filled with elongate, rod- to spindle-shaped, orange to brick-red granules.
b. The *eosinophil* has prominent small, round cytoplasmic granules that vary in color from bright red to pink depending on the species (Figure 49-2). In a few species the granules may appear lavender blue using Romanowsky-type stains. The eosinophil is not seen as frequently as the heterophil, and the granules of the eosinophil will stain differently than those of the heterophil within the same blood smear. Compared with other bird species, raptors tend to have slightly greater numbers of eosinophils in circulation.
c. The *basophil* has prominent small, round, deep-magenta to purple cytoplasmic granules and, unlike the mammalian basophil, has a round to oval, nonlobed nucleus (Figure 49-3). The contents of basophil granules can be dissolved by Romanowsky-type stains,

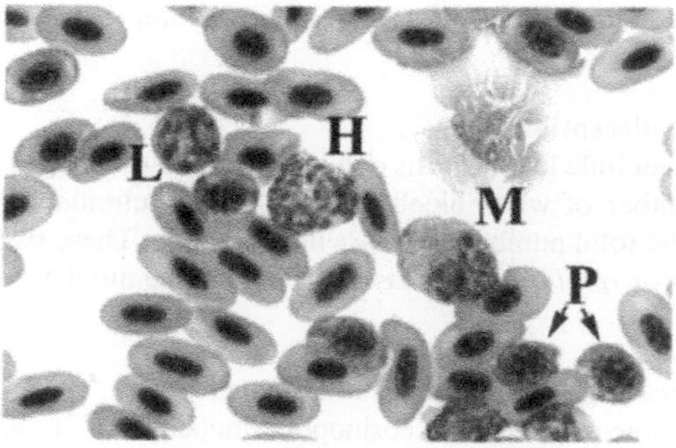

Figure 49-1 Blood smear from an Eclectus parrot. A heterophil *(H)*, lymphocyte *(L)*, monocyte *(M)*, and polychromatophils *(P; arrows)* are shown. (Wright's stain; original magnification 1000×.)

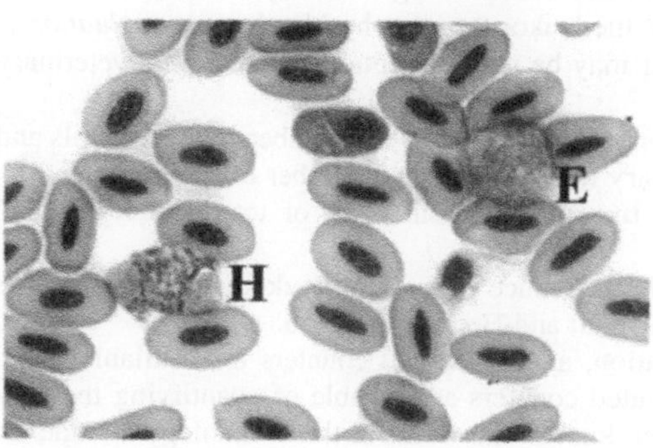

Figure 49-2 Blood smear from a Bald eagle. A heterophil *(H)* and an eosinophil *(E)* are shown. The heterophil has a lobulated nucleus with characteristic spindle-shaped cytoplasmic granules, and the eosinophil has a round nucleus and round granules. (Wright's stain; original magnification 1000×.)

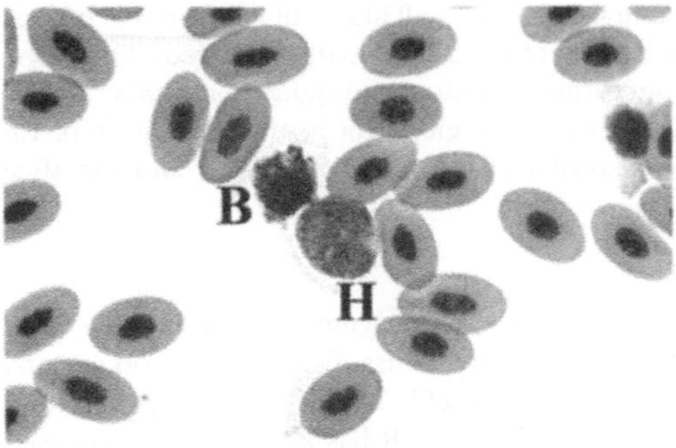

Figure 49-3 A basophil *(B)* and a heterophil *(H)* from an owl. (Wright's stain; original magnification 1000×.)

giving the basophil a foamy, vacuolated appearance with few granules, if any. Careful examination of these cells in a blood smear may reveal a few characteristic granules, particularly over the nucleus, helping to identify them as basophils.

d. The *monocyte* is similar to its mammalian counterpart. It is a large mononuclear cell with abundant cytoplasm and a round to oval to indented nucleus (see Figure 49-1). Monocytes lack the prominent cytoplasmic granules of the granulocytes but may contain fine, dustlike, pink granulation and small, clear vacuoles.

e. The *lymphocyte* is also morphologically similar to that of mammals and is the predominant leukocyte in some species of birds (see Figure 49-1). It is a mononuclear cell, with low to scant amounts of blue cytoplasm, high nuclear/cytoplasmic (N/C) ratio, and a round nucleus. Birds normally have small and larger lymphocytes in circulation. Care must be taken not to confuse the small lymphocytes with thrombocytes. Thrombocytes may be smaller, more oval, with a darker, more condensed nucleus, indistinct pale to nonstaining cytoplasm, and in contrast to lymphocytes, may readily clump in blood smears.

4. What are the most common leukocyte alterations?

The most common leukocyte alterations include leukocytosis and leukopenia. *Leukocytosis* refers to an absolute increase in the total number of white blood cells (WBCs) in circulation. *Leukopenia* refers to an absolute decrease in the total number of WBCs in circulation. These two alterations are the result of increases (*-cytosis* or *-philia*) or decreases *(-penia)* in the number of individual leukocyte cell types.

5. What are common methods of enumerating total numbers of leukocytes?

These methods include *indirect* (blood smear estimation, eosinophil Unopette 5877) and *direct* (Natt and Herrick's) methods. The Unopette system and Natt and Herrick's are labor intensive because they involve manual enumeration of cells using a hemocytometer.

a. Under ideal conditions, estimation of the leukocyte count by *blood smear evaluation* is not as accurate as other methods but may be the only option available in a veterinary practice.

b. The *eosinophil Unopette 5877 system* is used to quantify the numbers of heterophils and eosinophils, but estimation is necessary to determine total number of leukocytes.

c. *Natt and Herrick's method* allows the direct measurement of total leukocytes and erythrocytes.

d. Blood smear evaluation is required to produce differential leukocyte counts for the eosinophil Unopette 5877 and for the Natt and Herrick's method.

For faster, automated, direct quantification, automated cell counters are available based on flow cytometric technology. These automated counters are capable of quantifying the total number of leukocytes in avian blood. However, known drawbacks of this technology include the potential for including nucleated erythrocytes and thrombocytes in the leukocyte count and, generally, inconsistent automated differential cell counts. Manual examination of a blood smear is therefore essential when performing differential cell counts in conjunction with an automated cell counter. Flow cytometric technology is expensive and available primarily to commercial laboratories with the time, finances, and dedicated personnel to utilize and service the technology appropriately. As with any automated technology daily quality control/quality assurance measures must be in place to produce reproducible, accurate results. (For detailed discussion on leukocyte count techniques, see the Bibliography following Chapter 53.)

6. What causes heterophilia?

In general, *heterophilia* may be caused by the following three conditions, acting singly or in combination (Box 49-1):

a. *Physiologic leukocytosis* frequently results in transient heterophilia accompanied by normal or increased lymphocyte counts. It is often seen in young birds and birds not accustomed to handling. Physiologic leukocytosis is mediated by epinephrine release and sudden physical exertion.
b. *Corticosteroid release or administration* is characterized by transient heterophilia accompanied by lymphopenia. It is associated with trauma, pain, disease, stressful conditions, and exogenous glucocorticoid administration. A common term used for the characteristic leukogram changes associated with corticosteroids is *stress leukogram.*
c. *Inflammation* is an important cause of heterophilia in pet birds, resulting from both infectious and noninfectious causes.

Box 49-1 *Causes of Heterophilia in Birds*

Inflammation

Infectious

Mycobacterium spp.
Chlamydophila psittaci (formerly known as *Chlamydia psittaci*)
Miscellaneous bacterial infections and fungi

Noninfectious

Tissue trauma and necrosis (injury, surgery)
Foreign bodies
Egg yolk coelomitis
Neoplasms
Hemorrhage, hemolysis

Corticosteroids

Exogenous

Glucocorticoid administration

Endogenous ("stress")

Excessive handling, physical restraint, unfamiliar environment
Transportation, high density
Food restriction, disease

Physiologic Leukocytosis

Epinephrine mediated
Young excited birds
Sudden physical exertion

Chronic myelogenous leukemia is a rarely seen cause of neutrophilia in domestic animals, and to my knowledge, it is undescribed in pet birds.

7. How do physiologic leukocytosis, corticosteroids, and inflammation result in heterophilia?

a. Heterophil redistribution
b. Decreased egress from the circulation to tissues
c. Increased hematopoietic production

8. Describe the mechanism of heterophil redistribution.

The marginal pool (MP) is not sampled during routine blood collection and consists of heterophils within blood vessels but found rolling along endothelial surfaces or having temporarily ceased moving. Under the influence of corticosteroids, sudden exercise, or epinephrine, mammalian neutrophils and probably bird heterophils redistribute from the MP to the circulating pool (CP).

9. What causes decreased egress of heterophils from the peripheral blood?

Decreased egress for the peripheral blood to the tissues is believed to be primarily caused by the effects of corticosteroids and may be mediated by down-regulation of adhesion molecules on the surfaces of leukocytes or endothelial cells.

10. When does hematopoietic tissue increase production of heterophil precursors?

Increased hematopoietic production of heterophil precursors occurs when there is increased demand for heterophils in the peripheral tissues. Infection (e.g., pneumonia, enteritis, dermatitis), trauma, immune-mediated injury, infarction, and neoplasms may result in increased demand for heterophils. Chemical mediators released from inflammatory cells, infectious agents, and damaged tissue stimulate the bone marrow to increase production. In healthy birds, hematopoietic production occurs primarily in the bone marrow; however, during conditions of increased demand, granulopoiesis may occur in extramedullary sites (e.g., spleen, liver, kidney).

11. What are the expected complete blood count (CBC) findings in birds with heterophilia of physiologic leukocytosis?

Typically, in other domestic animals, absolute increases in neutrophils are mild to moderate in degree; with few exceptions, however, the magnitude of the heterophilia in multiple avian species with physiologic leukocytosis has not been well documented or reported in the literature. In general, leukocyte counts may be higher than 10,000 cells per microliter (μl). For example, nestling psittacines may have leukocyte counts of 20,000 to 40,000 cells/μl, with most of the leukocytes being mature heterophils. Other helpful CBC clues are that physiologic leukocytosis is associated with normal or increased numbers of lymphocytes and that no heterophil left shift or heterophil toxicity occurs.

12. What are the expected CBC findings in birds with heterophilia due to corticosteroid influence?

As with physiologic leukocytosis, the magnitude of heterophilia and leukocytosis in corticosteroid-induced leukograms may be mild to moderate in degree, with most leukocytes being mature heterophils (no left shift, no toxic changes). A defining characteristic is the presence of lymphopenia, which helps distinguish corticosteroid-induced changes from physiologic leukocytosis. CBC changes typical of corticosteroid-induced leukograms may be confounded by the presence of inflammation or myeloproliferative disease.

13. What are the expected CBC findings in birds with heterophilia of inflammatory disease?

Mild heterophilia may be the only abnormality in mild inflammatory disease. With increasing severity, left shift (increased presence of immature heterophils, e.g., band forms, metamyelocytes, myelocytes, promyelocytes), heterophil toxicity (cytoplasmic basophilia, abnormal vacuolation, abnormally shaped cytoplasmic granules, degranulation, large heterophils), and greater numbers of heterophils may be present and reflect a significant demand for heterophils in tissues. Monocytosis may also be observed. In severe inflammatory disease (e.g., chlamydophilosis, mycobacteriosis), total leukocyte counts may reach or exceed 100,000 cells/µl. Keep in mind that overwhelming inflammation may result in heteropenia with left shift and heterophil toxicity (see following questions). The numbers of lymphocytes may be decreased, normal, or increased with inflammatory diseases.

14. What are the predominant causes of heteropenia?

Heteropenia may be caused by the following three conditions, acting singly or in combination (Box 49-2):

a. Overwhelming inflammation resulting in excessive tissue demand for heterophils
b. Decreased bone marrow heterophil production
c. Endotoxemia or gram-negative bacterial infections resulting in heterophil redistribution

Box 49-2 ***Causes of Heteropenia in Birds***

Inflammation

Overwhelming bacterial inflammation
Viral infection

Decreased Heterophil Production

Adverse pharmacologic effects

- Cyclophosphamide
- Other known myelosuppressive drugs
- Fenbendazole: painted storks
- Doxycycline and piperacillin: one case in budgerigars

Myelophthisic syndromes

- Leukemia
- Multicentric lymphosarcoma

Heterophil Redistribution

Endotoxemia
Gram-negative bacterial infections

15. What is the most common cause of overwhelming inflammation?

Overwhelming inflammation is primarily caused by an overwhelming insult (infectious or noninfectious) that elicits massive inflammatory cytokine release and marked, sudden tissue demand for heterophils. The differential list should include, but should not be limited to, disseminated bacterial infections, coelomitis, severe enteritis, and massive tumor necrosis. Any inflammatory condition where the rate at which heterophils exit the circulation exceeds the rate of production by the bone marrow will produce heteropenia. Ultimately, if the demand for heterophils is decreased or bone marrow production is sufficiently augmented, heterophil numbers may increase to within reference intervals or may result in heterophilia.

16. What causes decreased bone marrow heterophil production?

Heterophil production abnormalities may be the result of destruction of heterophil precursors, hormonal/chemical suppression of granulopoiesis, or myelophthisic processes.

Destruction of heterophil precursors in birds may be caused by viral infection or adverse drug reactions (e.g., fenbendazole in painted storks, piperacillin and/or doxycycline in one budgerigar). Suppression of granulopoiesis may occur with hormonal treatment (progesterone) and other myelosuppressive therapy (cyclophosphamide, cancer chemotherapies, radiation). Myelophthisic processes, such as neoplastic disease (leukemia, lymphosarcoma), may infiltrate the bone marrow and displace hematopoietic precursors.

17. Other than inducing overwhelming inflammation, how can endotoxemia contribute to heteropenia?

In domestic animals, during endotoxemia and gram-negative bacterial infections, neutrophils redistribute from the CP to the MP. Redistribution of heterophils from the CP to the MP caused by endotoxemia may also occur in birds.

18. How can the initial CBC help to determine the cause of the heteropenia?

Although heteropenia may be the only hematologic abnormality, birds with inflammatory diseases may have inflammatory leukograms (left shift, heterophil toxicity). Birds with leukemia, myelosuppressive therapy, or idiosyncratic drug reactions may have pancytopenias. Atypical cells in circulation may indicate leukemia.

19. What causes lymphocytosis?

Lymphocytosis may be caused by the following three conditions, acting singly or in combination (Box 49-3):

a. *Physiologic leukocytosis* associated lymphocytosis is accompanied by heterophilia. It is often seen in young birds and birds not accustomed to handling. Physiologic leukocytosis is mediated by epinephrine release or sudden physical exertion.
b. *Chronic antigenic stimulation* may result in a greatly expanded circulating lymphocyte pool. It is seen mainly in patients with chronic inflammation (infectious or non-infectious origin). The most common causes of chronic inflammation in birds are infectious agents (viruses, fungi, parasites, bacteria).
c. *Lymphoproliferative disease* (leukemia, lymphosarcoma) may be accompanied by lymphocytosis that varies from mild to severe (>100,000 cells/μl). It is rarely seen in pet birds.

Box 49-3 *Causes of Lymphocytosis in Birds*

Physiologic Leukocytosis
Sudden physical exertion
Epinephrine release

Chronic Antigenic Stimulation
Infection (bacteria, fungi, viruses, parasites)
Vaccination

Lymphoproliferative Disease
Leukemia
Lymphosarcoma

20. How do physiologic leukocytosis, antigenic stipulation, and lymphoproliferative disease result in lymphocytosis?

a. *Redistribution of lymphocytes* from the MP to the CP occurs after brief physical exertion (e.g., attempting to avoid physical restraint) and is mediated primarily by epinephrine.

b. *Increased production of lymphocytes* may result from chronic antigenic or cytokine stimulation or from an autonomous clonal proliferation of neoplastic lymphocytes. Proliferation secondary to antigenic stimulation is an appropriate, controlled response resulting in a heterogeneous population of lymphocytes, whereas neoplastic proliferations will be excessive and uncontrolled.

21. What are the expected CBC findings in birds with lymphocytosis of physiologic leukocytosis?

The lymphocytosis is transient and frequently accompanied by mild to moderate heterophilia with no left shift or toxic change in heterophils. The magnitude of the lymphocytosis is mild to moderate. Lymphocytosis may be greater than the heterophilia, particularly in species with predominant lymphocyte numbers in health.

22. What are the expected CBC findings in birds with lymphocytosis of chronic antigenic stimulation?

The lymphocytosis may be mild to moderate. Lymphocytosis in one reported case in a crane was approximately 45,000 lymphocytes/µl. The magnitude of the lymphocytosis may overlap with that of physiologic leukocytosis or of early lymphoproliferative disease. An important difference is that the lymphocytosis of chronic inflammatory disease is not transient as in physiologic leukocytosis. Heterophilia with left shift or toxic change or monocytosis may accompany lymphocytosis of chronic inflammatory disease. Reactive lymphocytes may be seen in circulation. Vaccination (duck plague, pasteurellosis) in some species of birds produces lymphocytosis secondary to antigenic stimulation.

23. What are the expected CBC findings in birds with lymphocytosis of lymphoproliferative disease?

Lymphocytosis may be greater than that seen with lymphocytosis of physiologic leukocytosis or of chronic inflammatory disease, but these may overlap. The lymphocyte counts in a cockatoo and an Amazon with lymphoid leukemia were approximately 38,000 to 49,000 cells/µl. Lymphoid leukemia in other birds species (emus, ducks) may have lymphocyte counts as high as 200,000 cells/µl. Atypical-appearing lymphocytes may be present in circulation and serve as a clue to the presence of neoplastic disease; however, the lymphocytes may also appear morphologically normal. Serial CBCs may help in differentiating mild neoplastic lymphocytosis from that of physiologic leukocytosis or chronic inflammatory disease. Anemia or pancytopenia may also be present and suggest bone marrow infiltration.

24. What are causes of lymphopenia?

Lymphopenia is primarily caused by the following three conditions, acting singly or in combination (Box 49-4):

a. Corticosteroid release/administration
b. Inhibition of lymphocyte production
c. Acute infection

25. How do corticosteroids, inhibition of lymphocyte production, and acute infection result in lymphopenia?

The mechanisms in lymphopenia include lymphocyte redistribution, trapping of lymphocytes in lymphoid tissues, suppression of lymphocyte proliferation, and lymphocyte destruction.

26. Describe the mechanisms of lymphocyte redistribution and lymphocyte trapping in lymphoid tissues.

Corticosteroids (endogenous or exogenous) promote redistribution of lymphocytes from the CP to the MP and other locations (bone marrow, lymphoid tissues). Under the influence of

Box 49-4 *Causes of Lymphopenia in Birds*

Corticosteroids

Exogenous

Glucocorticoid administration

Endogenous ("stress")

Excessive handling, physical restraint, unfamiliar environment
Transportation, high density
Food restriction, disease

Other Causes

Adverse pharmacologic effects

- Cyclophosphamide
- Other known immunosuppressive drugs

Radiation
Acute infection (viruses, bacteria)
Toxins (ochratoxin A)

inflammatory cytokines released during acute inflammation, and sometimes in combination with endogenous corticosteroid release, lymphocytes may be redistributed from the CP to the MP or other locations (bone marrow, site of inflammation, lymphoid tissue). Inflammatory cytokines may also promote the temporary sequestration of lymphocytes in lymphoid tissues as part of the antigen presentation process.

27. Describe the mechanisms of suppression of lymphocyte proliferation and lymphocyte destruction.

Lymphoid tissue, as with bone marrow, is an actively proliferating tissue susceptible to interference by substances that inhibit proliferation. Cancer chemotherapies, toxins, radiation, cyclophosphamide, and extended corticosteroid exposure may directly inhibit or destroy lymphocyte production. Viruses that infect lymphocytes may also be cytolytic. Congenital defects in lymphocyte production are extremely rare in domestic animals and are not documented in birds.

28. How does acute infection lead to lymphopenia?

Lymphopenia secondary to acute infections is believed to result from a combination of corticosteroid-induced effects, lymphocyte redistribution, and perhaps interference with lymphocyte production. This has not been adequately investigated in birds.

29. What are the expected CBC findings in birds with lymphopenia due to corticosteroid influence?

Lymphopenia caused by corticosteroids is generally a transient event and may be accompanied by heterophilia with no left shift or heterophil toxic changes.

30. What are the expected CBC findings in birds with lymphopenia due to decreased lymphocyte production?

Most lymphosuppressive and myelosuppressive treatments may produce decreases in several hematopoietic cell lines, resulting in selective cytopenias or pancytopenia. If inflammation is concurrently present, the CBC may reflect changes indicative of inflammation (e.g., heterophilia, monocytosis, left shift).

31. What causes monocytosis?

Inflammatory disease, acute or chronic, is the predominant cause of *monocytosis* in pet birds; in the literature, however, monocytosis is most often associated with chronic inflammatory processes (Box 49-5). Inflammation due to chlamydophilosis, mycobacteriosis, aspergillosis, parasitism, and viral infections (vaccination for duck plague virus or avipoxvirus) may cause monocytosis. Other reported causes include zinc-deficient diets in chickens and corticosteroids (endogenous or exogenous).

Box 49-5 ***Causes of Monocytosis in Birds***

Inflammation

Acute or chronic; most often associated with chronic inflammation

Bacteria

- *Chlamydophila psittaci* (formerly known as *Chlamydia psittaci*)
- *Mycobacterium* spp.
- *Mycoplasma* spp.
- Other genera

Fungi (aspergillosis)

Viruses

- Vaccination (avipoxvirus, duck plague virus)
- Infectious bursal disease (chickens)

Parasites

Foreign bodies

Nutritional

Zinc deficiency (chickens)

Corticosteroids

Exogenous

Glucocorticoid administration

Endogenous ("stress")

Excessive handling, physical restraint, unfamiliar environment

Transportation, high density

Food restriction, disease

32. How does inflammation result in monocytosis?

Monocytosis of inflammatory disease is mainly caused by increased bone marrow production of monocyte precursors in response to inflammatory cytokines. Monocytosis associated with corticosteroid influence is likely caused by redistribution from the MP to the CP.

33. What are the expected CBC findings in birds with monocytosis of inflammatory disease?

Monocytosis may be accompanied by heteropenia, heterophilia, heterophil left shift, and toxic changes. Lymphocytosis may be present in cases of chronic inflammatory disease with antigenic stimulation. If corticosteroid influence is present, a lymphopenia may be seen.

34. What is the significance of monocytopenia?

Its clinical significance is not clear, but *monocytopenia* may be seen with experimental toxin administration (ochratoxin A in chickens, paraquat in quail).

35. What causes eosinophilia?

Eosinophilia in birds rarely occurs but may be associated with parasitism (mites, intestinal parasites, parasites with tissue migration). Experimental exposure to foreign antigens, *Pasteurella multocida* vaccination in chickens, and some toxins (e.g., malathion, aflatoxin) may induce eosinophilia in poultry (Box 49-6). Eosinophilia is usually caused by increased bone marrow production. Neoplastic proliferation of eosinophils is not known to occur in pet birds.

Box 49-6 *Causes of Eosinophilia in Birds*

Parasites
Foreign antigens
Toxins
- Malathion (quail)
- Aflatoxin (chickens)

Vaccination
- *Pasteurella multocida* (chickens)

36. What is the diagnostic plan for birds with eosinophilia?

Blood smear, skin, and fecal examinations should be performed to look for the presence of parasites. Diagnostic imaging techniques may be necessary for the identification of some parasites (air-sac mites).

37. How can blood smear evaluation help in determining the cause of eosinophilia?

Examination of a blood smear may reveal blood parasites or may confirm that eosinophils are indeed present and that these cells were not confused with heterophils.

38. What causes eosinopenia in birds?

Eosinopenia is difficult to document in birds without an absolute count because of the naturally low numbers present in circulation. As in mammals, eosinopenia may be caused by endogenous or exogenous corticosteroids (Box 49-7). Experimental exposure to chlorfenvinphos, trichlorphon, and furalozidone produces eosinopenia in some poultry species.

Box 49-7 *Causes of Eosinopenia in Birds*

Corticosteroids

Exogenous
Glucocorticoid administration

Endogenous ("stress")
Excessive handling, physical restraint, unfamiliar environment
Transportation, high density
Food restriction, disease

Toxins

Experimental Exposure (poultry)
Chlorfenvinphos
Trichlorphon
Furalozidone

39. What causes basophilia in birds?

Basophilia is rarely detected in birds but may be caused by severe tissue damage, inflammation, parasitism, severe stress (feed restriction, starvation), and toxin exposure, as with ingestion of mycotoxin or furazolidone (Box 49-8). Anecdotal reports suggest that basophilia may be seen with chlamydophilosis. Most of these causes have been documented in poultry. The exact mechanisms involved are unknown.

Box 49-8 *Causes of Basophilia in Birds*
Severe tissue damage and inflammation
Parasitism
Endogenous ("stress") corticosteroids: severe feed restriction
Experimental toxin exposure: mycotoxins, furazolidone

40. What causes basopenia in birds?

The cause and significance of *basopenia* in birds are unknown.

41. What leukemic diseases affect birds?

a. Lymphocytic leukemia and lymphosarcoma
b. Myelogenous leukemia, primarily of granulocytic origin

Leukemia (lymphoid, myeloid, erythroleukemia) is described most often in chickens, and most cases result from viral infection (herpesviruses, retroviruses). Leukemia has been described in other species of birds, but a viral etiology has not been found. Pet birds are rarely diagnosed with leukemic diseases, and most of the reported cases of leukemia have been of lymphoid origin. Granulocytic tissue tumors *(granulocytic sarcomas)* have been described in pet birds, but well-documented reports of granulocytic leukemia in pet birds are not readily available.

42. How can the signalment help in ranking the differential list for avian leukocyte abnormalities?

a. Physiologic leukocytosis, corticosteroid-induced leukograms, and inflammation may be seen in birds of any age, species, or gender; however, physiologic leukocytosis may be a common occurrence in young, excitable, or easily frightened birds.
b. Heterophilia or heteropenia caused by inflammatory disease may be seen in birds of any age or species.
c. Although rarely seen, adverse drug reactions may occur in birds of any age or species.
d. Neoplastic disease (leukemia, miscellaneous neoplasms) occurs with increased frequency in older birds and in some species more than others (e.g., poultry more than psittacines).

43. How can the history help in ranking the differential list for avian leukocyte abnormalities?

a. Birds with physiologic leukocytosis may have a history of brief physical exertion (e.g., avoidance of physical restraint).
b. Stress-induced leukograms caused by endogenous corticosteroids are seen in birds in unfamiliar or stressful environments (veterinary office); birds not accustomed to handling or confinement; birds that have been handled, confined, or physically restrained for extended periods; and sick patients. Birds with exogenous corticosteroid-induced heterophilia have a history of corticosteroid administration.

c. Birds with inflammatory disease may have a history of trauma, respiratory difficulty (e.g., pneumonia), abnormal defecation (e.g., enteritis, hepatitis), weight loss, a growing mass, unthrifty condition, poor husbandry, and recent surgery.
d. Birds with heteropenia may have a history of very recent drug administration (idiosyncratic drug reaction resulting in heterophil precursor destruction).
e. A history of administration of known myelosuppressive drugs suggests depression of leukocyte (heterophil, lymphoid) production.
f. Birds with leukemia and other neoplastic diseases may have a history of weight loss or unthrifty condition.

44. How can the physical examination help in ranking the differential list for avian leukocyte abnormalities?

a. Birds with physiologic leukocytosis as the only abnormality may be characterized by increases in heart rate, respiratory rate, and muscular activity with no evidence of other disease conditions.
b. Stressed birds may demonstrate abnormal behaviors, abnormal posture, self-mutilation, and plucking; these may be complicated by other disease conditions (e.g., trauma, infections, tumors).
c. Birds with inflammatory disease (acute or chronic) may present with a multitude of abnormalities, including trauma (self-inflicted, other); space-occupying lesions (e.g., abscesses, tumors); excessive chest movements or tail bobbing with or without open-mouth breathing (e.g., dyspnea associated with pneumonia, parasites); blood in stool (e.g., enteritis); fever, paresis, or paralysis (renal or reproductive tract abscesses and neoplasms); lameness; depression; distended or painful abdomen (e.g., egg yolk coelomitis), oculonasal discharge (rhinitis, conjunctivitis); poorly digested excreta; and hemorrhage.
d. Birds with neoplastic disease may have a multitude of abnormalities, some of which may be similar to those seen with inflammatory disease. Masses may be present.

45. What is the diagnostic plan for birds with leukocyte abnormalities?

The physical examination and clinical findings may help to focus on a particular organ system or anatomic location and to determine if additional diagnostic tests are needed. Peripheral blood smear evaluation, additional CBCs, and serum biochemical analysis should be obtained in persistently abnormal or ill birds. Additional diagnostic tests may be necessary, including bone marrow aspirate/biopsy (for leukemia), diagnostic imaging techniques, microscopic evaluation of cytologic specimens and tissue biopsies, microbiologic culture, molecular diagnostic techniques (for infectious agents), and serology.

46. How do imaging techniques assist in ranking differential diagnoses of leukocyte abnormalities in birds?

Imaging techniques such as radiography, ultrasonography, and endoscopic examinations help to detect organomegaly, foreign bodies (e.g., metal objects), effusions, masses, and pulmonary/air-sac abnormalities and to localize organ lesions for cytologic or biopsy sampling. Ultrasonography and endoscopic examinations may be limited by the bird's size. Specialized imaging techniques and equipment (computed tomography, fluoroscopy, contrast studies) may also be necessary but may be limited by patient size, expense, time, and equipment availability.

47. When are aspirates or surgical biopsies indicated in birds?

These techniques are indicated in avian patients with space-occupying masses, effusions, any organ abnormality (size, shape, consistency, location, echotexture), and any evidence of bone marrow disease. Excessive respiratory difficulty, bleeding tendencies, and excessive stress are contraindications for some of these procedures.

48. Describe the avian erythrocyte.

In Romanowsky-stained blood smears the avian erythrocyte (red blood cell, RBC) is a nucleated, elliptic cell with orange-pink cytoplasm. It is generally larger (10-15 micrometers [μm] in length) than mammalian erythrocytes. The nucleus is elliptic, condensed, and centrally positioned. Slight anisocytosis (difference in cell size) and poikilocytosis (difference in cell shape) may be normally seen in healthy birds. If seen with increased magnitude and frequency, however, these morphologic changes may indicate disease (e.g., anemia, dyserythropoiesis).

49. What are important factors to consider evaluating avian patients for erythroid disorders?

a. Erythroid morphology may be evaluated in fresh blood smears (no anticoagulant) or in smears of EDTA or heparinized blood.
b. Erythrocyte counts should be performed with EDTA or heparinized blood samples. *Caution:* EDTA may lyse ostrich RBCs on prolonged contact. Furthermore, if hematologic analysis and clinical chemistries are required with a small blood sample, heparinized blood (lithium heparin, *not* sodium heparin) is the best anticoagulant to maximize plasma volume for chemical analysis. EDTA, sodium heparin, and citrate will interfere with some clinical chemistry parameters.
c. Erythrocytes should be examined for the presence of anisocytosis, poikilocytosis, polychromasia, and intracellular parasites *(Plasmodium, Haemoproteus).*

50. How is red cell mass evaluated?

a. Red cell mass is evaluated by measuring the hematocrit (Hct), the percentage of whole blood composed of erythrocytes. Hct is measured easily and quickly by determining packed cell volume (PCV) after centrifugation of a small amount of blood.
b. Erythrocyte (RBC) count and hemoglobin (Hgb) concentration are additional indicators of red cell mass that are routinely provided by automated analyzers. Erythrocytes may be enumerated manually using Natt and Herrick's method or the Unopette 5850 system.
c. PCV of healthy pet birds should be 35% to 55%; however, because avian erythrocytes are larger than those of mammals, the erythrocyte count is relatively lower ($1.5\text{-}4.5 \times 10^6$ cells/μl). In normal, household or aviary pet birds, PCV may vary slightly between species and age groups. Nestlings up to 6 months of age may have slightly lower PCV, erythrocyte, and Hgb values.

51. Define MCV and MCHC.

Mean cell volume (MCV) is a measure of RBC volume and is routinely provided by most automated analyzers. *Mean corpuscular hemoglobin concentration* (MCHC) is a calculated value indicating the Hgb concentration within individual erythrocytes. Most automated analyzers provide it. These two erythrocyte measurements are used to characterize anemia and help determine the cause of the anemia. The utility of these indicators depends on the availability of a commercial laboratory or automated analyzer.

52. Define reticulocyte and polychromatophils.

Reticulocytes are immature erythrocytes that contain increased amounts of ribonucleic acids (RNA). Reticulocytes are visualized by staining erythrocytes with vital stains such as new methylene blue (NMB). Reticulocytes with greater amounts of RNA will be visualized as polychromatophils in Romanowsky-stained peripheral blood smears. Reticulocyte counts are a more sensitive method of detecting immature erythrocytes than polychromasia.

Polychromatophils are immature erythrocytes that contain increased amounts of RNA. They are visualized in Romanowsky-stained peripheral blood smears as erythrocytes with blue-staining cytoplasm. The more intense the blue color, the more RNA the polychromatophils contain, which is an indication of the degree of immaturity. Polychromatophils will appear as reticulocytes in smears of NMB-stained blood. Not every reticulocyte will be visualized as a polychromatophil in Romanowsky-stained blood smears because some reticulocytes may not contain enough RNA to be recognized as polychromatophils.

Healthy, nonanemic birds frequently have immature erythrocytes in circulation. Typically, 1% to 5% of a bird's erythrocytes are polychromatophils, versus about 2% to 10% reticulocytes. The relatively higher polychromasia and reticulocytosis in birds compared with mammals is hypothesized as being caused by the significantly shorter life span of avian erythrocytes (28-45 days).

53. Define anisocytosis and poikilocytosis.

Anisocytosis is variation in the size of erythrocytes. *Poikilocytosis* is the presence of abnormally shaped erythrocytes.

54. What is the most common erythrocyte abnormality in pet birds?

Anemia, characterized by decreased PCV, RBCs, and/or Hgb, is the most common erythrocyte abnormality in birds (Box 49-9). Birds with PCV of 35% or less are generally considered anemic. Erythrocytosis (increased red cell mass) is an uncommon finding in pet birds.

Box 49-9 *Causes of Anemia in Birds*

Regenerative Anemia

Blood loss (nonchronic)
- Trauma
- Coagulopathy
- Tumor or organ rupture
- Parasites

Hemolysis
- Parasites
- Toxins (lead, zinc)

Nonregenerative Anemia

Anemia of inflammation (acute/chronic, infectious/noninfectious)
Nutritional (iron deficiency)
Chronic external blood loss
Myelosuppressive treatment (cancer chemotherapy, radiation)
Hypothyroidism
Adverse pharmacologic effects (fenbendazole in storks)
Direct damage to erythroid precursors by infectious agents (e.g., viruses)
Diet-induced nephritis (chickens)
- High in protein
- High in calcium
- Deficient in vitamin A

55. How are anemias classified?

a. Presence or absence of a regenerative response
b. Size of RBCs, as measured by MCV and confirmed by blood smear evaluation
c. Amount of Hgb per cell, as measured by MCHC and confirmed by blood smear evaluation
d. Pathophysiologic mechanism leading to anemia

56. How is erythrocyte regeneration measured?

a. Numbers of reticulocytes: single best measure of erythroid regeneration
b. Numbers of polychromatophils (Figure 49-4; see also Figure 49-1): underestimates actual number of reticulocytes, but it is a quick, simple, and good indicator of regeneration
c. Erythroid hyperplasia in bone marrow

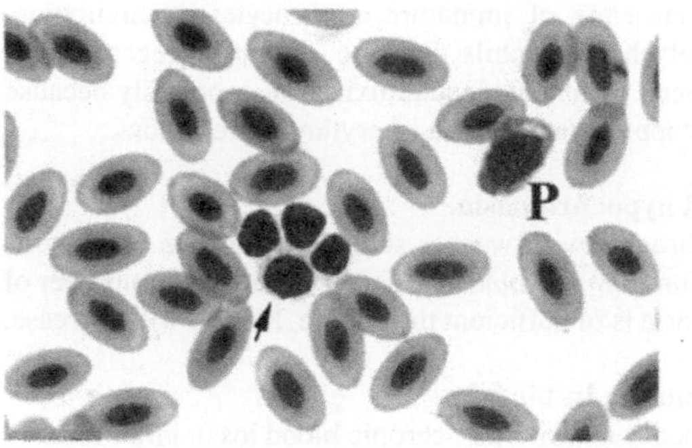

Figure 49-4 A group of thrombocytes *(arrow)* and a polychromatophil *(P)* from a Red Tail hawk. Thrombocytes can be identified by a colorless cytoplasm and a tendency to adhere to one another in blood smears. (Wright's stain; original magnification 1000×.)

57. What is the significance of increased reticulocytosis or polychromasia in birds?

Increased reticulocytosis or polychromasia (>5%-10% of erythrocytes) indicates an erythroid regenerative response to anemia. If this percentage is of adequate magnitude, bone marrow examination may not be necessary to determine if regeneration is present.

58. What is the significance of increased numbers of progressively immature erythroid precursors in birds?

During significant regenerative responses, binucleated erythrocytes, mitotic figures, and younger erythroid precursors (rubricytes, prorubricytes) may be seen in circulation associated with marked polychromasia. Younger erythroid precursors have increased amounts of deeper blue cytoplasm, larger round nuclei, and appear progressively rounder. If immature cells are present in circulation without proportionately greater numbers of polychromatophils, *erythroleukemia* (not reported in pet birds), or inappropriate release of precursors from the bone marrow (due to leukemia, lead intoxication, other toxins), should be considered. *Conure bleeding syndrome* is a condition in which affected birds have episodic bleeding and microscopic analysis shows a marked regenerative response, with high numbers of polychromatophils and immature erythrocytes. It has been referred to in the literature as "erythroleukemia," but there is no conclusive evidence of the cause (neoplastic or nonneoplastic) or nature of this disease (see Question 105).

59. Define microcyte, microcytosis, and microcytic.

a. *Microcyte* is an erythrocyte with decreased cell volume. Microcytes appear as small erythrocytes in peripheral blood smears.
b. *Microcytosis* refers to an increase in the numbers of microcytes in circulation.
c. *Microcytic* describes an anemia characterized by erythrocytes with decreased cell volume. If the microcytosis is of sufficient magnitude, MCV will decrease.

60. What is the significance of microcytosis in birds?

Microcytosis in pet birds may be seen with iron deficiency (rare), either nutritional or resulting from chronic blood loss, and in chicks experimentally treated with cyclophosphomide and infected with *Salmonella gallinarum.*

61. Define macrocyte, macrocytosis, and macrocytic.

a. *Macrocyte* is an erythrocyte with increased cell volume. Macrocytes appear as larger erythrocytes in peripheral blood smears.
b. *Macrocytosis* refers an increase in the numbers of macrocytes in circulation.
c. *Macrocytic* describes an anemia characterized by erythrocytes with increased cell volume. If the macrocytosis is of sufficient magnitude, MCV will increase.

62. What is the significance of macrocytosis in birds?

Macrocytosis is associated with the presence of immature erythrocytes in circulation, primarily polychromatophils. Although polychromatophils indicate erythroid regeneration, macrocytes and polychromasia may also be seen with acute lead intoxication, reportedly because of a regenerative response and possibly an inappropriate release of erythroid precursors.

63. Define hypochromic erythrocyte and hypochromasia.

A *hypochromic erythrocyte* is an erythrocyte with weakly staining cytoplasm and results from decreased intracellular Hgb concentration. *Hypochromasia* refers to an increased number of hypochromic erythrocytes. If the hypochromasia is of sufficient magnitude, MCHC will decrease.

64. What is the significance of hypochromasia in birds?

Hypochromasia is seen with iron deficiency (nutritional, chronic blood loss), inflammatory diseases, during regenerative responses (due to presence of polychromatophils), and reportedly in some cases of lead intoxication.

65. Is hyperchromasia an in vitro artifact?

Hyperchromasia, characterized by increased numbers of erythrocytes with high intracytoplasmic Hgb concentrations and measured by increased MCHC, is an artifact caused by in vitro or in vivo hemolysis. Other than suggesting that the blood sample is hemolyzed, hyperchromasia is of no clinical significance.

66. List the most common pathophysiologic mechanisms causing anemia in birds.

a. Blood loss
b. Hemolysis
c. Decreased erythrocyte production (nonregenerative anemias)

67. List causes and discuss significance of blood loss in birds.

a. Trauma: blunt force injury, fights, malicious injury, dog/cat bites
b. Inability to coagulate: congenital conditions (very rare), toxins (warfarin, aflatoxin from moldy food), viral infections (polyomavirus, Pacheco's disease virus, reovirus), severe liver disease, bacterial septicemia
c. Bleeding lesions: ulcers, intestinal bleeding secondary to damage from parasites, bleeding tumors, trauma and rupture of internal organs, vasculitis
d. Blood-sucking parasites (uncommon)

Birds in general tolerate acute blood loss well. Under experimental conditions, loss of 30% to 60% of blood volume in chickens and pigeons, respectively, does not produce hemorrhagic shock, and PCV values return to normal in 3 to 7 days. This has been specifically studied in pigeons and chickens but suggests that psittacines may have a similar capacity to respond to hemorrhage.

68. List some causes of hemolysis in birds.

a. Parasites: *Plasmodium* and *Aegyptianella* spp. are important etiologic agents. In contrast, *Haemoproteus* and *Leucocytozoon* generally do not induce hemolysis or adverse health effects unless infection is severe and bird is immunocompromised.

b. Toxins: aflatoxin, petroleum products, heavy metals (e.g., acute intoxication with lead, zinc), phenylhydrazine
c. Bacterial septicemia
d. Immune-mediated hemolytic anemia: rarely seen in birds

69. List and discuss infectious agents that cause blood parasitic diseases in birds (Figures 49-5 to 49-7).

a. Protozoa
 (1) *Plasmodium* spp.: gametocytes and multicellular schizonts generally found within erythrocytes but also in other blood cells
 (2) *Haemoproteus* spp.: gametocytes found within erythrocytes only (Figure 49-5)
 (3) *Leucocytozoon* spp.: gametocytes found within erythrocytes only (Figure 49-6)

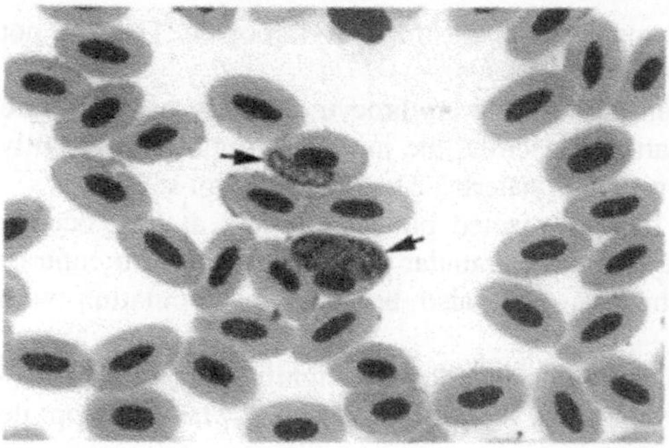

Figure 49-5 Blood smear from a dove infected with *Haemoproteus* spp. *(arrows)*. (Wright's stain; original magnification 1000×.)

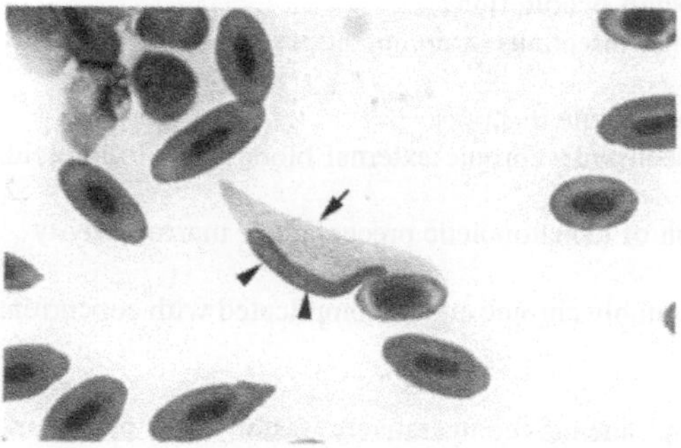

Figure 49-6 Blood smear from an owl infected with *Leucocytozoon* spp. A parasitized erythrocyte is shown *(arrow)*. The nucleus of the red cell is compressed to the edge of the erythrocyte *(arrowheads)*. In contrast to *Haemoproteus*, *Leucocytozoon* greatly distorts parasitized erythrocytes. (Wright's stain; original magnification 1000×.)

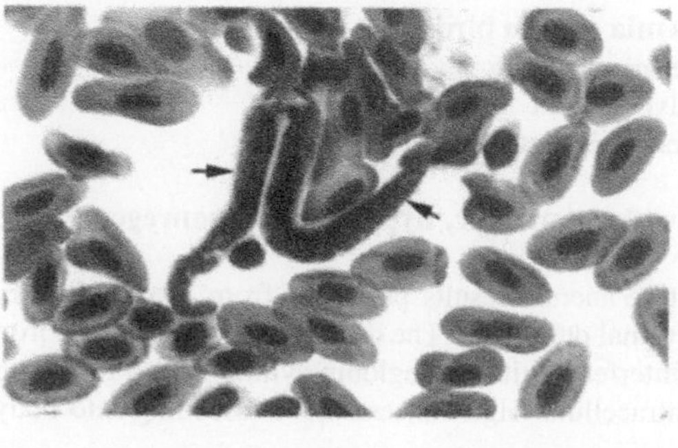

Figure 49-7 Blood smear from Common Murre with microfilariae in the blood *(arrows)*. (Wright's stain; original magnification 1000×.)

(4) *Atoxoplasma* spp.: sporozoites found within mononuclear leukocytes only
(5) *Trypanosoma* spp.: extracellular parasites

b. Rickettsia: *Aegyptianella* spp. (intraerythrocytic)
c. Nematodes: microfilariae (extracellular parasites) (Figure 49-7)

Blood parasitic infections are infrequently diagnosed diseases in captive-bred pet birds. Blood parasites are more likely to be seen in wild-caught pet birds and in wild birds. *Haemoproteus* spp., *Trypanosoma* spp., and some species of *Leucocytozoon* are generally considered nonpathogenic unless infections are severe and the bird is immunocompromised. *Plasmodium, Aegyptianella,* and *Atoxoplasma* spp. may cause significant morbidity and mortality. Microfilariae typically do not pose a problem, although the location of adult worms (e.g., pericardial sac) may affect the bird's health.

70. How are *Plasmodium, Haemoproteus, Leucocytozoon,* and *Aegyptianella* spp. differentiated?

a. *Leucocytozoon* spp. dramatically fill and distort parasitized erythrocytes. They do not produce granular pigment material or form schizonts.
b. *Haemoproteus* spp. do not dramatically distort the erythrocyte but may occupy more than 50% of the cytoplasm. They partially encircle the nucleus without significantly displacing it. They produce granular pigment material. They do not form schizonts.
c. *Plasmodium* spp. generally do not distort infected blood cells and at best occupy less than 50% of the cytoplasm. They produce granular pigment material. In contrast to *Haemoproteus,* multicellular schizonts may also be seen in circulation with *Plasmodium* spp.
d. *Aegyptianella* spp. form intracytoplasmic inclusions that are significantly smaller than *Plasmodium* and *Haemoproteus.* Described as *Anaplasma*-like, *Aegyptianella* spp. do not form granular pigment material.

71. What are causes of decreased erythrocyte production?

a. Inflammatory disease: acute or chronic, infectious or noninfectious
b. Myelosuppressive therapy: radiation
c. Adverse pharmacologic effects: fenbendazole in storks
d. Nutritional deficiencies: iron (also seen with chronic external blood loss), folic acid, starvation, other
e. Infectious agents: directed destruction of hematopoietic precursors or marrow cavity
f. Hypothyroidism
g. Toxins: aflatoxin, lead toxicity (presumably chronic and/or complicated with concurrent disease or inflammation)
h. Myelopthistic syndromes: leukemia

In these situations, birds will develop anemia comparatively faster than mammals, presumably because of the shorter avian erythrocyte life span.

72. What are the reported patterns of anemia seen in birds?

a. Microcytic, hypochromic, nonregenerative anemia
b. Macrocytic, hypochromic, regenerative anemia
c. Normocytic, normochromic, nonregenerative anemia

73. What conditions may be associated with microcytic, hypochromic, nonregenerative anemia in birds?

Microcytic, hypochromic, nonregenerative anemia results primarily from *iron deficiency* caused by chronic external blood loss or nutritional deficiency. The decreased availability of iron that occurs with *chronic external blood loss* interferes with hemoglobin synthesis and results in fewer, smaller erythrocytes with decreased intracellular Hgb concentration. Bleeding into body cavities (peritoneal cavity) should not result in this type of anemia because the erythrocytes and iron should be reutilized promptly. Loss of blood into the gastrointestinal tract is considered an external loss. Nutritional deficiency of iron is *not* a common cause of anemia in pet birds and is primarily seen in poultry. Chronic lead intoxication in mammals, and possibly birds, may occasionally result in a nonregenerative anemia.

74. What conditions may be associated with macrocytic, hypochromic, regenerative anemia in birds?

Macrocytic, hypochromic, regenerative anemia results from acute blood loss (single episode or a few episodes of bleeding, initial stages of chronic blood loss process) and may be seen in acute cases of lead intoxication.

Acute blood loss may be initially (within a few hours) characterized as normocytic and normochromic because the only change is loss of erythrocytes. As time progresses, a regenerative response is initiated, with release of larger (macrocytic) and immature (hypochromic) erythrocytes. Birds respond to blood loss significantly earlier (1-3 days) than mammals (several days).

In cases of *lead intoxication* the polychromasia, macrocytosis, and release of earlier stages of erythroid maturation may be caused by a combination of inappropriate release of erythroid precursors due to bone marrow damage and regeneration secondary to hemolysis. Lead intoxication may be diagnosed with blood assays for lead, δ-aminolevulinic acid dehydratase, and free erythrocytic protoporphyrin. Basophilic stippling of erythrocytes is not a common finding in pet birds intoxicated with lead.

75. What conditions may be associated with normocytic, normochromic, nonregenerative anemia in birds?

Normocytic, normochromic, nonregenerative anemia results from (a) acute blood loss immediately after a single episode of blood loss, (b) myelosuppression (bone marrow neoplasia, radiation), (c) starvation, and (d) anemia of inflammatory disease.

As indicated in Question 74, after *acute blood loss* the anemia may be normocytic and normochromic because it may be too early to detect an increase in polychromatophilic erythrocytes. *Myelosuppressive therapy* (radiation) and *starvation* may inhibit erythropoiesis without significant changes in the volume or Hgb concentration of erythrocytes. Myelopthistic processes may be severe enough that the erythropoietic precursors are replaced (leukemia, fibrosis).

76. What are the mechanisms leading to anemia of inflammatory disease in birds?

The pathogenesis of *anemia of inflammatory disease* (AID) is complex and mediated by inflammatory cytokines. Most investigations have focused on nonavian species, but the mechanisms likely apply to birds. The pathogenesis probably involves a combination of decreased erythrocyte survival and inhibition of erythropoiesis.

Traditionally, AID has been associated with chronic inflammatory disease (avian mycobacteriosis, aspergillosis, chlamydophilosis, gout); however, both acute and chronic inflammatory diseases will produce AID. Perhaps because of the short life span of avian erythrocytes, AID associated with chronic inflammatory conditions produces a more noticeable anemia. The exact cause(s) of decreased erythrocyte survival is not known; however, inhibition of erythropoiesis is likely caused by a combination of decreased iron availability/utilization, decreased erythropoietin production, and decreased response to erythropoietin.

77. How can the signalment help in ranking the differential list for avian anemia?

Anemia of any cause may occur in birds of any species, gender, or age. However, older birds may present with chronic inflammatory conditions (e.g., neoplasms, granulomatous pneumonia), and nestlings may present with poor nutrition and acute inflammatory conditions such as bacterial septicemias and trauma (e.g., gavage tube injury, crop burns).

78. How can the history help in ranking the differential list for avian anemia?

The history may be indicative of blood loss (trauma, visible hemorrhages in the skin, bloody stool, large tumor), inflammatory disease (dyspnea; space-occupying masses, e.g., abscess, neoplasm), erythrosuppression (recent drug administration, starvation), and toxin exposure (ingestion of lead-containing products, zinc-plated or zinc-containing objects, exposure to petroleum products).

79. How can the physical examination help in ranking the differential list for avian anemia?

The physical examination abnormalities include, but are not limited to, frank hemorrhage or hematomas, effusions, dyspnea (pneumonia), space-occupying masses, emaciation, skin disease, and parasites (e.g., mites).

80. Other than the presence of anemia, what are the expected complete blood count findings in avian anemic disorders?

a. Avian patients with inflammatory disease may have insignificant leukogram changes or may have multiple changes, including leukocytosis, leukopenia, heterophilia, heteropenia, heterophil left shift, heterophil toxicity, and monocytosis. The specific inflammatory leukogram pattern will depend on the type of inflammatory insult, severity, and duration.
b. Lymphopenia may occur if there is superimposed corticosteroid influence.
c. Lymphocytosis may be present in chronic inflammatory conditions caused by chronic antigenic stimulation or physiologic leukocytosis.
d. Although difficult to document, thrombocytopenia may occur.
e. Birds with blood loss anemia or hemolytic disease may have minimal or no additional complete blood count (CBC) abnormalities. Corticosteroid-induced changes or physiologic leukocytosis may be present. If the cause of blood loss is associated with inflammatory disease, the CBC may show more significant changes, as outlined above.

81. What is the diagnostic plan for birds with anemia?

Repeat CBCs and blood biochemical analysis may be necessary, although degree of anemia and size of the bird may limit additional blood sampling. If serial CBCs do not reveal regeneration, bone marrow examination may be necessary to determine if there is erythroid hyperplasia or any abnormality of erythropoiesis. Diagnostic imaging examinations, aspirates, and biopsies may be indicated to find foci of inflammation, bleeding, or neoplasia. Microbiologic culture and molecular analyses may also be helpful in diagnosing infectious causes.

82. How do imaging techniques assist in ranking differential diagnoses of anemia in birds?

See Question 46.

83. Define erythrocytosis.

Erythrocytosis refers to an increase in total red cell mass as measured by PCV, Hgb, and RBCs. Erythrocytosis rarely occurs in birds, and the pathophysiologic mechanisms are likely similar to those involved in mammals.

84. How is erythrocytosis classified?

a. *Relative* erythrocytosis due to hemoconcentration: does *not* represent a true increase in numbers of erythrocytes
b. *Primary* erythrocytosis: polycythemia vera
c. *Secondary* erythrocytosis: classified as appropriate or inappropriate

85. What laboratory changes in CBC and serum/plasma biochemistry would support hemoconcentration in birds?

Concurrent increases in PCV, Hgb, RBCs, protein (primarily albumin), and electrolytes (sodium and chloride) would support hemoconcentration. Uric acid may be increased in severe cases. The patient may be clinically dehydrated if water loss of sufficient magnitude. The absolute number of erythrocytes is not truly "increased," only concentrated.

86. Define primary erythrocytosis.

Primary erythrocytosis refers to *polycythemia vera,* a chronic myeloproliferative disorder of erythrocytes. Autonomous and orderly proliferation of the erythroid precursors results in greatly elevated numbers of mature erythrocytes. This contrasts with the immature erythroid precursors seen in other leukemic erythroid disorders (erythroleukemia [AML-A6], erythemic myelosis [M6Er]). Polycythemia vera has *not* been described in birds, but erythroid neoplastic diseases are seen in poultry.

87. What causes secondary erythrocytosis?

Secondary erythrocytosis results from conditions that lead to increased erythropoietin, erythropoiesis, and erythrocytosis. Secondary erythrocytosis is classified as follows:

a. *Appropriate* secondary erythrocytosis: increased erythropoietin production due to chronic hypoxic conditions (pulmonary disease, cardiac disease, high altitudes)

b. *Inappropriate* secondary erythrocytosis: caused by inappropriate production of erythropoietin (not in response to hypoxia). Although not reported in birds, benign or malignant neoplasms and renal cysts are causes of inappropriate production of erythropoietin in other domestic species.

88. What is the initial diagnostic plan for erythrocytosis in birds?

In avian erythrocytosis, blood smear evaluation, CBC, and serum/plasma biochemical analysis help to determine if there is hemoconcentration. If hemoconcentration is not supported, additional CBCs, biochemical analysis, blood gas determinations, and bone marrow aspirates may be necessary. Diagnostic imaging is necessary if pulmonary or renal disease is suspected. Hypoxemia or severe pulmonary disease with no evidence of dehydration supports secondary erythrocytosis. If available, blood gas analysis assists in documenting hypoxemia.

89. Describe avian thrombocytes.

Thrombocytes are small, round to sometimes elliptic, nucleated cells with scant amounts of very pale-blue to colorless cytoplasm and dense chromatin (see Figure 49-4). They may have small, pink-staining granules and tend to stick together in blood smear preparations. Quantifying thrombocytes numbers is difficult because of their tendency to clump together and the overlap in size with small lymphocytes. Generally, thrombocyte counts maybe obtained by the Natt and Herrick's method or by estimation obtained by microscopic examination of well-prepared blood smears; 20,000 to 30,000 thrombocytes per microliter is said to be an adequate number for most birds. These numbers translate to approximately 1 or 2 thrombocytes per 100-power oil immersion field.

90. How are thrombocytes differentiated from small lymphocytes?

When compared with small lymphocytes, thrombocytes tend to have darker staining nucleus, lower nuclear/cytoplasmic ratios, and very pale-blue to colorless cytoplasm. Generally, thrombocytes tend to clump. These clumps tend to be at the edge of the blood smear. It may help to look first for cells that are most consistent with thrombocytes, then compare these cells with the cells in question.

91. What is the most common disorder of avian thrombocytes?

Although rarely documented, *thrombocytopenia* is reportedly the most common disorder of avian thrombocytes. Thrombocyte function disorders have not been described in birds.

92. What causes thrombocytopenia in birds?

The most common reported cause of thrombocytopenia in birds is *bacterial septicemia.* Other causes may include viral infections (circovirus) and disseminated intravascular coagulopathy (DIC).

93. What mechanisms are involved in thrombocytopenia?

Thrombocytopenia involves increased utilization and destruction as well as decreased production of thrombocytes. Both mechanisms are likely involved in thrombocytopenia associated with bacterial septicemia. DIC results in an accelerated rate of platelet consumption.

94. How can the clinical history and physical examination suggest the presence of thrombocytopenia?

Petechial hemorrhages in the skin and mucosal surfaces and prolonged hemorrhage at an injection or venipuncture site strongly suggest the presence of thrombocytopenia. Concurrent coagulopathies involving other aspects of the clotting pathways may also be present.

95. What is the initial diagnostic plan in birds with thrombocytopenia?

Repeat blood smear evaluation may be necessary to confirm that the thrombocytopenia was not an artifact of poor cell distribution. If many thrombocytes are clumped and clustered in the feathered edge of the blood smear, an estimate of thrombocytes is not possible.

96. Briefly compare mammalian and avian hemostasis.

Avian hemostasis is significantly less understood than mammalian hemostasis because of technical difficulties (availability/variability of appropriate reagents/assays, assay optimization) and the apparent low frequency of hemostatic disorders in birds. It is known that in contrast to mammals, coagulation in birds depends primarily on the extrinsic pathway. The intrinsic pathway does not appear to play a major role in avian hemostasis.

97. Briefly describe the extrinsic pathway of coagulation.

Activation of the *extrinsic pathway* depends on contact of blood with tissue thromboplastin/tissue factor released from damaged tissues and activated endothelial cells. Factor III (Tissue Factor) complexes with and activates factor VII in the presence of calcium ions. The factor III-VII complex activates factor X in the presence of calcium ions and phospholipid. Factor X in turn activates the *common pathway.* Activation of the common pathway ultimately leads to formation and stabilization of the fibrin clot.

98. What laboratory test measures the activity of the extrinsic pathway of coagulation, and can it be used in birds as a routine diagnostic test?

Prothrombin time (PT) measures the activity of the extrinsic pathway. PT testing is primarily available in research laboratories and has been used to document coagulopathies in birds.

Practical use of PT measurement as a routine diagnostic test is greatly limited by technical limitations, expense, amount of work required to optimize the assay, and idiosyncrasies of avian plasma. For example, freezing avian plasma samples for transport to a laboratory may significantly increase PT results and render the test invalid.

99. Are tests of the intrinsic pathway of diagnostic use in birds?

Tests of the intrinsic pathway are likely to be of little clinical use because of its limited role in avian hemostasis.

100. List the known causes of avian hemostatic disorders.

a. Metabolic liver disease: hepatic lipidosis
b. Infectious agents: bacteria, viruses

c. Nutritional imbalances: vitamin K deficiency, vitamin E excess
d. Toxins: rodenticides, aflatoxin, ochratoxin, T-2 toxin
e. Idiopathic

101. How can metabolic liver disease result in a coagulopathy?

Severe impairment of the functional capacity of the liver will result in decreased synthesis of many proteins, including multiple hemostatic pathway factors. If the plasma coagulation factor concentration is sufficiently decreased, a coagulopathy will result. Severe metabolic liver disease, with the resultant hemorrhagic diathesis, is seen in chickens with hepatic lipidosis. Hepatic lipidosis is also seen in pet birds as a result of dietary caloric excess combined with nutritional deficiencies, and limited physical activity (parrots in all-seed diets). Hemorrhagic disease is seen in poultry with severe hepatic lipidosis.

102. How can infectious agents elicit coagulopathies?

Infectious agents may elicit coagulopathies by inducing severe impairment of liver function (hepatic necrosis) as well as thrombocytopenia and DIC.

Polyomavirus and Pacheco's disease virus (psittacid herpesvirus) severely damage the liver and are associated with hemorrhage. The pathogenesis of the hemorrhagic diathesis seen in these cases is likely a combination of impairment of hepatic synthesis of coagulation proteins and DIC. Poultry infected with *Salmonella* spp., *Escherichia coli,* and *Erysipelothrix rhusiopathiae* may develop DIC. Also, although not documented with controlled studies, psittacines with septicemia or endotoxemia could conceivably develop DIC.

103. What nutritional imbalances may result in coagulopathies?

Vitamin K deficiency is seen most often in poultry. Bleeding associated with vitamin E excess has occurred in pelicans and poultry but has not been described in pet birds.

104. Which toxins are known to cause coagulopathies in birds?

a. Anticoagulant rodenticides
b. Aflatoxin, ochratoxin, T-2 toxin

Anticoagulant rodenticides (brodifacoum, warfarin, diphacinone) are poisonous to birds and cause hemorrhages by inhibiting the synthesis of vitamin K–dependent hemostatic factors. Raptors are at highest risk for anticoagulant poisoning because they may consume other, poisoned animals. Aflatoxicosis is seen most often in poultry that consume moldy feed contaminated with *Aspergillus* fungi. *Aspergillus* spp. produce toxins that may lead to severe hepatic injury and decreased synthesis of clotting factors.

105. What is conure bleeding syndrome?

Conure bleeding syndrome is the term used for an idiopathic condition affecting some species of conures. Affected birds repeatedly and spontaneously bleed from multiple sites. Microscopic examination of blood smears reveals the presence of large numbers of polychromatophils and other earlier precursors. The cause is unknown, and it is not clear if the seemingly regenerative response associated with the clinical signs is neoplastic.

50. AVIAN BIOCHEMICAL ANALYSIS

1. What are some important principles to understand about the use of biochemical analysis in birds?

a. Current understanding of avian clinical biochemistry is in the beginning stages compared with knowledge of biochemical analysis in mammals.

b. Biochemical reference intervals can vary within and between species of birds. The variation may be caused by several factors, including differences in nutrition, environment/geography, instrumentation, methodology, number of animals examined, age, and quality of samples.

c. Although published data are available, thorough, peer-reviewed, controlled studies focused on normal reference intervals or on patterns associated with specific diseases are only available for a few species of pet birds.

d. Because of interspecies variations in analytes, published reference intervals (or those provided by the laboratory) from the species in question should be used as a *guide* and not as an absolute when interpreting biochemical data.

e. Plasma (lithium heparin plasma only) or serum may be used for avian biochemical testing. Plasma is recommended to harvest the maximum volume of sample fluid possible for analysis and to minimize artifacts related to prolonged contact with the cellular components of blood.

f. Plasma or serum should be promptly separated and analyzed to minimize artifacts.

2. How can in vivo or in vitro hemolysis affect biochemical parameters?

a. Direct interference with the measurement of analytes. The magnitude of interference with the measurement depends on the methodology and instrumentation used.

b. Release of erythrocyte contents that contribute to similar plasma/serum constituents (e.g., AST, LD). There is no direct interference with the actual measurement method. This effect is pronounced when erythrocytes contain higher concentrations of the constituent than the concentration present in plasma/serum.

c. Release of erythrocyte contents that contribute cofactors in biochemical reactions.

3. What are causes of hyperglycemia in birds?

a. Glucocorticoids: endogenous (stress), or exogenous

b. Epinephrine: excitement, "flight or fight response"

c. Diabetes mellitus: described in various psittacines

d. Egg yolk coelomitis: *transient* increases in glucose seen in affected cockatiels

e. ~72 hours of starvation in pigeons; not documented in other birds

Compared with mammals, birds have higher normal reference intervals for blood glucose concentrations, generally greater than 150 milligrams per deciliter (mg/dl) and reportedly as high as 800 mg/dl.

4. What are causes of hypoglycemia in birds?

Hypoglycemia may be seen with starvation (as short as 12 hours in some species of birds), decreased hepatic functional mass (diffuse severe hepatitis due to Pacheco's disease virus, polyomavirus, aflatoxicosis), intestinal parasitism, malnutrition, traumatic injury (described in raptors), enteritis, xylazine administration (documented only in chickens), intestinal malabsorption syndromes, bacterial septicemia (documented in poultry), and spiking mortality syndrome in chickens. Hepatic lipidosis may interfere with the ability of a bird to respond to decreasing glucose concentrations during fasting.

5. What biochemical tests are of use when evaluating the urinary system?

Uric acid analysis is used to evaluate the urinary system, and blood urea nitrogen (BUN) may be useful in detecting early renal disease some species of birds (pigeons).

Changes in other reported parameters (e.g., potassium, phosphorus) have been inconsistently associated with renal disease; however, further investigations are necessary. BUN and creatinine are typically very low in birds (below levels of detection by most methods) and are not routinely used as indicators of renal disease or dehydration in birds.

6. How are uric acid concentrations used in diagnosing kidney disease?

a. *Hyperuricemia* may be indicative of severe dehydration and severe renal disease (proximal tubular damage).
b. Uric acid is not a sensitive indicator of renal disease because it is primarily secreted in the proximal tubules, and the glomerular filtration rate (GFR) must be decreased at least 80% to detect increases in uric acid concentration.
c. In carnivorous birds (raptors, penguins), uric acid concentrations may increase significantly after feeding. Fasting for 24 hours is recommended when evaluation of kidney function is necessary in these species. Shorter fasting times may be necessary in ill individuals.
d. The association of hyperuricemia with renal disease is not always consistent because some birds with renal failure may have normal concentrations of uric acid.
e. Despite the drawbacks, uric acid is regarded as a useful marker of renal disease if reference intervals for the species in question are available.
f. If hyperuricemia is present, dehydration should be ruled out. Endoscopic examination and biopsy of the kidneys may be necessary to determine if renal disease is truly present and to further characterize the pathologic process.

7. Can urinalysis be of help in the diagnosis of renal disease in birds?

a. Urinalysis of a fresh, voided urine sample may be helpful in diagnosing avian renal disease. However, it is not often performed because of difficulty in obtaining a clean sample (no fecal contamination or urate crystals).
b. In general, noncontaminated urine from healthy birds should be negative to trace positive for protein (negative for ketones, glucose, hemoglobin), with a specific gravity between 1.005 and 1.020. The pH reportedly varies from 6.5 to 8.0, with some species of birds excreting more acidic urine. The sediment may contain squamous cells, spherical urate crystals, few bacteria, and less than three erythrocytes or leukocytes per high-power field (40× dry objective).
c. Yellow to green urine or urates (biliverdinuria) suggests liver disease.
d. Red urine suggests hemoglobinuria, which may occur with intravascular hemolysis (e.g., lead intoxication). However, red-brown discoloration of urine may be seen in healthy pet birds fed with feeds containing animal protein.

8. What are causes of renal disease in birds?

a. Infectious causes
   (1) Bacteria: hematogeneous spread or ascending infections from cloaca
   (2) Fungal: aspergillosis
   (3) Viral: most viral infections that target the kidney (e.g., avian polyomavirus) do not cause significant biochemical changes because birds may die before they demonstrate renal impairment. Some parrots may develop immune complex glomerulonephritis secondary to viral infection.

(4) Parasitic: most often seen in wild birds; however, the effect of these infections on renal function is unknown.

b. Toxic causes
   (1) Nephrotoxic compounds (aminoglycosides, others)
   (2) Dietary vitamin D excess produces metastatic mineralization and may lead to renal failure and gout.
   (3) Biliverdinuria: biliverdin may be toxic to the kidney; however, impairment of renal function has not been thoroughly documented.

c. Amyloidosis (ducks, geese, other wild and zoo birds)

d. Neoplasms: unknown if neoplasms involving kidneys will result in impairment of kidney function, but diffusely distributed neoplasms may destroy a significant portion of the kidneys.

e. Other causes
   (1) Severe sustained dehydration
   (2) High-cholesterol diet (pigeons)
   (3) Diet-induced nephritis (chickens)
      (a) High in protein
      (b) High in calcium
      (c) Deficient in vitamin A

9. What are some important principles to consider when discussing the hepatobiliary system in birds?

The goal of the examination of biochemical parameters (e.g., enzymes, bile acids) is to determine if hepatobiliary disease is present. *Hepatobiliary disease* is defined here as a pathologic process that results in hepatocellular injury and/or necrosis *and/or* interferes with liver function (e.g., decreased clearance of bile acids from blood). Both processes may occur simultaneously or as a consequence of each other.

A panel of biochemical parameters may help to determine if the structure or function of the liver is altered and what cellular component of the liver is diseased (hepatocytes, biliary system, or both). Unfortunately, alkaline phosphatase (ALP), a serum enzyme associated with bile ductular epithelium and cholestasis in mammals, is not specifically associated with biliary epithelium in birds. Gamma-glutamyltransferase (GGT) activity increases with liver disease, but its specificity for bile ductular epithelium and cholestasis in birds must be investigated further. Serum/plasma enzyme activity (AST, LD, CK; see Question 10) is primarily used to determine if hepatocellular injury is present and to help localize the disease process to a particular cell type (hepatocytes or myocytes). In domestic animals and birds, increased serum/plasma activity of some enzymes only occurs with reversible or with irreversible (necrosis/death) cell injury, whereas increased activity of other enzymes results from increased enzyme production.

To determine if there is interference with liver function, other biochemical tests are necessary. Liver function tests, such as serum/plasma bile acid concentration, are *not* specific for a particular hepatic cell type (hepatocytes vs. biliary epithelial cell) because they test the function of the liver as a whole.

10. What biochemical tests are useful in the evaluation of hepatocellular injury in birds?

a. Aspartate transaminase (AST): sensitive but nonspecific indicator of tissue injury (liver, skeletal muscle)

b. Lactate dehydrogenase (LD): nonspecific indicator of tissue injury

c. Glutamate dehydrogenase (GD): specific but nonsensitive indicator of severe hepatocellular injury (necrosis) in some psittacine species; not widely available

d. Creatine kinase (CK): sensitive and specific indicator of muscle injury

Other serum/plasma enzymes, including alanine transaminase (ALT) and sorbitol dehydrogenase (SDH), that correlate with hepatocellular injury in mammals are not routinely used in avian medicine. An important point to reemphasize is that *the correlation between the activity of all biochemical enzymes and hepatocellular injury is not entirely similar to what is known to occur in mammals and has only been studied in a few species of birds*. Therefore, further research into pet avian clinical enzymology is clearly needed.

11. How are changes in aspartate transaminase, lactate dehydrogenase, and creatine kinase interpreted?

a. Increased enzyme activities of AST and LD suggest hepatocellular injury. CK must be evaluated concurrently because changes in CK will indicate if there is *recent* or *ongoing* muscle injury. Muscle injury may result in increased AST and LD activity.
b. Clinical history should be considered; increased activity of AST, LD, and CK is expected if bird has known muscle injury.
c. Concurrent increases in the activities of AST, LD, and CK indicate that muscle injury is present and that superimposed hepatocellular injury *may* be present.
d. Because of the short half-life and quick clearance of CK and LD compared with AST (LD decreases fastest, followed by CK, then AST) in birds, a one-time finding of increased AST activity alone may indicate a one-time event of muscle injury or hepatocellular injury.
e. A one-time simultaneous increase in the activity of AST and LD, *without* a concurrent increase in CK activity, suggests acute or ongoing hepatocellular injury.
f. Persistently increased activities of AST and LD in repeat biochemical analysis without increases in CK activity suggest ongoing hepatocellular injury.
g. A *nonhemolyzed sample* is critical. Lysis of avian erythrocytes may result in increased activities of AST and LD simultaneously or individually.
h. Serial biochemical analysis over days may be much more informative and helpful than a one-point-in-time analysis.
i. Activities of AST and LD within the reference intervals do *not* rule out the presence of liver disease (e.g. decreased hepatic functional mass).
j. *Definitive diagnosis* of the specific disease condition (i.e., hepatitis, cancer) causing injury depends on histologic evaluation of a liver biopsy.

12. What are the general mechanisms leading to increased fasting serum/plasma bile acid concentration in birds?

Decreased biliary excretion of bile acids due to cholestasis (impaired bile flow) may be seen with obstruction of bile ducts caused by hepatitis, lipidosis, choleliths, hepatic fibrosis, cholangitis, neoplasms, and other causes. *Decreased removal of bile acids from the blood* may be seen with decreased hepatic functional mass resulting from diffuse liver disease or with portal vascular anomalies. These mechanisms have been studied extensively in humans and other mammals and likely apply to birds.

13. Is serum/plasma bile acid concentration useful in the diagnosis of hepatic dysfunction in birds?

Serum/plasma bile acid concentration may be a sensitive and specific indicator of avian hepatic dysfunction; however, further study and validation is necessary in pet birds. A fasted sample (<12 hours) is preferred because increases may occur after feeding in some birds and because the crop may store and release food after eating. Care should be taken with sick and small birds because they may become hypoglycemic if fasted for 12 hours or less.

Other biochemical abnormalities that may indicate or suggest the presence of hepatic dysfunction in domestic animals include, but are not limited to, hypoglycemia, hypoalbuminemia, and hypocholesterolemia. The difficulty in interpreting these changes alone is that they have not been validated in birds, are not sensitive indicators of dysfunction, and are not always specific for decreased liver function. Other nonhepatic diseases may elicit similar changes. Therefore, these changes must be interpreted together, as well as in conjunction with clinical and laboratory indicators of hepatobiliary disease. Other tests of liver function are described but typically are not routinely available to the practitioner or require increased labor (e.g., clearance tests).

14. List some of the causes of avian hepatic dysfunction.

a. Severe diffuse hepatitis: Pacheco's disease virus, polyomavirus, bacterial, other. Avian patients may die before any dysfunction is detected.
b. Hemochromatosis
c. Severe diffuse hepatic lipidosis
d. Hepatic fibrosis
e. Diffuse infiltration of the liver by neoplasms (lymphosarcoma, others)
f. Aflatoxicosis

15. Is the determination of bilirubin and biliverdin concentrations routinely used in avian medicine to diagnose cholestasis?

Serum/plasma bilirubin or biliverdin concentrations are not routinely used in avian medicine. Because birds lack biliverdin reductase, the enzyme that catalyzes the conversion of biliverdin to bilirubin, serum/plasma bilirubin concentrations are typically low compared with mammals. Although increases in bilirubin can be produced experimentally in some species of birds, it reportedly is of limited use clinically.

The use of serum/plasma biliverdin concentration has not been adequately explored as a potential diagnostic tool for detection of cholestasis in birds.

Other biochemical parameters of cholestasis in mammals (ALP, GGT) are not routinely utilized in avian medicine for the diagnosis of cholestasis. In birds, ALP activity correlates mainly with the presence of osteoblastic activity, and use of GGT to diagnose hepatobiliary disease in birds necessitates further study.

16. What causes increased triglyceride and cholesterol concentrations in birds?

a. Excessive dietary fat: all-seed diets in parrots
b. Obesity: seen in birds with severe hepatic lipidosis
c. Other factors/causes: gender, hormonal influences, xanthomatosis, egg yolk coelomitis, egg laying

17. What causes hypernatremia in birds?

a. Dehydration
b. Dietary excess: salt toxicity is often described in poultry and wild birds. Pet birds could be affected as well.

Other causes of hypernatremia in domestic animals have not been adequately investigated, but may also occur, in birds.

18. What causes hyponatremia in birds?

a. Overhydration: excessive water ingestion or IV administration of hypotonic fluids
b. Intestinal loss due to enteritis

Hyponatremia may also occur with hypoadrenocorticism (Addison's disease) in domestic animals. Although, natural cases of hypoadrenocorticism have not been well documented in birds, experimental adrenalectomy results in hyponatremia.

19. What causes hyperchloremia in birds?

a. Dehydration and/or heat stress
b. Metabolic acidosis: hyperchloremia may occur with acid-base imbalances in chickens, domestic animal species, and humans; however, this has not been adequately investigated in pet birds.

Other causes of hyperchloremia in domestic animals have not been adequately investigated, but may also occur, in birds.

20. What causes hypochloremia in birds?

a. Intestinal loss due to enteritis: parasitism (chickens infected with *Eimeria* spp.)
b. Metabolic alkalosis: hypochloremia may occur with experimental acid-base and nutritional imbalances in poultry and other domestic species; however, this has not been adequately investigated in pet birds.

Other causes of hypochloremia in domestic animals have not been adequately investigated, but may also occur, in birds.

21. What causes hyperkalemia in birds?

a. In vivo and in vitro hemolysis: avian erythrocytes contain high concentrations of potassium.
b. Delayed separation of plasma/serum from the cellular elements of blood (macaws)
c. Decreased urinary excretion due to renal disease

Other causes of hyperkalemia may include severe tissue necrosis, inorganic acidosis, renal obstruction, and renal disease. Hyperkalemia secondary to renal disease in birds has been described; however, hypokalemia may also occur. Further investigation is needed to determine how renal disease affects blood potassium concentrations. Experimental adrenalectomy results in hyperkalemia, but naturally occurring hypoadrenocorticism is not documented in birds. Both higher and lower concentrations of potassium have been documented when serum is compared with plasma, likely a result of species differences; delayed separation of plasma/serum from cellular elements of macaw blood increases potassium concentration by 30% within 4 hours, but delayed separation decreases potassium concentration in chickens.

22. What causes hypokalemia in birds?

a. Intestinal loss due to intestinal disease
b. Renal loss due to renal disease
c. Delayed separation of plasma/serum from cellular elements of blood (chickens, pigeons)
d. Decreased dietary intake
e. Metabolic alkalosis: hypokalemia may occur with acid base-imbalances in poultry and other domestic species; however, this has not been adequately investigated in pet birds.

Other causes of hypokalemia in domestic animals have not been adequately investigated, but may also occur, in birds.

23. What causes hypercalcemia in birds?

a. Vitamin D excess or toxicity
b. Excessive dietary calcium or calcium/phosphorus dietary imbalance: most often documented in poultry
c. Egg laying: primarily due to increases in protein-bound calcium
d. Egg binding
e. Egg yolk coelomitis

Most commercial analyzers determine total calcium (protein bound and ionized); however, determination of ionized calcium is possible with specialized instrumentation. Lipemia may falsely increase calcium concentration.

Other causes of hypercalcemia in domestic animals have not been adequately investigated, but may also occur, in birds.

24. What causes hypocalcemia in birds?

a. Idiopathic: seen primarily in African gray parrots. Feeding increased dietary calcium may partially compensate for hypocalcemia
b. Low serum albumin or total protein: decrease in protein-bound fraction

c. Dietary deficiency of vitamin D: exacerbated during egg laying
d. Calcium/phosphorus dietary imbalance: most often documented in poultry
e. Magnesium deficiency (chickens)
f. Experimental dietary excess of aluminum (chickens)
g. Acid-base imbalance induced by heat stress (chickens)
h. Moldy feed with oxalic acid (chickens)

Other causes of hypocalcemia in domestic animals have not been adequately investigated, but may also occur, in birds.

25. What causes hyperphosphatemia in birds?

a. Vitamin D toxicity
b. Calcium/phosphorus dietary imbalance: phosphorus in excess

Other causes of hyperphosphatemia in domestic animals have not been adequately investigated, but may also occur, in birds.

26. What causes hypophosphatemia in birds?

a. Calcium/phosphorus dietary imbalance: most often documented in poultry, rheas, and ostriches
b. Vitamin D deficiency
c. Phosphorus-binding compounds
d. Intestinal malabsorption: reported in poultry

Other causes of hypophosphatemia in domestic animals have not been adequately investigated, but may also occur, in birds.

27. List and discuss important considerations with regard to measurement of proteins in birds.

a. *Refractometry* is a simple, quick method for determination of *total plasma solids* (TPS), an indirect measure of the amount of the total protein concentration. In most clinical practice situations, TPS is an adequate method of protein concentration estimation. An important drawback, however, is that the higher blood concentrations of glucose and other plasma components found in pet birds may contribute significantly to the TPS value and therefore may lead to overestimation of the amount of protein in plasma.
b. When an accurate determination of protein concentration is necessary in birds, the *biuret method,* the method used by most commercial chemistry analyzers, is the method of choice for total protein determination.
c. Commercial analyzers often measure albumin concentration with dye-binding methods. Although these methods provide accurate measurements of albumin concentrations for most domestic species, the same may not be true for birds due to technical limitations. When determination of albumin concentration is necessary, determination by *electrophoretic methods* is reportedly the most accurate method currently available.
d. Quantification of the *globulin fraction of blood proteins* is generally obtained by subtracting the albumin concentration from the total protein (obtained by biuret method). Alternatively, the globulin fraction may be determined by protein electrophoresis.
e. *Protein electrophoresis* allows accurate determination of the various serum/plasma protein fractions: transthyretin (prealbumin), albumin, and alpha, beta, and gamma globulins. Protein electrophoresis is generally only available at commercial laboratories and is not considered a routine test.

28. What causes hypoproteinemia in birds?

a. Intestinal absorption/increased intestinal loss: intestinal parasites, diffuse severe enteritis, hemorrhage
b. Heat stress: most often described in poultry

c. Excessive fluid therapy
d. Protein-losing glomerulopathies: amyloidosis (ducks, other birds)
e. Inflammatory disease
f. Hypoalbuminemia due to hepatic insufficiency: viral infection, toxins
g. Chronic malnutrition

Other causes of hypoproteinemia in domestic animals have not been adequately investigated, but may also occur, in birds.

29. What causes hyperproteinemia in birds?

a. Dehydration
b. Egg laying: increases lipoproteins and other egg proteins
c. Some cases of hepatic insufficiency
d. Chronic antigenic stimulation: aspergillosis, chlamydial disease, other chronic inflammatory diseases, vaccination
e. Egg yolk coelomitis

Hepatic insufficiency and chronic antigenic stimulation may lead to hyperproteinemia because of an increase in globulins.

30. What causes hypoalbuminemia in birds?

Causes of hypoalbuminemia are similar to those that cause hypoproteinemia. In domestic animals, protein-losing glomerulopathies, inflammation (albumin is negative acute phase reactant protein), and hepatic insufficiency tend to result in greater albumin loss than globulin (alpha, beta, gamma) loss. Severe hepatic insufficiency and severe protein-losing nephropathies may progress to a point where there are decreased concentrations of globulins in the blood.

31. What causes hyperalbuminemia?

Dehydration is the most common cause of hyperalbuminemia.

32. What causes increases in the alpha and beta fractions of globulin as detected in protein electrophoretograms?

Increases in the alpha and beta fractions of globulin are generally associated with inflammatory disease.

33. What does increased fibrinogen concentration indicate in birds?

Increased fibrinogen concentration may be seen during inflammatory diseases, such as bacterial and fungal infections. The use of fibrinogen as an indicator of inflammation is well documented in most domestic animals. Some studies indicate fibrinogen increases with inflammation in birds, but further investigation is needed. If plasma is used in electrophoresis, fibrinogen (an acute-phase reactant protein) will migrate in the beta region. Fibrinogen may be determined semiquantitatively by the heat precipitation method.

34. Are serum lipase and amylase useful in the detection of pancreatitis in birds?

Serum lipase and amylase are not routinely used in avian medicine for the diagnosis of pancreatitis in birds. The significance of these parameters in avian disease requires further investigation. Pancreatic biopsy is currently the best method to diagnose pancreatitis.

35. Is blood gas analysis used routinely in avian clinical practice?

Blood gas analysis is not routinely used in avian clinical practice. Blood samples used for blood gas analysis must be cooled and analyzed immediately after collection to minimize oxygen consumption and metabolism in erythrocytes. Avian erythrocytes consume oxygen several times faster than mammalian erythrocytes, which adversely affect blood gases. This situation requires that the practitioner have in-house blood gas analysis instrumentation.

Most investigations of blood gas and acid-base status have been conducted in poultry and not in pet birds. In general, birds appear to respond in a manner similar to mammals in regard to blood gas responses.

51. REPTILIAN HEMATOLOGY

1. How are reptilian blood cells different from the blood cells of mammals?

Reptilian blood cells are similar to mammalian blood cells in some aspects but differ significantly in others, particularly morphology. As in mammals, reptilian blood cells include erythrocytes, leukocytes, and thrombocytes (platelets), all of which are easily evaluated by examination of air-dried, Romanowsky-stained blood smears.

2. What are some important principles to understand about the identification of reptilian leukocytes by blood smear evaluation?

a. Proper identification of leukocytes depends on familiarity with the morphology of leukocytes and the species of reptile, prompt processing of the blood sample, quality of the blood smear, and staining techniques used to visualize the leukocytes.

b. Fresh blood (no anticoagulant) and heparin anticoagulated blood samples are both satisfactory for use in the identification of leukocytes, but fresh blood smears are preferred. EDTA causes lysis of erythrocytes in multiple reptile species so its use as an anticoagulant is not recommended. When cell enumeration is required, it is best to keep samples at a cool temperature when shipping. Long transit times may result in inaccurate leukocyte counts, abnormal morphology, or hemolysis.

c. Gaining familiarity with leukocyte morphology requires frequent examination of blood samples from normal and sick patients of various species. Morphology of cells and staining affinity of cytoplasmic granules vary between species of reptiles.

d. Use of consistent staining techniques and methods are important to avoid excessive variation in cell staining and to ensure consistent and accurate leukocyte identification.

e. Formalin fumes, even if the source is a few feet away, will alter cellular proteins in such a way that the staining intensity and affinity of leukocytes will be altered. Blood smears should be kept away from formalin sources and stained promptly.

f. If a blood smear must be stored for longer periods, for later examination or for archiving, immersion oil should be removed with appropriate solvents, and the slide permanently coverslipped.

3. What are some important considerations in evaluating leukocyte responses in reptiles?

a. Leukocyte parameters vary greatly between species of reptiles.

b. Within a species, significant differences may result from temperature, photoperiod, season of the year, gender, and age. The degree of variation may be marked in reptiles and is greater than in mammals and birds.

c. Few controlled clinical studies specifically address leukocyte reference intervals and leukocyte patterns associated with specific disease conditions. Information often originates from individual case reports and anecdotal accounts.

d. Absolute numbers of leukocytes are more diagnostically accurate than relative percentages of leukocytes. Whenever possible, a total leukocyte count should be performed.

e. Because of all these factors, available reference intervals should be used as a *guide* and not as a rigid standard.
f. Pathophysiologic mechanisms and causes that lead to changes in the reptilian leukogram are generally believed to be similar to those in mammals and birds.
g. Practitioners should develop in-house reference intervals for the species of reptiles most frequently seen in their practice. This may help interpret differences in reference intervals caused by the uniqueness of the local pet reptile population, environment, temperature, and other factors.

4. Describe the various reptilian leukocytes.

The *heterophil* is the predominant leukocyte in health in some reptiles and predominates in many disease conditions, as discussed in the following questions. In most species of reptiles (chelonians, crocodilians, snakes, some lizards) the nucleus is round to oval, although the nucleus is lobulated in a few lizards (e.g., Green iguana). The heterophil of most reptile species has a cytoplasm that is densely packed with elongate, rod- to spindle-shaped, orange to brick-red granules that may partially obscure the nucleus (Figure 51-1). In other species the granules may not be as numerous.

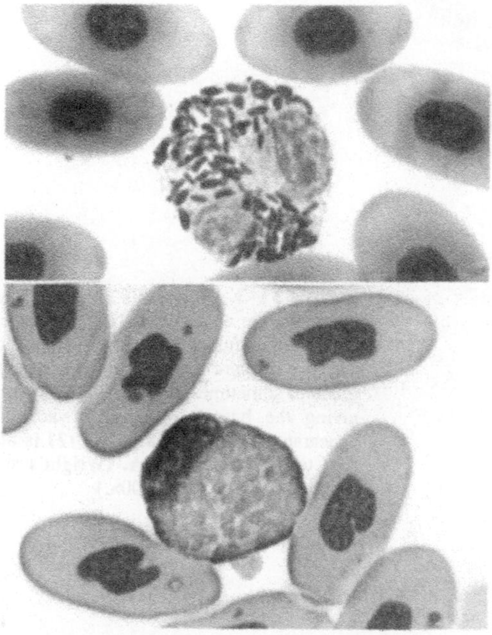
A
B

Figure 51-1 Mature heterophils from a Green iguana (**A**) and a ball python (**B**). In contrast to the lobulated nucleus of iguana heterophils, the mature heterophil from snakes and other reptiles is characterized by a round to oval nucleus. (Wright's stain; original magnification 1000×.)

The *eosinophil* has prominent round, small cytoplasmic granules that vary in color from bright red to pink depending on the species (Figure 51-2). In a few species (e.g., Green iguana) the granules may appear lavender blue in color using Romanowsky-type stains. One must keep in mind that the granules of the eosinophil will stain differently than those of the heterophil within the same blood smear.

The *basophil* has prominent, small, deep-magenta to purple, round cytoplasmic granules and, unlike the mammalian basophil, has a round to oval, nonlobed nucleus (Figure 51-3). The contents of basophil granules can be dissolved by Romanowsky-type stains, giving the basophil a foamy, vacuolated appearance with few granules, if any. Careful examination of these cells in

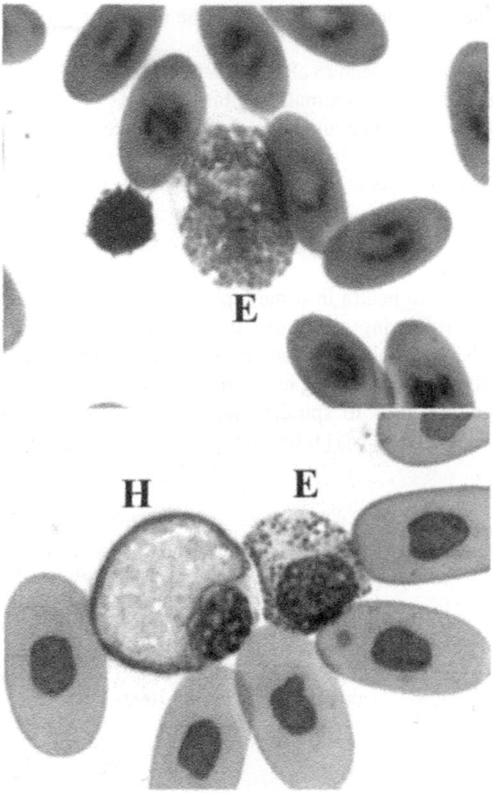

A
B

Figure 51-2 Eosinophils *(E)* from a Green iguana **(A)** and a snake **(B).** In general, reptilian eosinophils have a round nucleus and round to oval granules. The color of the granules varies between species. In the iguana the granules of the eosinophil stain lavender blue with Romanowsky-type stains. In other reptiles the granules may be eosinophilic/pink. A mature heterophil *(H)* is adjacent to the eosinophil from the snake. (Wright's stain; original magnification 1000×.)

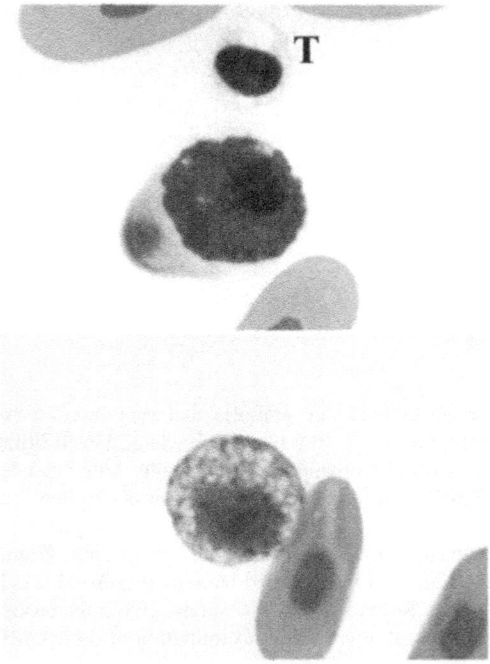

A
B

Figure 51-3 Basophils from a snake. Basophils are characterized by a cytoplasm that is packed full of deep purple granules that partially obscure the nucleus **(A).** Basophil granules sometimes dissolve during staining, giving the basophil a foamy, vacuolated appearance **(B).** A thrombocyte *(T)* is adjacent to the basophil in **A.** (Wright's stain; original magnification 1000×.)

a blood smear may reveal a few characteristic granules, particularly over the nucleus, helping to identify them as basophils. Some species of reptiles (e.g., turtles) may have naturally high numbers of circulating basophils.

The *monocyte* is similar to its mammalian counterpart. It is a large mononuclear cell with abundant cytoplasm and a round to oval to indented nucleus (Figure 51-4). Cytoplasmic vacuolation may be seen. The *azurophil* is morphologically similar to the monocyte and is unique to some species of reptiles (snakes, iguanas). Some species of snakes in particular have greater numbers of azurophils than other reptiles. The azurophil is generally regarded as a cell of monocytic origin that contains numerous fine, red intracytoplasmic granules. The granules may be numerous enough to impart a red color to the cytoplasm.

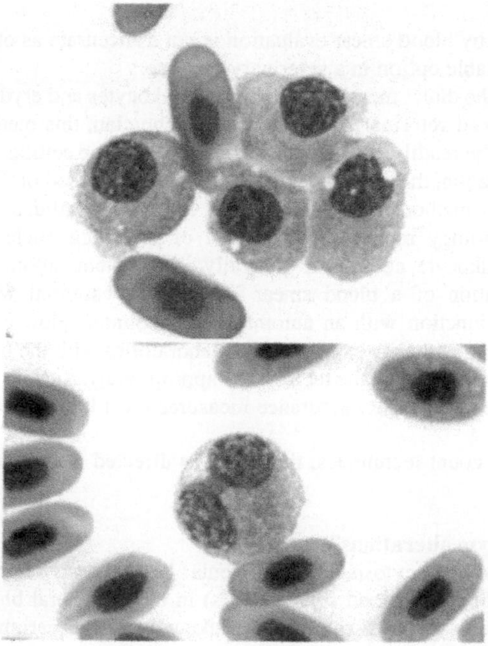

A

B

Figure 51-4 Azurophils from a snake **(A)** and a monocyte from a Green iguana **(B)**. Azurophils, generally regarded to be of monocytic origin, are round, mononuclear cells with round to oval nuclei and numerous dustlike, fine, pink cytoplasmic granules. The pink granules are not evident in this monochrome image. The reptilian monocyte **(B)** is similar to the mammalian monocyte. (Wright's stain; original magnification 1000×.)

The *lymphocyte* is also morphologically similar to that of mammals. It is the predominant leukocyte in many species of reptiles (up to 80% of circulating lymphocytes). The lymphocyte is a mononuclear cell, with low to scant amounts of blue cytoplasm, high nuclear/cytoplasmic ratio, and a round nucleus (Figure 51-5). Reptiles normally have small and larger lymphocytes in circulation. Care must be taken not to confuse the small lymphocytes with thrombocytes. Thrombocytes may be smaller, more oval, with a darker, more condensed nucleus and indistinct, pale to nonstaining cytoplasm, and in contrast to lymphocytes, may readily clump in blood smears.

5. What are common methods of enumerating total numbers of leukocytes?

Leukocyte enumeration methods include *indirect* methods (blood smear estimation, eosinophil Unopette 5877 system) and *direct* methods (Natt and Herrick's). Natt and Herrick's method is more labor intensive because it involves manual enumeration of cells using a hemocytometer. Some authors do not recommend the use of the eosinophil Unopette 5877 system in reptiles because of discrepancies with the Natt and Herrick's method. The discrepancies may be greater in species with normally low heterophil counts.

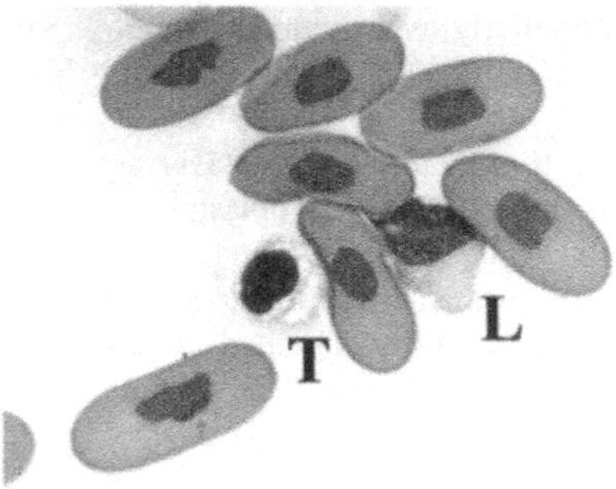

Figure 51-5 Thrombocyte *(T)* and lymphocyte *(L)* from a snake. Notice the colorless cytoplasm of the thrombocyte compared with the darker cytoplasm of the lymphocyte. (Wright's stain; original magnification 1000×.)

a. Estimation of the leukocyte count by blood smear evaluation is not as accurate as other methods but may be the only available option in a veterinary practice.
b. Natt and Herrick's method allows the direct measurement of total leukocytes and erythrocytes. In the hands of an experienced veterinarian or veterinary technician, this method produces accurate results and can be readily performed in a clinical practice setting.

For faster, automated, direct quantification, there are automated cell counters based on flow cytometric technology. Unfortunately, this methodology has not been adequately validated in reptiles. Known drawbacks of this technology include the potential of including nucleated erythrocytes and thrombocytes in the leukocyte count and generally inconsistent automated differential cell counts. Manual examination of a blood smear is therefore essential when performing differential cell counts in conjunction with an automated cell counter. Flow cytometric technology is expensive and available primarily to commercial laboratories with the time, finances, and dedicated personnel to utilize and service the technology appropriately. As with any automated technology, daily quality control and quality assurance measures must be in place to produce reproducible, accurate results.

For detailed discussion on leukocyte count techniques, the reader is directed to the list of references.

6. What are the most common leukocyte alterations?

The most common alterations include leukocytosis and leukopenia. *Leukocytosis* refers to an absolute increase in the total number of white blood cells (WBCs) in the peripheral blood. *Leukopenia* refers to an absolute decrease in the total number of leukocytes in the peripheral blood. These two alterations are the result of increases (*-cytosis* or *-philia*) or decreases *(-penia)* in the number of individual leukocyte cell types.

7. What causes heterophilia in reptiles?

Heterophilia in reptiles may be caused by the following two conditions, acting singly or in combination (Box 51-1):

a. *Corticosteroid release* or *administration* is characterized by heterophilia accompanied by lymphopenia in most animals. It may be associated with trauma, pain, disease, stressful conditions, and exogenous glucocorticoid administration. A common term used for the characteristic leukogram changes associated with corticosteroids is *stress leukogram.*
b. *Inflammation* is an important cause of heterophilia in pet reptiles and results from infectious and noninfectious causes.

The reptile's response to these conditions may be modified by other factors, such as temperature and season of the year. Increased numbers of dysplastic or immature heterophils may be seen in cases of granulocytic leukemia, but mature heterophilia caused by chronic myelogenous leukemia is not documented in reptiles. Physiologic leukocytosis is another cause of heterophilia/neutrophilia in animals, but whether it occurs in reptiles is not known.

Box 51-1 *Causes of Heterophilia in Reptiles*

Inflammation

Infectious

Atypical myoobacteriosis
Mycoplasma (alligators)
Miscellaneous bacterial infections/abscesses
Fungal infections

Noninfectious

Tissue trauma/necrosis
- Traumatic injuries
- Ischemia
- Renal disease
- Surgery

Foreign bodies
Neoplasms

Corticosteroids

Exogenous

Glucocorticoid administration

Endogenous ("stress")

Excessive handling, physical restraint, unfamiliar environment
Transportation, high density
Food restriction, disease

8. How do corticosteroids and inflammation result in heterophilia?

The mechanisms leading to heterophilia include heterophil redistribution, decreased egress from the circulation to tissues, and/or increased hematopoietic production.

9. Describe the mechanism of heterophil redistribution.

The marginal pool (MP) is not sampled during routine blood collection and consists of heterophils within blood vessels but found rolling along endothelial surfaces or having temporarily ceased moving. Under the influence of corticosteroids, sudden exercise, and epinephrine, mammalian neutrophils and perhaps reptile heterophils redistribute from the MP to the circulating pool (CP).

10. What causes decreased egress of heterophils from the peripheral blood in reptiles?

Decreased egress for the peripheral blood to the tissues is believed to result primarily from the effects of corticosteroids and may be mediated by down-regulation of adhesion molecules on the surfaces of leukocytes or endothelial cells.

11. When does hematopoietic tissue increase production of heterophil precursors in reptiles?

Increased hematopoietic production of heterophil precursors occurs when there is increased demand for heterophils (e.g., inflammation) in the peripheral tissues. Infection (pneumonia, enteritis, dermatitis), trauma, infarction, and neoplasms may result in increased demand for heterophils. Chemical mediators released from inflammatory cells, infectious agents, and damaged tissue stimulate the bone marrow to increase production. In healthy reptiles, hematopoietic production occurs primarily in the bone marrow. During conditions of increased demand, however, granulopoiesis may occur in extramedullary sites, such as the spleen, liver, and kidney.

12. What are the expected complete blood count findings in reptiles with heterophilia caused by corticosteroid effects?

The complete blood count (CBC) changes typical of corticosteroid-induced leukograms in other species have not been extensively studied in reptiles. However, a few studies indicate that heterophilia may occur with "stress" and exogenous glucocorticoids. Changes may be confounded by the presence of inflammation or environmental effects (e.g., low temperature).

13. What are the expected CBC findings in reptiles with heterophilia of inflammatory disease?

Mild heterophilia may be the only CBC abnormality in mild inflammatory disease. With increasing severity, left shift (increased presence of immature heterophils, e.g., band forms, metamyelocytes, myelocytes, promyelocytes; Figure 51-6), heterophil toxicity (cytoplasmic basophilia, abnormal vacuolation, abnormally shaped cytoplasmic granules, degranulation, large heterophils), and greater numbers of heterophils may be present and reflect a significant demand for heterophils in tissues. Monocytosis or azurophilia may also be observed. Overwhelming inflammation may result in heteropenia with left shift and heterophil toxicity (see Question 15). The number of lymphocytes may be decreased, normal, or increased with inflammatory disease. Environmental factors (e.g., temperature) may also influence the magnitude of the changes.

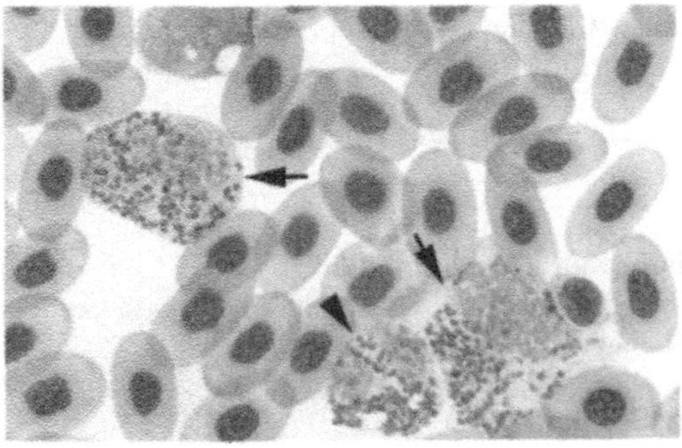

Figure 51-6 Blood smear from a Green iguana with a heterophil left shift. Three heterophils are shown. Two immature heterophils with round nuclei *(arrows)* and one mature heterophil with a lobulated nucleus *(arrowhead)* are shown. Notice also the rounding of granules and cytoplasmic vacuolation.

14. What are causes of heteropenia in reptiles?

Heteropenia may be caused primarily by overwhelming inflammation resulting in excessive tissue demand for heterophils (Box 51-2).

Box 51-2 *Causes of Heteropenia in Reptiles*

Inflammation

Overwhelming bacterial infection
Viral infection
Fungal infection

Other Possible Causes

Myelophthisic syndromes (leukemia, lymphosarcoma)
Myelosuppressive therapies (radiation, cancer chemotherapies)
Heterophil redistribution caused by endotoxemia or gram-negative bacterial infections

In other domestic animals and birds, myelophthistic syndromes (leukemia, lymphosarcoma), endotoxemia or gram-negative bacterial infections, and other causes may result in heteropenia. Although it is likely that the same causes occur in reptiles, this has not been adequately investigated.

15. What is the most common cause of overwhelming inflammation?

Overwhelming inflammation is caused primarily by an overwhelming insult (infectious most commonly) that elicits massive inflammatory cytokine release and marked, sudden tissue demand for heterophils. The differential list should include, but should not be limited to, disseminated bacterial infections, abscesses, fungal infections, viral infections, coelomitis, pneumonia, severe enteritis, and massive tumor necrosis. Any inflammatory condition where the rate at which heterophils exit the circulation exceeds the rate of production by the bone marrow will produce heteropenia. Ultimately, if the demand for heterophils is decreased or bone marrow production is sufficiently augmented, heterophil numbers may increase to within reference intervals or may result in heterophilia.

16. What causes decreased bone marrow heterophil production?

In domestic animals, decreased production of granulocytic precursors may be the result of direct destruction of precursors, suppression of granulopoiesis, or myelophthisic processes. The mechanisms leading to decreased heterophil production have not been well studied in reptiles, but it is assumed that similar mechanisms may play a role. It is known that radiation therapy can result in leukopenia in some species of reptiles. Likewise, myelophthisic processes, such as neoplastic disease (leukemia, lymphosarcoma), may infiltrate the bone marrow, displace hematopoietic precursors, and can result in heteropenia.

17. How can the initial complete blood count help to determine the cause of heteropenia in reptiles?

Although heteropenia may be the only hematologic abnormality, reptiles with inflammatory diseases may have inflammatory leukograms (left shift, heterophil toxicity, monocytosis/azurophilia). Reptiles with leukemia may have marked increases in the total numbers of leukocytes (>200,000 cells/µl), undifferentiated cells, and individual cell types (e.g., lymphocytes). Atypical cells in circulation (e.g., lymphoblasts, undifferentiated cells) may be present in leukemic patients. Reptilian patients exposed to radiation or other myelosuppressive treatments may have pancytopenias.

18. What causes lymphocytosis in reptiles?

Lymphocytosis may be caused by the following two conditions, acting singly or in combination (Box 51-3):

a. *Chronic antigenic stimulation* may result in a greatly expanded circulating lymphocyte pool. It is seen most often in veterinary patients with inflammatory disease (infectious or noninfectious). The most common causes of chronic inflammation in reptiles are infectious agents (viruses, fungi, parasites, bacteria).

b. *Lymphoproliferative disease* (leukemia, leukemic lymphosarcoma) may be accompanied by lymphocytosis that varies from mild to severe (>100,000 cells/µl). Atypical cells may be present in circulation. Although not a common disease of reptiles, lymphoproliferative is the most frequently encountered type of leukemic disease.

Physiologic leukocytosis is another cause of lymphocytosis in animals, but whether this occurs in reptiles is unknown. Environmental influences and nutritional status may affect lymphocytes numbers.

Box 51-3 *Causes of Lymphocytosis in Reptiles*

Chronic Antigenic Stimulation

Infectious/Inflammatory

Bacteria
Fungi
Viruses
- Inclusion body disease

Parasites

Lymphoproliferative Disease

Leukemia
Lymphosarcoma

19. How do antigenic stimulation and lymphoproliferative disease result in lymphocytosis?

Both chronic antigenic stimulation and lymphoproliferative disease result in *increased lymphocyte production and proliferation.* Antigenic stimulation results in heterogeneous/polyclonal lymphocyte expansion, while lymphoproliferative disease represents an autonomous clonal proliferation of neoplastic lymphocytes.

20. What is inclusion body disease?

Inclusion body disease (IBD) is disease of boid snakes (pythons, boas) believed to be caused by a retrovirus. IBD may result in significant lymphocytosis (>30,000 cells/µl) in early stages of the disease. Intracytoplasmic inclusions may rarely be seen within lymphocytes in circulation. It is unclear whether the lymphocytosis results from chronic antigenic stimulation or from a clonal proliferation directly induced by the virus.

21. What are the expected CBC findings in reptiles with lymphocytosis of chronic antigenic stimulation?

Heteropenia, heterophilia with left shift or toxic change, and monocytosis or azurophilia may accompany lymphocytosis associated with inflammatory disease in reptiles. Reactive lymphocytes may be seen in circulation. As mentioned, IBD may be associated with marked increases in lymphocyte numbers.

22. What are the expected CBC findings in reptiles with lymphocytosis of lymphoproliferative disease?

Lymphocytosis of lymphoproliferative disease may be greater than that associated with inflammatory disease, but the two conditions may overlap. The lymphocyte counts in some reptile cases of lymphoproliferative disease have been greater than 176,000 cells/µl. Atypical-appearing lymphocytes may be present in circulation and serve as a clue to the presence of neoplastic disease; however, the lymphocytes may appear morphologically normal. Serial CBCs may be of help differentiating mild neoplastic lymphocytosis from that of inflammatory disease. Anemia or pancytopenia may also be present and suggest bone marrow infiltration.

23. What causes lymphopenia in reptiles?

The causes of *lymphopenia* in reptiles have not been extensively studied. It is known, however, that environmental influences (low temperatures, malnutrition, hibernation), corticosteroid release ("stress") or administration, concurrent disease (renal failure, fibropapillomatosis in green turtles, parasitism, viral infection), and therapeutic irradiation for cancer may be associated with decreases in the number of circulating and tissue lymphocytes (Box 51-4). In reptiles the specific mechanisms that lead to lymphopenia in these conditions are for the most

Box 51-4 *Causes of Lymphopenia in Reptiles*

Malnutrition
Low environmental temperature
- Poor husbandry
- During hibernation

Concurrent disease
- Renal disease
- Parasitism
- Viral infection

Hormones
- Exogenous glucocorticoid administration
- Endogenous ("stress") corticosteroid release
- Exogenous testosterone

Radiation therapy and cancer chemotherapy

part *presumed* to be similar to those that lead to lymphopenia in domestic animals and birds: lymphocyte redistribution, trapping of lymphocytes in lymphoid tissues, suppression of lymphocyte proliferation, and lymphocyte destruction.

24. What are the mechanisms of lymphocyte redistribution and lymphocyte trapping in lymphoid tissues?

In domestic animals, corticosteroids (endogenous or exogenous) promote the redistribution of lymphocytes from the CP to MP and other locations (bone marrow, lymphoid tissues). Under the influence of inflammatory cytokines released during acute inflammation, and sometimes in combination with endogenous corticosteroid release, lymphocytes may be redistributed from the CP to MP or other locations (bone marrow, site of inflammation, lymphoid tissue). Inflammatory cytokines may also promote the temporary sequestration of lymphocytes in lymphoid tissues as part of the antigen presentation process.

25. What are the mechanisms of suppression of lymphocyte proliferation and lymphocyte destruction?

As with bone marrow, lymphoid tissue is an actively proliferating tissue susceptible to interference with proliferation. Cancer chemotherapies, radiation, and extended corticosteroid exposure will directly inhibit or destroy lymphocyte production in reptiles and other animals. Concurrent disease, malnutrition, and low temperatures (due to poor husbandry or during hibernation) may result in very low numbers of lymphocytes in lymphoid or hematopoietic tissues. Viruses that infect lymphocytes may also be cytolytic. Congenital defects in lymphocyte production are extremely rare in domestic animals and are not documented in reptiles.

26. How does acute infection lead to lymphopenia in reptiles?

In other animals and presumably in reptiles, lymphopenia secondary to acute infection is believed to result from a combination of corticosteroid-induced effects, lymphocyte redistribution, and perhaps interference with lymphocyte production.

27. What are the expected CBC findings in reptiles with lymphopenia caused by corticosteroid effects?

In other domestic animals and birds, lymphopenia due to corticosteroids is generally a transient event and may be accompanied by increases in the numbers of heterophils (no left shift or heterophil toxic changes). Limited studies suggest the same may be true in some species of reptiles.

28. What are the expected CBC findings in reptiles with lymphopenia due to decreased lymphocyte production?

In animals and presumably in reptiles (one documented case in a Boa constrictor), many lymphosuppressive and myelosuppressive treatments may produce decreases in several hematopoietic cell lines resulting in selective cytopenias or pancytopenia.

29. What causes monocytosis or azurophilia in reptiles?

Inflammatory disease, acute or chronic, is the predominant cause of *monocytosis* or *azurophilia* in reptiles; in the literature, however, either condition is most often associated with chronic inflammatory processes (Box 51-5). Inflammation due to bacterial infections, mycotic infections, parasitism, viral infections, foreign bodies, tissue damage, and neoplasms may cause monocytosis or azurophilia.

Box 51-5 *Causes of Monocytosis/Azurophilia in Reptiles*

Acute inflammation

Chronic inflammation (most often)

- Bacteria
- Fungi
- Parasites
- Viruses
- Foreign bodies
- Tissue damage
- Neoplasia

30. How does inflammation result in monocytosis or azurophilia?

Monocytosis or azurophilia of inflammatory disease is most often caused by increased bone marrow production of monocyte precursors, probably in response to inflammatory cytokines and antigenic stimulation.

31. What are the expected CBC findings in reptiles with monocytosis or azurophilia of inflammatory disease?

Monocytosis may be accompanied by heteropenia, heterophilia, heterophil left shift and/or toxic changes. Lymphocytosis may be present in cases of inflammatory disease/antigenic stimulation. If corticosteroid influence is present, a lymphopenia may be seen.

32. What is the significance of monocytopenia or azuropenia?

The clinical significance of monocytopenia/azuropenia is unknown in reptiles.

33. What causes eosinophilia and basophilia in reptiles?

Eosinophilia and *basophilia* in reptiles may be associated with parasitism and other diseases.

34. What is the diagnostic plan for reptiles with eosinophilia and basophilia?

Blood smear and skin, oral, and fecal examinations should be performed to identify the presence of parasites in reptiles with eosinophilia or basophilia.

35. How can blood smear evaluation help in determining the cause of eosinophilia and basophilia?

Examination of a blood smear may reveal blood parasites or may confirm that eosinophils are indeed present and that these cells were not confused with heterophils.

36. What is the significance of eosinopenia and basopenia in reptiles?

The significance of *eosinopenia* and *basopenia* is unknown in reptiles.

37. What leukemic diseases affect reptiles?

Lymphocytic leukemia and leukemic lymphosarcoma are more frequently reported in reptiles than myelogenous leukemia (granulocytic and monocytic).

38. How can the signalment help in ranking the differential list for leukocyte abnormalities in reptiles?

a. Inflammation and corticosteroid-induced leukograms may be seen in reptiles of any age, species, or gender.

b. Heterophilia or heteropenia due to inflammatory disease may be seen in reptiles of any age or species.

c. Neoplastic disease (leukemia, miscellaneous neoplasms) occurs with increased frequency in older reptiles but may be seen at any age.

39. How can the history help in ranking the differential list for leukocyte abnormalities in reptiles?

a. "Stress-induced" leukograms caused by endogenous corticosteroids may be seen in reptiles in unfamiliar or stressful environments (veterinary office); reptiles not accustomed to handling or confinement; reptiles that have been handled, confined, or physically restrained for excessively long periods; and reptiles that are. Reptiles with exogenous corticosteroid–induced heterophilia will have a history of corticosteroid administration.

b. Reptiles with inflammatory disease may have a history of trauma, respiratory difficulty (pneumonia), abnormal defecation (enteritis, hepatitis), weight loss, a growing mass, unthrifty condition, poor husbandry, and recent surgery.

c. History of therapy with a known myelosuppressive agent suggests depression of leukocyte production.

d. Reptiles with leukemia and other neoplastic diseases may have a history of weight loss or unthrifty condition.

40. How can the physical examination help in ranking the differential list for leukocyte abnormalities in reptiles?

Reptiles with inflammatory disease (acute or chronic) may present with a multitude of abnormalities, including trauma, space-occupying lesions (abscesses, tumors), open-mouth breathing (dyspnea associated with pneumonia), blood in stool (enteritis), paresis or paralysis, distended or painful abdomen, oculonasal discharge (rhinitis, conjunctivitis), and hemorrhage.

Reptiles with neoplastic disease also may have many abnormalities, some of which are similar to those seen with inflammatory disease. Masses may be present.

41. What is the diagnostic plan for reptiles with leukocyte abnormalities?

The physical examination and clinical findings may help in focusing on a particular organ system or anatomic location and in determining if additional diagnostic tests are needed. Peripheral blood smear evaluation, additional CBCs, and serum biochemical analysis should be obtained in persistently abnormal or ill reptiles. Additional diagnostic tests may include diagnostic imaging techniques, microscopic evaluation of cytologic specimens and tissue biopsies, microbiologic culture, molecular diagnostic techniques (for infectious agents), and serology.

42. How do imaging techniques assist in ranking differential diagnoses of leukocyte abnormalities in reptiles?

Imaging techniques (radiography, ultrasonography, endoscopic examinations) help to detect organomegaly, foreign bodies (e.g., metal objects), effusions, masses, and pulmonary abnormalities and to localize organ lesions for cytologic or biopsy sampling. Ultrasonography and endoscopic examinations may be limited by the reptile's size. Specialized imaging techniques and equipment (computed tomography, fluoroscopy, contrast studies) may also be necessary but may be limited by patient size, expense, time, and equipment availability.

43. When are aspirates or surgical biopsies indicated in reptiles?

These techniques are indicated in reptiles with space-occupying masses, effusions, any organ abnormality (size, shape, consistency, location, echotexture), and evidence of bone marrow disease. Excessive respiratory difficulty, bleeding tendencies, and excessive stress are contra-indications for some of these procedures.

44. Describe the reptilian erythrocyte.

In Romanowsky-stained blood smears the reptilian erythrocyte (red blood cell, RBC) is a nucleated, elliptic cell with orange-pink cytoplasm. Reptilian RBCs are larger than mammalian erythrocytes. The nucleus is elliptic, condensed, and centrally positioned. Although slight aniso-cytosis and poikilocytosis (see Question 49) may normally be seen in healthy reptiles, if seen with increased magnitude and frequency, these morphologic changes may indicate disease (anemia, regeneration, severe inflammation).

45. What are important factors to consider evaluating reptiles for erythroid disorders?

a. Erythroid morphology may be evaluated in fresh blood smears (no anticoagulant) or smears of heparinized blood.
b. Erythrocyte counts should be performed with heparinized blood samples.
   (1) EDTA may lyse reptilian RBCs on prolonged contact.
   (2) If hematologic analysis and clinical chemistries are needed out of a small blood sample, heparinized blood (lithium heparin, *not* sodium heparin) is the best anti-coagulant to maximize plasma volume for chemical analysis.
   (3) EDTA, sodium heparin, and sodium citrate may interfere with some clinical chemistry measurements.
c. Erythrocytes should be examined for the presence of anisocytosis, poikilocytosis, polychromasia, and intracellular parasites.

46. How is red cell mass evaluated in reptiles?

Red cell mass is evaluated by measuring the hematocrit (Hct), the percentage of whole blood composed of erythrocytes. Hct is measured easily and quickly by determining the packed cell volume (PCV) after centrifugation of a small amount of blood. PCV of healthy pet reptiles should be between 20% and 40%, but the significant species differences must be taken into account when evaluating reptiles.

The erythrocyte (RBC) count and hemoglobin (Hgb) concentration are additional indicators of red cell mass that are routinely provided by automated analyzers. Erythrocytes may be enumerated manually using Natt and Herrick's method or the Unopette system. Reptiles have lower numbers of circulating erythrocytes than mammals and birds. In general, the number of erythrocytes varies among different reptile groups (lizards > snakes > turtles). Species with larger erythrocytes tend to have lower erythrocyte counts. The erythrocyte mass may vary with season, age, environmental factors, and gender.

47. Define MCV and MCHC.

Mean cell volume (MCV) is a measure of red cell volume and is routinely provided by most automated analyzers. *Mean corpuscular hemoglobin concentration* (MCHC) is a calculated value indicating how much Hgb concentration is within individual erythrocytes, as provided by most automated analyzers.

These two erythrocyte measurements are used to characterize anemia and to help determine the cause of the anemia in domestic animal species and birds. The use of these indicators to classify anemias in reptiles has not been adequately investigated. It is generally assumed, however, that these indicators may be used in a manner similar to that used in other animal species.

48. Define reticulocyte and polychromatophils.

Reticulocytes are immature erythrocytes that contain increased amounts of ribonucleic acids (RNA). They are visualized by staining erythrocytes with vital stains such as new methylene blue (NMB). Reticulocytes with greater amounts of RNA will be visualized as polychromatophils in Romanowsky-stained peripheral blood smears. Reticulocyte counts are a more sensitive method of detecting immature erythrocytes than polychromasia.

Polychromatophils are immature erythrocytes that contain increased amounts of RNA. They are visualized in Romanowsky-stained peripheral blood smears as erythrocytes with blue staining cytoplasm. The more intense the blue color the more RNA they contain, which is an indication of the degree of immaturity. Polychromatophils will appear as reticulocytes in smears of NMB-stained blood. Not every reticulocyte will be visualized as a polychromatophil in Romanowsky-stained blood smears since some reticulocytes may not contain enough RNA to be recognized as polychromatophils. Polychromatophils may be seen in low numbers in the peripheral blood of healthy reptiles, and may be found with increased frequency in young reptiles.

49. Define anisocytosis and poikilocytosis.

Anisocytosis is variation in the size of erythrocytes. *Poikilocytosis* is the presence of abnormally shaped erythrocytes. Minimal to mild poikilocytosis and anisocytosis may normally be seen in healthy reptiles; however, an increased number of erythrocytes with variation in size and shape is abnormal and supports the presence of disease.

50. What is the most common erythrocyte disorder in reptiles?

Anemia, characterized by decreased PCV, RBCs, and/or Hgb, is the most common erythrocyte disorder in reptiles (Box 51-6).

Box 51-6 ***Causes of Anemia in Reptiles***

Acute blood loss
- Trauma
- Coagulopathy
- Tumor or organ rupture
- Parasites

Chronic external blood loss*

Hemolysis
- Parasites

Anemia of inflammation (acute/chronic, infectious/noninfectious)

Nutritional causes
- Starvation
- Malnutrition

Myelosuppressive treatment
- Radiation

*Hypochromic erythrocytes may be seen.

51. What are some morphologic abnormalities of reptilian erythrocytes?

Erythrocyte morphologic abnormalities seen in the peripheral blood of reptiles include irregular nuclear shape, mitotic figures, and binucleation. These may be seen with malnutrition, starvation, and regenerative responses, emergence from hibernation, and/or inflammation. Other morphologic abnormalities that could occur in reptiles include hypochromic erythrocytes and basophilic stippling. The presence of hypochromic erythrocytes (pale-staining erythrocytes with decreased Hgb content) suggests iron deficiency from malnutrition or chronic external blood loss. Basophilic stippling reportedly may be seen in reptiles with regenerative responses, iron deficiency, and lead intoxication.

52. How are anemias classified in reptiles?

Anemias are classified according to the presence or absence of a regenerative response and the pathophysiologic mechanism leading to anemia. Evaluation of reptile anemias using other parameters (size of RBCs by MCV, amount of Hgb/cell by MCHC) has not been adequately investigated.

53. How is erythrocyte regeneration measured?

a. Numbers of reticulocytes: single best measure of erythrocyte regeneration
b. Numbers of polychromatophils: underestimates actual number of reticulocytes, but it is a quick, simple, and good indicator of regeneration
c. Erythroid hyperplasia in bone marrow

54. What is the significance of increased reticulocytosis or polychromasia in reptiles?

Increased reticulocytosis or *polychromasia* indicates an erythroid regenerative response to anemia and blood loss. If the condition is of sufficient magnitude, bone marrow examination may not be necessary to determine if regeneration is present. Reportedly, increased polychromasia may also be seen during shedding in reptiles.

55. What is the significance of increased numbers of progressively immature erythroid precursors in reptiles?

During significant regenerative responses, binucleated erythrocytes, mitotic figures, and younger erythroid precursors (rubricytes, prorubricytes) may be seen in circulation associated with marked polychromasia. Irregular nuclear shape, mitotic figures, and binucleation may also be seen during strong regenerative responses. Younger erythroid precursors have increased amounts of deeper blue cytoplasm, larger round nuclei, and appear progressively rounder. If immature cells are present in circulation without proportionately greater numbers of polychromatophils, erythroid neoplasms (not described in reptiles) and inappropriate release of precursors from the bone marrow (from leukemia, other causes) should be considered.

56. List pathophysiologic mechanisms causing anemia in reptiles.

a. Blood loss
b. Hemolysis
c. Decreased erythrocyte production (nonregenerative anemias)

57. List causes of blood loss in reptiles.

a. Trauma: injuries (blunt force, malicious, rodent induced), fights
b. Bleeding lesions: ulcers, intestinal bleeding secondary to damage caused by parasites, bleeding tumors, trauma and rupture of internal organs
c. Blood-sucking parasites

58. What causes hemolysis in reptiles?

Hemolysis is not routinely documented in reptiles, although protozoal hemoparasites and iridovirus may be causes. Other causes of hemolysis in domestic animals and birds (e.g., toxins, incompatible blood transfusions) have not been adequately investigated in reptiles.

59. What are some blood parasitic diseases of reptiles?

a. Nematodes: microfilariae (Figure 51-7, *A*)

b. Protozoa: various species (Figure 51-7, *B*). Most protozoal organisms are within erythrocytes, but some occur within leukocytes and some are free from cells (see Bibliography following Chapter 53 for more information).

c. Other organisms: *Chlamydia* and poxviruses (monocytes); iridoviruses (erythrocytes)

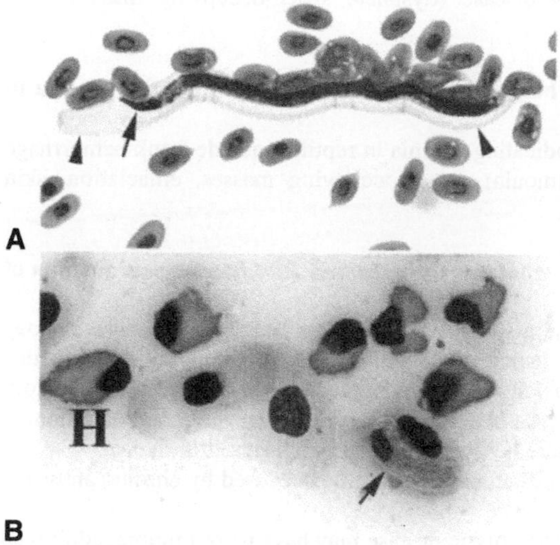

Figure 51-7 Peripheral blood from a panther chameleon (**A**) and a turtle (**B**). A *Folayella furcata* microfiliaria is shown in the peripheral blood image from the chameleon. Notice the sheath *(arrowhead)* that covers the microfiliaria *(arrow)*. An intraerythrocytic Haemogregarine is shown in the peripheral blood image from the turtle *(arrow)*. Heterophils *(H)* are also shown. (Diff-Quik; original magnification 500× [**A**] and 1000× [**B**].)

Blood parasites may be seen more often in wild or wild-caught pet reptiles and pet reptiles housed outside. Most parasitic diseases do not pose a health threat, but some may lead to hemolytic anemia and other problems, particularly if other concurrent diseases and immunosuppression are present.

60. What are possible causes of decreased erythrocyte production in reptiles?

a. Inflammatory disease (acute or chronic, infectious or noninfectious)

b. Nutritional deficiencies (starvation, malnutrition)

c. Myelosuppression (radiation, myelopthistic processes, e.g., leukemia)

Since reptile erythrocytes have a long life span in circulation (600-800 days), nonregenerative anemia could take significantly longer to develop in reptiles compared with mammals and birds.

61. What are the mechanisms leading to anemia of inflammatory disease in reptiles?

The pathogenesis of *anemia of inflammatory disease* (AID) is complex and mediated by inflammatory cytokines. Investigations have focused on other animal species, but the mechanisms could apply to reptiles. The pathogenesis likely involves a combination of decreased erythrocyte survival and inhibition of erythropoiesis.

Traditionally, AID has been associated with chronic inflammatory disease; however, both acute and chronic inflammatory diseases will produce AID in multiple animal species. Although the exact cause(s) of decreased erythrocyte survival is not known, inhibition of erythropoiesis likely results from a combination of decreased iron availability and utilization, decreased erythropoietin production, and decreased response to erythropoietin.

62. How can the signalment help in ranking the differential list for anemia in reptiles?

Anemia of any cause may occur in reptiles of any species, gender, or age. However, older reptiles may present with chronic inflammatory conditions (neoplasms), and neonates may present with poor nutrition and inflammatory conditions (e.g., bacterial septicemias, abscesses, trauma).

63. How can the history help in ranking the differential list for anemia in reptiles?

The reptile's history may indicate blood loss (trauma, visible hemorrhages in the skin, bloody stool, large tumor), inflammatory disease (dyspnea, space-occupying masses, e.g., abscess, neoplasm), and malnutrition.

64. How can the physical examination help in ranking the differential list for anemia in reptiles?

Physical examination abnormalities indicating anemia in reptiles include frank hemorrhage or hematomas, effusions, dyspnea (pneumonia), space-occupying masses, emaciation, skin disease, and parasites (mites).

65. Other than the presence of anemia, what are the expected CBC findings in anemia of reptiles?

a. Reptiles with inflammatory disease may have insignificant leukogram changes or may have multiple changes, including leukocytosis, leukopenia, heterophilia, heteropenia, heterophil left shift, heterophil toxicity, and monocytosis. The specific inflammatory leukogram pattern will depend on type of inflammatory insult, severity, and duration.
b. Lymphopenia may be present if there is superimposed corticosteroid influence.
c. Lymphocytosis may be present in inflammatory conditions caused by chronic antigenic stimulation.
d. Reptiles with blood loss anemia or hemolytic disease may have no or minimal additional CBC abnormalities.

66. What is the diagnostic plan for reptiles with anemia?

Repeat CBCs and blood biochemical analysis may be necessary, although additional blood sampling may be limited by degree of anemia and size of the patient. If serial CBCs do not reveal the presence of regeneration, bone marrow examination may be necessary to determine if there is erythroid hyperplasia or any abnormality of erythropoiesis. Diagnostic imaging examinations, aspirates, and biopsies may be indicated to find foci of inflammation, bleeding, or neoplasia. Microbiologic culture and molecular analysis may also help in diagnosing infectious causes.

67. How do imaging techniques assist in ranking differential diagnoses of anemia in reptiles?

See Question 42.

68. Describe reptilian thrombocytes.

Thrombocytes are small, round to sometimes elliptic, nucleated cells with scant amounts of very pale-blue to colorless cytoplasm and dense chromatin (see Figures 51-3 and 51-5). Thrombocytes may have small, pink-staining granules and tend to stick together in blood smear preparations. Quantifying or estimating number of thrombocytes is difficult because they tend to clump together and they overlap in size with small lymphocytes. Generally, thrombocyte counts may be obtained by the Natt and Herrick's method or by estimation through microscopic examination of well-prepared blood smears. The adequate number of thrombocytes that healthy reptiles should possess has not been adequately investigated.

69. How are thrombocytes differentiated from small lymphocytes?

Compared with the small lymphocyte, thrombocytes tend to have darker staining nucleus, lower nuclear/cytoplasmic ratios, and very pale-blue to colorless cytoplasm. Generally, thrombocytes tend to clump. These clumps tend to be at the edge of the blood smear. It may help to look first for cells that are most consistent with thrombocytes, then compare these cells with the cells in question. Activated thrombocytes may have vacuolated cytoplasm. Special cytochemical stains may help differentiate thrombocytes from lymphocytes; for example, thrombocytes stain with periodic acid–Schiff (PAS), but lymphocytes do not stain with PAS.

70. What is the most common disorder of reptilian thrombocytes?

Disorders of thrombocytes have not been adequately investigated in reptiles, but thrombocytopenia would be expected to occur in reptiles as in other species. Some species of protozoal parasites may infect reptilian thrombocytes.

71. What is known of reptilian hemostasis?

Very little is known of reptilian hemostasis compared with other domestic animal species and birds. Currently, routine assessment of reptilian hemostasis is not practical.

52. REPTILIAN BIOCHEMICAL ANALYSIS

1. What are some important principles to understand about the use of biochemical analysis in reptiles?

a. Current understanding of reptilian biochemical changes in disease is less than the knowledge of biochemical changes in birds and mammals, primarily because of the lack of scientific studies on reptilian biochemistry.
b. Biochemical reference intervals can vary greatly within and between species of reptiles (even more so than in birds). This variation may be caused by several factors, including differences in nutrition, environment/geography, instrumentation, methodology, number of animals examined, age, and quality of samples.
c. Contamination of blood samples with lymph fluid may occur and will affect biochemical results.
d. Because of interspecies variations in analytes, published reference intervals (or those provided by the laboratory) should be used as a *guide* and not as an absolute when interpreting biochemical data.
e. Plasma (lithium heparin plasma only) should be used for reptile biochemical analysis. Heparinized plasma maximizes the available sample volume for analysis and minimizes artifacts related to prolonged contact with the cellular components of blood. Plasma should be promptly separated and analyzed.

2. How can in vivo or in vitro hemolysis affect clinical chemistry parameters?

a. Direct interference with the measurement of analytes (e.g., hemoglobin interference with optical measurements). The magnitude of interference with the measurement depends on the methodology and instrumentation used.
b. Release of erythrocyte contents that contribute to similar plasma/serum constituents (e.g., AST, LD). There is no direct interference with the actual measurement method.

This effect is pronounced when erythrocytes contain higher concentrations of the constituent than the concentration present in plasma/serum.

c. Release of erythrocyte contents that contribute cofactors in biochemical reactions.

3. What are causes of hyperglycemia in reptiles?

a. Glucocorticoids: endogenous ("stress") or exogenous; may be associated with concurrent diseases such as infections

b. Diabetes mellitus: few cases described

Glucose concentrations vary due to age, feeding, wild versus captive status, nutritional status, and environmental conditions. For example, juvenile iguanas have higher plasma glucose concentrations than adults, but the same is not true for mugger crocodiles.

4. What are causes of hypoglycemia in reptiles?

Hypoglycemia is primarily seen with starvation, anorexia, and malnutrition. Other reported conditions that could result in hypoglycemia include liver disease, septicemia, and endocrinopathies.

5. What biochemical tests are of use when evaluating the urinary system?

Uric acid, calcium, and phosphorus concentrations are used to evaluate the urinary system.

BUN and creatinine concentrations are typically low and variable in most species of reptiles and are not routinely used as indicators of renal disease in reptiles. However, BUN concentration may increase with dehydration, which may assist in conserving body water in desert reptiles.

6. How are uric acid concentrations used in diagnosing kidney disease?

a. *Hyperuricemia* may indicate severe dehydration or severe renal disease.

b. Uric acid is not a sensitive indicator of renal disease because it is primarily secreted in the proximal tubules, and the glomerular filtration rate (GFR) must be decreased significantly to detect increases in uric acid concentrations. Some reptiles with renal failure may have normal concentrations of uric acid because functional impairment may not be of sufficient magnitude to produce increased uric acid concentration.

c. In carnivorous reptiles, uric acid concentrations may increase significantly after feeding and peak a day after a meal. This increase reportedly should not exceed 15 mg/dl in healthy individuals.

d. Despite the drawbacks, uric acid is regarded as a useful marker of renal disease if reference intervals for the species in question are available.

e. If hyperuricemia is present, dehydration should be ruled out. Endoscopic examination and biopsy of the kidneys may be necessary to determine if renal disease is truly present and to further characterize the pathologic process.

7. How are calcium and phosphorus concentrations used in diagnosing kidney disease?

a. In renal disease, urinary excretion of phosphorus may decrease and result in increased plasma concentration.

b. Plasma calcium/phosphorus ratio less than 1.0 suggests renal disease.

c. Renal disease is also suggested when the product of calcium and phosphorus concentration is greater than 55 mg/dl. However, this is not a reliable indicator of renal disease in adult female iguanas.

d. In adult female iguanas (and perhaps other female reptiles) the product of calcium and phosphorus concentrations may exceed 100 mg/dl. Calcium and phosphorus concentrations are typically elevated during egg development.

8. Can urinalysis be of use in the diagnosis of renal disease in reptiles?

As in birds, urinalysis is not a routine laboratory test in reptile medicine because of the difficulty in obtaining a clean sample without urate crystals or fecal material.

9. What are causes of renal disease in reptiles?

a. Infectious causes: bacteria, protozoal parasites
b. Toxic causes
   (1) Nephrotoxic compounds (e.g., aminoglycosides)
   (2) Dietary vitamin D excess produces metastatic mineralization and may lead to renal failure and gout.
c. Poor husbandry
   (1) Nutritional: herbivorous reptiles may consume diets excessively high in animal protein or containing excessive concentrations of vitamin D.
   (2) Long-term exposure to low temperatures may inhibit uric acid secretion and may complicate dehydration and a poor diet.
d. Sustained dehydration

10. What are some important principles to consider when discussing the hepatobiliary system in reptiles?

Current understanding of plasma bile acid and enzymatic changes (e.g., sensitivity, specificity, plasma half-life) as a result of hepatobiliary disease in reptiles is greatly inadequate and requires further careful investigation.

Current practice is to interpret changes in plasma enzyme activities in a manner similar to that in mammals and birds. This approach has not been adequately validated with any controlled scientific study.

11. What clinical chemistry tests may be useful in the evaluation of hepatobiliary disease in reptiles?

a. Aspartate transaminase (AST): sensitive but nonspecific indicator of tissue injury (liver and skeletal muscle)
b. Lactate dehydrogenase (LD): nonspecific indicator of tissue injury
c. Creatine kinase (CK): sensitive and specific indicator of muscle injury

A few studies indicate that liver tissue activities of gamma-glutamyltransferase (GGT), alkaline phosphatase (ALP), and alanine transaminase (ALT) are low, and their use in detecting hepatocellular injury or cholestasis has not been adequately investigated. The use of bile acids, bilirubin, and biliverdin concentrations for diagnosis of hepatobiliary disease in reptiles has not been adequately investigated and is not routinely practiced.

12. How are changes in plasma aspartate transaminase, lactate dehydrogenase, and creatine kinase interpreted?

a. Increased enzyme activities of AST and LD suggest hepatocellular injury. CK must be evaluated concurrently because changes in CK activity will indicate if there is *recent* or *ongoing* muscle injury. Tissue injury (e.g., muscle injury) may result in increased activities of AST and LD.
b. Clinical history should be considered. For example, if muscle injury is known to be present or has occurred within the previous day (injection, trauma, major surgery involving muscle tissue), increases in AST, LD, and CK should be expected.
c. Concurrent increases in the activities of AST, LD, and CK indicate that muscle injury is present and that superimposed hepatocellular injury *may* be present. Monitoring the patient with repeat biochemical analyses over a few days may be helpful in determining if hepatocellular injury was a contributory factor.
d. Persistently increased activities of AST and LD in repeat biochemical analyses without increases in CK activity suggest that ongoing hepatocellular injury may be present.
e. A *nonhemolyzed sample* is critical. Lysis of reptile erythrocytes may result in increased activities of AST and LD.

f. Serial biochemical analyses over days may be much more informative and helpful than a one-point-in-time analysis.
g. Activities of AST and LD within the reference intervals do *not* rule out the presence of liver disease (e.g., decreased hepatic functional mass).
h. *Definitive diagnosis* of the specific disease condition (e.g., hepatitis, cancer) causing injury depends on histologic evaluation of a liver biopsy.

13. What types of hepatobiliary diseases occur in reptiles?

a. Infectious disease
   (1) Viruses: herpesvirus, adenovirus
   (2) Protozoa: *Entamoeba invadens,* others
   (3) Bacteria: various
   (4) Fungi: various
b. Metabolic disease: hepatic lipidosis
c. Neoplastic disease: hepatoma, hepatocellular carcinoma, cholangioma, cholangiocarcinoma, lymphosarcoma, others
d. Other diseases
   (1) Idiopathic fibrosis
   (2) Biliary hyperplasia

14. What is the significance of increased triglyceride and cholesterol concentrations in reptiles?

Increased triglyceride and cholesterol concentrations are associated with egg laying in females and may be seen in reptiles with hepatic lipidosis. Postprandial increases in triglycerides and cholesterol are seen in some species of reptiles.

15. What causes hypernatremia or hyperchloremia in reptiles?

Dehydration causes hypernatremia and hyperchloremia in reptiles. Other causes in domestic animals have not been adequately investigated, but may also occur, in reptiles.

16. What causes hyponatremia or hypochloremia in reptiles?

A reported cause of hyponatremia is intestinal loss due to enteritis. Other causes of hyponatremia and hypochloremia in domestic animals have not been adequately investigated, but may also occur, in reptiles.

17. What causes hyperkalemia in reptiles?

a. In vivo and in vitro hemolysis: reptile erythrocytes contain abundant potassium.
b. Decreased urinary excretion due to renal disease: an inconsistent finding that has not been thoroughly investigated in reptiles.

Other causes of hyperkalemia in domestic animals have not been adequately investigated, but may also occur, in reptiles.

18. What causes hypokalemia in reptiles?

a. Intestinal loss due to intestinal disease
b. Decreased food intake and anorexia

Other causes of hypokalemia in domestic animals have not been adequately investigated, but may also occur, in reptiles.

19. What causes hypercalcemia in reptiles?

a. Vitamin D excess or toxicity
b. Excessive dietary calcium
c. Egg laying: primarily due to increases in protein-bound calcium

Most commercial analyzers determine total calcium (protein bound and ionized); however, determination of the biologically active ionized calcium is possible with specialized instrumentation. Other causes of hypercalcemia (parathyroid diseases, paraneoplastic syndromes) in domestic animals have not been adequately investigated, but may also occur, in reptiles.

20. What causes hypocalcemia in reptiles?

a. Dietary deficiency of vitamin D or calcium
b. Calcium/phosphorus imbalance

Other causes of hypocalcemia in domestic animals have not been adequately investigated, but may also occur, in reptiles.

21. What causes hyperphosphatemia in reptiles?

a. Vitamin D toxicity
b. Dietary excess of phosphorus
c. Renal disease
d. Hemolysis
e. Egg laying

Other causes of hyperphosphatemia in domestic animals have not been adequately investigated, but may also occur, in reptiles.

22. What causes hypophosphatemia in reptiles?

Dietary deficiency of phosphorus causes hypophosphatemia in reptiles. Other causes of hypophosphatemia in domestic animals have not been adequately investigated, but may also occur, in reptiles.

23. List and discuss important considerations in measurement of proteins in reptiles.

a. *Refractometry* is a simple, quick method for determination of *total plasma solids* (TPS), an indirect measure of the amount of total protein. In most clinical practice situations, TPS is an adequate method of plasma protein concentration estimation.
b. When an accurate determination of protein concentration is necessary in reptiles, the *biuret method,* the method used by most commercial chemistry analyzers, is likely the method of choice for total protein determination in reptiles.
c. Commercial analyzers often measure albumin concentration with dye-binding methods. These methods provide accurate measurements of albumin concentrations for most domestic species. It is generally assumed that the same methods are useful in reptile species. Electrophoretic methods may also be used to measure albumin concentration.
d. Quantification of the *globulin fraction of blood proteins* is generally obtained by subtracting the albumin concentration from the total protein concentration (obtained by biuret method). Alternatively, the globulin fraction may be determined by protein electrophoresis.
e. *Protein electrophoresis* allows the accurate determination of the various serum/plasma protein fractions: transthyretin (prealbumin), albumin, and alpha, beta, and gamma globulins. Protein electrophoresis is generally only available at commercial laboratories and is not typically considered a routine test.

24. What causes hypoproteinemia or hypoalbuminemia in reptiles?

Causes of hypoproteinemia may include decreased intestinal absorption and increased intestinal loss (intestinal parasites, diffuse severe enteritis, hemorrhage), protein-losing renal disease, hypoalbuminemia due to hepatic insufficiency, and chronic malnutrition. Some of these conditions have not been adequately documented in reptiles.

25. What causes hyperproteinemia in reptiles?

Causes of hyperproteinemia may include dehydration, egg laying (due to increases in lipoproteins and other egg proteins), and chronic antigenic stimulation. Chronic antigenic stimulation may lead to hyperproteinemia due to increases in globulins.

26. What causes hyperalbuminemia in reptiles?
Dehydration is likely the most common cause of hyperalbuminemia in reptiles.

27. What causes increases in the alpha and beta fractions of globulin as detected in protein electrophoretograms?
Increases in the alpha and beta fractions of globulin in other animals are generally associated with inflammatory diseases.

28. Are serum lipase and amylase useful for detecting pancreatitis in reptiles?
Serum lipase and amylase activities are not routinely used in reptile medicine for the diagnosis of pancreatitis. The significance of these parameters in reptile disease requires further investigation. Pancreatic biopsy is currently the best method to diagnose pancreatitis or pancreatic neoplasia.

29. Is blood gas analysis used routinely in reptile practice?
Blood gas analysis is not routinely used in reptile practice. However, limited research in lizards suggests that reptiles may respond to respiratory acid-base disturbances in a manner similar to mammals.

53. AVIAN AND REPTILIAN CYTOPATHOLOGY

1. What are some important principles to understand about the use of cytology in avian and reptilian medicine?

a. Cytologic examination of fluids, tissues, and lesions is a quick, inexpensive, and effective tool available to bird and reptile practitioners.
b. Cytologic examination is very useful in the evaluation of living and deceased birds and reptiles.
c. Proper identification of disease processes depends on good-quality preparations (well spread, not too thick) and familiarity with normal cytology of various tissues.
d. Development of a consistent staining technique with use of Romanowsky-type quick stains is critical for the proper identification of cells, extracellular substances, and organisms. Staining affinity of cytoplasmic granules and other structures may vary with the staining kit and staining technique.
e. Formaldehyde liquid and fumes will distort the staining affinity of cells, organisms, and extracellular substances. Exposure of an unstained slide to formaldehyde must be prevented at all times.
f. If a cytologic preparation must be stored for long periods, for later examination or for archiving, immersion oil should be removed with appropriate solvents and the slide permanently coverslipped.

2. List samples typically used for cytologic examination.

a. Fine-needle aspirates
b. Impression smears

c. Scrapings
d. Swab preparations
e. Lavages
f. Fecal smears

3. List disease processes that can be diagnosed with cytology.

a. Neoplasms
b. Inflammation
c. Infectious diseases
d. Degenerative conditions
   (1) Hepatic lipidosis
   (2) Hemochromatosis/hemosiderosis
   (3) Gout

4. List the types of specimens, abnormalities, and lesions that can be sampled for cytologic examination.

a. Ulcers
b. Masses
c. Crusts
d. Exudates
e. Fluids
f. Discoloration
g. Feces
h. Any tissue/organ with or without visible abnormalities

5. How does one determine what constitutes a normal finding when sampling tissues?

One must gain familiarity with the normal cytology of various tissues. This can be accomplished only by the frequent examination of tissue samples from veterinary patients (healthy and ill) and from fresh carcasses. Although time consuming and labor intensive, samples obtained from fresh carcasses allow examination of internal tissues that would be difficult or dangerous to sample in a live animal.

When sampling a specific tissue or an organ system, one should think about the types of cells that are at these sites. For example, a normal tracheal lavage should contain ciliated respiratory epithelial cells, mucus, and none to very low numbers of inflammatory cells. Squamous epithelial cells may also be seen and are usually contaminants from the oral cavity or from the syrinx (birds). Increased numbers of heterophils indicate inflammatory disease.

Abnormal findings are supported by detecting normal-appearing cells in the wrong location, abnormal-appearing cells in any location, organisms in tissues that should not contain the organisms, and abnormal extracellular material in any location.

6. What are the initial steps involved in evaluation of a cytologic sample?

a. Determine if the samples are of good cellularity. A poorly cellular sample may not be diagnostically useful depending on the site examined. For example, cellularity is expectedly low in a normal tracheal wash; however, a liver aspirate of good diagnostic quality should contain high numbers of hepatocytes available for evaluation.
b. Use sedimentation and cytocentrifugation techniques to concentrate fluids and washes of low cellularity. For estimation of cellularity, however, a direct fluid smear must be evaluated.
c. Determine if cytologic characteristics of the tissue sampled are normal or abnormal.
d. If the samples are not normal, decide if the changes seen represent a neoplastic, hyperplastic, or inflammatory pathologic process.

7. What is neoplasia, and how is it identified in cytologic samples?

Neoplasia refers to an autonomous (not caused by external stimulus) increase in the numbers of tissue cells.

Neoplasia generally is identified by the presence and often the predominance of tissue cells with mild to marked nuclear and cellular pleomorphism (Box 53-1). The more pronounced the magnitude of pleomorphism, the greater is the likelihood of neoplasia and malignancy. Inflammation *may* be present, particularly if the neoplasm is ulcerated or ruptured. A common dilemma in some cytologic samples is how to differentiate inflammation secondary to neoplasia from *tissue dysplasia* secondary to inflammation.

Numerous types of neoplasms in all organ systems have been described in reptiles and birds.

Box 53-1 *Cytologic Criteria for Malignancy*

Nuclear Criteria*

- Anisokaryosis: variation in nuclear size
- Multinucleation: particularly important if anisokaryosis present within same cell
- Karyomegaly: exceedingly large nuclei
- Variation in shape, size, and uniformity of nucleoli: giant or abnormally shaped nucleoli
- Increased number of mitotic figures: particularly important in tissues that do not have many mitotic figures (most tissues except bone marrow)
- Abnormal morphology of mitotic figures

Cytoplasmic Criteria

- Anisocytosis: variation in cell size
- Exceedingly large cells
- Variation in cell shape

*Most reliable criteria.

8. List the different tumor types and describe general guidelines on their differentiation.

a. *Carcinoma:* cohesive, round to polygonal epithelial cells, generally with abundant cytoplasm and round to oval nuclei. If the neoplasm is of glandular origin, structures reminiscent of tubules or acini may be present. Carcinomas usually exfoliate well.

b. *Sarcoma:* elongate-spindle to plump-spindle, discrete mesenchymal cells with variable amounts of cytoplasm and oval to elongate nuclei. Depending on the specific tissue of origin, extracellular matrix may be seen in close association with the neoplastic cells. Sarcomas usually do not exfoliate well.

c. *Discrete round cell tumors:* discrete, round cells with variable amounts of cytoplasm and round to oval nuclei. Depending on the cell type, cytoplasmic granules may be present (mast cells). These tumors usually exfoliate well.

d. *Unknown tissue origin:* cytologic characteristics do not readily identify the tissue of origin.

9. What is tissue dysplasia, and how is it identified in cytologic samples?

Tissue dysplasia refers to *reversible* and atypical morphologic changes in cells that occur in response to inflammation or irritation.

Tissue dysplasia may be identified in cytologic samples in association with variable amounts of inflammation and is cytologically characterized by minimal to moderate nuclear and cytoplasmic pleomorphism (see Box 53-1). The more intense the inflammatory process, the more pronounced may be the dysplastic changes.

10. How does one differentiate between neoplasia with secondary inflammation and inflammation with secondary tissue dysplasia?

Because both dysplasia and neoplasia may share morphologic changes, such as cellular and nuclear pleomorphism, *dysplasia* secondary to inflammation must be differentiated from *neoplasia* with secondary inflammation. Typically, when dysplastic cellular changes are caused only by inflammation, the inflammatory process predominates, and the dysplastic changes are not excessive. When neoplasia is present in association with inflammation, the magnitude of the cellular and nuclear pleomorphism is usually greater than the intensity of the inflammatory process. Neoplastic cells usually (but not always) predominate in such samples.

In some cases, cytologic differentiation between dysplasia caused by inflammation and neoplasia may not be possible, and histologic examination is required.

11. What is hyperplasia, and how is it identified in cytologic samples?

Hyperplasia refers to an increase in the numbers of tissue cells in response to a known or unknown stimulus (dependent growth). It is accompanied by *hypertrophy,* an increase in cell size and cell function.

Hyperplasia may be caused by hormones or local release of inflammatory cytokines, or it may be idiopathic. Hyperplasia may be seen in multiple tissues with or without the presence of inflammation. Hyperplastic cells may exhibit dysplastic changes, particularly when associated with inflammation. Hyperplastic cells without an inflammatory component may be cytologically difficult to differentiate from normal cells. The only clue may be the presence of very high numbers of normal-appearing cells in a sample site that is usually characterized by lower cellularity.

In some cases, cytologic differentiation between well-differentiated neoplasia and hyperplasia may not be possible, and histologic examination is required.

12. What are the cytologic characteristics of inflammation in birds and reptiles?

The hallmark of inflammation is the presence of inflammatory leukocytes in cytologic samples. Heterophils, macrophages, multinucleated giant cells, lymphocytes, plasma cells, eosinophils, and basophils may be present singly or in combination. The proportion of each inflammatory cell type depends on the inciting cause and duration of the lesion.

13. What is the significance of heterophilic inflammation?

Heterophils predominate (>80% of inflammatory cells) in *heterophilic inflammation* and indicate acute or recent inflammation. They begin to accumulate in tissues within 3 hours of the inflammatory insult. Heterophils are frequently seen in lesions caused by many types of bacteria (with the notable exception of *Mycobacterium*). Heterophil degeneration may be detected if bacteria (primary or secondary infection) are part of the inflammatory process (Figure 53-1).

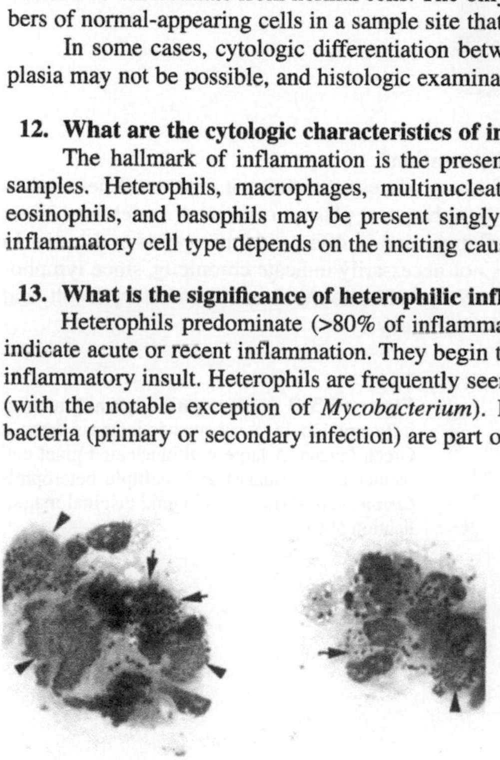

Figure 53-1 Aspirate of a subcutaneous mass from a Green iguana depicting intact and degenerate heterophils *(arrowheads)* with extracellular and intracellular bacteria *(arrows).* (Wright's stain; original magnification 1000×.)

14. What is heterophil degeneration?

Heterophil degeneration is characterized by multiple nuclear and cytoplasmic changes that are *unrelated* to heterophil toxicity. Degenerate heterophil changes are caused by released bacterial toxins *at the site* of inflammation or infection. These toxins alter the cell and nuclear membrane permeability, primarily causing swelling and vacuolation (Figure 53-2; see also Figure 53-1). Bacteria may be present within heterophils. If degenerate changes are seen, examine the slide carefully for the presence of bacteria within heterophils or in the extracellular space. Degeneration is characterized by the following:

a. Cytoplasmic vacuolation and foaminess
b. Nuclear swelling and chromatin hyalinization (chromatin will appear more eosinophilic and smooth)
c. *Karyorrhexis* (nuclear fragmentation into numerous, variably sized fragments)
d. *Karyolysis* (lysis of the nucleus)

Karyorrhexis and karyolysis are generally seen with severe heterophil degeneration.

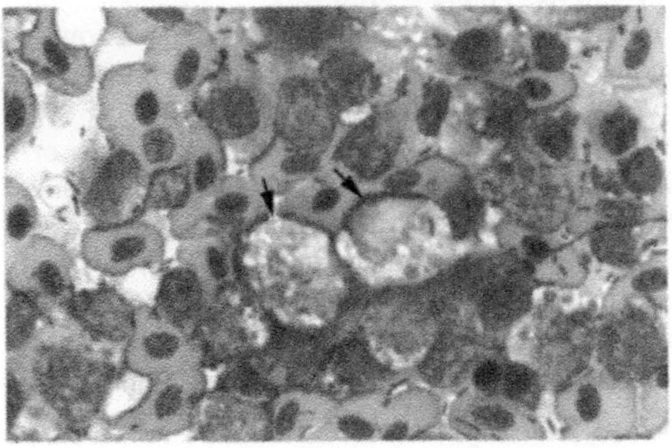

Figure 53-2 Impression smears of the epicardial surface from an African Gray parrot hatchling that died of sepsis. Degenerate heterophils *(arrows)* and numerous extracellular bacteria are shown. Bacterial fibrinous epicarditis was diagnosed by histology. (Wright's stain; original magnification 1000×.)

15. What is the significance of mixed inflammation?

Mixed inflammation refers to an inflammatory process containing a mixture of heterophils (at least 50% of leukocytes), macrophages, lymphocytes, plasma cells, and sometimes, giant multinucleated cells (Figure 53-3). Mixed inflammation is often seen in reptiles and birds. In reptiles, as in birds, mixed inflammation does not necessarily indicate chronicity, since lymphocytes and macrophages may migrate to tissues within a few hours of an inflammatory insult, and multinucleated giant cells form within hours to a few days.

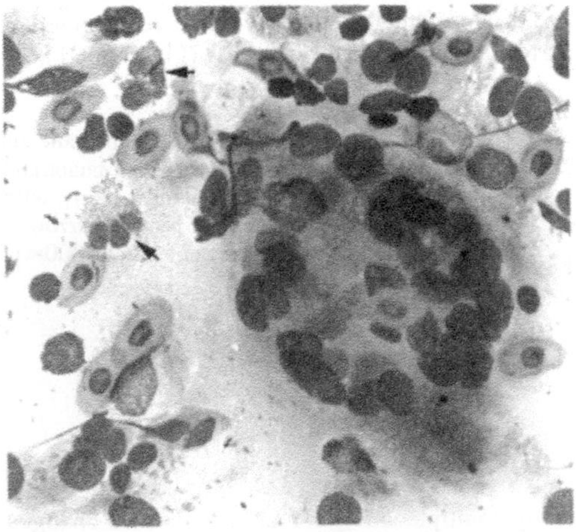

Figure 53-3 Heterophilic granulomatous inflammation in a subcutaneous mass from a Green iguana. A large multinucleated giant cell (center of the image) and multiple heterophils *(arrows)* are shown. (Diff-Quik; original magnification 500×.)

16. What is the significance of a predominantly macrophagic inflammatory process with or without multinucleated giant cells?

The presence of macrophages and multinucleated giant cells does not necessarily indicate a chronic (several weeks to months) inflammatory process. Conditions in reptiles often associated with a predominantly *macrophagic inflammatory process* with or without multinucleated giant cells (granulomatous inflammation) include *Mycobacterium* infection (Figure 53-4), fungal infection, and foreign bodies; xanthomatosis occurs in birds. In contrast to mammals, this type of inflammation may also be seen with many inflammatory conditions, such as bacterial abscesses (birds, reptiles), histomoniasis (turkeys), and chlamydophilosis (birds).

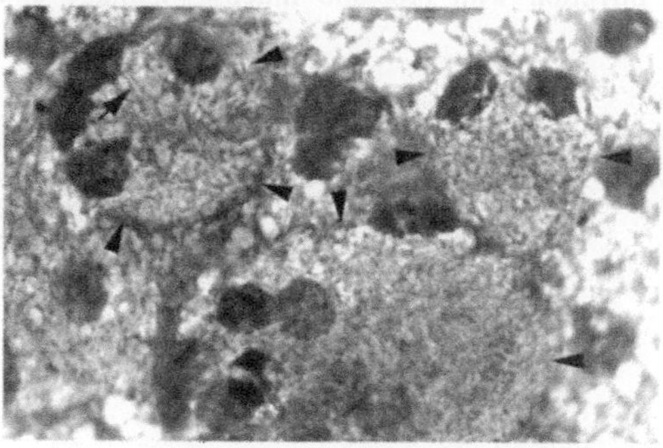

Figure 53-4 Impression smears of the mucosal intestinal surface of an Amazon parrot that died with disseminated mycobacteriosis. Multiple multinucleated giant cells *(arrowheads)* packed full of numerous nonstaining, rod-shaped mycobacteria *(arrow)* are shown. (Diff-Quik; original magnification 1000×.)

Granulomatous inflammation is another term often used to describe mixed inflammatory reactions consisting primarily of numerous macrophages with multinucleated giant cells. These reactions may contain variable numbers of lymphocytes and plasma cells.

17. When is the presence of bacteria expected, and when is it an abnormal finding?

a. In general, a *heterogeneous* population of bacteria is expected in very high numbers from fecal and cloacal cytologic samples and in lower numbers from the oral cavity, crop (birds), and esophagus. Bacteria may be seen on the surface of squamous epithelial cells in tracheal washes due to contamination from the oral cavity.

b. In organs where bacteria are expected (oral cavity, digestive tract), the presence of a *monotonous* or *homogeneous* population of bacteria suggests an abnormal overgrowth.

c. In any anatomic location, the presence of inflammatory cells with intracellular bacteria is an abnormal finding and suggests the inflammatory reaction is in response to an active infectious process (primary or secondary infection).

d. The finding of bacteria in organs or tissues that should not contain bacteria (e.g., liver, lungs, air sacs) represents an abnormal finding.

18. How is cytology used in the diagnosis of bacterial infections?

The main advantage of cytology is that, if present in sufficient numbers, bacteria may be quickly and easily visualized (see Figures 53-1, 53-2, and 53-4). A primarily heterophilic or a mixed inflammatory process (with neutrophil predominance) is seen with most bacterial infections, and heterophil degeneration may be an important feature. The inflammatory reaction to mycobacteria consists of macrophages with or without multinucleated giant cells. Mycobacteria do not stain with Romanowsky-type stains and are seen as negative-staining rod-shaped structures within macrophages and giant cells and in the extracellular space (see Figure 53-4). Acid-fast stains are necessary to visualize the organisms.

19. When is the presence of a fungus expected, and when is it an abnormal finding?

Finding fungal organisms (yeasts, hyphae, fruiting bodies) should be considered an abnormal finding in any tissue or organ from a bird or a reptile. In *birds,* very infrequently seen spherical to oval-shaped yeasts (1 or 2 yeasts per one or two 100×-objective oil immersion fields) in the absence of inflammation may be seen in samples from the upper alimentary tract, feces, and cloaca. Many consider the finding of these low numbers of yeasts in birds to be of no clinical significance.

Greater numbers of yeasts, with or without budding, in the upper alimentary tract, feces, and cloaca are an important finding and indicate yeast overgrowth (Figure 53-5). The presence of hyphae associated with yeasts, with or without budding, in the same anatomic locations mentioned above suggests severe infection with probable mucosal damage and invasion.

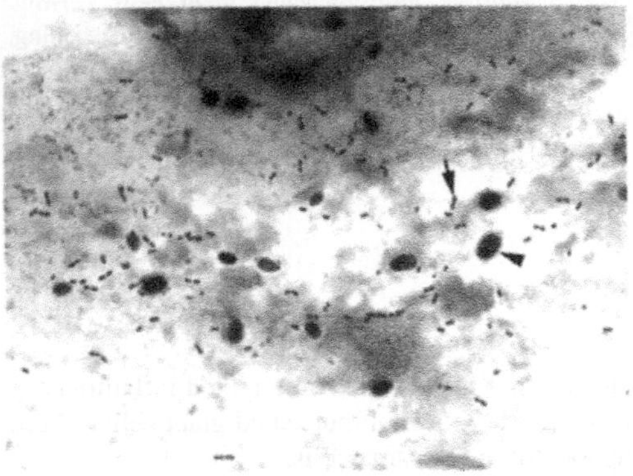

Figure 53-5 Fresh fecal smear from an Amazon parrot with yeast overgrowth. Numerous bacteria *(arrow)* and oval yeasts *(arrowhead)* are shown. (Diff-Quik; original magnification 1000×.)

20. How is cytology used in the diagnosis of fungal infections?

a. The main advantage of cytology is that, if present in sufficient numbers, fungi may be easily visualized.
b. The inflammatory reaction to fungi in tissue consists primarily of macrophages and multinucleated giant cells (granulomatous inflammation), with variable numbers of heterophils and other inflammatory cells.
c. Fungi may be seen in tissue as yeasts and hyphae. In those species that form hyphae in tissue (e.g., *Aspergillus*), fruiting bodies may be present and help identify the fungus.
d. The specific morphology of yeasts varies depending on the infecting fungus, but characteristics to look for include the presence of a capsule *(Cryptococcus),* type of budding (broad vs. narrow base), and size of the yeast.
e. The specific morphology of hyphae vary with the fungus, but characteristics to look for include pigmentation, branching, type of branching (dichotomous vs. nondichotomous), approximate angle of branching (right angles vs. other), hyphae thickness and uniformity (parallel-sided cell walls) and presence or absence of fruiting bodies and other structures (Figure 53-6).

21. When is the presence of protozoa expected, and when is it an abnormal finding?

In birds and reptiles, finding protozoal organisms (sporozoites, cysts, trophozoites, merozoites, oocysts) is an abnormal finding in most organs or tissues. However, the presence of some flagellates and ciliates in the stool of reptiles is not always correlated with clinical disease. Infected individuals may serve as carriers and may present with disease if immunosuppressed because of other diseases or conditions.

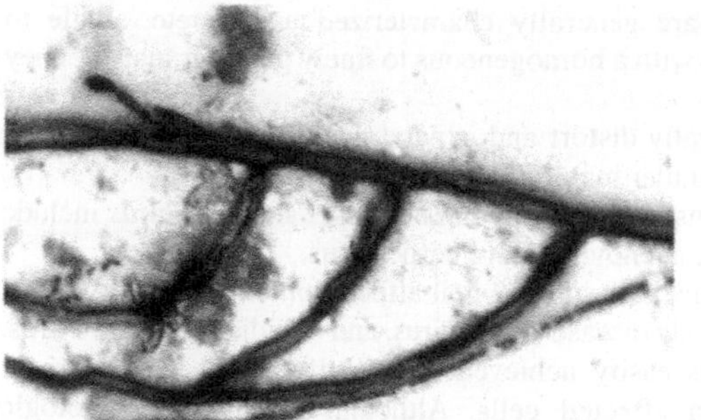

Figure 53-6 Impression smear of caseous material from the oral cavity of a Bearded Dragon lizard. Numerous branching, septate hyphae were seen and are shown in the image. (Wright's stain; original magnification 1000×.)

22. How is cytology used in the diagnosis of protozoal infections?

a. The main advantage of cytology is that, if present in sufficient numbers, protozoal organisms may be easily visualized (Figure 53-7).
b. The inflammatory reaction to protozoa may vary from nonexistent (*Giardia* in gastrointestinal tract) to heterophilic to a mixed inflammatory process with or without abundant necrotic material.
c. *Trichomonas, Sarcocystis,* and *Giardia* organisms are seen in samples from pet and wild birds.
d. Intestinal protozoa other than *Giardia* are not usually seen in pet birds but are seen in wild birds and poultry.
e. *Entamoeba invadens,* coccidia, and other protozoa are often seen in reptiles.
f. Morphology of the organisms depends on the specific protozoal agent, but characteristics to look for include number and location of nuclei, flagella, location and number of flagella, shape of organisms, and presence of a cyst wall. With intestinal protozoa it is helpful to determine the combination and number of merozoites and sporocysts per oocyst.
g. Blood protozoa may be encountered during cytologic evaluation of tissues resulting from blood contamination or presence of tissue stages.

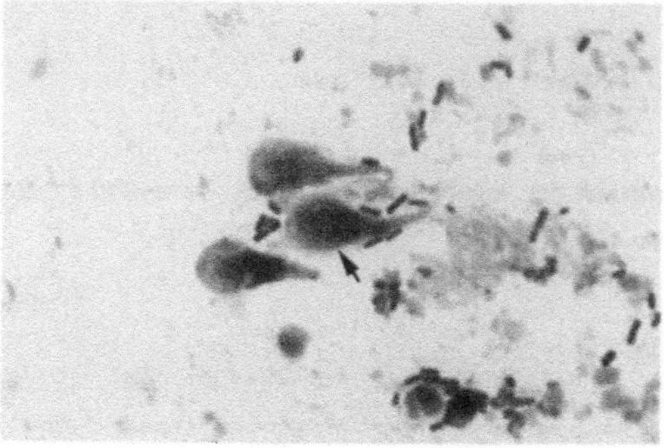

Figure 53-7 Three *Giardia* spp. throphozoites *(arrow)* in a fresh fecal smear from a budgerigar with loose stools. *Giardia* throphozoites are characterized by a pyriform shape, two prominent nuclei, and flagella (not shown). (Diff-Quik; original magnification 1000×.)

23. When is the presence of viral inclusions expected, and when is it an abnormal finding?

Viral inclusions (cytoplasmic or nuclear) are an abnormal finding in any tissue of birds or reptiles.

24. How is cytology used in the diagnosis of viral infections in birds and reptiles?

a. *Viral inclusions* may rarely be seen by cytologic examination of affected tissues.

b. *Intracytoplasmic viral inclusions* are generally characterized as discrete, single to multiple structures of variable sizes with a homogeneous to finely granular matrix. They may also appear as vacuoles.
c. *Intranuclear viral inclusions* generally distort and expand nuclei and are identified as hyaline, homogeneous to finely granular material within the nucleus.
d. Viruses that may form cell inclusions in tissue and that affect pet and wild *birds* include poxvirus, polyomavirus, circovirus, adenovirus, and herpesvirus.
e. Viruses that may form cell inclusions in tissue and that affect *reptiles* include poxvirus, herpesvirus, adenovirus, inclusion body disease (IBD) virus, and ophidian paramyxovirus.
f. Cytologic diagnosis of poxvirus is easily achieved by identifying the characteristic intracytoplasmic inclusions within affected cells. Although presumptive cytologic diagnosis of viral infections other than poxvirus is possible, diagnosis is most often made using histopathologic examination.

25. How is cytology used in the diagnosis of helminth infections in birds and reptiles?

a. Routine cytologic examination of tissues, masses, and feces may reveal various life stages of helminths. One should keep in mind that the use of cytology is generally not the most sensitive method of diagnosing helminth infections.
b. Adult filarids produce blood microfilariae that may be found in cytologic preparations due to the presence of peripheral blood.
c. Fecal smears, tracheal washes, aspirates, and upper gastrointestinal samples may reveal the presence of helminth eggs or larvae (Figure 53-8).

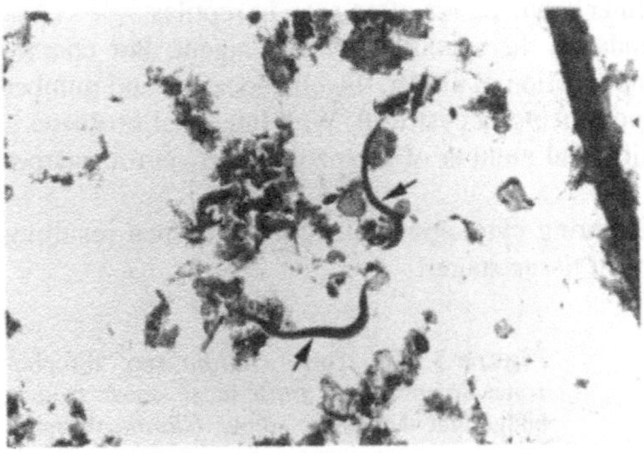

Figure 53-8 Fecal smear from a salamander infected with *Rhabdias* spp. lungworms. Two *Rhabdias* spp. larvae are shown *(arrows)*. Although the sample is not from a reptile, the image demonstrates the benefits of cytologic examination of feces. (Wright's stain; original magnification 100×.)

26. List some diseases of the avian integument for which cytology may be useful in the diagnosis (Box 53-2).

a. Xanthoma/xanthomatosis
b. Neoplasms
c. Bacterial, viral, fungal and parasitic infections
d. Foreign body reactions

Box 53-2 *Avian and Reptilian Integumentary Diseases with Diagnostic Role for Cytology*
Xanthoma/xanthomatosis (birds)
Neoplasms: various
Bacterial, viral (poxvirus), fungal, and parasitic infections
Foreign body reactions

27. Describe xanthoma and xanthomatosis.

Xanthomas are nonneoplastic swellings or masses cytologically characterized by accumulations of lipid-filled macrophages, giant cells, and extracellular cholesterol crystals with or without fibrosis. Xanthomas are usually found in the integument but may be found in other locations. The cholesterol crystals are visualized in cytologic preparations as angular, rectangular, negative-staining structures in the extracellular space.

Xanthomatosis is the term used when multiple xanthomas are present. Xanthomatosis is generally associated with increased serum cholesterol and triglycerides and is often seen in birds.

28. What neoplasms of the avian integument can be diagnosed cytologically?

Most neoplasms of the avian integument can be diagnosed cytologically. Although multiple types of tumors have been identified in birds, common neoplasms include the following:

a. Lipomas: often seen in pet birds, particularly budgerigars
b. Epithelial tumors
   (1) Squamous cell carcinoma: often seen in fowl, but can occur in many species of birds
   (2) Papilloma: may consist primarily of cytologically normal squamous cells
c. Sarcomas
   (1) Fibrosarcoma
   (2) Liposarcoma
d. Discrete round cell tumors
   (1) Lymphosarcoma: frequently seen in fowl with avian leukosis, but may be seen in any species of bird
   (2) Melanomas

For detailed cytologic descriptions of these and other tumors, see the Bibliography at the end of this chapter.

29. What bacterial infections of the avian integument can be diagnosed cytologically?

Mycobacterium spp. do not stain with Romanowsky-type stains (see Figure 53-4). They appear as negative-staining structures within macrophages and multinucleated giant cells. Miscellaneous types of bacteria can also be diagnosed cytologically.

30. What viral infections of the avian integument can be diagnosed cytologically?

Poxvirus produces intracytoplasmic inclusions that distend infected squamous cell and displace the nucleus paracentrally (Figure 53-9). Poxviral lesions consist of small, crusty areas to discrete masses and are most often seen in the oral cavity and the unfeathered skin. A mixed inflammatory process may be seen.

Other viruses affecting the skin of birds include *circovirus,* such as psittacine beak and feather disease (PBFD) virus, and *polyomavirus,* such as budgerigar fledging disease (BFD)

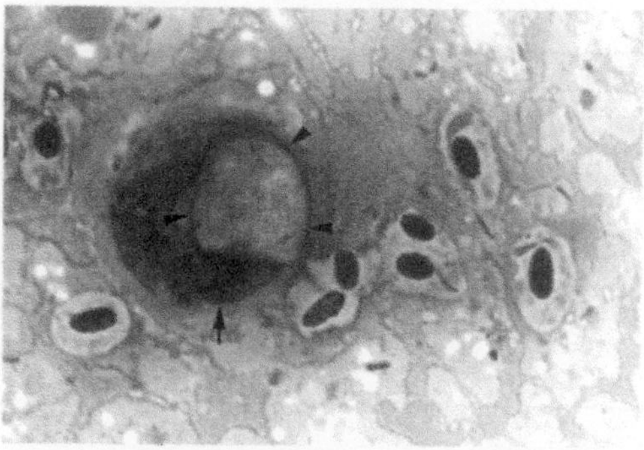

Figure 53-9 Impression smear of a mass in the beak of a Sanderling (a shorebird). One swollen squamous epithelial cell with a single, round, intracytoplasmic poxvirus inclusion *(arrowheads)* is shown. The nucleus is displaced to the edge of the cell *(arrow).* (Diff-Quik; original magnification 1000×.)

virus. Although these viruses may form prominent intranuclear inclusions, diagnosis is often obtained by histopathology and not by cytology.

31. What fungal infections of the avian integument can be diagnosed cytologically?

Any fungus infecting the avian integument that stains with Romanowsky stains and that is present in sufficient numbers may be diagnosed cytologically. If organisms are not seen, the inflammatory process (primarily macrophages and multinucleated giant cells) should produce a high degree of suspicion for a fungal etiology.

32. What parasitic infections of the avian integument can be diagnosed cytologically?

Mites are diagnosed cytologically in birds. *Knemidokoptes* species are most often seen in budgerigars and poultry. Mites may be detected in unstained scrapings made from the typical crusty lesions. Some *trematodes* may form subcutaneous cysts in passerine and gallinaceous birds. Fine-needle aspirates would consist of the typical operculated trematode eggs (see following questions on alimentary tract).

33. What are the cytologic characteristics of foreign body reactions in birds?

The inflammatory reaction is primarily macrophagic with multinucleated giant cells. Heterophils may be detected with secondary bacterial infections. The foreign body may be evident cytologically (plant material, keratinaceous debris).

34. When is cytologic examination of the alimentary tract useful in birds?

Cytologic examination is of use when evaluation of the oral cavity, crop, upper intestinal content, cloacal samples, and feces is necessary.

35. List the indications for obtaining cytologic samples from the alimentary tract in birds.

a. Crusts
b. Masses
c. Ulcers
d. Excessive mucus or exudates
e. Dysphagia
f. Regurgitation
g. Delayed crop emptying
h. Diarrhea
i. Bloody stool

36. List some diseases of the alimentary tract in birds for which cytology may be useful in the diagnosis (Box 53-3).

a. Bacterial infections
b. Poxvirus

Box 53-3 *Avian and Reptilian Alimentary Diseases with Diagnostic Role for Cytology*
Bacterial infections: overgrowth
Poxvirus: oral cavity of birds
Parasitic infections: trichomoniasis, giardiasis, other intestinal protozoa, helminths
Fungal infections: candidiasis, other fungi
Neoplasia
Hypovitaminosis A

c. Parasitic infections
   (1) Trichomoniasis
   (2) Giardiasis
   (3) Other intestinal protozoa
   (4) Helminths
d. Fungal infections (candidiasis)
e. Neoplasia
f. Hypovitaminosis A

37. Can bacterial overgrowth be diagnosed cytologically in birds?

a. Bacterial overgrowth of the upper and lower alimentary tract may be *strongly suspected* cytologically by the presence of numerous, morphologically similar bacteria in Romanowsky-stained smears.
b. Gram-stained smears assist in the diagnosis by confirming that the bacteria present in the samples are of the same Gram stain status. Use of Romanowsky-type stains will *not* assist in the determination of Gram stain status.
c. Overgrowth of *Clostridium* spp. may be strongly suspected in cases of diarrhea, if the characteristic "safety pin" spores are present on fecal smears.

38. What are the cytologic characteristics of intestinal mycobacteriosis in birds?

Romanowsky-stained impression smears and scrapings of intestinal mucosa will reveal macrophages and giant cells distended with numerous rod-shaped, negative-staining organisms in avian mycobacteriosis. Variable numbers of columnar intestinal epithelial cells may be present. Acid-fast stains are necessary to visualize the organisms (see Figure 53-4).

39. How do oral poxviral lesions differ from integumentary poxviral lesions in birds?

Cytologically, oral and integumentary poxviral lesions are similar. Grossly, the oral lesions ("wet pox") may be more caseous and fibrinous in appearance.

40. Describe the cytologic characteristics of avian trichomoniasis.

a. Trichomonads (*Trichomonas* spp.) are irregularly oval to round (8-14 μm in diameter) protozoan organisms characterized by a single nucleus, anterior flagella, undulating membrane, and an axostyle. The cytoplasm is basophilic.
b. The nucleus is located toward one end of the organism and typically stains eosinophilic.
c. The flagella extend from the end of the organism (location of nucleus) into the extracellular space.
d. The intracellular axostyle typically stains eosinophilic and extends in a straight line from the area of the nucleus toward the end of the organism, opposite the end where the flagella are located.
e. An undulating membrane is present to one side of the organism.
f. Infections are often found in the upper alimentary tract but may also occur in the respiratory tract.
g. A mixed inflammatory cell reaction is most often associated with the organisms.
h. Although trichomoniasis may occur in any bird species (e.g., budgerigars, cockatiels), it is most often reported in pigeons and raptors.
i. Unstained wet-mount sample preparations are best in demonstrating the motile, flagellated organisms.

41. Describe the cytologic characteristics of avian giardiasis.

Giardia spp. are protozoan parasites affecting the lower alimentary tract of birds. Trophozoites are approximately 10 to 20 μm × 5 to 15 μm in size and are characterized by a pear-shaped body, two nuclei, flagella, a disk-shaped structure, and basophilic cytoplasm. They may be detected in fecal smears and cloacal swabs. *Giardia* cysts may also be seen and are characterized by a round shape, four nuclei, and the absence of flagella. They measure approximately 10 to 14 μm × 8 to 10 μm in size (see Figure 53-7).

42. Describe the cytologic characteristics of intestinal coccidian infections in birds.

Coccidian life stages can be detected in fecal smears or in intestinal scrapings if present in sufficient numbers. Merozoites, schizonts, macrogamonts, microgametes, and oocysts may be readily identified in mucosal scrapping or impression smears. Disseminated intestinal coccidial infection can also occur in birds. Organisms may be identified in multiple extraintestinal tissues (blood, lungs, liver, spleen). Intestinal coccidia are most often encountered in poultry and wild birds.

43. Is cytology useful in the diagnosis of alimentary tract helminth infections in birds?

Helminth eggs and larvae may be seen in direct smears of fecal material, and crop lavages (see Figure 53-8). Cytology is limited by its low sensitivity of detection.

Collyriclum faba is a trematode that may form subcutaneous cysts in the cloacal opening of passerine and gallinaceous birds. Aspiration of these cysts may reveal numerous operculated, pigmented eggs.

44. Describe the cytologic characteristics of avian candidiasis.

Candida spp. are round to oval, basophilic yeasts approximately 3 to 4 μm in diameter (see Figure 53-5). *Candida* organisms proliferate primarily by budding; however, hyphae may form in severe infections with invasion of the mucosal surface. Although very low numbers of yeasts may be seen in clinically normal birds, high numbers of yeasts, prominent budding, and hyphae formation indicate severe infections.

Candidiasis is associated with poor diets (all seed), immunosuppression, and concurrent alimentary tract diseases. Candidiasis is frequently seen in pet birds. *Candida* organisms may be found in samples from the oral cavity, crop, cloaca, and feces. Some dietary supplements may contain yeasts that, if fed to birds, will be present in fecal samples and must be ruled out from true yeast overgrowth.

45. Describe the cytologic characteristics of avian gastric yeasts.

Avian gastric yeasts are large, rod-shaped, elongate, and gram-positive yeasts. Staining characteristics in Romanowsky-stained smears are variable, but avian gastric yeasts may stain pale pink with small, round, pink nuclei (Figure 53-10). They are associated with severe weight loss in canaries and psittacines (budgerigars, cockatiels). The proposed name for this yeast is *Macrorhabdus ornithogaster.*

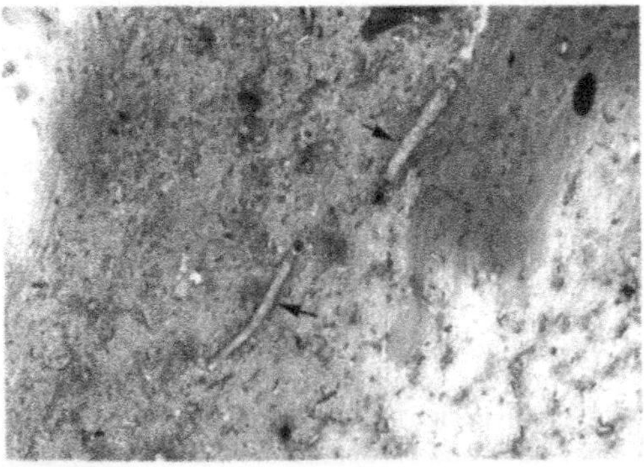

Figure 53-10 Two large, rod-shaped avian gastric yeasts *(arrows)* and numerous extracellular bacteria are shown in a fresh fecal smear from a cockatiel. (Wright's stain; original magnification 1000×.)

46. What neoplasms of the alimentary tract can be diagnosed cytologically in birds?

a. Papilloma: oral, esophageal, and cloacal; consist primarily of normal-looking squamous cells. Definitive diagnosis requires histologic examination.
b. Squamous cell carcinoma of oral cavity, esophagus, and crop (uncommon)
c. Other neoplasms (e.g., leiomyosarcoma, carcinoma) may be seen in the provetriculus, ventriculus, and intestines.

47. Describe the cytologic appearance of cutaneous lesions associated with hypovitaminosis A in birds.

The cells in the cutaneous lesions mainly consist of large numbers to dense aggregates of normal-appearing, keratinized, squamous epithelial cells. Inflammation and organisms are not present unless an infection (fungal, bacterial) is superimposed. The cytologic characteristics are not specific for hypovitaminosis A, but if accompanied by the appropriate clinical findings, the cytologic characteristics can suggest the disease.

48. List some diseases of the liver in birds for which cytology may be useful in the diagnostic process (Box 53-4).

a. Inflammation of any cause (bacterial, fungal, parasitic)
b. Hepatocellular degeneration
c. Neoplasia (metastatic or primary)
d. Hemosiderosis and hemochromatosis
e. Amyloidosis

Box 53-4 *Avian and Reptilian Liver Diseases with Diagnostic Role for Cytology*
Inflammation of any cause: bacterial, fungal, protozoal, viral
Hepatocellular necrosis: may be associated with viral infection
Hepatocellular degeneration: lipidosis, glycogen accumulation
Bile stasis
Neoplasia: metastatic or primary
Hemosiderosis/hemochromatosis (birds primarily)
Amyloidosis (birds primarily)

49. List some infectious causes of inflammation in the liver of birds.

a. *Mycobacterium* spp.
b. *Chlamydophila psittaci* spp. (found within macrophages)
c. *Histomonas meleagridis* (primarily turkeys and other poultry species)
d. Viruses: most produce intranuclear inclusions that may be seen cytologically; however, the diagnosis is most often obtained by histologic examination.
   (1) Pacheco's disease virus (Psittacid herpesvirus)
   (2) Avian polyomavirus
   (3) Adenovirus
e. Other miscellaneous bacteria, fungi, and helminths
f. Tissue stages of hemoparasites *(Haemoproteus, Plasmodium)* may be seen in the liver with or without associated inflammation.

50. Describe the cytologic appearance of hepatocellular degeneration in birds.

When hepatocytes accumulate lipid *(hepatic lipidosis),* the cytoplasm will have variable numbers of clear, round, variably sized, sharply demarcated vacuoles. The vacuoles are clear because the lipid is washed out during fixation. The vacuoles may distort the hepatocytes to the point of displacing the nucleus. When hepatocytes accumulate glycogen or when organelles swell *(hydropic degeneration),* the cytoplasm appears foamy and lighter staining without clear vacuoles. Hepatocytes may have both types of cytoplasmic changes.

51. What causes hepatocellular degeneration in birds?

The multiple causes of hepatocellular degeneration include toxins, metabolic diseases, hypoxia, infectious agents, and poor nutrition (high-fat diets in pet birds). For example, cockatoos (umbrella and Moluccan), and blue and gold macaw neonates reportedly develop hepatic lipidosis if overfed with hand-fed formula.

Nonpathologic hepatocellular lipid accumulation, without the presence of clinical signs or inflammation, may be a normal finding in very young ducklings and geese (<1 week old). This subsides as the yolk sac is reabsorbed.

52. What neoplasms of the liver may be diagnosed cytologically in birds?

a. Carcinomas: hepatocellular, cholangiocarcinoma, metastatic
b. Sarcomas: hemangiosarcoma, others
c. Discrete round cell tumors: lymphosarcoma

Hyperplasia and benign tumors of hepatocytes and bile duct cells are difficult to diagnose cytologically and are usually diagnosed by histologic examination.

53. What is the difference between hemosiderosis and hemochromatosis?

Hemosiderosis describes increased iron (hemosiderin) accumulation in tissue cells (hepatocytes, macrophages, other tissues) *without* the presence of tissue damage. Hemosiderosis may occur in any species of bird and may progress to hemochromatosis in some species. Hemosiderosis without architectural damage may result from hemolytic disease but may also be idiopathic.

Hemochromatosis describes increased iron accumulation in tissue cells (hepatocytes, macrophages) *with* concurrent tissue damage (inflammation, fibrosis). The tissue damage is believed to result from the accumulation of iron. Hemochromatosis is often seen in mynah birds *(Gracula religiosa),* Rhamphastidae (toucans), Sturnidae (birds of paradise), and quetzals but may occur in any species of bird.

Mynah birds, toucans, birds of paradise, and quetzals have a predisposition to hemosiderosis and hemochromatosis. The cause of this predisposition is likely multifactorial and may include excessive dietary iron, species characteristics, and other, unknown causes.

54. What are the cytologic characteristics of hemosiderosis and hemochromatosis?

In hemosiderosis and hemochromatosis, hepatocytes and macrophages with increased amounts of intracellular iron may have golden-brown to gray, granular pigment within the cytoplasm (Figure 53-11). Hemosiderin accumulation in hemochromatosis is very prominent in hepatocytes.

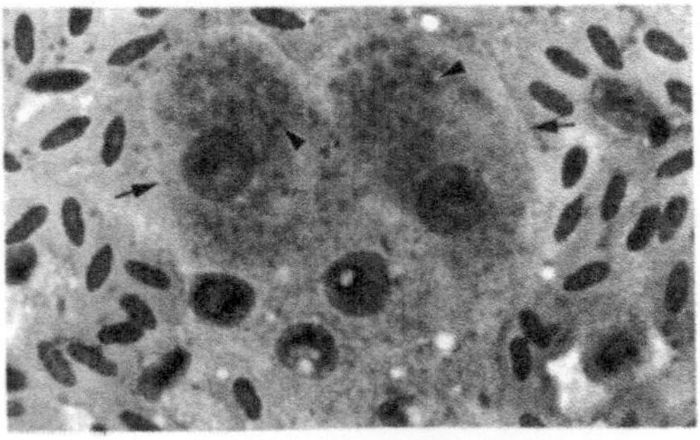

Figure 53-11 Impression smear from the liver of a Mynah bird with hepatic hemochromatosis. Hepatocytes *(arrows)* with intracellular granular deposits of hemosiderin *(arrowheads)* are shown. (Diff-Quik; original magnification 1000×.)

Inflammation (heterophils, lymphocytes, macrophages) is seen in hemochromatosis. Although difficult to find, fibrosis may be seen cytologically as increased numbers of spindle-shaped mesenchymal cells. Inflammation must be differentiated from extramedullary hematopoiesis.

55. What are the cytologic characteristics of amyloidosis?

If present in sufficient quantities, *amyloid* may be seen in cytologic preparations as extracellular, amorphous, eosinophilic to basophilic, globular to fibrillar material. Because the appearance of this material in Romanowsky-stained preparations is not specific for amyloid, Congo red stain may be used to determine if suspicious extracellular material is amyloid. Green birefringence under polarized light indicates the material is amyloid. Amyloidosis is frequently seen in Anseriformes (ducks, geese), gulls, shorebirds, and birds in zoologic collections.

Cytologic identification of amyloidosis has *not* been described in birds but has been described in domestic animals and humans. Diagnosis is most frequently obtained by histologic examination.

56. List some diseases of the renal system in birds for which cytology may be useful in the diagnostic process (Box 53-5).

a. Infections/inflammation
   (1) Bacteria (miscellaneous)
   (2) Fungi: aspergillosis
   (3) Parasites: protozoa, helminths
b. Neoplasia
   (1) Renal carcinomas (often seen in budgerigars)
   (2) Embryonal nephroma (often seen in budgerigars)
   (3) Lymphosarcoma
   (4) Metastatic tumors
c. Gout
d. Amyloidosis may be seen in ducks and geese as part of systemic disease.
e. Inflammation, infectious agents, and tubular casts may be seen in urine sediment.

Box 53-5 *Avian and Reptilian Kidney Diseases with Diagnostic Role for Cytology*
Bacterial, viral, fungal and parasitic infections
Neoplasia: renal carcinomas, lymphosarcoma, embryonal nephroma (birds), other neoplasms
Amyloidosis (birds primarily)
Renal gout

57. Describe the cytologic appearance of embryonal nephroma in birds.

Because of their "primitive" origin (less differentiated, thus "embryonal"), neoplastic cells may have an *epithelial* (cohesive, polygonal clusters) or a *mesenchymal* (spindle-shaped, noncohesive) appearance. It may be difficult if not impossible to determine the differentiation of some neoplastic cells.

Embryonal nephromas sometimes produce extracellular, pink, fibrillar to amorphous, extracellular matrix. This material will be intimately associated with the neoplastic cells and may represent cartilaginous matrix or osteoid.

58. Describe the cytologic appearance of renal gout in birds.

In addition to the cuboidal to polygonal, tubular epithelial cells, *gout* samples will contain aggregates of extracellular, eosinophilic, fine, needle-shaped crystals that may be associated with a mixed inflammatory infiltrate. Urate crystals are birefringent under polarized light. The typical spherical, refractile, nonstaining, variably sized urate crystals routinely seen in urine and cloacal swabs should not be confused with the thin, needle-shaped urate crystals typically seen in gout. Lesions associated with gout may also be seen in various organs, particularly joints.

59. When is cytologic evaluation of the respiratory system useful in birds?

Cytologic examination is of use when the clinical signs suggest respiratory disease (dyspnea, nasal discharge) in birds. Diagnostic samples include the following:

a. Nasal swabs (Figure 53-12)
b. Tracheal lavage
c. Bronchoalveolar lavage
d. Air sac swabs and lavages
e. Postmortem imprints and scrapings

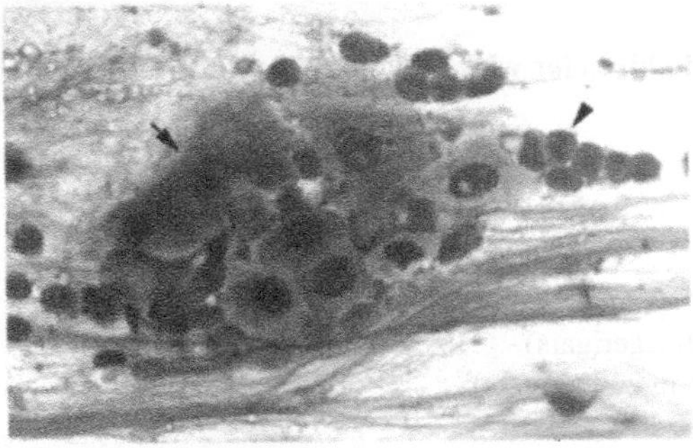

Figure 53-12 Smear of a swab sample from the nasal cavity of a Sun conure with nasal discharge. Squamous epithelial cells *(arrows)* and numerous small lymphocytes *(arrowheads)* are shown. (Diff-Quik; original magnification 500×.)

60. List some diseases of the respiratory system in birds for which cytology may be useful in the diagnostic process (Box 53-6).

a. Infectious agents: bacteria, fungi, protozoa
b. Neoplasms: primary or metastatic (rarely seen)
c. Helminth infections may be detected cytologically (eggs, larvae) but are rarely seen in pet birds.

Box 53-6 *Avian and Reptilian Respiratory Diseases with Diagnostic Role for Cytology*
Infectious agents: bacteria, fungi, protozoa, helminths (eggs or larvae may be seen) Neoplasms: primary or metastatic (rarely seen)

61. What bacterial agents may be encountered in respiratory infections in birds?

a. *Mycobacterium* spp.
b. *Chlamydophila psittaci* spp.
c. *Mycoplasma* spp.
d. Spiral-shaped bacteria (Figure 53-13)
e. Miscellaneous bacteria

62. Describe the cytologic characteristics of chlamydial infections.

Chlamydophila psittaci organisms are difficult to detect and will present as intracellular aggregates of small, blue to pink, coccoid organisms (elementary or reticulate bodies) within

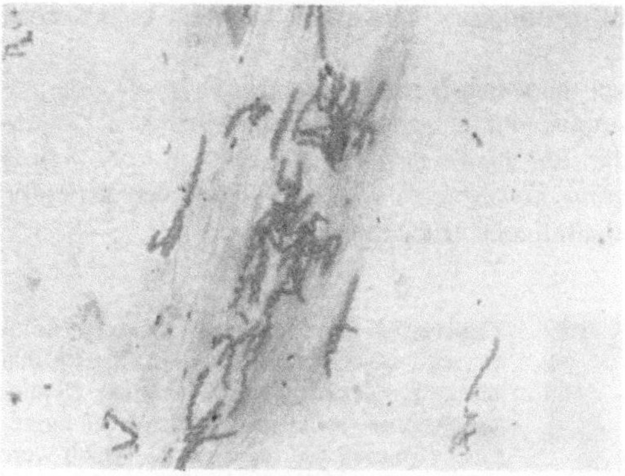

Figure 53-13 Smear of a swab sample from the nasal cavity of a Lovebird. Numerous spiral-shaped bacteria are shown. (Diff-Quik; original magnification 1000×.)

macrophages. Sometimes the organisms occur within epithelial cells. The inflammatory reaction varies from heterophilic to mixed to macrophagic. Elementary bodies (~0.3 μm; infectious stage) are smaller than the reticulate bodies (~1 μm; proliferative stage). The organisms may be confused with *Mycoplasma* because of similar size (~0.3 μm) and appearance. *Mycoplasma* organisms are extracellular bacteria found on the surface of epithelial cells and macrophages.

Macchiavello's and Gimenez stains may be used to facilitate the identification of *Chlamydophila psittaci;* however, *Mycoplasma* and Rickettsiae may stain similarly. Therefore, other specific tests (culture, molecular diagnostic techniques) must be used to identify the organisms definitively. *Chlamydophila psittaci* spp. cause disease throughout the respiratory tract and in other tissues.

63. What is the significance of spiral-shaped bacteria in choanal and nasal swabs from psittacines?

The significance of spiral-shaped bacteria is unknown. However, these bacteria have been detected in birds with some mild clinical signs of respiratory disease (sneezing, nasal discharge). The spiral-shaped bacteria stain lightly basophilic or may stain poorly with Romanowsky stains (see Figure 53-13).

64. List some of the fungal diseases that may affect the respiratory tract of birds.

a. *Aspergillus* is implicated in most cases of mycotic respiratory disease in birds.
b. *Candida albicans* is not a common cause but is seen as part of disseminated disease.
c. *Cryptococcus neoformans* and other fungi are infrequently described in clinical cases.

65. Describe the cytologic characteristics of avian aspergillosis.

Aspergillus grows in tissues as hyphae accompanied by a mixed to a macrophagic and granulomatous inflammatory reaction. Hyphae are septate, nonpigmented, and basophilic, with parallel-sided cell walls and dichotomous branching (successive forking into two branches) at approximately 45-degree angles. The hyphae may not stain well. Conidiophores (fruiting body) bearing conidia may be found and help identify the fungal hyphae as *Aspergillus*. Conidia may be confused with small yeasts. Pigmented hyphae (brown pigmentation) are indicative of other species of fungi.

66. List some of the protozoal diseases that affect the respiratory tract of birds.

a. *Sarcocystis falcatula*
b. *Trichomonas* spp.
c. *Cryptosporidium* spp. (chickens)

67. Describe the cytologic characteristics of pulmonary *Sarcocystis falcatula* infection in birds.

Postmortem scrapings of pulmonary tissue may reveal mostly blood with small elongate ("banana-shaped") merozoites singly or in groups with minimal to no inflammation (Figure 53-14). An eosinophilic nucleus is present within the merozoites. The cytologic morphology is not specific for *S. falcatula* because *Toxoplasma gondii* may stain similarly. Histologically, meronts and merozoites are found within endothelial cells of the lung.

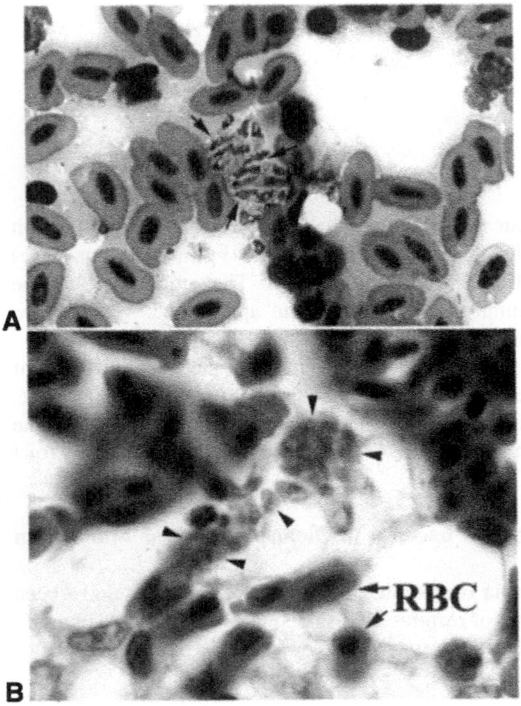

Figure 53-14 Scraping (**A**) and histologic section (**B**) from an Amazon parrot that died of *Sarcocystis falcatula* infection. Cytologic preparations contained rarely seen aggregates of merozoites (*arrows,* **A**), which were within endothelial cells in tissue sections of the lung (*arrowheads,* **B**). *RBC,* Red blood cells. (**A,** Wright's stain; original magnification 1000×. **B,** Hematoxylin and eosin; original magnification 400×.)

S. falcatula infection is frequently fatal, and affected birds may die suddenly or with few clinical signs. Infection results from contamination with opossum feces infected with *S. falcatula* sporocysts.

68. List and briefly discuss the cytologic significance of some viral infections that affect the respiratory system of birds.

a. Herpesvirus
b. Poxvirus
c. Paramyxovirus

Some of these viruses form cytoplasmic or nuclear inclusions that may be seen cytologically; however, a diagnosis is most often reached with histologic examination. Mixed inflammatory reactions may be seen with these viruses. Syncytial cell formation is seen with some herpesviral respiratory infections of birds.

69. List cytologic characteristics of normal coelomic fluid in birds.

a. Clinically normal birds should have minimal to no collectable fluid in the coelomic cavity.

b. Cytologically, the fluid is of low cellularity and consists primarily of macrophages and mesothelial cells.
c. Mesothelial cells are found singly or in cohesive clusters. They are polygonal to round cells with abundant basophilic cytoplasm and round to oval, finely stippled nuclei. Nuclear and cytoplasmic pleomorphism is minimal to nonexistent.
d. Macrophages appear as round to oval, mononuclear cells with intracytoplasmic vacuoles and round to oval to sometimes indented nuclei.
e. If peripheral blood contamination has occurred, there should be no inflammatory reaction or erythrophagocytosis. Thrombocytes may be present.

70. Describe the cytologic changes that characterize mesothelial cell reactivity or dysplasia in birds.

Reactive mesothelial cells are characterized as follows:
a. Round shape
b. Increased amounts of cytoplasm
c. Increased cytoplasmic basophilia
d. Increased nuclear and cytoplasmic pleomorphism
e. Prominent nucleoli
f. Vacuolation, binucleation, mitotic figures, and fibrillar pink cytoplasmic margins may be seen.

Reactive mesothelial cell changes result from inflammatory or irritant processes in the coelomic cavity. The more intense the inflammatory or irritant process, the more reactive may be the mesothelial cells. Extremely reactive mesothelial cells may be difficult to differentiate from carcinoma or mesothelioma cells. Caution is needed when diagnosing neoplasia if inflammation is present in the sample.

71. List some diseases of the coelomic cavity in birds for which cytology may be useful in the diagnostic process (Box 53-7).

a. Infectious diseases
   (1) Miscellaneous bacteria spread from systemic infections, penetrating trauma, and ruptured intestines.
   (2) Heterophilic inflammatory reaction with heterophil degeneration is primarily seen.
b. Irritating substances
   (1) Yolk coelomitis: may have a superimposed bacterial component
   (2) Urinary leakage (rarely seen)
c. Hemorrhage
d. Neoplasms

Box 53-7 ***Avian and Reptilian Coelomic Diseases with Diagnostic Role for Cytology***

Infectious agents: bacteria, fungi, protozoa
Irritating substances: yolk coelomitis, urates
Hemorrhage
Neoplasms (various)

72. Describe the cytologic characteristics of yolk coelomitis.

Marked amounts of basophilic, spherical to amorphous yolk material. This material is likely protein because the lipid portion is dissolved by the fixative found in most staining kits. Acutely in yolk coelomitis, minimal inflammation may occur. Over time, a mixed inflammatory reaction may be present. Macrophages may be greatly vacuolated due to the presence of intracytoplasmic lipid. Reactive mesothelial cells may be seen. A superimposed bacterial component may be present.

73. Describe the cytologic characteristics of urinary leakage in birds.

Examination of acute leakage will reveal the typical spherical, variably sized, refractile, and nonstaining urate crystals without significant inflammation. Longer-standing lesions may contain inflammatory cells.

74. Describe the cytologic characteristics of hemorrhage in birds.

Acutely, the only cytologic change with avian hemorrhage may be the presence of high numbers of erythrocytes and leukocytes, with an erythroid/leukocyte ratio and leukocyte distribution similar to those of peripheral blood. Thrombocytes are typically not present unless hemorrhage is ongoing. Hemorrhage that has been present for longer periods will elicit an inflammatory reaction. Within hours, macrophages may be seen internalizing erythrocytes (erythrophagocytosis), and if present longer, macrophages may contain intracytoplasmic evidence of erythrocyte degradation (hemosiderin, hematoidin crystals).

75. Describe the cytologic characteristics of avian erythropoiesis.

Avian erythropoiesis is similar to mammalian erythropoiesis, with the notable differences of the oval shape of later stages of erythrocytes and the retention of the nucleus in mature erythrocytes. Erythrocyte precursors are classified as rubriblasts, prorubricytes, rubricytes, and polychromatophils. As the cells mature, the following changes are seen:

a. The cytoplasm changes from basophilic to eosinophilic due to progressive hemoglobin accumulation in the cytoplasm.
b. Cell size decreases.
c. Cell shape and nuclear shape change from round to oval.
d. Nucleus condenses and is darker staining.

In the normal bone marrow the later stages should predominate over the earlier stages.

76. Describe the cytologic characteristics of avian granulopoiesis.

Avian granulopoiesis is similar to mammalian granulopoiesis. Granulocytic precursors are classified as myeloblast, promyelocyte, myelocyte, metamyelocyte, and band granulocyte, followed by the mature granulocyte. As the cells mature, the following changes are seen:

a. Cytoplasmic basophilia decreases.
b. Cell size decreases.
c. Nucleus condenses, is darker staining, and lobulates (heterophils, eosinophils), although not to the degree seen in mammals.
d. Primary granules (granules typical of each granulocyte) are first evident in promyelocytes. Heterophils have both the orange primary granules (round at this point) and the large magenta-purple granules. The other granulocytes have only the primary granules.
e. The primary granules in all cells increase in number as the cell matures.
f. The primary granules of the heterophil progressively change from round to spindle shaped as the heterophil matures.

77. Describe the cytologic characteristics of avian thrombopoiesis.

Thrombopoiesis in birds is different from that in mammals. Thrombocytes develop from thromboblasts, not from megakaryocytes. As thrombocyte precursors mature, the following changes are seen:

a. Cells progressively decrease in size.
b. Cytoplasm is less basophilic to colorless.
c. Nucleus condenses.
d. Small eosinophilic granules may be seen in mature thrombocytes.

78. How are changes in the erythroid or myeloid compartment evaluated in birds?

Changes in the erythroid and myeloid compartments should be interpreted in light of the peripheral blood changes, and are interpreted in a manner similar to mammalian bone marrow evaluation. (For more detailed discussion, see the Bibliography and other reference books on domestic animal cytology and bone marrow interpretation.)

79. Other than thrombocyte, erythroid, and myeloid precursors, list cells that may be seen in low numbers in avian bone marrow smears.

a. Lymphocytes and plasma cells
b. Osteoblasts
c. Osteoclasts

80. Other than bone marrow hyperplasia or hypoplasia, what other processes may be identified cytologically in avian bone marrow smears?

Both lymphoid leukemia and myeloid leukemia are often seen in poultry and primarily result from viral infections (Box 53-8). Pet birds are rarely diagnosed with leukemia (usually lymphoid). Metastatic neoplasia may also be identified on bone marrow smears. Infectious processes (e.g., fungal or bacterial infections) are not specifically described in birds but are seen in other species.

Box 53-8 *Avian and Reptilian Bone Marrow Diseases with Diagnostic Role for Cytology*
Neoplasms: leukemia, metastatic
Infectious agents: bacteria, fungi, microfilaria
Hematopoietic disorders: hyperplasia, hypoplasia

81. List some diseases of the eyes and conjunctiva in birds for which cytology may be useful in the diagnostic process (Box 53-9).

a. Infectious diseases
   (1) Bacteria: *Mycobacterium* spp., *Chlamydophila psittaci, Mycoplasma* spp., other miscellaneous bacteria
   (2) Fungi (miscellaneous)
   (3) Viruses: avian poxvirus
   (4) Parasites: mites (*Knemidokoptes* spp.)
b. Neoplastic diseases
   (1) Periorbital/intraocular tumors (lymphosarcoma, others)
   (2) Conjunctival tumors
c. Hypovitaminosis A

Box 53-9 *Avian and Reptilian Ocular and Conjunctival Diseases with Diagnostic Role for Cytology*
Infectious agents: bacteria, fungi, poxviruses, mites
Neoplasms (various)
Hypovitaminosis A

82. List some important diseases of avian joints in which cytology would be useful in the diagnostic process (Box 53-10).

a. Gout: extracellular, needlelike, elongate, fine urate crystals are accompanied by a granulomatous inflammatory reaction similar to that seen in gout in other tissues, such as the kidneys (Figure 53-15).

b. Infections: miscellaneous bacteria induce a heterophilic inflammatory reaction. Heterophil degeneration and phagocytosed bacteria may be seen.

Box 53-10 *Avian and Reptilian Joint Diseases with Diagnostic Role for Cytology*
Gout
Infectious agents: bacteria

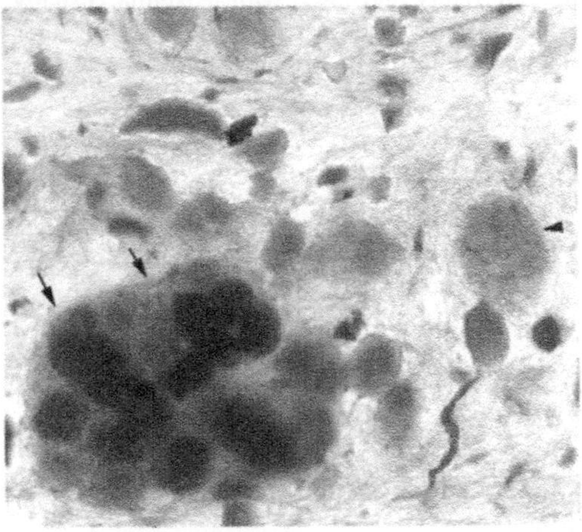

Figure 53-15 Aspirate of a swollen joint from a cockatiel. Marked amounts of extracellular, fibrillar, crystalline urates *(arrowhead)* and a multinucleated giant cell *(arrows)* are shown. (Diff-Quik; original magnification 600×.)

83. List some diseases of the pericardium in birds for which cytology may be useful in the diagnostic process.

a. Infections
   (1) Bacterial: *Mycobacterium* spp., other miscellaneous bacteria
   (2) Fungal (miscellaneous)

b. Gout: accumulation of urate crystals in the pericardial sac

Antemortem diagnosis of these diseases is possible by examination of pericardial fluid samples obtained by endoscopic examination. However, diagnosis of avian pericardial disease is most often reached after postmortem examination.

84. List some diseases of the spleen in birds for which cytology may be useful in the diagnostic process.

a. Infections
   (1) Bacterial: *Chlamydophila psittaci,* other miscellaneous bacteria
   (2) Viral: avian polyomavirus intranuclear inclusions are sometimes seen in the spleen and could be identified cytologically.
   (3) Parasitic: tissue stages of hemoparasites *(Plasmodium, Leukocytozoon, Haemoproteus)*

b. Neoplasms: lymphosarcoma, other neoplasms

85. List some diseases of the central nervous system in birds for which cytology may be useful in the diagnostic process.

a. Infections
   (1) Bacterial: *Mycobacterium* spp., other miscellaneous bacteria
   (2) Fungal: *Aspergillus* spp., other miscellaneous fungi
b. Xanthomatosis: may affect the brain
c. Neoplasms: primary tumors, metastatic tumors

Currently, cytologic examination of central nervous system lesions in birds primarily occurs at necropsy.

86. List some diseases of the reproductive system in birds for which cytology may be useful in the diagnostic process.

a. Infections: miscellaneous bacterial infections
b. Neoplastic disease: budgerigars tend to develop primary ovarian and testicular tumors. The cytologic characteristics are similar to those of mammals.

87. List some diseases of the exocrine pancreas in birds for which cytology may be useful in the diagnostic process.

a. Neoplasia: pancreatic adenocarcinoma, ductular carcinoma
b. Inflammation: acute pancreatic necrosis, viral-induced inflammation, inflammation secondary to coelomitis

88. List some diseases of the endocrine system where cytology may be useful in the diagnostic process.

a. Infectious disease (very rare)
b. Neoplasms: pituitary adenoma is the most common endocrine tumor of birds.

In general, endocrine tumors and other conditions of endocrine organs are not common in birds. Diagnosis is most often reached by histopathologic examination of postmortem tissues.

89. Is postmortem (necropsy) examination of avian blood smears useful?

Postmortem examination of blood smears is a useful tool in the diagnosis of some avian blood diseases, particularly if autolysis is not severe. Blood can be collected from the heart and large blood vessels. Blood parasites (microfilariae, intracellular protozoa, bacteria), polychromasia, and leukemic cells can be detected microscopically.

It is important to remember that after death of the bird, intracellular parasites may escape from parasitized cells and may be found extracellularly. Also, individual morphology of cells may be adversely affected by even mild autolysis (swelling of nuclei and cytoplasm, cytoplasmic blebbing).

90. List some diseases of the reptile integument for which cytology may be useful in the diagnostic process (see Box 53-2).

a. Neoplasms
b. Bacterial, viral, fungal, and parasitic infections
c. Foreign body reactions

91. What neoplasms of the reptile integument can be diagnosed cytologically?

Most neoplasms of the reptile integument can be diagnosed cytologically. Although multiple types of tumors have been identified in reptiles, common neoplasms include the following:

a. Epithelial tumors
   (1) Squamous cell carcinoma
   (2) Sarcomas
   (3) Fibrosarcoma

b. Discrete round cell tumors
   (1) Lymphosarcoma
   (2) Melanomas/melanochromatophoroma

For detailed cytologic descriptions of these and other tumors, see the Bibliography.

92. What bacterial infections of the reptile integument can be diagnosed cytologically?

Any bacterial abscess or granuloma of reptiles can be diagnosed cytologically.

93. What viral infections of the reptile integument can be diagnosed cytologically?

Poxvirus produces intracytoplasmic inclusions that distend infected squamous cell and displace the nucleus paracentrally. Poxviral lesions consist of small, crusty areas to discrete masses and are most often seen in the oral cavity. A mixed inflammatory process may be seen. Poxvirus has been reported in caimans and crocodiles.

Other viruses affecting the skin of reptiles include *herpesvirus* and *papillomavirus*. Although these viruses may form prominent intranuclear inclusions in tissue, diagnosis is often obtained by histopathology and not by cytology.

94. What fungal infections of the reptile integument can be diagnosed cytologically?

Any fungus infecting the reptile integument that stains with Romanowsky stains and is present in sufficient numbers may be diagnosed cytologically (Figures 53-16 and 53-17). If organisms are not seen, the inflammatory process (primarily macrophages and multinucleated giant cells) should produce a high degree of suspicion for a fungal etiology.

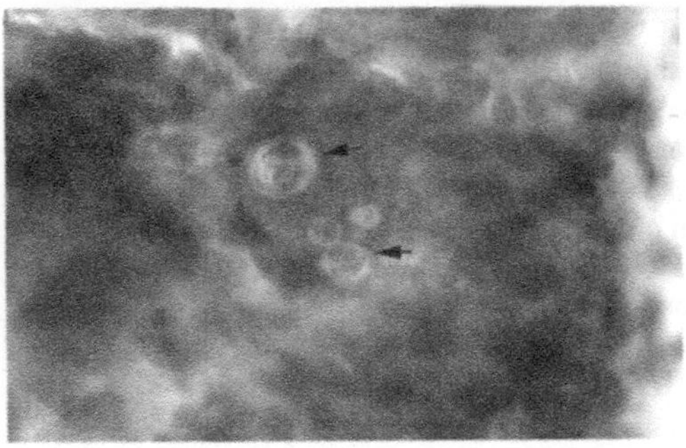

Figure 53-16 Aspirate of a subcutaneous mass from a snake. Multiple round to oval budding yeasts are shown *(arrows). Geotrichum candidum* was cultured from the lesion. (Original magnification 1000×.)

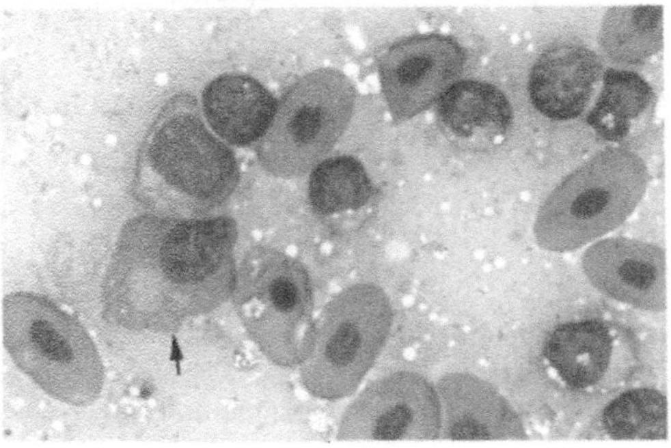

Figure 53-17 Aspirate of a subcutaneous mass from the snake in Figure 53-16. Multiple small lymphocytes and a plasma cell *(arrow)* are shown. (Wright's stain; original magnification 1000×.)

95. What parasitic infections of the reptile integument can be diagnosed cytologically?

Mites may be detected in unstained scrapings made from lesions. Larvae from subcutaneous filarids may be seen in blood smears or tissue aspirates.

96. What are the cytologic characteristics of foreign body reactions in reptiles?

Cytologic characteristics of foreign body reactions in reptiles are similar to those of birds; see Question 33.

97. When is cytologic examination of the alimentary tract useful in reptiles?

Cytologic examination is of use in reptiles when evaluation of the oral cavity, upper intestinal contents, cloacal samples, and feces is necessary.

98. List the indications for obtaining cytologic samples from the alimentary tract in reptiles.

a. Crusts
b. Masses
c. Ulcers
d. Excessive mucus or exudates.
e. Dysphagia
f. Regurgitation
g. Diarrhea
h. Bloody stool

99. List some diseases of the alimentary tract in reptiles for which cytology may be useful in the diagnostic process (see Box 53-3).

a. Bacterial infections
b. Parasitic infections
   (1) Amoeba
   (2) *Cryptosporidium*
   (3) Other intestinal protozoa: *Giardia* spp., ciliates, other flagellates
   (4) Helminths
c. Fungal infections
d. Neoplasia

100. Can bacterial overgrowth be diagnosed cytologically in reptiles?

Cytologic diagnosis of bacterial overgrowth in reptiles is similar to that in birds; see Question 37, *a* and *b*.

101. Describe the cytologic characteristics of intestinal coccidian infections in reptiles.

a. Coccidian life stages can be detected in fecal smears or in intestinal scrapings if present in sufficient numbers.
b. Merozoites, schizonts, macrogamonts, microgametes, and oocysts may be readily identified in mucosal scrapping or impression smears (Figure 53-18).
c. Disseminated intestinal coccidial infection can also occur. Organisms may be identified in multiple extraintestinal tissues (blood, lungs, liver, spleen).

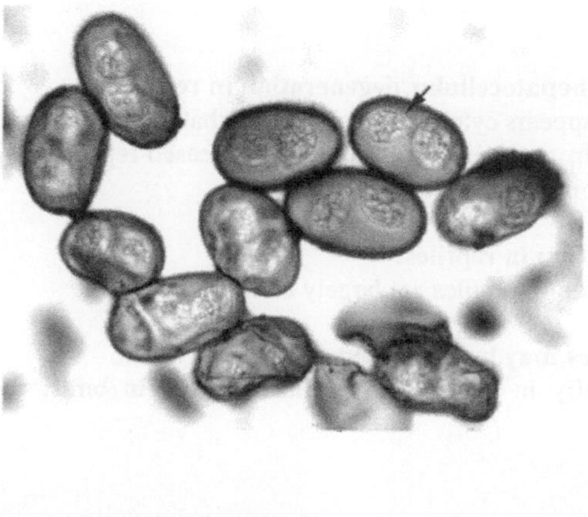

Figure 53-18 Fecal smear from a Veiled chameleon with a severe *Isospora* spp. infection. Multiple oocysts, each with two sporocysts *(arrow)* are shown. (Diff-Quik; original magnification 1000×.)

102. Is cytology useful in the diagnosis of alimentary tract helminth infections in reptiles?

Helminth eggs may be seen in direct smears of reptile fecal material, particularly in heavy infestations (Figure 53-19). Cytology is limited by the low sensitivity of detection. In carnivorous reptiles, helminth eggs originating from rodent prey may be seen in fecal samples and must be differentiated from reptilian parasites (see Figure 53-18).

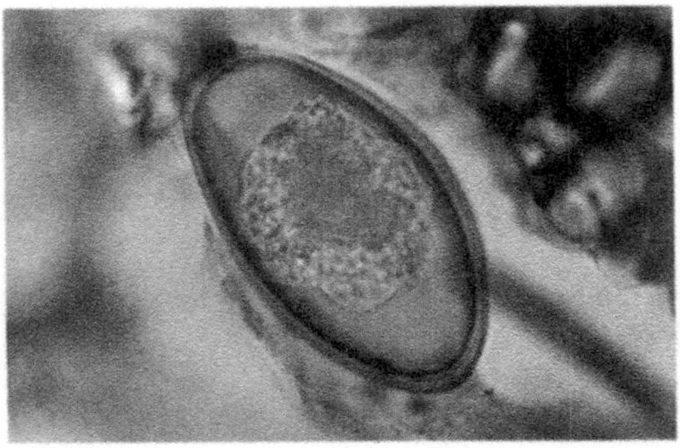

Figure 53-19 Fecal smear from a Bearded Dragon lizard. A pinworm egg is shown. (Diff-Quik; original magnification 1000×.)

103. What neoplasms of the reptile alimentary tract can be diagnosed cytologically?

Leiomyosarcoma, fibrosarcoma, adenocarcinoma, and squamous cell carcinomas are some of the neoplasms that may be seen in reptiles and diagnosed cytologically.

104. List some diseases of the liver in reptiles for which cytology may be useful in the diagnostic process (see Box 53-4).

a. Inflammation of any cause: bacterial, fungal, parasitic
b. Hepatocellular degeneration: lipidosis
c. Neoplasia: metastatic or primary

105. List some infectious causes of inflammation in the liver of reptiles.

a. *Chlamydophila psittaci:* found within macrophages
b. *Entamoeba invadens*
c. Viruses: diagnosis most often obtained by histologic examination
   (1) Herpesvirus
   (2) Adenovirus
d. Other miscellaneous bacteria, fungi, and helminths
e. Tissue stages of hemoparasites (protozoa, microfilariae) may be seen in the liver with or without associated inflammation.

106. Describe the cytologic appearance of hepatocellular degeneration in reptiles.

Hepatocellular degeneration in reptiles appears cytologically similar to that in birds (Figure 53-20); see Question 50. Cytologic imprints from the liver of healthy and diseased reptiles may contain numerous melanophores and melanin pigment.

107. What causes hepatocellular degeneration in reptiles?

The causes of hepatocellular degeneration in reptiles are largely unknown.

108. What neoplasms of the liver in reptiles may be diagnosed cytologically?

Liver neoplasms diagnosed cytologically in reptiles are similar to those in birds; see Question 52.

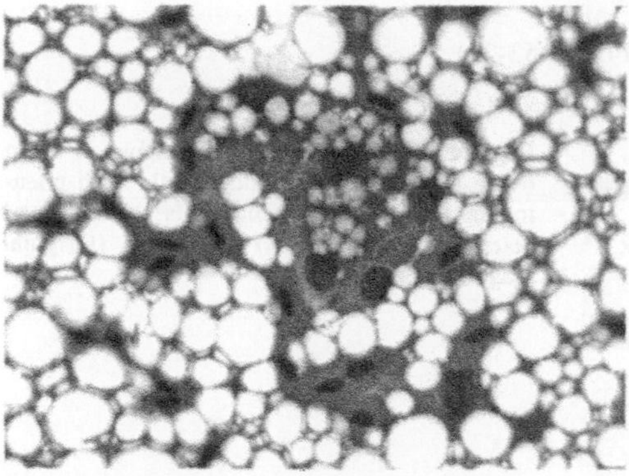

Figure 53-20 Impression smear of the liver of a Bearded Dragon lizard with hepatic lipidosis. An aggregate of degenerate, vacuolated hepatocytes and numerous extracellular clear spaces (lipid) are shown in the center of the image. (Wright's stain; original magnification 500×.)

109. List some diseases of the reptile renal system for which cytology may be useful in the diagnostic process (see Box 53-5).

a. Infections/inflammation
   (1) Bacteria (miscellaneous)
   (2) Fungi
   (3) Parasites: protozoa
b. Neoplasia
   (1) Renal carcinomas, adenocarcinomas
   (2) Lymphosarcoma
   (3) Metastatic tumors
c. Gout
d. Inflammation, infectious agents, and tubular casts may be seen in urinary sediments.

110. Describe the cytologic appearance of renal gout in reptiles.

Renal gout in reptiles appears cytologically similar to that in birds; see Question 58. Again, the typical spherical, refractile, nonstaining, variably sized urate crystals routinely seen in urine and in cloacal swabs (Figure 53-21) must not be confused with the thin, needle-shaped urate crystals typically seen in gout (see Figure 53-15).

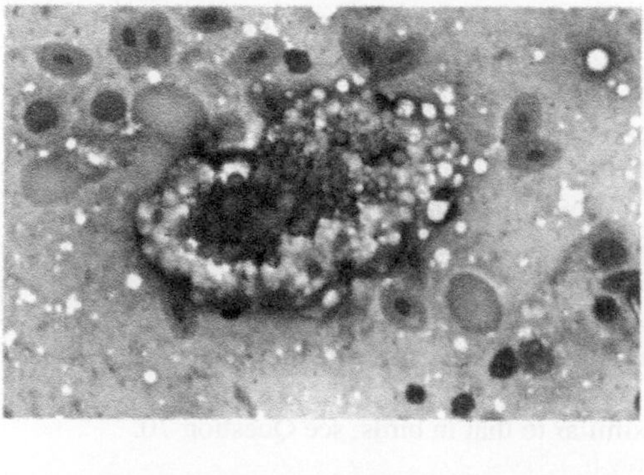

Figure 53-21 Impression smear of a kidney from an Ornate Uromastyx lizard. An aggregate of urate crystals typical of those found in the urine of healthy birds and reptiles is shown. (Wright's stain; original magnification 500×.)

111. When is cytologic evaluation of the respiratory system useful in reptiles?

Cytologic examination is of use when the clinical signs (e.g., dyspnea, nasal discharge) suggest respiratory disease in the reptile. Diagnostic samples include the following:

a. Nasal swabs
b. Tracheal lavage

c. Bronchoalveolar lavage
d. Postmortem imprints and scrapings (Figure 53-22)

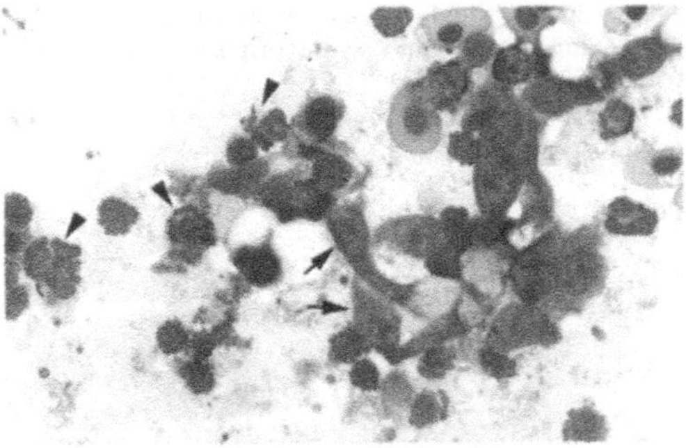

Figure 53-22 Impression smear of lung tissue from a Red Ear Slider turtle with pneumonia. Columnar epithelial cells *(arrows)* and heterophils *(arrowheads)* are shown. (Original magnification 500×.)

112. List some diseases of the respiratory system in reptiles for which cytology may be useful in the diagnostic process (see Box 53-6).
a. Infectious agents: bacteria, fungi, protozoa
b. Neoplasms: primary or metastatic (rarely seen)
c. Helminth infections: eggs, larvae of lungworms

113. List bacterial agents that may be seen with respiratory infections in reptiles.
a. *Mycobacterium* spp. (uncommon)
b. *Mycoplasma* spp.: chelonians
c. Miscellaneous bacteria

114. List some of the fungal diseases that may affect the respiratory tract of reptiles.
a. *Aspergillus* spp.
b. *Candida albicans*
c. *Cryptococcus neoformans* and other fungi have not been frequently described in clinical cases.

In general, fungal respiratory infections are uncommon in reptiles.

115. What are some viral infections that affect the respiratory system of reptiles?
Herpesvirus and *ophidian paramyxovirus* affect the reptile respiratory system. Some of these viruses form cytoplasmic or nuclear inclusions that may be seen cytologically; however, a diagnosis is most often reached with histologic examination.

116. Describe the cytologic characteristics of normal coelomic fluid in reptiles.
The cytologic characteristics of coelomic fluid of reptiles are similar to those of birds; see Question 69.

117. Describe the cytologic changes that characterize mesothelial cell reactivity or dysplasia in reptiles.
Mesothelial cell reactivity in reptiles is similar to that in birds; see Question 70.

118. List some diseases of the coelomic cavity in reptiles for which cytology may be useful in the diagnosis (see Box 53-7).
a. Infections
(1) Miscellaneous bacteria spread from systemic infections, penetrating trauma, and ruptured intestines.

(2) Heterophilic inflammatory reaction with heterophil degeneration is primarily seen.

b. Hemorrhage
c. Neoplasms
d. Yolk coelomitis (Figure 53-23)

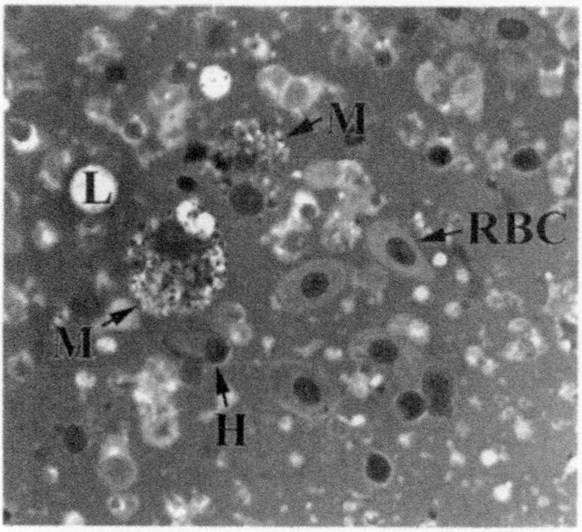

Figure 53-23 Coelomic fluid smear from a Monitor lizard with yolk coelomitis. Foamy, vacuolated macrophages *(M)*, red blood cells *(RBC)*, a heterophil *(H)*, and numerous extracellular lipid vacuoles *(L)* are shown in a dark-staining proteinaceous background. (Original magnification 600×.)

119. Describe the cytologic characteristics of hemorrhage in reptiles.
Hemorrhage in reptiles appears cytologically similar to that in birds; see Question 74.

120. Describe the cytologic characteristics of reptile erythropoiesis.
Reptile erythropoiesis is similar to mammalian and avian erythropoiesis; see Question 75.

121. Describe the cytologic characteristics of reptile granulopoiesis.
Reptile granulopoiesis is similar to mammalian and avian granulopoiesis; see Question 76.

122. How are changes in the erythroid or myeloid compartment evaluated in reptiles?
Evaluation of erythroid/myeloid compartment changes in reptiles is similar to that for birds; see Question 78.

123. Other than thrombocyte, erythroid, and myeloid precursors, what cells may be seen in low numbers in reptile bone marrow smears?

a. Lymphocytes and plasma cells
b. Osteoblasts
c. Osteoclasts

124. Other than bone marrow hyperplasia or hypoplasia, what other processes may be identified cytologically in reptile bone marrow smears (see Box 53-8)?

a. Leukemia: lymphoid, myeloid (granulocytic, monocytic); both are seen in reptiles.
b. Metastatic neoplasia
c. Infectious agents (Figure 53-24)

125. List some diseases of the eyes and conjunctiva in reptiles for which cytology may be useful in the diagnostic process (see Box 53-9).

a. Bacterial infection: miscellaneous bacteria
b. Fungal infection: miscellaneous fungi

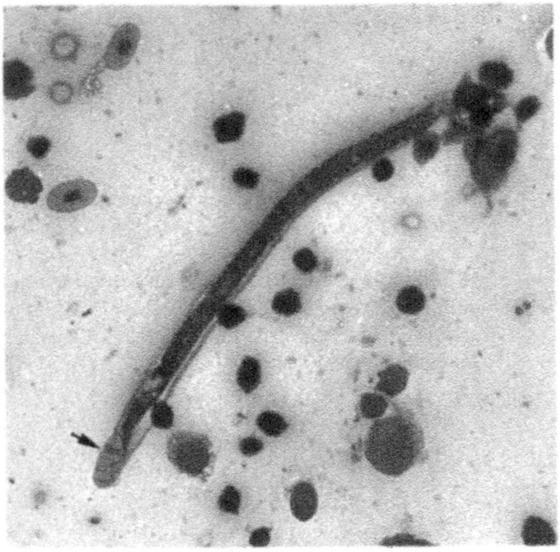

Figure 53-24 Impression smear of the bone marrow from a Panther chameleon infected with *Folayella furcata*. A microfilaria with a prominent sheath *(arrow)* is shown. (Original magnification 500×.)

c. Viral infection: reptile poxvirus in crocodiles and caimans (seen infrequently)
d. Parasitic infection: mites

126. List some important diseases of reptile joints for which cytology would be useful in the diagnostic process (see Box 53-10).

a. Gout: extracellular, needle-like, elongate, fine urate crystals accompanied by a granulomatous inflammatory reaction similar to that seen in gout in other tissues such as the kidneys (see Figure 53-15).
b. Infections: miscellaneous bacteria induce a heterophilic inflammatory reaction. Heterophil degeneration with phagocytosed bacteria is primarily seen.

127. List disease of the pericardium in reptiles for which cytology may be useful in the diagnostic process.

a. Gout in reptiles may be diagnosed by postmortem cytologic analysis showing the accumulation of urate crystals in the pericardial sac.
b. Pericarditis—bacteria and fungi may be seen cytologically.

128. List some diseases of the central nervous system in reptiles for which cytology may be useful in the diagnostic process.

a. Infections
   (1) Bacterial: miscellaneous bacteria.
   (2) Fungal: miscellaneous fungi
b. Neoplastic: primary tumors, metastatic tumors

Currently, cytologic examination of central nervous system lesions in reptiles primarily occurs at necropsy.

129. List some diseases of the reproductive system in reptiles for which cytology may be useful in the diagnostic process.

a. Infections: miscellaneous bacteria
b. Neoplasms: ovarian adenocarcinoma, interstitial cell tumor, seminoma, granulosa cell tumor, sarcoma

Cytologic characteristics of reproductive system neoplasms in reptiles would be expected to be similar to those seen in other domestic animals and birds.

130. List some diseases of the exocrine pancreas in reptiles for which cytology may be useful in the diagnostic process.

a. Neoplasia: pancreatic adenocarcinoma
b. Inflammation

131. Is postmortem (necropsy) examination of reptile blood smears useful?

As for birds, postmortem examination of reptile blood smears is useful in the diagnosis of some blood diseases; see Question 89.

It is important to remember that after death of the reptile, intracellular parasites may escape from parasitized cells and may be found extracellularly. Also, individual morphology of cells may be adversely affected by even mild autolysis (swelling of nuclei and cytoplasm, cytoplasmic blebbing).

Avian and Reptilian Clinical Pathology

BIBLIOGRAPHY

Benson KG, Murphy JP, MacWilliams P: Effects of hemolysis on plasma electrolyte and chemistry values in the common green iguana *(Iguana iguana), J Zoo Wildl Med* 30:413-415, 1999.

Bounous DI, Stedman NL: Normal avian hematology: chicken and turkey. In Feldman BF, Zinkl JG, Jain NC, editors: *Schalm's veterinary hematology,* ed 5, Baltimore, 2000, Lippincott, Williams & Wilkins, pp 1147-1154.

Campbell TW: *Avian hematology and cytology,* ed 2, Ames, 1995, Iowa State University Press.

Campbell TW: Clinical pathology. In Mader DR, editor: *Reptile medicine and surgery,* Philadelphia, 1996, Saunders, pp 248-257.

Campbell TW: Cytology. In Rithchie BW, Harrison GJ, Harrison LR, editors: *Avian medicine: principles and applications,* Lake Worth, Fla, 1994, Wingers Publishing, pp 199-222.

Campbell TW: Hemoparasites. In Mader DR, editor: *Reptile medicine and surgery,* Philadelphia, 1996, Saunders, pp 379-381.

Campbell TW: Normal hematology of psittacines. In Feldman BF, Zinkl JG, Jain NC, editors: *Schalm's veterinary hematology,* ed 5, Baltimore, 2000, Lippincott, Williams & Wilkins, pp 1155-1160.

DeHert P, Ducatelle R, Lepoudre C, et al: An epidemic of fatal hepatic necrosis of viral origin in racing pigeons *(Columba livia), Avian Pathol* 24:475-483, 1995.

Divers SJ: Reptilian liver and gastrointestinal testing. In Fudge AM, editor: *Laboratory medicine: reptile and exotic pets,* Philadelphia, 2000, Saunders, pp 205-209.

Divers SJ: Reptilian renal and reproductive disease diagnosis. In Fudge AM, editor: *Laboratory medicine: reptile and exotic pets,* Philadelphia, 2000, Saunders, pp 217-222.

Espada Y: Avian hemostasis. In Feldman BF, Zinkl JG, Jain NC, editors: *Schalm's veterinary hematology,* ed 5, Baltimore, 2000, Lippincott, Williams & Wilkins, pp 552-555.

Fudge AM: Avian blood sampling and artifact considerations. In *Laboratory medicine: avian and exotic pets,* Philadelphia, 2000, Saunders, pp 1-8.

Fudge AM: Avian complete blood count. In *Laboratory medicine: avian and exotic pets,* Philadelphia, 2000, Saunders, pp 9-18.

Fudge AM: Avian cytodiagnosis. In *Laboratory medicine: avian and exotic pets,* Philadelphia, 2000, Saunders, pp 124-132.

Fudge AM: Avian liver and gastrointestinal testing. In *Laboratory medicine: avian and exotic pets,* Philadelphia, 2000, Saunders, pp 47-55.

Fudge AM: Avian metabolic disorders. In *Laboratory medicine: avian and exotic pets,* Philadelphia, 2000, Saunders, pp 56-60.

Fudge AM: Disorders of avian erythrocytes. In *Laboratory medicine: avian and exotic pets,* Philadelphia, 2000, Saunders, pp 28-34.

Fudge AM, Joseph V: Disorders of avian leukocytes. In Fudge AM, editor: *Laboratory medicine: avian and exotic pets,* Philadelphia, 2000, Saunders, pp 19-17.

Garner MM, Homer BL, Jacobson ER, et al: Staining and morphologic features of bone marrow hematopoietic cells in desert tortoises *(Gopherus agassizii), Am J Vet Res* 57:1608-1615, 1996.

Halliday BE, Silverman JF, Finley JL: Fine-needle aspiration cytology of amyloid associated with nonneoplastic and malignant lesions, *Diagn Cytopathol* 18:270-275, 1998.

Harr KE: Clinical chemistry of companion avian species: a review, *Vet Clin Pathol* 31:140-151, 2002.

Harr KE, Alleman AR, Dennis PM, et al: Morphologic and cytochemical characteristics of blood cells and hematologic and plasma biochemical reference ranges in green iguanas, *J Am Vet Med Assoc* 218:915-921, 2001.

Hawthorne TB, Bolon B, Meyer DJ: Systemic amyloidosis in a mare, *J Am Vet Med Assoc* 196:323-325, 1990.

Hochleithner M: Biochemistries. In Rithchie BW, Harrison GJ, Harrison LR, editors: *Avian medicine: principles and applications,* Lake Worth, Fla, 1994, Wingers Publishing, pp 223-245.

Irizaary-Rovira A, Wolf A, Bolek M: Blood smear from a wild-caught Panther chameleon *(Furcifer pardalis), Vet Clin* Pathol 31(3):129-132, 2002.

Jacobson ER: Reptilian viral diagnostics. In Fudge AM, editor: *Laboratory medicine: avian and exotic pets,* Philadelphia, 2000, Saunders, pp 229-235.

Jacobson ER, Telford SR: Chlamydial and poxvirus infections of circulating monocytes of a flap-necked chameleon *(Chamaeleo dilepsis), J Wildl Dis* 26:572-577, 1990.

Jenkins JR: Avian metabolic chemistries, *Semin Avian Exotic Pet Med* 3:25-32, 1994.

Jones MP: Avian clinical pathology, *Vet Clin North Am Exotic Anim Pract* 2:663-687, 1999.

Knotek Z, Hauptman K, Knotková Z, et al: Renal disease haemogram and plasma biochemistry in green iguana, *Acta Vet Brno* 71:333-340, 2002.

Kolmstetter C, Carpenter JW, Ernst S: What is your diagnosis? *J Avian Med Surg* 9:195-197, 1995.

Kreuder C, Irizarry-Rovira AR, Janovitz EB, et al: Avian pox in sanderlings from Florida, *J Wildl Dis* 35:582-585, 1999.

Lance VA, Elsey RM: Plasma catecholamines and plasma corticosterone following restraint stress in juvenile alligators, *J Exp Zool* 283:559-565, 1999.

Latimer KS, Bienzle D: Determination and interpretation of the avian leukogram. In Feldman BF, Zinkl JG, Jain NC, editors: *Schalm's veterinary hematology,* ed 5, Baltimore, 2000, Lippincott, Williams & Wilkins, pp 417-432.

Latimer KS, Goodwin MA, Davis MK: Rapid cytologic diagnosis of respiratory cryptosporidiosis in chickens, *Avian Dis* 32:826-830, 1988.

Lumeij JT: Avian clinical biochemistry. In Kaneko JJ, Harvey JW, Bruss ML, editors: *Clinical biochemistry of domestic animals,* ed 5, San Diego, 1997, Academic Press, pp 857-883.

Lumeij JT: Avian clinical enzymology, *Semin Avian Exotic Pet Med* 3:14-24, 1994.

MacNeill AL, Uhl EW, Kolenda-Roberts H, Jacobson E: Mortality in a wood turtle *(Clemmys insculpta)* collection, *Vet Clin Pathol* 31:133-136, 2002.

Mader DR: Normal hematology of reptiles. In Feldman BF, Zinkl JG, Jain NC, editors: *Schalm's veterinary hematology,* ed 5, Baltimore, 2000, Lippincott, Williams & Wilkins, pp 1126-1132.

Mader DR: Reptilian metabolic disorders. In Fudge AM, editor: *Laboratory medicine: reptile and exotic pets,* Philadelphia, 2000, Saunders, pp 210-216.

Morrisey JK: Blood transfusions in exotic species. In Feldman BF, Zinkl JG, Jain NC, editors: *Schalm's veterinary hematology,* ed 5, Baltimore, 2000, Lippincott, Williams & Wilkins, pp 855-860.

Murray MJ: Reptilian blood sampling and artifact considerations. In Fudge AM, editor: *Laboratory medicine: avian and exotic pets,* Philadelphia, 2000, Saunders, pp 185-192.

Nordberg C, O'Brien RT, Paul-Murphy J, Hawley B: Ultrasound examination and guided fine-needle aspiration of the liver in Amazon parrots (*Amazona* species), *J Avian Med Surg* 14:180-184, 2000.

Phalen DN: Avian renal disorders. In Fudge AM, editor: *Laboratory medicine: avian and exotic pets,* Philadelphia, 2000, Saunders, pp 61-68.

Pierson FW: Laboratory techniques for avian hematology. In Feldman BF, Zinkl JG, Jain NC, editors: *Schalm's veterinary hematology,* ed 5, Baltimore, 2000, Lippincott, Williams & Wilkins, pp 1145-1146.

Powers LV: Avian hemostasis. In Fudge AM, editor: *Laboratory medicine: avian and exotic pets,* Philadelphia, 2000, Saunders, pp 35-46.

Rae M: Avian endocrine disorders. In Fudge AM, editor: *Laboratory medicine: avian and exotic pets,* Philadelphia, 2000, Saunders, pp 76-89.

Raskin RE: Reptilian complete blood count. In Fudge AM, editor: *Laboratory medicine: avian and exotic pets,* Philadelphia, 2000, Saunders, pp 193-197.

Redrobe S, MacDonald J: Sample collection and clinical pathology of reptiles, *Vet Clin North Am Exotic Anim Pract* 2:709-730, 1999.

Rosskopf WJ: Disorders of reptilian leukocytes and erythrocytes. In Fudge AM, editor: *Laboratory medicine: avian and exotic pets,* Philadelphia, 2000, Saunders, pp 198-204.

Schmidt RE, Reavill DR: Reptilian surgical pathology. In Fudge AM, editor: *Laboratory medicine: reptile and exotic pets,* Philadelphia, 2000, Saunders, pp 236-242.

Stockham SL, Scott MA: Enzymes. In *Fundamentals of veterinary clinical pathology,* Ames, 2002, Iowa State University Press, pp 433-460.

Stockham SL, Scott MA: Liver function. In *Fundamentals of veterinary clinical pathology,* Ames, 2002, Iowa State University Press, pp 461-486.

Telford SR Jr: Diagnosis of reptilian protozoal infections. In Fudge AM, editor: *Laboratory medicine: avian and exotic pets,* Philadelphia, 2000, Saunders, pp 236-242.

Tyler RD, Cowell RL, Baldwin CJ, Morton RJ: Introduction. In Cowell RL, Tyler RD, Meinkoth JH, editors: *Diagnostic cytology and hematology of the dog and cat,* ed 2, St Louis, 1999, Mosby, pp 1-19.

INDEX

Page numbers followed by f indicate figures; t, tables; b, boxes.

B

C

D

H

M

Q

R

S

T

U

Printed and bound by CPI Group (UK) Ltd, Croydon, CR0 4YY
03/10/2024
01040848-0012